Microvascular
Injury

Volume 7 in the Series

Major Problems in Dermatology

ARTHUR ROOK, MA, MD, FRCP

Consulting Editor

OTHER MONOGRAPHS IN THE SERIES

PUBLISHED

Warin and Champion: **Urticaria**
Noble and Somerville: **Microbiology of Human Skin**
Rajka: **Atopic Dermatitis**
Alexander: **Dermatitis Herpetiformis**
Ridley: **The Vulva**
Cunliffe and Cotterill: **The Acnes**

FORTHCOMING

Lyell and Arbuthnott: **Staphylococci and the Skin**

Microvascular Injury

Vasculitis, Stasis and Ischaemia

T. J. RYAN, MA, BM, BCh(Oxon.), FRCP

*Consultant Dermatologist, Department of Dermatology,
The Slade Hospital and the Radcliffe Infirmary, Oxford*

With contributions by

M. W. KANAN, MB, ChB (Cairo), MRCP, DPhil (Oxon.)

Honorary Consultant Dermatologist, Radcliffe Infirmary, Oxford

G. W. CHERRY, BA

Graduate Student, University of Oxford, Oxford

1976

W. B. Saunders Company Ltd   London · Philadelphia · Toronto

W. B. Saunders Company Ltd: 1 St. Anne's Road
Eastbourne, East Sussex BN21 3UN

West Washington Square
Philadelphia, Pa. 19105

833 Oxford Street
Toronto, Ontario M8Z 5T9

Library of Congress Cataloging in Publication Data

Ryan, Terence John.
  Microvascular injury.

  (Major problems in dermatology ; 7)
  1. Blood-vessels — Diseases. I. Cherry, George,
joint author. II. Kanan, Wajdi, joint author.
III. Title. IV. Series. [DNLM: 1. Blood-vessels —
Injuries. 2. Skin diseases. 3. Vascular diseases.
W1 MA492S v.7 / WG500 R989m]
RC691.R9   616.1'3   76-4252
ISBN 0-7216-7858-0

Printed at The Lavenham Press Ltd, Lavenham, Suffolk, England.

Print No: 9 8 7 6 5 4 3 2 1

Foreword

A variety of factors have determined the selection of subjects for monographs in this series. The rapid growth of knowledge of some uncommon but important diseases makes it impossible for a general textbook of acceptable length to provide a comprehensive account, such as the laboratory worker or research-minded clinician requires. Some diseases have not attracted the attention they deserve because they fall uneasily into the boundary zone between two or more of the conventional medical specialities. Other diseases have been illuminated by research in newly developed laboratory sciences, work which is often largely unfamiliar to many of the clinicians who are called upon to care for these patients.

The spectrum of diseases to which this book is devoted qualifies for inclusion in this series on all these grounds. Collectively these diseases are by no means uncommon, but they may first present in the clinics of any one of a wide range of specialists. A very large amount of fundamental research on the microcirculation under physiological and pathological conditions has greatly increased our insight into the processes underlying these diseases, but has so far made relatively little impact on the average clinician. We are fortunate that Dr Terence Ryan of Oxford has devoted himself for some years to this field of research, and in the light of a very comprehensive knowledge of the widely scattered literature, and of his own clinical and laboratory work, is particularly well placed to survey the present state of our understanding of a fascinating group of diseases, the theoretical interest of which extends even beyond their very considerable practical importance.

Cambridge, 1976   Arthur Rook

Preface

Vasculitis is surely one of the most difficult problems in medicine. It comes within the experience of most doctors several times a year and always presents diagnostic difficulties. Prognosis and management are also difficult. In writing this book I have attempted to explain vasculitis. To do so the problem has been broadened so that vasculitis is defined somewhat loosely as microvascular injury. Such injury is caused by various physical, infective and immunological processes and it was not intended to give a complete account of these but merely to devote a chapter to each and to indicate how they fit into our understanding of blood vessel responses. Minor injury to vessels often produces only temporary leaking, while severe injury so often causes obstruction to blood flow that it has been necessary to include information about its consequences — urticaria and ischaemic necrosis. Much attention has been given to the background or constitutional defects which determine how the vessel reacts to injury and repairs itself.

This approach has meant that disease entities as such have received no special attention but hopefully the index will help the reader to find information about every significant type of vasculitis that has been given a name. I am well aware that the practising dermatologist may find it difficult to find the answer required for a particular patient where physical signs have been given one of the many names used to describe vasculitis. This book is a personal view of mechanisms and to some extent morphology is absorbed rather than delineated.

The preparation for this book began during my medical studies twenty years ago when the then Nuffield Professor, Leslie Witts, suggested that I present a patient with cryoglobulinaemia at a grand round. Later, as House Physician to Sir George Pickering, blood vessels were always in mind. Renwick Vickers' interest in vasculitis meant that, as his Registrar in Dermatology, I was encouraged to collect considerable material for the main theme of vasculitis and the blood supply of the skin for the 1966 joint meeting of the British Association of Dermatology and Société Française de Dermatologie held in Oxford. Much of the clinical material in this book has been generously provided by Renwick Vickers.

Perhaps the single most exciting moment in my education in this field was a first view of blood flow and blood vessels in the hamster cheek pouch chamber. Gordon Sanders was responsible for this and I am grateful to him for introducing me to the multidisciplinary world of the British, American and European Microcirculation Societies.

Many colleagues have worked full-time on blood vessels and vasculitis with myself as an intermittent onlooker, and I gladly acknowledge the contributions of Amal Kurban, Robert Turner, Kioshi Nishioka, Rodney Dawber, Katherine Grice, George Cherry, Julia Ellis and Wajdi Kanan. Writing papers with Peter Copeman, George Cherry and Wajdi Kanan has been the most valuable experience because between us we have enjoyed many hours trying to analyse both old and new concepts. I hope that the frequent references to Peter Copeman will be sufficient acknowledgement of his influence. I am indebted to the Royal College of Physicians of Australia and particularly to Dr Ken Paver and Professor Ron Penney for allowing me to talk almost non-stop for two days at a workshop on vasculitis in Sydney in November 1973 when I began to put pen to paper.

Thanks to Arthur Rook I have had the opportunity to write about my favourite subject and by his early reading of the manuscript some of the nonsense was eliminated. Thanks to John Mitchell, the actual writing has been made less worrying because I have always known that there was a 'guardian angel' reading the manuscript with marvellous care and ridding it of all its worst grammatical errors. My secretary, Mrs Margo Cook, has done a splendid job of typing. My wife Anne has spent many hours working on the references and the index — both boring jobs — and I am grateful to her for not complaining. I am indebted to Bill Schmitt and Margaret Pettifer of W. B. Saunders for their help in preparing the manuscript.

Finally, I would like to acknowledge two years' support from the Wellcome Trust for a technician who, whilst working on viscosity and fibrinolysis, provided much previously unpublished data on which to base Chapters 9 and 10. The work on the nose described in Chapter 9 was supported by the Medical Research Council.

Oxford, 1976   T. J. Ryan

Acknowledgements

The author is grateful to the following journals for allowing him to reproduce material: *Acta Dermato-venereologica* (Figures 9.7, 9.8, 10.10, 13.1, 14.5 and 15.1; Table 13.2), *American Journal of Clinical Pathology* (quote from Pearl Zeek's paper, 1952), *American Journal of Medical Science* (Table 8.3), *American Journal of Medicine* (Table 10.1), *American Journal of Pathology* (Figure 4.19), *American Journal of Physiology* (Figure 11.6), *Archives of Dermatology* (Table 14.7), *Archives of Internal Medicine* (quote from Wolff's 1970 paper; Tables 11.1 and 15.5), *Bibliotheca Anatomica* (Tables 15.6, 15.7 and 15.8), *British Journal of Dermatology* (Figures 3.9, 3.16, 4.17, 7.2, 9.9, 9.10a, 12.15, 12.16, 12.18, 14.5, 14.7, 14.8 and 15.1; Tables 1.1, 1.2, 3.1, 3.2, 6.1, 7.2, 12.1, 14.1 and 15.1), *British Medical Journal* (quote from Osler's paper, 1914; Figures 7.6, 12.19 and 13.3), *Dermatologica* (Figure 9.4a), *International Journal of Dermatology* (Figure 1.1), *Journal of Investigative Dermatology* (Figure 4.28), *Lancet* (Figure 10.9; Tables 9.2, 14.6 and 15.3), *Medicine* (Tables 8.1 and 11.2 to 11.11), *Pathologica Europeae* (Figures 9.12 and 9.14), *Philippine Journal of Science* (Figure 9.11), *Plastic and Reconstructive Surgery* (Figure 5.2), *Practitioner* (Table 6.2), *Revue Canadienne de Biologie* (Figure 6.2), *Seminars in Hematology* (Table 7.3), and *Thrombosis et Diathesis Haemorrhagica* (quote from McKay's paper, 1973).

The author is also grateful to the following publishers: Academic Press (Figures 3.15 and 4.18 were taken from *Physiology and Pathophysiology of the Skin*), Blackwell Scientific Publications (Table 13.1 was taken from *Textbook of Dermatology*), Butterworths (Figure 7.5 was taken from Wright's *Radiological Diagnosis of Lung and Mediastinal Tumours*), Excerpta Medica (Table 8.4 was taken from *A Guide to Drug Eruptions*), and the Medical and Technical Publishing Company (Table 7.5 was taken from *Immunological Aspects of Skin Disease*).

Many individuals and organisations have kindly lent photographs and tables: Dr Martin Black (Figures 3.3 and 4.30), Bristol Royal Infirmary (Table 15.2), Professor Brodthagen (Figures 10.10, 13.1 and 15.1), Dr David Brown (Figure 6.4), Professor Watson Buchanan (Figure 13.3), Dr P. Copeman (Figures 10.2, 10.3, 12.4, 12.15 and 14.1; Table 12.1), Dr R. Cormone (Figure 14.10), Dr Michael Dunnill (Figure 14.3), Dr Robin Eady (Figure 10.4), Dr P. Emerson (Figure 14.5), Professor George Findlay

(Figures 8.5 and 13.7), Dr Benjamin Golcman (Figure 9.6, a and b), Mr Alf Gunning and Dr Alan Sharp (Figure 8.9), Dr Mark Hewitt (Figure 11.7), Dr R. Holemans (Figure 11.6), Professor T. Jansen (Figure 15.7), Dr Tony Leatham (Figures 14.8 and 14.9), Dr Colin MacDougall (Figures 8.6 and 8.9, b and c), Dr H. Maricq (Figures 12.3a and 14.4), the Medical Illustration Department, the Radcliffe Infirmary, Oxford (Figure 1.5), Mrs Dianne Shelby (Figure 12.5), Dr Sydney Truelove (Figure 3.19), Professor C. Wong (Figure 3.15), and Dr F. Wright (Figures 7.5, 14.1 and 14.2).

Finally the author wishes to thank those authors who have allowed him to use material from their published works: Agle (Table 11.1), Aldo (Table 15.5), Amjad (Figure 12.19), Bartak (Figure 4.17), Bruinsma (Tables 8.4 and 8.5), Cameron (Figure 7.6), Carlson (Table 15.3), Colman (Table 10.1), Cream (Figure 7.2), Gocke (Table 8.2), Grey (Table 7.3), Grice (Table 15.1), Haim (Tables 13.2 and 13.3), Holti (Tables 15.6, 15.7 and 15.8), Jablonska (Table 7.5), McKay (quote in chapter 10), Michaelsson (Table 14.7), Palmer (Table 6.2), Ratnoff (Tables 11.2 to 11.11), Shillitoe (Table 9.2), Wilhelm (Table 6.2), Williamson (Table 4.19), Wolff (quote in Chapter 11), Yoshikawa (Table 8.1).

Contents

Introduction

In 1914 Sir William Osler, writing from Oxford, described the 'visceral lesions of purpura and allied conditions'. Sixty years later, writing from the same hospital about patients from the same towns and villages, the present writer finds greater agreement with Osler than with any other author. Osler clearly stated that the lesions were due to red blood corpuscles, to serum alone, or to both, exuding from the blood vessels. He then went on to describe purpura, urticaria, erythema, ischaemia, necrosis and various combinations of visceral lesions, as well as triggers, idiosyncrasies, genetic diseases such as hereditary angio-oedema, and the effects of exposure to heat and cold.

This book is about injury to the small blood vessels of the skin (Tables I.1 and I.2) and it attempts to explain the rashes resulting from the exudative process. The consequences of such injury include swelling of endothelial cells, increased vascular permeability and leakiness, varying degrees of leucocyte infiltration, fibrinoid change, bleeding and occlusion by clot formation within the vessels. The resulting skin lesions range from slight local redness through transient or more long-lasting swelling to haemorrhage or ischaemic necrosis. When deep, such lesions are often nodular.

Urticaria, intravascular coagulation and ischaemia often are discussed in the same terms as vasculitis, and therefore this book is not so much a monograph on micro-vascular injury or on 'vasculitis' as a description of blood vessel reactions and coagulation disorders associated with a wide range of inflammatory processes. A broad view is taken of the latter because a mild inflammatory reaction to micro-injury overlaps with a normal physiological response, and the more severe reactions result in ischaemia and coagulation. Such reactions are often provoked by repeated minor insults to the vessel wall, which result in paralysis and exhaustion of repair mechanisms, as is demonstrated in the Shwartzman phenomenon (see Chapter 10). However, the injury herein described is directed primarily against the vessel and not against the organ supplied, as would be the case, for instance, in a hair follicle infected by staphylococci or *Trichophyton verrucosum*.

During the past ten years, workers in the field of transplantation have noted changes in blood supply similar to those in vasculitis. George Cherry (see Chapter 5) and Wajdi

Table I.1. Vasculitis, stasis and ischaemia: the themes and subjects covered in this monograph.

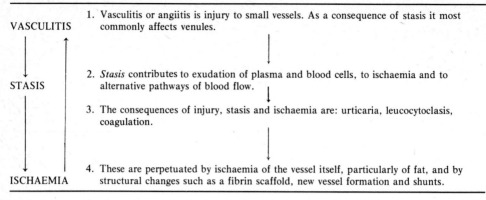

VASCULITIS

1. Vasculitis or angiitis is injury to small vessels. As a consequence of stasis it most commonly affects venules.

STASIS

2. *Stasis* contributes to exudation of plasma and blood cells, to ischaemia and to alternative pathways of blood flow.

3. The consequences of injury, stasis and ischaemia are: urticaria, leucocytoclasis, coagulation.

ISCHAEMIA

4. These are perpetuated by ischaemia of the vessel itself, particularly of fat, and by structural changes such as a fibrin scaffold, new vessel formation and shunts.

Kanan (see Chapter 9) have conducted similar studies on the skin and nose; and so similar is the pathology of transplanted skin to that of vasculitis that their studies have been incorporated in this text. In addition, data on the pathology of stasis have been included in order to draw attention to the similarities in thrombophlebitis, gravitational stasis and vasculitis.

The authors have merely applied to the injured vessel much of the information in the literature on normal vessels. Variations in the anatomy and reactivity, or in the effect of the psyche, are important whatever the state of the vessel, and in the context of these there is often no clear dividing line between physiology and inflammation.

Table I.2. Vascular injury.

Vascular injury is a combination of:

Noxious trigger, e.g.		Constitutional defect
Immune complexes		Altered reactivity
Infective agents	plus	Prepared site
Drugs		The anatomy of stasis
Food		Pathergic tissue
		Locus minores resistentiae

This book is not concerned with detailed descriptions of such rashes and histopathology as have been described previously in texts on vasculitis (or angiitis). The reasons for this omission should become apparent in Chapters 1 and 2, for here are described the muddling and inconclusive arguments between many very distinguished authors who, without our present knowledge of mechanisms, have attempted to classify individual patients in morphological terms on the basis of physical signs. In so doing they have merely created a literature and a jargon which have made dermatology incomprehensible to workers in other fields. There are no clear divisions between the various rashes caused by injury to blood vessels. Whenever more than one expert on rashes is asked to give an opinion and to classify any one rash, complete agreement is rare. In Chapters 3 and 4 the eruptions are discussed in general terms without attempting to name each variation. Studies on transplanted skin in Chapter 5 and on the nose in Chapter 9 are used to explain the physical signs and the pathology of such rashes.

The authors are primarily interested in blood vessels, and it is therefore to be hoped that those who are not dermatologists will be able to understand this text. Thus, 'ulcers of the skin due to small vessel block as a consequence of exposure to cold' is a description that, if written on a pathological request form, a consultation slip or a treatment chart, should awaken the interest of a haematologist or a nurse and encourage them to greet the patient with more understanding than they would if the only information provided consisted of terms such as erythrocyanosis crurum frigidarum, micropapular chilblains of Hutchinson, livedo reticularis or cutaneous polyarteritis nodosa. It should not be necessary for one's colleagues to learn jargon, nor do the authors wish to perpetuate it, and they would be pleased if non-dermatologists or surgeons concerned with transplantation, for instance, could read this book and find the language similar to their own.

In Chapters 1 to 4 a spectrum of vascular responses to injury is described, ranging from the physiological, through urticaria and vasculitis, to vessel necrosis, ischaemia and coagulation. There is a point of overlap at which the endothelial response to injury switches from maximal stimulation to irreversible disintegration.

The literature on vasculitis since the beginning of the nineteenth century is a record of the classification of those physical signs which are not easily classified because of variability in their intensity, depth and distribution in the skin. As will be seen in Chapter 1, there were important starting points like Willan (1808) on purpura, Kussmaul and Maier (1866) on periarteritis nodosa, and Bazin (1861) on deep nodules of the lower leg. Thereafter the literature is characterised by fashionable ideas about syphilis, tuberculosis, foci of infection, allergy and autoimmunity. Those with special interests in chest diseases, renal diseases, histopathology, cryoglobulins, clotting or fibrinolysis introduced new biases into the classification, and by incorporating studies on skin flaps and/or the nose we are introducing still further aspects. From time to time, the word 'spectrum' has been used as a means of avoiding artificial subdivisions of disease, and over the years a spectral view of morphology has developed; however, classification by separation into major and minor subheadings is more suitable for underlying mechanisms.

In other chapters current concepts of inflammation, coagulation and fibrinolysis are discussed, and several skin diseases illustrate these very well. It is hoped that a few basic scientists will be interested to read how problems of permeability and cellular infiltration are commonplace in a dermatology clinic.

Today, the physician's task is not so much to give a morphological label to a patient's vasculitis but to recognise from the clinical picture that the patient's vessels are excessively permeable and leak, or are overwhelmed by a leucocyte infiltrate, coagulation or bleeding. In addition, he should have some knowledge of the triggers of such injury and how to detect them, and he should understand how constitutional controlling factors determine the way the vessels react and how noxious agents are localised, as is exemplified by studies of the nose described in Chapter 9. For the most part, the physician will be treating a reaction to injury; this is often peculiar to the individual, being partly inherent and partly acquired or learned by either the tissues or the entire organism. With such knowledge, the patient can be treated more intelligently than is the case when, for instance, a diagnosis of polyarteritis nodosa is glibly made, and the currently listed therapy for that particular malady is liberally prescribed.

Injury and its consequences are usually focal but may be diffuse. When a disease affects more than one organ it is referred to as *complicated,* but when it is focal and involves only a few organs it is called *limited.* Using this terminology it can be said that many of the syndromes resulting from microvascular injury are merely an admixture of focal with complicated pathology. An important factor which determines where the pathology is manifest and therefore the characteristics of the mixture is a proliferative and leaky vessel.

In a previous monograph Ryan (1973) has discussed a spectrum of vascular morphology ranging from atrophy to hypertrophy. The two ends of the spectrum are illustrated in Figure I.1. The behaviour of injured vessels described in this monograph features mostly towards the right of that spectrum. It is a proliferating, leaking and fibrinolytically exhausted vessel sitting in a fibrin latticework; it has a positive electric charge on its internal surface and is drained by a hypertrophic and hypoxic tissue. The blood vessels contain slow flowing viscous blood and this encourages neutrophil diapedesis.

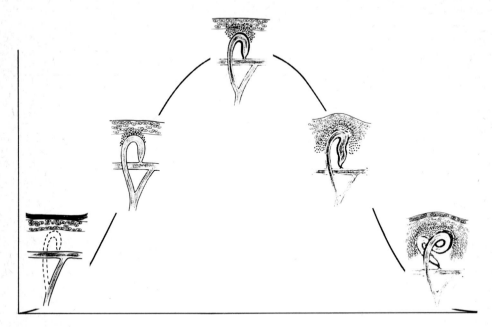

Figure. I.1. Frequency of distribution of different types of upper dermal vasculature. The commonest pattern is featured at the peak of the curve. Atrophy lies to the left and hypertrophy and hyperplasia to the right.

This is a characteristic not only of vasculitis but also of neoplasia, psoriasis and wound healing (Ryan, 1976). Epithelial tissues cause this reaction when they are injured, when they have increased metabolic requirements or when they undergo acute degeneration, as in ischaemia. It is a pattern of compensated hypoperfusion observed in shock and at certain sites of permanent venous stasis, such as the liver, the anterior nose or adipose tissue. These and similar tissues are consequently more vulnerable to acute deprivation of blood supply. Much of this monograph is concerned with those circumstances which make the skin similarly susceptible.

References

Bazin, E. (1861) *Extrait des Leçons Théoriques et Cliniques sur la Scrofule,* Paris. p. 146.
Kussmaul, A. & Maier, R. (1866) Ueber eine bisher nicht beschriebene eigenthümliche Arterien erkrankung (Periarteritis nodosa), die mit Morbus Brightii und rapid fortschreitender allgemeiner Muskellähmung einhergeht. *Deutsches Archiv für klinische Medizin,* **1,** 484.
Osler, W. (1914) The visceral lesions of purpura and allied conditions. *British Medical Journal,* **i,** 517.
Ryan, T. J. (1973) In *Physiology and Pathophysiology of the skin,* Vol. 2 (Ed.) Jarrett, A. London: Academic Press.
Ryan, T. J. (1976) Proceedings of Twenty-fifth Annual Symposium on the Biology of Skin. *Journal of Investigative Dermatology,* in press.
Willan, R. (1808) In *Cutaneous Diseases.* London: J. Johnson.

1. Nineteenth Century Observations

Most reviews of urticaria and vasculitis begin with an historical appreciation, the purpose being to support the particular classification, interpretation or jargon favoured by the reviewer. Our forefathers' writings on diseases make enjoyable reading — their descriptions of morphology were, like the Old Testament, beautifully written, and they were unsurpassed in their recognition and classification of physical signs. Yet, were they alive today, many of these writers would admit that the persisting use of their terminology is impeding a mechanistic and realistic approach to dermatology. Furthermore, they would agree that their conclusions were often wrong, being based on only a small fraction of the knowledge available to us about the mechanisms operating in disease. After all, they wrote in terms of physical signs which are merely patterns produced by reactions and do not necessarily designate disease entities. In fact, it is only now becoming possible to name diseases after the disorders of function that often produce the pathology and provide an explanation of the rash.

Classification: 'lumping' and 'splitting'

During the past 20 years, there has been much discussion of the relative merits of 'lumping' and of 'splitting' the classic and the more recently described features of skin disease. 'Lumping' was necessarily used during the great period of classic description when skin manifestations such as purpura or bullae were first outlined. 'Splitting' is a natural sequel to 'lumping' and helps to relate morphology to pathogenesis at a time when understanding of underlying mechanisms is particularly poor. This is why physicians have inevitably given new names to the reaction patterns and physical signs of their patients whenever they have differed from the classic descriptions.

The literature on vasculitis is confusing just because many authors have split off particular reaction patterns which others have subsequently attempted to absorb into a parent group. 'Splitting off' usually results in the coining of a new name, and a huge vocabulary is thereby gradually amassed, to the dismay of the uninitiated who have to

1

Table 1.1. Cutaneous angiitis: descriptive terms.

	References
1. Primarily affecting the skin	
Haemorrhagic microbids	Miescher, 1946
Arteriolitis allergica	Ruiter, 1952
Mono-, bi-, tri- and pentasymptom complexes	Gougerot and Blum, 1950
Nodular dermal allergids	Gougerot and Duperrat, 1954
Dermatitis nodularis necrotica	Werther, 1910; Duemling, 1930
Facial granuloma with eosinophilia	Cobane, Straith and Pinkus, 1950
Erythema elevatum diutinum	Hutchinson, 1888; Radcliffe Crocker and Williams, 1894
Idiopathic lethal granulomas of midline facial tissues	McBride, 1897
Cutaneous polyarteritis nodosa	Lindberg, 1932
2. Affecting skin and other systems	
Allergic angiitis	Churg and Strauss, 1951
Leucocytoclastic angiitis	Winkelmann and Ditto, 1964
Allergic vasculitis	Lever, 1967; Wilkinson, 1965
Purpura or peliosis rheumatica	Ruiter, 1956
Anaphylactoid or Schönlein—Henoch purpura	See Table 1.2
Acute febrile neutrophilic dermatosis	Sweet, 1964
3. Primarily systemic disorders	
Wegener's granulomatosis	Wegener, 1939
Allergic granulomatosis	Churg and Strauss, 1951
Pathergic granulomatosis	Fienberg, 1955
Non-infectious necrotising granules	
Hypersensitivity angiitis	Zeek, 1952
Necrotising angiitis	Zeek, 1952
Hypersensitivity type of periarteritis nodosa	Zeek, 1952

wade through it. This dermatologists' jargon creates a barrier for the non-dermatologist which he could well do without. The confusion engendered by this jargon is illustrated in Tables 1.1 and 1.2 in which the various names given to vasculitis, urticaria and erythema perstans are listed.

'Splitting' is designed to show that a particular pattern of disease is an entity differing significantly from related patterns in its morphology, behaviour, causation, prognosis and treatment. In dermatology, however, such criteria are rarely defined with a strictness sufficient to promote general agreement. This deficiency stems from a concentration on morphology which is not a reliable guide to causation, prognosis and

Table 1.2. Synonyms of Schönlein—Henoch purpura.

Schönlein's purpura (1839)
Henoch's purpura (1874)
Osler's syndrome (1914)
Anaphylactoid purpura (Glanzmann, 1916)
Allergic purpura
Purpura rheumatica (e.g. by Ruiter, 1956)

also
Non-thrombocytopenic purpura
Acute vascular purpura
Vascular anaphylactoid purpura
Primary purpura, purpura simplex
Urticarial purpura

treatment. Why this is so is discussed more fully in Chapter 3, but the chief reason is that morphology is no respecter of mechanisms. It certainly was a misfortune that our forefathers had little knowledge of these mechanisms.

Clearly, then, once it is accepted that morphology is unreliable in this respect, much of the past literature becomes valueless and the debates which every author on vasculitis includes in discussion become mere chat about obsolete jargon.

The separation of dermatology from general medicine

The confusion over vasculitis terminology is a product of the last 50 years, aggravated by the fact that dermatology, during the last century, has become divorced from general medicine, founding its own societies and producing its own specialist journals and reference books.

As a result, even in the late 1950s, physicians seeking help with the management of a patient with urticaria, vasculitis, purpura or necrosis would be disappointed even by the major medical textbooks. In Cecil and Loeb's (1959) or in Price's (1956) *Textbook of Medicine,* for example, the only sections remotely covering such processes would be devoted either to polyarteritis nodosa or to Schönlein—Henoch purpura.

Likewise, it was a mere 25 years or so ago that books on dermatology began to include discussions on some aspects of vascular disease in general medicine. The twelfth edition of Roxburgh, for instance, was the first to include Schönlein—Henoch purpura, although at the same time purely dermatological concepts such as nodular vasculitis as a subheading of Bazin's disease were described. In the *Handbook of Diseases of the Skin* by Sutton (1949) little space was devoted to non-thrombocytopenic purpuras, although a classification based on aetiology and drawn from medical texts was used.

By the 1960s, dermatologists could formulate names for most patterns of skin disease. General physicians, however, were not interested in such pursuits, yet when they found their own texts lacking detail in this respect, they readily accepted the dermatologists' ability to recognise the most minute variation in physical signs.

Early description and comments (Willan, Hebra)

The debate on classification of vascular diseases of the skin began almost as soon as the nineteenth century authors started to classify and to introduce descriptive terms.

According to Hebra (1868), cutaneous diseases produced by extravasation of blood had been briefly mentioned by Hippocrates but the exact meaning of a few of his statements had been disputed by several subsequent writers. Hebra suggested that prior to the sixteenth century all diseases of the skin had been referred to as leprosy, but that thereafter "they were constantly brought into relation with either syphilis or scorbutus". He pointed out that purpura was not fully established as an entity until the nineteenth century when several writers were concerned with it, mainly in relation to infectious diseases.

Willan (1808) had described purpura simplex, purpura haemorrhagica, purpura urticans and purpura contagiosa (Figure 1.1). Purpura simplex occurred in patients who were not ill, although they sometimes were pale and languid and complained of limb pains. The petechiae were sometimes preceded for a day or two by a general, red efflorescence. Purpura contagiosa, by contrast, was a severe illness caused probably by disease such as typhus, malaria or meningococcal septicaemia. Purpura urticans affected the legs, arms and heart and was accompanied by ankle oedema. The lesions were rounded elevations which gradually increased in size and subsided 24 hours after they had appeared, by which time livid spots were seen. Clearly, Willan was observing the same rash as had concerned Heberden (1802) and would later concern Schönlein (1837), Henoch (1874) and subsequent writers describing anaphylactoid purpura or allergic vasculitis.

(452)

O R D E R III.

V. P U R P U R A.

―――――――

THE title Purpura, or Efflorefcentia purpurata, has been applied to papulous eruptions on the fkin, to different forms of Rafhes*, and to the purple eruption which often occurs in malignant Feverst. Riverius is, I believe, the firft author who makes a diftinction be-tween Purpura and petechial Fevers : he obferves, Nullum dari fignum harum febrium verè pathognomo-nicum,—nedum bubonem, aut carbunculum, in verè peftilenti,—neque maculas purpureas in Febre malignâ, quamvis illa a pluribus medicis purpurata nominetur ;

* To the Red-gum, by Etmuller :
    To the Scarlatina, by Schultzius and Juncker; and in the Ephemerides Act. Nat. Cur. &c :
    To the Measles, by Hafenreffer, II. 4. and Morton, Pyretolog. Appendix :
    To the Miliaria, Lichen, and Nettle Rash, by Juncker, Hoffman, &c. and in Act. Nat. Cur.

    † Sennertus, Lib. V. Porchon, Traitè du Pourpre, a Paris, 1688. Sauvages, Nos. Med. &c.

                                                                cum

Figure 1.1. The opening paragraph in the chapter on purpura by Willan (1808), in which he makes a distinction between purpura and the petechiae of infectious diseases.

To illustrate aptly an attempt to classify the unclassifiable, the following quotation from Hebra's *Diseases of the Skin* is given:

"When afterwards the artificial systems of classification which came into vogue in all natural sciences were adopted in dermatology, it was found difficult to arrange *petechiae;* so that each author placed them in a different position. Plenck ranges them among the "spots" as *maculae lividae;* Peter Frank puts them among exanthems, while ecchymomata are included in the class "Impetigines". Biett who frankly gave up the attempt to carry out a consistent principle of classification, placed purpura, lupus and syphilis together in one class, with no common character except that they could not be arranged in any other divisions. Willan and Bateman reckon purpura among the Exanthemata, and distinguished several varieties which we shall have to speak of further on. Wilson who follows them in other respects, has removed it to the class of Maculae. Alibert and Rayer, who tried to establish a more natural system of classification, arranged cutaneous haemorrhages in a special class which the former writer calls 'Haematoses', subdividing it into 'Petechiae and Pelioses'.''

During the hundred years since Hebra wrote this, classification has become even more complex because it is now recognised that purpura may be associated with urticaria, deep nodules, the syndrome of polyarteritis nodosa or intravascular coagulation.

Peliosis and purpura — the superficial lesion (Schönlein and Henoch) (Table 1.3)

When Schönlein (1837) described peliosis rheumatica in patients with inflammation of the joints, he was writing for readers who were familiar with the description by Werlhof (1775) of a girl who had severe nosebleeds, haematemesis and widespread intracutaneous haemorrhages — a clinical picture similar to that seen sometimes in smallpox and almost certainly a syndrome caused by disseminated intravascular coagulation or thrombocytopenia. The disease described by Schönlein was a much milder one than that which Werlhof reported. In fact, his description is more in keeping with a toxic erythema: "The spots are small, the size of a lentil, a millet seed, bright red, not elevated above the skin, disappearing on pressure of the finger; they become gradually a dirty brown, yellowish, the skin over the spot appears somewhat branny, the eruption comes by fits and starts, often throughout several weeks. Every slight change in temperature, for instance going around in a room that is a little cooled off, can produce a new eruption''. Schönlein, comparing his patients' disease to that of Werlhof's, emphasised that peliosis was bright red, never blue or livid.

Henoch (1874) devoted himself exclusively to the study of the disease in children and, described joint and intestinal symptoms which clearly had a haemorrhagic basis with "sometimes large ecchymoses (in two cases) and in the other two (first and third), they had only a characteristic form of circumscribed, small light red spots, like those of an exanthema, which were not above the level of the skin and did not disappear on pressure''. These early descriptions were of purpura; for deeper, nodular lesions one must refer initially to erythema nodosum, described first by Willan (1808), and then turn to Bazin (1861).

Table 1.3. Willan—Schönlein—Henoch purpura.

Age and sex	More common in boys
Site	Lower extremities and buttocks, occasionally on forearms and trunk
Lesions	Erythematous weal followed by purpuric papule; may become bullous or ulcerate
Associated findings	Pain and swelling in knees and ankles; epigastric pain and melaena; rarely nephritis
Histology	Vascular endothelium shows swelling and degeneration. Perivascular infiltrate of fragmented neutrophils

Author's view
The spectrum of urticaria, vasculitis and coagulation or thrombosis occurring in all age groups and due to a variety of injurious agents or impaired protective and repair mechanisms in the walls of capillaries and venules.

Erythema induratum — the deep lesion (Bazin) (Table 1.4)

Bazin (1861) described "red indurated plaques from which, with digital pressure, the redness disappears momentarily, soon to return. One feels an induration on the skin and in the skin which reaches more or less deeply into the subcutaneous tissues. The redness, which is more or less dark, quite often violaceous and more marked in the centre, blends insensibly at the periphery with the normal colour of the skin. There is no itching in these plaques; digital pressure on them causes scarcely any pain".

Table 1.4. Erythema induratum (Bazin's disease), a nodular form of vasculitis.

Age and sex	Young and adult females
Site	Calves bilaterally
Lesions	One or several deep, non-tender, bluish-red, subcutaneous nodules that ulcerate or are absorbed, leaving depressed, atrophic scars. Lesions persist for months
Associated findings	Internal focus of tuberculosis
Laboratory findings	Tuberculin test positive
Histology	Lower dermis and subcutis show panarteritis and phlebitis with fat necrosis, a non-specific inflammatory infiltrate and caseous tubercles. Difficult to demonstrate tubercle bacilli

Author's view
The spectrum of delayed urticaria, vasculitis and coagulation or thrombosis occurring predominantly in females, especially in the legs, and due to a variety of injurious agents or impaired protective repair mechanisms in venules. Ischaemic necrosis of fat and the arterial wall is a late but common event.

"This affection is observed commonly on the legs, more often perhaps in females than males. I have often found it on the legs of young laundresses, young women with all the attributes of scrofulous corpulence and ruddiness. Its site of predilection is the lateral and lower part of the leg. At times one sees it located a little above the heel, along the Achilles tendon. Finally, one may also see it on the face, and I have seen it alternating with scrofulus ophthalmia in that region".

Arterial disease (Kussmaul and Maier)

Kussmaul and Maier (1866) described periarteritis nodosa in the days when the practice of medicine differed so much from that of today that doubt must be cast on the validity of subsequent attempts to fit their description into any classification of vasculitis.

Their first patient was a young man recently treated for scabies and imprisoned for begging. After his death, students rapidly dissected his body as an anatomical exercise, much to the consternation of the authors who then had to take specimens for analysis. They reported worm infestation (Figure 1.2) since the internal organs in particular were riddled with immature filarial-like objects each up to 13 mm in length "similar to that sometimes found in horses". It was only subsequently that they decided to report the case in more detail (Figure 1.3) leaving the worms unexplained but concentrating on their findings in the vasculature.

The patient had a history of nephritis, acute in onset and characterised by thirst, frequency of micturition, oliguria and an albumin-laden urine containing some red cells and casts. These symptoms were followed by severe paralysis, by pain in most muscles of the body and by some peripheral neuropathy. Histologically there was gross hypertrophy and some degeneration of the media and adventitia of the small arteries.

They were writing at a time when arterial disease was often syphilitic, death was frequently due to tuberculosis, changes in smooth muscle were commonly due to typhoid, and peripheral neuropathies were a consequence of diphtheria. Trichiniasis also was common. For this reason they were in fact recording some unusual features, in

VII.

Aneurysma verminosum hominis.

Vorläufige Nachricht

von

Prof. A. Kussmaul und Prof. R. Maier.

Figure 1.2. The chapter heading from the first volume of *Deutsches Archiv für klinische Medizin* in which Kussmaul and Maier described worm infestation in their patient.

particular the smallness of the affected arteries and the absence of gross diarrhoea, chest disease or evidence of trichiniasis.

Kussmaul and Maier's account and drawings leave no doubt that they were describing arteries (Figure 1.4) and that capillaries and veins were not affected. Most of the lesions, a few dozen per square inch, were isolated small nodules involving the vessels and were no larger than poppy seeds. Some, however, especially in the skin of the abdomen and chest, became palpable shortly before death. Bifurcations were usually involved. There also were odd clinical features such as persistent opisthotonos. The microscopic changes in the media seemed to consist primarily of hypertrophy and hyperplasia of smooth muscle. There was little to suggest hypersensitivity angiitis or intravascular coagulation, as has been noted in some later descriptions of polyarteritis nodosa.

XXIII.

Ueber eine bisher nicht beschriebene eigenthümliche Arterienerkrankung (Periarteritis nodosa), die mit Morbus Brightii und rapid fortschreitender allgemeiner Muskellähmung einhergeht.

Von

Prof. A. Kussmaul und R. Maier

in Freiburg i. Br.

Hierzu Taf. III—V.

Krankengeschichte.

Figure 1.3. The chapter heading from the first volume of *Deutsches Archiv für klinische Medizin* in which Kussmaul and Maier described the same patient as in Figure 1.2 but now refer to periarteritis nodosa and Bright's disease.

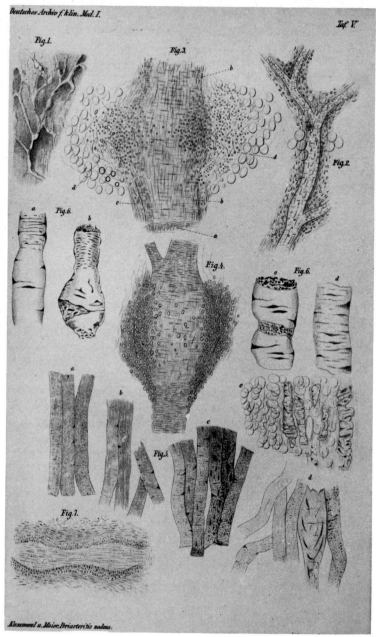

Figure 1.4. Illustration of the pathology in the first description of periarteritis nodosa. 'Figure 1' shows arterial disease but the other illustrations are difficult to interpret.

Their second case did not come to postmortem but had a biopsy of the gastrocnemius. The patient was aged 28 and presented with muscle pain, fever and widespread paralysis. There was facial oedema and albuminuria which later cleared. Loss of sensation was not a feature but the muscle paralysis persisted for several months. The muscle biopsy showed none of the nodular arterial changes seen in the first case, but microscopic changes were noted in the small vessels which, in view of their location in the calf of someone who had been bedridden and paralysed for several months, may not have represented primary arterial disease.

As no other significant descriptions were written during the nineteenth century, twentieth century dermatologists based their classification on these two cases, returning to them repeatedly.

Osler and later elaborations

Osler saw many patients with purpura. His descriptions of those who presented at the Radcliffe Infirmary, Oxford, would apply equally well to cases seen there at the present time (Figure 1.5). These clear descriptions, written in the language of general physicians, emphasise that there is a class of disease affecting blood vessels which shows polymorphism — urticaria, purpura and necrosis.

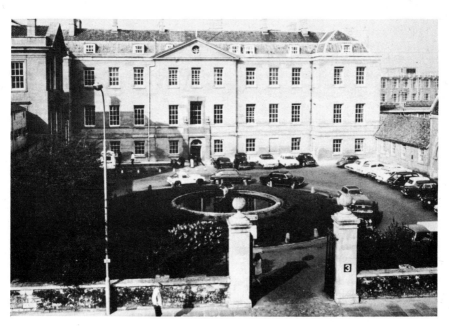

Figure 1.5. The Radcliffe Infirmary, 1975. The patients described in this monograph and those described by William Osler (1914) came from the villages and towns of Oxfordshire and were examined and recorded in this building.

Osler (1914) published from Oxford *The Visceral Lesions of Purpura and Allied Conditions* which ignored terminology to such an extent that it has been quoted very little by subsequent writers obsessed with classification. Discussing the character of the skin lesions, he wrote: "all are exudative, in which the blood element — either the red blood corpuscles alone, the serum alone or both combined — pass out of the vessels". He described purpura on its own, with swelling (purpura urticans), or associated with urticarial weals or angio-oedema. Under the same heading he included erythema which could be diffuse, localised or associated with swelling; in fact, he outlined a reaction pattern ranging from toxic erythema to erythema nodosum and erythema multiforme. Bullae, necrosis and ulceration, which were thought to result from a very intense localised infiltrate of blood and serum, could occur even in the erythema of chilblains, so common in the occupants of the large Victorian houses of north Oxford.

Osler emphasised in particular the variety of lesions, and the fact that some patients had only a single acute attack whilst others had repeated episodes in which the lesions might differ from one outbreak to the next.

The visceral lesions were described in detail under cerebral, ocular, gastrointestinal, renal and cardiac complications, and it is clear that these patients seen at the Radcliffe Infirmary were suffering from a spectrum of disease ranging from urticaria through various patterns of purpura and vasculitis to disseminated intravascular coagulation. Osler listed many triggers including viral and bacterial infection, idiosyncrasy to drugs and foods, serum sickness, hereditary factors (especially in angio-oedema), snake venom, and exposure to cold or heat.

Polyarteritis nodosa — a diagnosis too frequently made (Table 1.5)

Perhaps because Osler did not give a specific name to the spectrum of disorders he was describing, textbooks of medicine did not find a place for them and remained of little value to the physician searching for help in making a diagnosis. Even Osler's textbook seems not to have incorporated all this information in any one section. Moreover, even 40 to 50 years later, the present author as a houseman at Osler's hospital had to search through all the texts to find a diagnosis that might fit a patient suffering from hypertension, peripheral neuropathy and a rash; only in the section on polyarteritis nodosa could descriptions be found of the bizarre manifestations of this class of disorder. By then, polyarteritis nodosa had become the term applied to the type of patient described by Osler in his 1914 paper. How this came about was well reviewed by Pearl Zeek in 1952.

During the period from 1866 to 1900, polyarteritis nodosa clearly described a disease affecting arteries smaller than the aorta and its main branches. There was no question of an arteriolitis, capillaritis or venulitis. The clinical description stressed palpable changes in peripheral arteries, which was an important distinction at a time when syphilitic

Table 1.5. 'Peri'- and polyarteritis nodosa.

Periarteritis nodosa: 19th century view
A disease of arteries in young men; palpable nodules due to aneurysms. Rupture of arteries, embolism and thrombosis affects all organs except lungs.

Polyarteritis nodosa: 20th century view

Age and sex	Most frequent in males aged 20 to 50 years
Site	Skin lesions may occur anywhere on body, sometimes along course of arteries
Lesions	Non-specific urticaria, erythema multiforme, erythema nodosum, purpura; subcutaneous nodules becoming bullous, pustular or necrotic
Associated findings	Malaise, joint pains, muscle tenderness, hypertension, peripheral neuropathy, abdominal pain, intermittent fever, coronary sclerosis; melaena; hypertensive retinitis, nodular lesions of retinal arteries
Laboratory findings	Eosinophilia, leucocytosis, mild hypochromic anaemia, haematuria, albuminuria, and oval fatty bodies in urine
Histology	Skin and muscle biopsy diagnostic. Shows necrosis and acute inflammation of media of small arteries and occasionally veins, with occlusion, thrombosis, aneurysm formation and scarring

Author's view
Ischaemia of arterial walls secondary to hypertension, distal capillaritis or distal thrombosis. Most of the 20th century features are capillary and venular. Immune complexes or toxins first affect capillaries and veins and are found in arterial walls following necrosis from ischaemia.

involvement of the large arteries was so common. Because benign and malignant hypertension were, at that time, not understood, and since neither the malignant variety nor polyarteritis nodosa involved the pulmonary arteries, it was later debated whether polyarteritis nodosa might be secondary to hypertension. The histologically recognised features included necrosis of the media and adventitia with intravascular thrombosis, and recanalisation of thrombosed vessels was described. The following passage is taken from Zeek (1952):

"Thus at the turn of the century, periarteritis nodosa was generally considered a rare but distinct disease entity, which could be differentiated from syphilis, and which, in its fatal stage, was characterised at autopsy by readily visible, nodular lesions at the points of branching of small and medium sized muscular type arteries. The lesions were frequently widespread throughout the body, except in the lungs and brain. They were thought to begin as foci of fibrinoid necrosis and inflammation in the media or adventitia, and were prone to result in localised ruptures of the media or with the formation of small aneurysms. Capillaries were never involved and veins only occasionally by spread from contiguous arteries. The aetiology was unsolved but was generally thought to be an unidentified toxic or infectious agent. However, one investigator (Meyer, 1878) had suggested a possible relationship between fluctuating hypertension and the lesions of polyarteritis nodosa, even before modern tools for the measurement of blood pressure were available".

From 1900 to 1925 one moved into the era of foci of infection and to the beginning of the era of allergy. As animals seemed to develop a similar disease in response to infection, much effort was spent on investigating this possibility but failed to prove the point. In the meantime Arthus (1903) described changes in vascular morphology resulting from the reaction between non-toxic agents and hypersensitive vessels, and around this concept of hypersensitivity a considerable literature began to evolve.

The study of increasingly small arteries and venules

The more frequent use of the microscope and the interest in hypersensitivity encouraged a concept of subclinical microscopic polyarteritis which included a much wider range of pathology affecting vessels. As smaller and ever smaller vessels were studied, they were found to be involved in clinical syndromes which, if not identical to Kussmaul and Maier's disease, were certainly similar to it. Furthermore, the smaller the vessel studied, the more closely the picture resembled that observed by Arthus (1903).

Important in a negative sense was the complete lack of interest in venules and veins. This was probably because Starling's (1896) concept of the balance between hydrostatic and osmotic pressure was at that time learned by every doctor in training, and therefore arteries and capillaries were regarded as the effective vasculature, veins being considered as mere capacity vessels channelling the blood rather inefficiently back to the heart.

Now, of course, it is known that venules and capillaries are the main site for the Arthus and the Shwartzman phenomena and also for fluid exchanges, and that, in terms of Osler's diseases of exudation, these vessels and not arteries are involved. This advance in understanding is described in detail in Chapter 12.

As concepts of vasculitis tended to incriminate smaller vessels, histopathologists inevitably began to study a size of vessel equivalent to arterioles and venules. It was only natural, however, that in the histological examination of polyarteritis nodosa it was always assumed that the vessels being studied were increasingly small arteries, because in light microscopy the histopathology of venules and arterioles, when inflamed, are indistinguishable; in any case, inflamed venules in skin resemble small arteries (see Chapter 4).

Polyarteritis nodosa became such a familiar term that there was a tendency to rename the vascular lesions found in rheumatic fever and in serum sickness. Furthermore, by the early 1940s, very small vessels had been included in the picture of polyarteritis nodosa, and Rich (1942), studying the lesions in sulphonamide sensitivity, described them too as polyarteritic:

"The necroses in these minute focal areas appear to develop as a result of damage to minute arterioles and capillaries. In the present case the abundance of lesions in vessels of this calibre provided an exceptional opportunity to observe that these little focal inflammatory infiltrations develop immediately about a necrotic, minute vessel."

In the light of modern knowledge it seems likely that when interest is shifted to increasingly small vessels, one necessarily begins to scrutinise a range of pathology which encompasses the exudative small vessel lesions described by Willan, Schönlein, Henoch and Osler and which may be due to a number of triggers including allergy, infection and physical factors such as stasis or cold.

Pearl Zeek (1952) believed that the early descriptions of polyarteritis nodosa included many cases of malignant hypertension. However, Kussmaul and Maier's patients with severe paralysis but with neither headache nor cardiomegaly seem difficult to place in this way, yet equally they did not have the histology of an Arthus phenomenon or of disseminated intravascular coagulation.

Present-day dermatologists are so aware of the many variations on these earlier descriptions that it is difficult to know how to incorporate them into our present classifications. For instance, should Henoch's name be retained for a disease in children merely because he was a paediatrician? Or should the disorder described by Schönlein be classified as a purpura? And the use of Bazin's name is equally difficult to justify, for at first he recorded neither tenderness nor ulceration; in fact, he gave no details which would have helped to confirm that his patients had tuberculosis, and of course he lived before that disease could be confirmed bacteriologically. Should one, in fact, give names to these disorders on the basis either of descriptions of single cases or of later writings by the same authors or even of later interpretations? How can one avoid the descriptive terms illustrated in Tables 1.1 and 1.2?

In conclusion, it can be seen that many authors during the past 200 years have classified, reclassified and decried classification on a morphological basis. The time has come to abandon the attempt and to concentrate on mechanisms, for only now are we beginning to have sufficient knowledge to make such classifications rational. Morphology can be more completely expressed in pathological terms while pathology can be shown to be based on function, which is open to analysis. We are more fortunate than our forebears in this respect, for, as Arthur Rook pointed out in another volume in this series (Warin and Champion, 1974), they were just as aware of the difficulties and the need for an improved classification but had less information at their disposal.

There is a real need for a generic name for these diseases. Copeman (1975) comes near to providing the term that most closely fits the subject of this monograph. He uses the term 'venulitis'.

References

Arthus, M. (1903) Injections répétées de sérum de cheval chez le lapin. *Compte Rendu de la Société de Biologie,* **55,** 817.

Bazin, E. (1861) *Extrait des Leçons Théoriques et Cliniques sur la Scrofule.* p. 146.

Cecil, R. L. & Loeb, R. F. (1959) *A Textbook of Medicine.* Philadelphia: W. B. Saunders.

Churg, J. & Strauss, Lotte (1951) Allergic granulomatosis, allergic angiitis and periarteritis nodosa. *American Journal of Pathology,* **27,** 277.

Cobane, J. H., Straith, C. L. & Pinkus, H. (1950) Facial granulomas with eosinophilia. Their relation to other eosinophilic granulomas of the skin and to reticulo granuloma. *Archives of Dermatology,* **61,** 442.

Copeman, P. W. M. (1975) Cutaneous angiitis. *Journal of the Royal College of Physicians of London*, **9**, 103.
Copeman, P. W. M. & Ryan, T. J. (1970) The problems of cutaneous angiitis with reference to histopathology and pathogenesis. *British Journal of Dermatology*, **81**, 2.
Duemling, W. W. (1930) Dermatitis nodularis necrotica. Report of a case and review of the literature. *Archives of Dermatology and Syphilology*, **21**, 229.
Fienberg, R. (1955) Editorial. Pathergic granulomatosis. *American Journal of Medicine*, **19**, 829.
Gairdner, D. (1948) The Schonlein—Henock syndrome (anaphylactoid purpura). *Quarterly Journal of Medicine*, **17**, 95.
Glanzmann, E. (1916) Beiträge zur kinntnis der purpura im Kindesalter. *Jahrbuch für Kinderheilkunde*, **83**, 271.
Gougerot, H. & Blum, P. (1950) Un nouveau cas de trisymptôme on plutot pentasymptôme. *Bulletin de la Société Française de Dermatologie et de Syphiligraphie*, **57**, 336.
Gougerot, H. & Duperrat, B. (1954) The nodular dermal allergids of Gougerot. *British Journal of Dermatology*, **66**, 283.
Heberden, W. (1802) *Commentaries on the History and Cure of Diseases*, 3rd edition. pp. 395-397. London: Payne.
Hebra, F. (1868) *Diseases of the Skin*, Volume II, p. 404. London: The New Sydenham Society.
Henoch, E. H. (1874) Über eine eigenthümliche form von purpura. *Berliner klinische Wochenschrift*, **11**, 641.
Hutchinson, J. (1888) On two remarkable cases of symmetrical purple congestion of the skin in patches, with induration. *British Journal of Dermatology*, **1**, 10.
Kussmaul, A. & Maier, R. (1866) Ueber eine bisher nicht beschriebene eigenthümliche Arterien erkrankung (Periarteritis nodosa), die mit Morbus Brightii und rapid fortschreitender allgemeiner Muskellähmung einhergeht. *Deutsches Archiv für klinische Medizin*, **1**, 484.
Lever, W. F. (1967) *Histopathology of the Skin*. Philadelphia: J. B. Lippincott.
Lindberg, K. (1932) Uber eine subkutane form der Periarteritis nodosa mit langwierigem verlauf. *Acta Medica Scandinavica*, **77**, 455.
McBride, P. (1897) Idiopathic lethal granulomas of the midline facial tissues. Quoted by Alexader, B. R. in *Archives of Dermatology*, **79**, 390.
Meyer, P. (1878) Ueber Periarteritis nodosa oder multiple Aneurysmen de mit kleineren Arterien. *Virchows Archiv für pathologische Anatomie*, **74**, 277.
Miescher, G. (1946) Uber kutane formen der Periarteritis nodosa. *Dermatologica*, **92**, 225.
Osler, W. (1914) The visceral lesions of purpura and allied conditions. *British Medical Journal*, **i**, 517.
Price, F. W. (1956) *Price's Textbook of the Practice of Medicine* (Ed.) Hunter, D. Oxford: Oxford University Press.
Radcliffe Crocker, H. & Williams, C. (1894) Erythema elevatum diutinum. *British Journal of Dermatology*, **6**, 33.
Rich, A. R. (1942) The role of hypersensitivity in periarteritis nodosa, as indicated by seven cases developing during serum sickness and sulphonamide therapy. *Bulletin of the Johns Hopkins Hospital*, **71**, 375.
Roxburgh, A. C. (1961) *Roxburgh's Common Skin Disease*, 12th edition (Ed.) Borrie, P. London: H. K. Lewis.
Ruiter, M. (1952) Cutaneous forms of periarteritis nodosa. *Nederlandische Tijdschrift, Geneesk*, **96**, 794.
Ruiter, M. (1956) Purpura rheumatica, allergic cutaneous arteriolitis, a type of. *British Journal of Dermatology*, **68**, 16.
Schönlein, J. L. (1837) Peliosis rheumatica (pelcircumsc). In *Allgemeine und specielle Pathologie und Therapie*, 3rd edition, Volume 2, p. 48. Quoted from a translation of the lectures given to his students. Reported in *Allgemeine und specielle Pathologie und Therapie*, 4th edition, Volume 2 (1839) p. 42. St. Gallen: Comptoir.
Starling, E. H. (1896) On the absorption of fluids from the connective tissue spaces. *Journal of Physiology*, **19**, 312.
Sutton, R. L. (1949) *Handbook of Diseases of the Skin* (Ed.) Sutton, R. L. & Sutton, R. L. Jr. p. 453. London: Henry Kimpton.
Sweet, R. D. (1964) An acute febrile neutrophilic dermatosis. *British Journal of Dermatology*, **76**, 349.
Warin, R. P. & Champion, R. H. (1974) *Urticaria*. London: W. B. Saunders.
Wegener, F. (1939) Ueber eine eigenartige rhinogene Granulomatose mit besonderer Beteiligung des Arteriensystems und der Nieren. *Beiträge zur pathologischen Anatomie und zur allgemeinen Pathologie*, **102**, 36.
Werlhof, P. G. (1775) *Morbus Maculosus Haemorrhagicas, Opera Omnia*. Hanover: Helwing. 748 pp.
Werther (1910) Quoted by Duemling, W. W.
Wilkinson, D. S. (1965) Some clinical manifestations and associations of "allergic" vasculitis. *British Journal of Dermatology*, **77**, 186.
Willan, R. (1808) In *Cutaneous Diseases*. London: J. Johnson.
Winkelmann, R. K. & Ditto, W. B. (1964) Cutaneous and visceral syndromes of necrotising "allergic" angiitis. A study of 38 cases. *Medicine* (Baltimore), **43**, 59.
Zeek, P. M. (1952) Periarteritis nodosa. A critical review. *American Journal of Clinical Pathology*, **22**, 777.

2. Twentieth Century Elaboration and The Naming of Physical Signs

Variations in the morphology of skin lesions are as important to the dermatologist as are the differences between crepitations, rhonci and rales to the chest physician, or third heart sound and a split second sound to the cardiologist. The significance of a particular collection of physical signs continues to be discussed.

Copeman (1975) has recently re-introduced the views of Heberden on this topic with the following quotation: "There is a great variety of cutaneous disorders . . . Several of the appearances here mentioned have been distinguished among the ancient physicians by peculiar names: there is great difficulty, though happily not much use, in ascertaining the appearances to which these names were appropriated; for this reason the ancient divisions and titles of cutaneous diseases are very little regarded by the moderns . . . Many morbid appearances of the skin are judged to be proofs of a diseased constitution, rather than merely local disorders of the part which is afflicted with them." Concepts such as cutaneous polyarteritis nodosa, nodular vasculitis, and the 'Chöffler Train' are outlined in this chapter to illustrate the morphologist's dilemma.

Cutaneous polyarteritis nodosa

This subject has been bedevilled by much conflicting information. Thus Ketron and Bernstein (1939) reviewed 200 cases of polyarteritis nodosa in the literature and calculated a 25 per cent incidence of skin involvement, whereas others (Borrie and Stansfeld, 1966) have called this figure meaningless and have emphasised that skin involvement is rare in the classic disorder. Again, on the one hand, the first patient of Kussmaul and Maier (1866) developed, late in the disease from which he eventually died, some palpable rather than visible subcutaneous nodules on his trunk, and on the other, Lindberg (1931, 1932), in describing two patients with subcutaneous nodules whom he had observed for four and nine years respectively, emphasised a cutaneous form of the disease with a good prognosis.

It is against this background of uncertainty that one must place the concept of cutaneous polyarteritis nodosa, a disorder which, in the minds of some authors, has become associated with a bluish reticulate pattern on the skin, termed livedo reticularis (Borrie, 1972), while others (Braverman, 1970; Copeman and Ryan, 1971; Ryan and Wilkinson, 1972) would prefer to associate reticulate patterns on the skin with capillary and venous phenomena.

The clinical distinction and possibly also the histological distinction between this cutaneous and a deeper nodular eruption — nodular vasculitis — is not always easy, especially when involvement of small vessels and leucocytoclastic angiitis are included in the concept of polyarteritis nodosa. Nodules, however, were considered diagnostic by Lamb (1914). These can be the size of a hazelnut, but usually are impalpable (Keil, 1938); they either disappear in a few days or last for months (Miller and Daley, 1946), and they may even resemble erythema nodosum (Klotz, 1917; Spiegel, 1936; Vining, 1938; Miescher, 1946).

The types of rash seen include urticaria, often accompanied by or followed by purpura (Cohen, Kline and Young, 1936; Spiegel, 1936; Grant, 1940), papulo-bullous lesions (Debré et al, 1928), vesicles (Grant, 1940), or erythema multiforme (Osler, 1914; Hutinel, Coste and Arnaudet, 1930; Spiegel, 1936; Grant, 1940) and this varied picture makes nonsense of a purely arterial concept of the disease. Similarly oedema, when present, may be due to congestive cardiac failure, acute nephritis or dermatomyositis and is likewise not purely arterial in origin but implies a capillary and venous injury which may be a primary event in the pathogenesis.

Fine and Meltzer (1969) have grouped, on clinical and histological grounds, sub-acute nodular migratory panniculitis, nodular vasculitis, erythema induratum, erythema nodosum migrans and chronic erythema nodosum. As their description includes disease patterns that others might call cutaneous polyarteritis nodosa, the range of associated lesions could be very wide.

Lyell and Church (1954) drew attention to livedo reticularis as mentioned in early descriptions of syphilis and tuberculosis and emphasised that this is a chronic condition appearing in protracted disease. They described three cases, two with livedo reticularis and one with purpura. The histology described an angiitis involving small vessels in the dermis and accompanied by leucocytoclasis, fibrous thickening of deeper vessels and recanalisation of thrombi. The purpura was accompanied by a prolonged prothrombin time and by Factor VII deficiency (see also Chapter 13).

Several authors have emphasised an association of purpura gangrenosum with polyarteritis nodosa. Furthermore, as consumption of clotting factors, exudation of platelets and fibrin, and thrombosis are so often features of polyarteritis nodosa, there is every justification for believing that disseminated or local intravascular coagulation underlies many of the lesions mentioned in the early descriptions of the disease; this is discussed in Chapter 10.

In recent years, Borrie (1972) has promoted the use of the term cutaneous polyarteritis nodosa for what he believed to be a specific clinical and histological entity comprising subcutaneous nodules with an arteritis in the subcutis and usually with livedo reticularis in the affected area; the site of predilection is the lower legs. Bradford et al (1962) termed a somewhat similar picture livedo reticularis with nodules. Borrie reviewed 102 cases seen at St Bartholomew's Hospital which had been diagnosed as polyarteritis nodosa, and found that in 18 patients skin lesions had been present. Histology of the skin showed eczema in one of these patients and leucocytoclastic angiitis in four. Twelve, however, presented a remarkably uniform clinical and histological picture in which the only tissues affected were skin, muscle and peripheral nerves. Histologically there was fibrinoid necrosis of vessels lying in the superficial subcutis; also, infiltration by polymorphonuclear leucocytes was frequent and leucocytoclasis was sometimes present.

Unusual for arterial disease but quite compatible with venous pathology, despite necrosis of vessels, was a total absence of infarction.

Borrie believed that this should be recognised as a specific pattern because of its benign prognosis. An alternative view is that nodular vasculitis is an adequate term under which to group these patterns, and that subdivisions, if any, should be based on pathogenic factors, not on morphology. Certainly, clear evidence of primary arterial disease is singularly lacking in most relevant publications, and venous rather than arterial pathology is often the more likely cause. In the human leg, moreover, chronic venous pathology is rarely a consequence of severe systemic disease, but often results from a local thrombotic process, and if arterial pathology does occur, it is usually caused by ischaemia, hypertension or coagulation and does not merit consideration as a disease entity (see Chapter 13). However, for a debate about nodular forms of vasculitis one must refer chiefly to French and American literature.

References

Borrie, P. (1972) Cutaneous polyarteritis nodosa. *British Journal of Dermatology*, **87**, 87.
Borrie, P. & Stansfeld, A. (1966) Cutaneous vasculitis. In *Modern Trends in Dermatology* (Ed.) Mackenna, R. M. B. p. 167. London: Butterworths.
Bradford, W. D., Cook, C. D. & Vawter, G. F. (1962) Livedo reticularis: A form of allergic vasculitis. Report of three cases. *Journal of Pediatrics*, **60**, 266.
Braverman, I. M. (1970) *Skin Signs of Systemic Disease*. p. 203. Philadelphia: W. B. Saunders.
Cohen, M. B., Kline, B. S. & Young, A. M. (1936) Clinical diagnosis of periarteritis nodosa. *Journal of the American Medical Association*, **107**, 1555.
Copeman, P. W. M. (1975) Cutaneous angiitis. *Journal of the Royal College of Surgeons*, **9**, 103.
Copeman, P. W. M. & Ryan, T. J. (1971) Cutaneous angiitis patterns of rashes explained by i) flow properties of blood ii) anatomical disposition of vessels. *British Journal of Dermatology*, **85**, 205.
Debré, R., Leroux, R., LeLong, M. & Gauthier-Villars, P. (1928) La première observation française de périartérite noueuse. *Archives de Médecine des Enfants*, **31**, 325.
Fine, R. M. & Meltzer, H. D. (1969) Chronic erythema nodosum. *Archives of Dermatology*, **100**, 33.
Grant, R. T. (1940) Observations on periarteritis nodosa. *Clinical Science*, **4**, 245.
Heberden, W. (1802) *Commentaries on the History and Cure of Diseases*, 3rd edition, pp. 395-397. London: Payne.
Hutinel, J., Coste, F. & Arnaudet, A. (1930) Péri-artérite noueuse de Kussmaul forme spléno-intestinale. *Archives de Médecine des Enfants*, **33**, 355.
Keil, H. (1938) Rheumatic subcutaneous nodules and simulating lesions. *Medicine* (Baltimore), **17**, 261.
Ketron, L. W. & Bernstein, J. C. (1939) Cutaneous manifestations of periarteritis nodosa. *Archives of Dermatology and Syphilology*, **40**, 929.
Klotz, O. (1917) Periarteritis nodosa. *Journal of Medical Research*, **37**, 1.
Kussmaul, A. & Maier, R. (1866) Ueber eine bisher nicht beschriebene eigenthümliche Arterien Erkrankung (Periarteritis nodosa), die mit Morbus Brightii und rapid fortschreitender allgemeiner Muskellähmung einhergeht. *Deutsches Archiv für klinische Medizin*, **1**, 484.
Lamb, A. R. (1914) Periarteritis nodosa; a clinical and pathological review of the disease with a report of two cases. *Archives of Internal Medicine*, **14**, 481.
Lindberg, K. (1931) Ein Beitrag zur kenntis der periarteriitis nodosa. *Acta Medica Scandinavica*, **76**, 183.
Lindberg, K. (1932) Uber eine subkutane form der periarteriitis nodosa mit langwierigem verlauf. *Acta Medica Scandinavica*, **77**, 455.
Lyell, A. & Church, R. (1954) The cutaneous manifestations of polyarteritis nodosa. *British Journal of Dermatology*, **66**, 335.
Miescher, G. (1946) Über kutane formen der periarteriitis nodosa. *Dermatologica*, **92**, 225.
Miller, H. G. & Daley, R. (1946) Clinical aspects of polyarteritis nodosa. *Quarterly Journal of Medicine*, **15**, 255.
Osler, W. (1914) The visceral lesions of purpura and allied conditions. *British Medical Journal*, **i**, 517.
Ruiter, M. (1953) A case of allergic cutaneous arteriolitis. *British Journal of Dermatology*, **66**, 174.
Ryan, T. J. & Wilkinson, D. S. (1972) Cutaneous vasculitis (angiitis). In *Textbook of Dermatology* (Ed.) Rook, A., Wilkinson, D. S. & Ebling, F. J. G. p. 920. Oxford: Blackwell Scientific Publications.
Spiegel, R. (1936) Clinical aspects of periarteritis nodosa. *Archives of Internal Medicine*, **58**, 993.
Vining, C. W. (1938) Case of periarteritis nodosa with subcutaneous lesions and recovery. *Archives of Disease in Childhood*, **13**, 31.

The deeper nodular lesions

These were first mentioned by Gougerot when he described 'a chronic indeterminate septicaemia with endocarditis', characterised by small dermal nodules, erythemato-papular elements and purpura, quoted by Gougerot and Duperrat (1954). Then, as the endocarditis was found to be an inconstant feature he altered the description to "a chronic indeterminate septicaemia with the triple lesions: purpura, erythema multiforme and nodules" (Gougerot, 1932). When septicaemia could not be proved this description became inappropriate, and the disease pattern was renamed 'maladie trisymptômique'. Gradually 'septicaemia' became replaced by 'allergides' and the syndrome became known as 'nodular dermal allergides' (Gougerot, 1951).

Gougerot and Duperrat (1954) agreed that when Ruiter (1953) used the term 'allergic arteriolitis' he was dealing with exactly the same condition. They emphasised the three variants: monosymptôme, consisting only of nodules; bisymptôme, with nodules and purpura or with nodules and urticaria; tetra or 'pentasymptôme', when the eruption comprises not only urticaria, purpura and nodules, but also bullae, necrotic ulcers and/or residual pigmentation. They were prepared to diagnose the condition on histological evidence alone without seeing the patient; and they agreed with Ruiter that the histology was distinct. Thus the stage was set for the subsequently fashionable histological classification exemplified by an important paper by Winkelmann and Ditto (1964).

Gougerot and Duperrat's inclusion of nodules, which, as they declared, were often at the junction of the dermis and the hypodermis, meant that the disease they were describing overlapped with nodular vasculitis defined by Montgomery, O'Leary and Barker (1945) as involving "primarily the legs, characterised by the presence of nodules and sometimes by ulceration, and which is associated with varying degrees of involvement of the blood vessels and with fibrosis".

Just as septicaemia was not the solution to all of Gougerot's problems in an era largely concerned with foci of infection, so tuberculosis failed to account completely for the picture described by Bazin (1861) at a time when the mycobacterium was not even isolated and yet was killing millions. Indeed, some later authors (Audry, 1898; Galloway, 1899, 1913) doubted its tuberculous aetiology altogether, while Whitfield (1901) blamed the cold and fat legs.

Montgomery, O'Leary and Barker (1945) introduced the term 'nodular vasculitis' partly in a negative sense since it was applied to patients who clearly had not got tuberculosis, chilblains, erythema nodosum, or thrombophlebitis or other changes due to chronic venous stasis. They saw the condition partly from a histopathological stand-point: vasculitis with varying degrees of thickening and obliteration of veins and arteries and with fibrosis, collections of foreign body giant cells and atrophy involving the fat but without forming definite tubercles. Montgomery later reviewed the progress of his concept and wished it to be preserved, albeit as a rather vague entity, for it was of value in distinguishing the clearly defined conditions from those chronic inflammatory nodules of the legs due to 'other causes'.

On clinical as well as histological grounds, Fine and Meltzer (1969) preferred to group nodular vasculitis, erythema induratum, sub-acute nodular migratory panniculitis, and erythema nodosum migrans under the one term chronic erythema nodosum.

Wilkinson (1954) also reviewed the vascular basis of some nodular eruptions of the legs and did so in a helpful way because it emphasised that in some patients the major factor is a reaction to cold, in others it is a combination of cold and tuberculosis and in yet others, phlebitis and thrombosis are predominant. In a few cases hypertension was important. Thus began a period during which English writers searched for a more mechanistic classification embracing thrombosis, stasis, cold, hypertension, bacterial infection and allergy.

Dermatologists have perhaps made too sharp a distinction between nodular vasculitis and thrombophlebitis, but the same can be said for many other overlapping syndromes, including thrombophlebitis migrans and Behçet's syndrome.

The position of erythema nodosum is not at all clear. It is of course most commonly manifested as a single episode of bilateral, tender, erythematous nodules. However, the less symmetrical forms commonly seen in gastroenterological units are liable to have clinical features found in pyoderma gangrenosum, Behçet's disease or panniculitis.

Involvement of fat in inflammation is the basis of a further nosological debate. As panniculitis is often associated with thrombophlebitis and sometimes also with arterial changes, it can be seen why Pierini, Abulafia and Wainsfield (1965) were prepared to group erythema induratum, periarteritis nodosa and idiopathic lipogranulomatous hypodermatitis in the same histological group. Moreover, when such a patient is also febrile, the disease may immediately be reclassified by some as Weber—Christian's non-suppurative panniculitis. Even autoerythrocytic sensitisation, otherwise known as psychogenic purpura, has been discussed under panniculitis in a textbook by Pinkus and Mehregan (1969).

Erythema nodosum-like lesions, thrombophlebitis and nodular vasculitis also occur in association with the triad of oral and genital ulceration with iritis described by Behçet (1937), and when any or all of these three features are missing, there is left a group of patients with a chronic, predominantly venous disease which is virtually unclassifiable (see Chapter 13). For instance, an association of erythema nodosum and superficial vein involvement of the dorsum of the hand has been described by Delaney and Leppard (1974).

The overlap between the concepts of polyarteritis nodosa and of nodular vasculitis is illustrated by Ruiter (1953). While looking at histological sections of so-called cutaneous polyarteritis nodosa, he noted a syndrome in which the smaller vessels, particularly those of the corium, bore the brunt of the allergic inflammatory reaction. In the medium-sized vessels of the muscular type the changes were insignificant or absent and did not resemble the cutaneous allergic vasculitis type of reaction usually found in polyarteritis nodosa. Because he was thinking in terms of polyarteritis it was inevitable that Ruiter should call these vessels 'still smaller arteries or arterioles' though in fact he may well have been observing small venules.

In the author's experience, migratory forms of erythema nodosum (Figure 2.1) of the type described by Baverstedt (1968) do have clinical features suggestive of local venous thrombosis, and in the case illustrated in Figure 3.8 changes in the blood supported a diagnosis of disseminated intravascular coagulation, although no thrombosis was detected in the veins of adequately deep biopsies. Sometimes, however, there is a florid granuloma in the vessel wall, which is a feature seen in some chronic intravascular coagulation syndromes.

Ruiter was impressed by such aetiological factors as a haemolytic streptococcal sore throat and a raised antistreptolysin titre, or a dramatic recurrence of disease on taking butobarbitone. He was also struck by the fact that the histology resembled an Arthus response and that there was often a distinctly anaphylactoid urticarial nature to the lesion.

Opposed to classification on clinical grounds because of the large number of variants, he said of Gougerot: "After having started with a 'monosymptom' he has at the moment already arrived at a 'pentasymptom'" (Ruiter, 1953).

He pointed out at the same time that the histological changes manifest themselves clinically in the form of erythema (hyperaemia), papules (dermal infiltration), vesicles, pustules, maceration (exudation) and predominantly superficial necrosis, urticarial oedema, cutaneous haemorrhages, pigmentation and telangiectasis.

Similarities between his cases and those previously described as purpura rheumatica and allergic granulomatosis caused him (Ruiter, 1954a) to suggest that his histological term 'allergic cutaneous arteriolitis' might be used to cover all these groups, including those described by Schönlein (1837) and later by Churg and Strauss (1951).

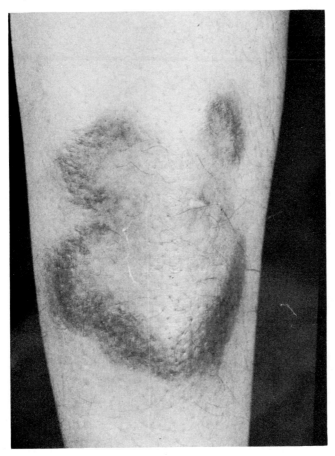

Figure 2.1. Erythema nodosum migrans. The inflammatory edge of this full skin thickness lesion has taken two to three weeks to spread to this size. Healing is taking place in the centre.

In a letter criticising an article by Gougerot and Duperrat (1954) entitled "The nodular dermal allergides of Gougerot", he (Ruiter, 1954b) wrote: "In general, I am convinced of the fundamental value of clinical morphology in dermatological diagnosis; but the polymorphism and variability of the eruptions concerned have led me to wonder if a valuation predominantly based on clinical morphological characteristics might not prove to be unsatisfactory and I have therefore abandoned that method of approach". A similar opinion was voiced by Cream, Gumpel and Peachey (1970) in a discussion of Schönlein—Henoch purpura in the adult:

"The clinical picture depends on the extent and site of the small vessel involvement and histological appearances may depend on such variables as the age of the lesion and the cut of the section. It is also apparent that the findings in a given patient may vary from site to site if multiple simultaneous biopsies are obtained. In our patients no particular form of rash could be picked out as being especially prone to occur without systemic involvement and we feel there is little to be gained at present by attempting to subdivide and classifying what is probably a spectrum of disease on the basis of minor clinical and histological appearances".

On the other hand there is a dilemma to be overcome when physicians clearly recognise a variant. For instance, most British dermatologists recognise a somewhat nodular and pustular lesion heavily infiltrated with neutrophils and associated with fever that characterises one of the more recently delineated syndromes (Sweet, 1964). Should one perpetuate it or regard it, as do some German authors (Heise, 1971), as merely part of the spectrum of erythema multiforme and erythema elevatum diutinum? Case 4 in Sweet's original series had ulcerative colitis, and Figure 2.2, which is from a recently observed case of Crohn's disease of the large bowel, illustrates how this syndrome may merge into pyoderma gangrenosum (see also Pegum (1974) and Chapter 13).

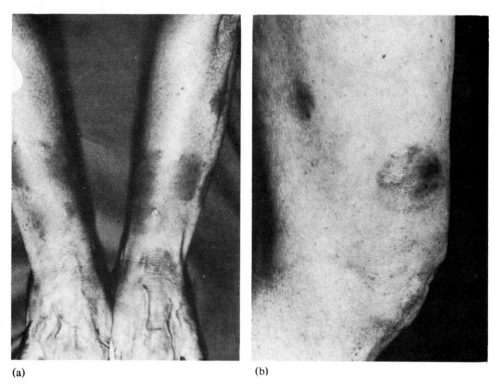

(a)   (b)

Figure 2.2. Acute erythema with pustules developing in the centre affecting arms (a) and legs (b) associated with fever and neutrophilia. The patient also had Crohn's disease of the colon, mucosal ulceration and iritis.

If one returns to the period when the term polyarteritis nodosa began to be applied to small vessels, one finds that the term vasculitis seemed barely to exist and that classifications of purpura, though provided, were not accompanied by adequate descriptions of non-thrombocytopenic or of non-scorbutic forms. Therefore those who described the cutaneous manifestations of blockage of, or exudation from, small vessels did so under the heading polyarteritis nodosa. Today the term vasculitis is used for a pattern of morphology which may have more to do with capillaries and venules than with arteries, often has little association with hypertension and, in dermatological practice, may well not be systemic. It is a pattern which cannot be clearly distinguished from the small vessel disease described by Ruiter or Gougerot, and which forms a spectrum of disease ranging from urticaria to disseminated intravascular coagulation. It has localised or limited, systemic or complicated forms and, while the vessels involved are much smaller than those originally described, there are still difficulties in classifying morphology which in some cases involves very small vessels and in others involves larger ones.

Throughout this volume the term spectrum is used to cover the complete range of exudative pathology, but it may be extended to include physiological permeability at one end and intravascular coagulation and ischaemia at the other. In this respect papers by Taylor and Jacoby (1949) and Melczer and Venkei (1947) are relevant. Both emphasised the diagnostic value of a prolonged bleeding time in polyarteritis nodosa and the 1949 paper postulated a common aetiology for purpura fulminans, post-scarlatinal purpura and gangrene, purpura necroticans and polyarteritis nodosa. This theme is pursued in this monograph and no clear dividing line is made between these various manifestations of local intravascular coagulation, gangrene and phagedenic ulceration.

References

Audry, C. (1898) Étude de la lésion de l'érythème induré. *Annals de Dermatologie et de Syphiligraphie,* **3,** 209.
Baverstedt, E. (1968) Erythema nodosum migrans. *Acta Dermato-venereologica,* **48,** 381.
Bazin, E. (1861) *Extrait des Leçons Théoriques et Cliniques sur la Scrofule.* p. 146.
Behçet, H. (1937) Uber die rezidivierende aphthose durch ein virus verursachte Geschwure am Mund, am Auge und an den Genitalien. *Dermatologische Wochenschrift,* **105,** 1152.
Churg, J. & Strauss, L. (1951) Allergic granulomatosis, allergic angiitis and periarteritis nodosa. *American Journal of Pathology,* **27,** 277.
Cream, J. J., Gumpel, J. M. & Peachey, R. D. G. (1970) Schönlein—Henoch purpura in the adult. A study of 77 adults with anaphylactoid or Schönlein—Henoch purpura. *Quarterly Journal of Medicine,* **34,** 461.
Delaney, T. J. & Leppard, B. (1974) Erythema nodosum with superficial vein involvement. *British Journal of Dermatology,* **90,** 205.
Fine, R. M. & Meltzer, H. D. (1969) Chronic erythema nodosum. *Archives of Dermatology,* **100,** 33.
Galloway, J. (1899) A case of probable Bazin's disease; in a girl of 13, and a localised congestion of the nose in a little boy of 7, the patients being brother and sister. *British Journal of Dermatology,* **11,** 206.
Galloway, J. (1913) Case of erythema induratum, giving no evidence of tuberculosis. *British Journal of Dermatology,* **25,** 217.
Gougerot, H. (1932) Septicémie chronique indéterminée caractérisée par des petits nodules dermiques ('dermatitis nodularis non necroticans') elements erythemato-papuleux purpura. *Bulletin de la Société Française de Dermatologie et de Syphiligraphie,* **39,** 1192.
Gougerot, H. (1951) Allergides nodulaires dermiques. *Minerva Dermatologica,* **26,** 39.
Gougerot, H. & Duperrat, B. (1954) The nodular dermal allergides of Gougerot. *British Journal of Dermatology,* **66,** 283.
Heise, H. (1971) Akute febrile neutrophile dermatose oder erythema exsudativum multiforme. *Dermatologische Monatsschrift,* **157,** 278.
Melczer, N. & Venkei, T. (1947) Uber die hautformen der periarteriitis nodosa. *Dermatologica,* **94,** 214.
Montgomery, H., O'Leary, P. A. & Barker, N. W. (1945) Nodular vascular diseases of legs; erythema induratum and allied conditions. *Journal of the American Medical Association,* **128,** 335.
Pegum, J. (1974) Discussion of Goldin, D. & Wilkinson, D. S. Pyoderma gangrenosum and chronic myeloid leukaemia. *Proceedings of the Royal Society of Medicine,* **67,** 1240.
Pierini, L. E., Abulafia, J. & Wainfield, S. (1965) Las hypodermitis. *Archives of Argentinian Dermatology,* **15,** 1.
Pinkus, H. & Mehregan, A. H. (1969) *A Guide to Histopathology.* p. 194. London: Butterworths.
Ruiter, M. (1953) A case of allergic cutaneous vasculitis (arteriolitis allergica). *British Journal of Dermatology,* **65,** 77.
Ruiter, M. (1954a) Some further observations on allergic cutaneous arteriolitis in which the author describes two cases that have granulomatous diseases as well as cutaneous vasculitis. *British Journal of Dermatology,* **66,** 174.
Ruiter, M. (1954b) Letter. *British Journal of Dermatology,* **66,** 459.

Schönlein, J. L. (1837) Peliosis rheumatica (pelcircumsc). In *Allgemeine und specielle Pathologie und Therapie,* 3rd edition, Volume 2, p. 48. Quoted from a translation of the lectures given to his students. Reported in *Allgemeine und specielle Pathologie und Therapie,* 4th edition, Volume 2, p. 42. St. Gallen: Comptoir.

Sweet, R. D. (1964) An acute febrile neutrophilic dermatosis. *British Journal of Dermatology,* **76,** 349.

Taylor, A. W. & Jacoby, N. M. (1949) Acute polyarteritis nodosa in childhood. *Lancet,* **ii,** 792.

Whitfield, A. (1901) Nature of the disease known as erythema induratum scrofulosorum. *British Journal of Dermatology,* **13,** 323.

Wilkinson, D. S. (1954) The vascular basis of some nodular eruptions of the legs. *British Journal of Dermatology,* **66,** 201.

Winkelmann, R. K. & Ditto, W. B. (1964) Cutaneous and visceral syndromes of necrotising or "allergic" angiitis. A study of 38 cases. *Medicine* (Baltimore), **43,** 59.

Respiratory tract involvement

The purely arterial diseases described by early authors did not involve the lungs, but as smaller and smaller vessels began to be studied the spectrum of disease moved into a different order of pathology — a more exudative one.

It is not surprising that this move resulted in increasing numbers of reports of systemic disease involving the lungs. Kussmaul and Maier (1866), as Zeek (1952) suggested, may have been looking at a generalised disease due to systemic hypertension and, consequently, sparing the lungs. Zeek therefore proposed that polyarteritis nodosa is a multi-system disease which is usually associated with hypertension, lasts several months to a year or more, and affects the small and medium-sized muscular type of arteries found near hila of viscera, in striated muscle and near peripheral nerves. Associated lesions such as rupture of aneurysms and vascular obstruction are, in her view, sequelae of hypertension, and the more intravascular coagulation is a feature, the less exudation there will be; this theme is developed in Chapter 10. It is notable that the ischaemia which often terminates vasculitis in most tissues is not often found in the upper respiratory tract.

Burton and Burton (1972) have recently reviewed pulmonary eosinophilia associated with vasculitis and extravascular granulomata. They described a spectrum ranging from benign pulmonary eosinophilia with asthma to the severe necrosis of the upper respiratory tract described by Wegener (1939). Three classic descriptions have initiated this particular debate:

1. Loffler (1932) described a benign, transient eosinophilic infiltration of the lungs caused usually by *Ascaris* infestation, and with asthma as a predominant feature.

2. Churg and Strauss (1951) described 13 patients with a clinical syndrome comprising severe asthma, fever and eosinophilia; in addition, bloody diarrhoea, haematuria, purpura, arthralgia and peripheral neuropathy were usual. The histological picture included fibrinoid necrosis of arterial walls. There were also extravascular (usually extravenous) epithelioid and giant cell granulomata; the latter often began as an extravascular exudate, became eosinophil abscesses and then necrosed and incited alteration of the collagen. It is significant that infarction and adherent mural thrombi were also encountered.

This disease process therefore includes a fierce exudation mainly from venules with fibrin deposition and the formation of eosinophilic abscesses which excite a secondary macrophage response and are walled off by collagen and epithelioid cells. The vessels supplying the area are blocked by thrombi, but even in the absence of thrombus formation, the arterial walls are liable to necrose.

Braverman (1970) has pointed out that the asthma usually remits before the onset of the vasculitis, and this feature will be explained in Chapters 3 and 10. It supports the concept of a switch from an exudative to an obstructive phase of vascular pathology as one moves through a spectrum ranging from excessive fibrinolysis to impaired fibrinolysis and coagulation.

3. Wegener (1939) described a syndrome comprising granulomatous ulcers of the upper and lower respiratory tract, a rapid progression producing disseminated vasculitis, granulomata and, in the late stages, renal involvement. Bleeding and vascular occlusion are features of the granulomata and, as Reed et al (1963) emphasised, the syndrome overlaps with polyarteritis nodosa and pyoderma gangrenosum. Venous thrombosis is a frequent accompaniment and can be quite independent of the granulomata (see Chapter 13).

Burton and Burton (1972) have reported and discussed intermediate cases, and have demonstrated the ridiculous state of affairs that present-day classification has produced, by introducing the 'Chöffler Train' as a name for the spectrum 'Löffler—Chöffler—Churg—Chegener—Wegener syndromes'. They state that "until advances in our knowledge of the aetiology of these conditions result in a rational resolution of the imbroglio, we feel that the scheme we have outlined may serve to emphasise the possible relationship between these syndromes and the fluidity of their boundaries".

In an effort to place the whole subject on a mechanistic rather than a morphological basis, one may suggest that the 'Chöffler Train' is the counterpart in the lungs of the spectrum of exudative pathology seen in the skin that ranges from physiological responses through urticaria and vasculitis to intravascular coagulation.

The spectrum of pulmonary granulomatosis branches in the direction of lymphoma well delineated by Liebow (1973). The exact relationship of midline granuloma or Wegener's granulomatosis to sarcomata of the reticuloendothelial system or immunological systems is difficult to ascertain and is discussed in Chapter 13. Attempts by Liebow (1973) to provide a useful classification have resulted in further subdivisions and terms such as lymphomatoid granulomatosis and necrotising sarcoid have been created.

References

Braverman, I. M. (1970) *Skin Signs of Systemic Disease.* p. 203. Philadelphia: W. B. Saunders.
Burton, J. L. & Burton, P. A. (1972) Pulmonary eosinophilia associated with vasculitis and extravascular granulomata. *British Journal of Dermatology,* **87,** 412.
Churg, J. & Strauss, L. (1951) Allergic granulomatosis, allergic angiitis and periarteritis nodosa. *American Journal of Pathology,* **27,** 277.
Kussmaul, A. & Maier, R. (1866) Ueber eine bisher nicht beschriebene eigenthümliche Arterien erkrankung (periarteritis nodosa), die mit Morbus Brightii und rapid fortschreitender allgemeiner Muskellähmung einhergeht. *Deutsches Archiv für klinische Medizin,* **1,** 484.
Liebow, A. A. (1973) Pulmonary angiitis and granulomatosis. *American Review of Respiratory Disease,* **108,** 1.
Loffler, W. (1932) Zur differential Diagnose der lungenin filtrierungen uber fluchtige Succedan-Infiltrate (mit Eosinophile). *Beitrage zur Klinik der Tuberkulose,* **79,** 368.
Reed, W. B., Jensen, A., Konwaler, B. E. & Hunter, D. (1963) The cutaneous manifestations in Wegener's granulomatosis. *Acta Dermato-venereologica,* **43,** 250.
Wegener, F. (1939) Ueber eine eigenartige rhinogene Granulomatose mit besonderer Beteiligung des Arterien-systems und der Nieren. *Beitrage zur pathologischen Anatomie und zur allgemeinen Pathologie,* **102,** 36.
Zeek, P. M. (1952) Periarteritis nodosa. A critical review. *American Journal of Clinical Pathology,* **22,** 777.

3. Factors Determining the Clinical Picture

Teaching medical students to recognise disease by examining the skin is a useful exercise for both student and tutor. Students see the lesions but do not have the vocabulary to describe them. They select lesions for description that the teacher would prefer to ignore because they are not diagnostic and cannot be fitted into the narrow confines of classic description. Indeed many rashes have to be squeezed into the diagnostic register and they consequently tend to be remembered only by their classical lesions, all other features of the eruption being forgotten.

While writing this book the author has attempted to abandon morphological and pathological boundaries and to describe a process (Table I.1) that in any one lesion may be intermittent or continuous, perpetuated, exacerbated, or blocked and eliminated. In a few patients these morphological changes occur uniformly and simultaneously in all lesions, but in most no such uniformity exists.

Whatever the nature of the trigger, be it an immune complex or a bacterial toxin, the type of lesion produced depends on the subsequent host reaction. This is a process of removal and repair, in which enzyme and cellular activity are intimately involved. As these are to a large extent dependent on the individual's constitution rather than on extraneous influences, the patterns of response they produce can be grossly abnormal as a result of genetic disturbances. This occurs, for example, if there is an inborn absence of an inhibitor, as in hereditary angio-oedema or a failure of digestion by a neutrophil, as in chronic granulomatous disease.

Whether or not the response to an injurious agent takes the form of urticaria, vasculitis or disseminated intravascular coagulation, and whether or not the eruption is acute, chronic, recurrent, limited or extensive, depends as much on the reactions within the host as on the nature of the noxious agent (Table I.2). The host response is the product of an interaction between thousands of factors each with a significant part to play in maintaining or restoring a balance (see Chapter 6). Thus it is rare for the ultimate disease process to depend on the quality and quantity of the initial noxious agent.

A rider to this way of thinking is the fact that a constitutional defect often determines why, under the same circumstances, one person develops a rash from a drug reaction, another does not, and yet another develops a different disease. A further rider is that, for the most part, we are unaware of the many injurious agents constantly attacking us, for when we are in good health, our constitution can deal with them effectively.

To apportion blame to triggering and to constitutional factors is difficult, but since one does not detect noxious triggers when one's constitution is instantly detoxicating them, and one is usually unaware of their presence, it is probable that they are not as harmful or blameworthy as is sometimes suggested.

THE MORPHOLOGY OF EXUDATION

Osler (1914) described a very wide range of clinical syndromes in his report on the visceral lesions of purpura. His clear descriptions remind one of the cases within one's own experience, though his descriptions were not confused by twentieth century terminology. He rightly emphasised that the common denominator was exudation from blood vessels, whether of serum or red cells. The skin lesions he described were of four types: purpura, effusion, erythema and necrosis. His details of these (Osler, 1914) are given below.

"From the anatomical standpoint four lesions are met with in the cases under consideration. All are exudative, in which the blood elements — either the red blood corpuscles alone, the serum alone, or both combined — pass out of the vessels."

Purpura

"This, the most common lesion, is either simple or associated with swelling, purpura urticans, and with oedema of the hands and feet or about the joints, particularly the knees and elbows. The larger areas may be capped with bullae — purpura bullosa. There are cases in which the vesicular character of the purpura is very striking. A man aged 34 was admitted in his fourth severe attack of purpura. The backs of his hands were covered with simple purpura; just below the right elbow was a fresh eruption of blebs looking like herpes, some on hyperaemic, some on purpuric bases. Two inches above the left condyle was a patch of pearly vesicles, solid, not on a reddened base; above the joint of the other elbow was a raised bulla 2 cm by 7 mm with haemorrhagic contents. Over the right second rib were two patches of pemphigoid purpura, one 2 by 3 cm, the other 1½ cm in length. Practically all varieties of purpura are seen, reaching to the severest grade or morbus maculosus Werlhofii."

Effusion

"Effusions of serum alone, forming the ordinary weals of urticaria or the patches of angio-neurotic oedema, are the next in frequency of occurrence. The clinical features may be those of ordinary urticaria or of angio-neurotic oedema."

Erythema

"Erythema, either diffuse and with or without swelling, or localised, as in the common form of erythema exudativum multiforme; sometimes patches have the appearance of erythema nodosum. In Case XIII (*British Journal of Dermatology,* Volume 12) of my series a patient had attacks of violent colic for months without skin lesions, and then was admitted with a typical attack of erythema multiforme on hands, forearms, face; on the legs some of the patches were exactly like erythema nodosum."

Necrotic areas

"When a localised infiltration of blood and serum is very intense in a patch of considerable size, bullae form and the superficial layers of the skin necrose, leaving an open ulcer. This is more frequently seen in the severer types of purpura, with large serous exudation, but it may occur in intense erythema, as in that most typical of all varieties, chilblains."

"There are two outstanding clinical features — first, the recurrence of attacks at long or short intervals over periods ranging from a few months to many years, and secondly, the morphological inconstancy of the skin lesions. In Willan's case, purpura, angio-neurotic oedema, and necrotic sloughs were present in one attack. Within a few weeks the patient may run the gamut of a skin atlas — purpura, oedema, exudative erythema, pemphigoid lesions, etc.; or in the same individual followed for many years the skin lesions may differ in the different attacks. Very many of my reported cases followed for years have shown these polymorphic characters."

"Even the unusually stable, hereditary form of angio-neurotic oedema may present erythematous lesions of the worst type. For years I had correspondence with a Mrs W., aged 54, of California, a victim of aggravated angio-neurotic oedema of 20 years standing; a case illustrating how terrible the disease may be. Her mother had the same affection. The attack began when she was 27, after the birth of her second child. Oedema would come on at any time, anywhere, accompanied with severe vomiting, often of blood. Tea, coffee, or strawberries would bring on an attack within three hours. The face and throat were much affected. The attacks usually began with red spots like weals on the cheeks. The outlines of the neck would be obliterated. She came into hospital, October 4th 1904, in an attack with infiltration of the inner side of the left arm and elbow, with black and blue spots, and the right arm enormously oedematous, with a vivid erythema extending up and down the arm. There was no fever, no enlargement of the spleen, no albumin in the urine. A specially interesting thing was to find that this patient belonged to the New Jersey family of hereditary angio-neurotic oedema, which I described in 1888 (*American Journal of the Medical Sciences,* April 1888). She was the great-great-granddaughter of the man aged 92 (who had been taken as a boy to see the famous Benjamin Rush) who so kindly worked out for me the family history. It is worth noting that another member of this family had had her appendix removed for the colic associated with oedema, and two had died of oedema of the glottis."

This long quotation is included to illustrate a stage in the history of dermatology when purpura and urticaria were thought of as related, when a physician could write authoritatively on skin morphology and when the fact that a rash could vary in different regions of the body and from day to day was clearly recognised. The particular morphology and pattern of the rash was not given much significance and did not achieve the diagnostic importance of, for instance, the terms maladie trisymptôme or penta-symptôme of the French School (see page 17).

Copeman and Ryan (1970) have outlined reasons for not paying too much attention to morphology (see Table 3.1). Morphology of a rash is a poor guide to the nature of the underlying disease and to prognosis and treatment. In fact, a simple look at the way in which the rash is produced will show that it does not necessarily give any clear indication of what disease underlies it. The physician must be able to recognise purpura, effusion,

Table 3.1. Reasons why morphology is misleading.

1. The various morphological patterns are not disease entities but the end-result of complex pathological processes. Rashes are often signs of systemic diseases such as lupus erythematosus, rheumatoid arthritis, Hodgkin's disease or adenocarcinoma.
2. No single clinical or histopathological pattern of cutaneous angiitis is consistently a feature of any malady. Any one pattern may be seen in more than one named disease.
3. The individual lesions of any single eruption may appear very different in different parts of the skin at the same time. Urticarial, erythematous, vesicular, purpuric and necrotic lesions can be seen in the same patient at the same time or may appear in succession at different stages of the disease.
4. Fibrinoid and many other features of vasculitis are not present in every lesion or even in every case.
5. Neither the capillary nor the venule nor the artery is the sole primary site of pathology in any variety of vasculitis.

erythema and necrosis but, having done so, he must then continue his investigations along lines which are independent of the pattern of the rash and not spend too much time discussing whether a particular variant is more significant than another.

In all these lesions the initial injury to the vessel produces both a reaction and efforts to repair damage; these two responses determine what the eruption looks like. In other words the morphology of the rash is decided much more by the idiosyncrasies of the local constitution than by the exact nature of the trigger. In the description of morphology that follows, Siemens' (1958) *General Diagnosis and Therapy of Skin Diseases* has been a useful guide.

THE INTENSITY OF THE INJURY

All reactions to injury depend to some extent on the intensity and the duration of the initial insult. A mild insult to the vessel wall produces a transient increase in its permeability (Wilhelm, 1971) and adhesiveness to leucocytes; a more severe injury will cause fibrin and platelets to build up on its wall and promote leucocyte diapedesis; an even more severe injury will cause death of endothelium and damage to the surrounding vessel wall. In Figure 3.1 the spectrum of urticaria, vasculitis and intravascular coagulation is illustrated. It can be seen that, in general, the milder micro-injuries produce the most transient lesions, including urticaria, while vasculitis and intravascular coagulation result from more prolonged and intense injury.

Patients with meningococcal septicaemia or those with circulating immune complexes, as in lepromatous leprosy, may have a mixture of lesions, some of which consist of very transient erythema or swelling, while others are more prolonged and ultimately become purpuric or even necrotic. The more intense the initial response or the greater the oedema, the more likely are blebs of initially clear fluid to result (Figure 3.2). Later, large blisters often contain dark blood and are associated with necrosis of the epidermis and upper dermis.

An injury to a vessel wall that produces only a mild reaction and does not interfere too much with blood flow is likely to attract white cells into the surrounding tissues after they have adhered to the endothelium. However, a sudden total occlusion of the vessel will prevent white cells flowing into the area. The difference in pathology here is therefore simply one of cellularity but it must be interpreted logically. Thus, when authors discuss disseminated intravascular coagulation they often equate cellularity with inflammation and consider that the pathology of clotting is non-inflammatory compared to that of vasculitis. But in this monograph vasculitis and thrombosed vessels are both considered to be a response to injury and therefore both are 'inflammatory'.

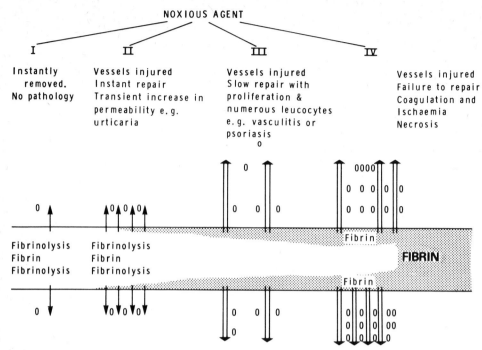

Figure 3.1. Spectrum of urticaria, vasculitis and ischaemia. From left to right there are increasing amounts of fibrin and exudation of serum and cells. At the far right, relative acellularity is a consequence of complete cessation of flow. Types I—IV represent not only a gradient of response but could represent a mild to severe injury, type I being the least noxious agent.

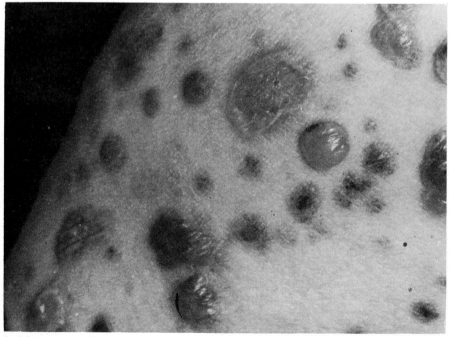

Figure 3.2. Acute vasculitis in a middle-aged woman presenting with more than one morphology. This figure shows clear blisters.

A significant difference between vasculitis and thrombosis is in the recruitment and contribution of the leucocyte in general and of the neutrophil in particular. So far as morphology is concerned 'vasculitis' shows more of the cardinal signs of inflammation — swelling, pain, heat and redness — throughout the lesion, whilst the ischaemia of intravascular coagulation may show only cyanosis followed by the changes of increasing necrosis, and only at the edge of these changes are the cardinal signs of inflammation in evidence. Slowly developing infarction, however, is often acellular, as exemplified by the papule of malignant atrophic papulosis (Figure 3.3).

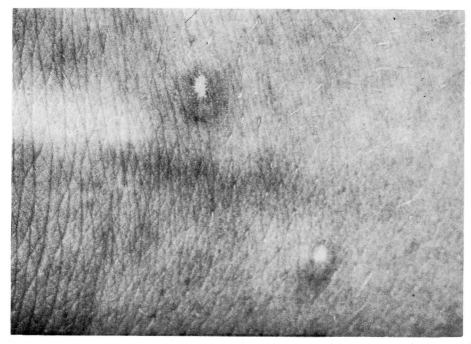

Figure 3.3. Degos' malignant atrophic papulosis. Note central white scar surrounded by dilated blood vessels (see also Figure 4.30 for histology).

TIMING FROM ONSET

Effusions in the skin are on the whole more transient than purpura. Urticaria should, therefore, not be diagnosed if a weal-like lesion proves to be a fixed entity lasting several days. But such interpretations require some knowledge of the time of onset and the duration of the lesions; thus one's first impressions often have to be modified by a subsequent and more detailed history or observation. The lesion of anaphylactoid purpura, for example, in which effusion precedes the purpura, may on its first appearance be urticarial (Figure 3.4), but it later becomes purpuric and still later it may in some instances become necrotic. The more urticarial the lesion, the more often the name Schönlein—Henoch purpura is used, while the presence of necrosis is more often taken to justify the term allergic vasculitis.

Urticarial lesions often take only two to three minutes to form, as is the case in cholinergic urticaria, but in those instances when they ultimately become purpuric, the

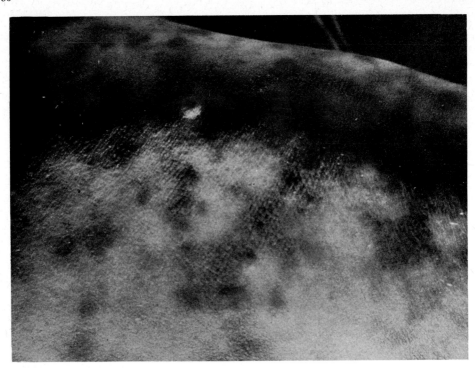

Figure 3.4. Urticarial skin lesions in a patient who for many years suffered from a particularly urticarial form of purpura. The dark areas are purpuric.

weal develops in one or two hours and becomes purpuric over a two to six-hour period. Necrosis, on the contrary, does not occur within such a short period but is more usually the product of a progressive two or three-day-old lesion. As lesions may crop eratically over many days or years, it can be seen that a rash is more likely to be polymorphic either in the initial phases of a severe acute disorder, such as during the first day of a meningococcal septicaemia, or in the later phases of a chronically erupting vasculitis secondary to circulating immune complexes. Chronicity in disease with varied rates of repair and healing tends to give rise to these polymorphic types of rashes. On the other hand a completely monomorphic rash of acute onset is very common on the first day of an attack of urticaria.

Injury to the epidermis provoking a vascular response takes time to produce its effects. For instance, the upper dermal reaction to epidermal injury takes six to eight hours to produce a picture suggestive of vasculitis, whereas that due to direct deposition of circulating immune complexes localised by pressure or suction can be obvious within one hour.

When immune complexes or bacterial endotoxin are involved they are much more likely to produce disease in areas of reduced resistance, in sites of reticuloendothelial paralysis or in the presence of extreme vascular stasis. Present concepts of the Shwartzman reaction are relevant in this context (see Chapter 10), for if those mechanisms essential to the removal of noxious influences and repair are inhibited by an initial insult, then a subsequent insult will result in a pathological response. This effect is produced by the pathology of venous stasis in the legs, which is one of the commonest factors encouraging the production of pathological responses to circulating noxious agents. Furthermore, a history of trauma at a site where there have been subsequent repeated episodes of vasculitis is very common. Therefore, the appearance of a lesion at a particular site may be due to a previous alteration of the local anatomical or functional constitution. For similar reasons preferential selection of cutaneous scars has been recorded for lesions of all types of vasculitis.

DEPTH OF ERYTHEMA AND URTICARIA

Depth is one of the most important factors determining the pattern and symptoms of a rash, affecting it in various ways. Very superficial acute lesions tend to sting like nettles, mid-dermal lesions tend to itch, while deep lesions are often tender. Superficial effusions tend to be transient. The converse is not necessarily true, for presumably a transient increase in permeability such as occurs in cholinergic urticaria would not be recognised in deeper tissues. Nevertheless, deep effusions are largest, last longer and give a more uniform contour and histological picture (Schneider and Undeutsch, 1965).

Inflammation affecting deeper vessels produces nodules or swellings which are usually tender rather than itchy or stinging. Delayed pressure urticaria, erythema nodosum, thrombophlebitis and nodular vasculitis are examples.

The erythemas tend to be superficial rashes which, if transient, are caused primarily by direct vascular injury but, if they are prolonged, epidermal injury is usually playing a large part in their causation (Figure 3.5). Erythema is a cardinal sign of inflammation and when acute it has a bright red hue, but in chronic conditions it is more livid and often mixed with brown, producing a dirty red or brown colour. The brown component arises from haemosiderin or melanin deposition and sometimes from infiltrates,

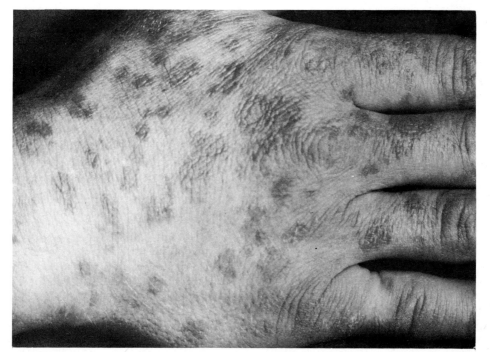

Figure 3.5. Erythema causes minimal swelling and does not interfere with normal line markings in the skin. Erythema induced by exposure to sunlight in an unduly sensitive patient.

particularly epithelioid or giant cell infiltrates. Erythema is often the longest lasting sign of dermatitis and may not vanish for weeks or months.

Erythemas also result from vasodilatation as in the flush of emotion or fever when they are bright red; those that result from passive hyperaemia or congestion of venules are characteristically darker with a bluish tint. The term livid or violaceous is commonly applied to such a colour which is usually associated with a cool skin. When redness of the skin is caused by permanent dilatation and elongation of the visible vessels, the term telangiectasis is used. Some such lesions are composed of greatly coiled vessels (Figure 3.6) running perpendicular to the skin, as in the lesions surrounding atrophie blanche (see Figure 12.7, page 283); others are seen in the fine linear horizontal vessels arising

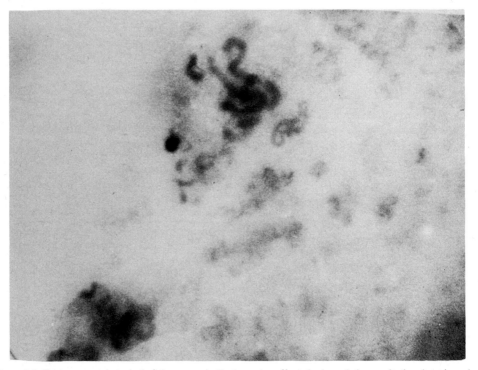

Figure 3.6. Tortuous vessels typical of those seen in the lower leg affected adversely by gravitational stasis and atrophie blanche. The photograph is taken through a Wild M.5 microscope and represents 0.3 mm² of the skin surface.

from the subpapillary venous plexus, as in arborising telangiectasia of the legs (Figure 12.8, page 284). Aneurysmal dilatation of papillary or subpapillary vessels produces a dotted pattern as in angioma serpiginosum or sometimes in acrocyanosis (Figure 3.7).

The colour of the lesion and the degree to which dilated vessels may show through the skin surface may be modified by surface exudate, scales or upper dermal oedema. The centre of a weal, for example, is often blanched by oedema fluid in spite of the fact that the vessels contributing to it are dilated. Erythemas may be any size, and the small, spotted, disseminated erythemas called roseolas may be located at points where arterioles bring blood to the skin or they may lie peripheral to the central arteriole at sites where capillary-venous stasis allows organisms, infective agents, immune complexes or other agents to sludge out.

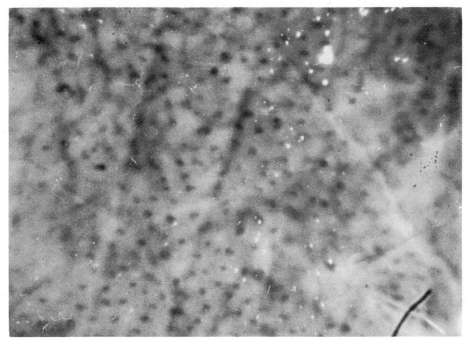

Figure 3.7. The dots in this figure are the dilated peaks of papillary vessels in the skin of a patient with acrocyanosis.

Raised lesions may be produced by the accumulation of fluid in the skin, by an increase in the number or size of infiltrating cells or cellular products such as collagen, or by the advent of a secondary epidermal or adnexal hypertrophy. A weal consists of circumscribed oedema of the skin produced by the escape of blood plasma through the vessel wall. It can be imitated by intradermal injection of liquids. Its pathogenesis explains its rapid development and disappearance, usually within a matter of hours. Its size may vary greatly, but only exceptionally is it so small that it can be confused with a papule. For the most part it expands quickly to form a coin-sized disc, but it may become larger, exceeding the size of the hand. At the height of its development, the edges of the lesion are well-defined, forming round or polycyclic figures. In the larger weals the centre is no higher than the edge and is, in fact, frequently depressed due to central regression. However, if the subcutis participates in the oedema, more rounded swellings develop, some of which are larger than a hen's egg and have vague edges. Generally a weal feels firm and is non-pitting, but if the oedema involves areas with very loose cutis and subcutis such as the eyelids, lips and genitalia, then prominent spherical, somewhat translucent and often very disfiguring swellings develop. These lesions are moderately soft, and the pit left by the pressure of a fingertip flattens only slowly. Such oedematous lesions, or angio-oedema, are often associated with weals, since *both weals and angio-oedema represent the same fundamental pathological process.*

Weals may have the colour of normal skin, but they may be redder if the superficial blood vessels are dilated, or paler if the vessels are compressed by the accumulation of extravasated fluid in the tissues. The once popular terms such as urticaria hyperaemica or erythematosa, or urticaria rubra and urticaria anaemica have no pathological significance and any attempt to name or to subclassify diseases by such morphological variations is no longer in favour.

Sometimes a weal develops into a blister; it commonly does so in reactions to insect bites, especially when these are on the lower legs (Figure 3.8a). The erythemas similarly may blister, as in erythema multiforme, dermatitis herpetiformis or pemphigoid. When bullae form in vasculitis they often are associated with infarction and central necrosis and consequently tend to be centrally depressed or umbilicated (Figure 3.9).

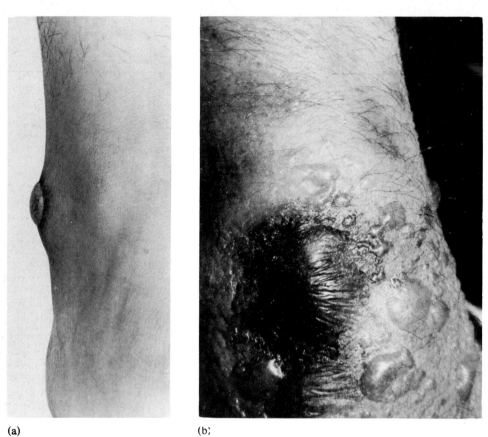

(a)   (b)

Figure 3.8. (a) Blister of ankle following an insect bite. Dependent sites are more likely to develop blisters from infarction as in (b) disseminated intravascular coagulation.

DEPTH OF PAPULES AND NODULES

Papules have a more variable morphology. As their shape depends on the depth of the underlying cellular infiltrate it is possible to estimate the site of this increased cellularity from the appearance of the papule. Thus, superficial papules are plateau-like with sharp edges, whereas deep-seated ones are hemispherical with indistinct borders. In many inflammatory processes the amount of horizontal and vertical spread of the infiltrate is so variable that some lesions remain superficial and well-defined while others are deeper and ill-defined. The deeper, ill-defined nodular lesion is less likely to be diagnosed by direct observation alone, and when seen without a history to indicate its acuteness or chronicity, its differential diagnosis is large and includes a carbuncle, erythema

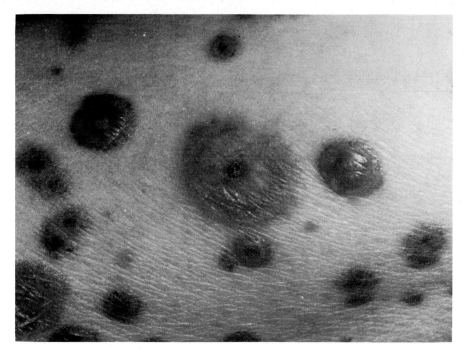

Figure 3.9. Central necrosis of an area of vasculitis often produces 'target' or umbilicated lesions. From the same patient as in Figure 3.2, taken at the same session.

nodosum, nodular vasculitis, insect bite, factitial, a halogen-induced or coumarin reaction, a coagulopathy, a deep mycotic infection, necrobiosis lipoidica or ischaemia.

Inflammation of the deep dermis and subcutaneous tissues often begins as a nodule, spreads into a plaque (Figure 3.10), develops a central depression and then progresses to form a large atrophic sclerosed area of skin with a surrounding ridge of thickened, slightly tender inflammatory tissue. The more rapidly evolving of these patterns resemble erythema nodosum while those that evolve more slowly resemble localised scleroderma. Various names are used for this disorder — migrating sub-acute nodular hypodermatitis (Vilanova and Pinol), erythema nodosum migrans (Baverstedt) or atrophic erythema nodosum (Rothman—Makai syndrome). Essentially there is inflammation of or in the fat with some inevitable involvement of the venous vasculature of the adjacent deep dermis. Infarction of fat sometimes leads to its liquefaction and extrusion through the dermis. More often the repair process simply leads to fibrosis of the affected areas (see Chapter 4).

As indicated in Chapter 6 there are broadly two types of inflammatory response in the skin:
1. Response due to epidermal injury which tends to result in prolonged injury to capillaries in the upper dermis.
2. Response due to injury which spares the epidermis and produces a more intense but transient increase in permeability of the vessels in the mid-dermis.

The depth in the skin of the inflammatory response depends on the site of the injury — whether epidermal or subepidermal — and is determined by the influence of epithelial breakdown products diffusing through the upper dermis. Such a pattern of response in which the end-result depends on the combined effects of epithelial and of direct endothelial injury applies equally to the adnexal tissues, although in practice acute

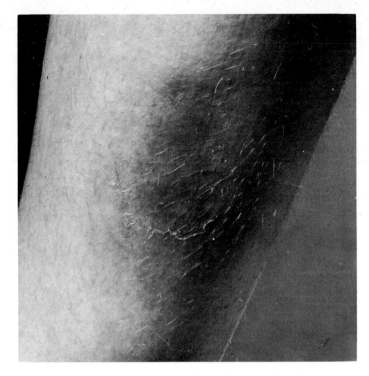

Figure 3.10. Slightly depressed non-tender lump in the lower leg of a teenage girl, related to cold exposure. This is the typical appearance of deep dermal or subcutaneous pathology.

primary injury to the hair follicle, sweat gland or sebaceous gland is rarer than injury to the surface epidermis.

It is commonly suggested that vasculitis, by definition, consists of a primary injury to the vessel. In practice, however, small vessels form a unit with the tissues they supply, and injury affects all parts of this unit (Ryan, 1973). Such epithelial—endothelial interaction is, in fact, very significant in upper dermal vasculitis and in papular urticaria.

This interplay can be seen in the effects of differing reactions to injury. An exudative response in papular urticaria can cause secondary epidermal hypertrophy; whereas in other circumstances gross extravasation of red cells into the dermal papilla can inhibit epidermal growth. In fact, the difference in the patterns of the diseases described by Schönlein and Henoch may have depended on this fact alone. Peliosis rheumatica of Schönlein (see page 5) was only mildly purpuric and branny scaling was associated, whereas the clearly purpuric lesions described by Henoch (page 5) were not associated with scaling.

A notable difference between a superficial papillary lesion and a deeper lesion is the ability of the former to rid itself of noxious agents by extrusion. Necrotic or granulomatous tissue in the papilla can be excreted by a process that has been termed 'catharsis' (Malak and Kurban, 1971). Deeper granulomas and necrotic tissue cannot be cleared so easily and tend therefore to produce more chronic lesions of the type described by Bazin (1861) as erythema induratum and other disorders which can be broadly included within the term nodular vasculitis (see Tables 1.2 and 1.4, Chapter 1).

Involvement of fat similarly tends to produce a deep chronic lesion. Necrotic fat is not easily disposed of and like all indigestible material tends to incite a chronic granulomatous and giant cell histology (see Chapter 4).

Polymorphism is most often a feature of dynamic processes, i.e. ones that evolve and regress, like most of the diseases discussed in this book. But it also results from cropping of lesions, as often occurs in papular urticaria or purpura in which a fresh lesion invariably looks different from one that is a few days old. It can also be a product of regional variation; for example, more extravasation of blood occurs in lesions of the lower leg than elsewhere, and discoid lupus erythematosus is more destructive on the face than on the trunk.

On the other hand, certain diseases in which one expects to see polymorphism, such as erythema multiforme or dermatitis herpetiformis, can be monomorphic, and then diagnosis by strict adherence to classical descriptions often has to be modified; in fact, should a physician dogmatically describe the classic features of a disease to a group of students, he may well find himself forced to play down an atypical feature during the discussion of any one patient.

One of the smallest lesions visible to the naked eye is a thrombosed papillary vessel or a papillary haemorrhage. Most purpuric lesions of the Schönlein—Henoch type can be seen to be made up of many such small bleeds or blocks if closely inspected (Copeman and Ryan, 1971). Such bleeding occurs from the peaks and the venous arm of the papillary vessel. The splinter haemorrhage or a thrombus in the nail fold are good examples of the way in which the skin extrudes a damaged papilla as soon as it ceases to support effectively the epidermis (Figures 3.11, a and b, and 3.12).

TYPE OF VESSEL

The anatomy of the skin is such that the capillaries are most densely distributed in the upper dermis and around the hair roots and sweat glands. The blood drains from the upper dermal capillaries into venules that are deeper and very numerous, far outnumbering arterioles (Ryan, 1973). Normally, arterioles are not found in the upper dermis, and true arteries are a feature of the deeper dermis and the subcutis. Consequently, true capillaritis is the most superficial of disorders whilst arteritis is relatively deep. Because 'sludging out' of noxious agents circulating in the blood occurs most readily in venules, it is there that immune complexes, bacterial endotoxin and the like produce their pathology. Such venular pathology is enhanced at sites where venous stasis is encouraged by gravitational effects or by cold and this accounts for some regional differences in pathology (Chapter 12).

As will be described in Chapter 4 there is no sure way of distinguishing histologically between small arteries and small veins if they have been injured for more than 24 to 48 hours, but there are a number of reasons for believing that most vascular pathology begins in capillaries and venules, which accounts for its early anatomical distribution. However, when an artery supplies only blocked capillaries and venules, or when vasoconstriction is extreme, as in hypertension, or if there is arteriolar block caused by embolisation or intravascular coagulation, the consequent arterial ischaemia has to be taken into account. As the smooth muscle in the walls of arterioles and arteries readily undergoes necrosis, it is particularly sensitive to such ischaemia (see Chapter 4). This change, which occurs predominantly in the deep dermis and subcutis, also arises when there is systemic hypertension, local hypertension due to arteriovenous shunting, or evidence of intravascular clotting or obstruction with or without destruction of the capillary and venular bed (see Chapter 13).

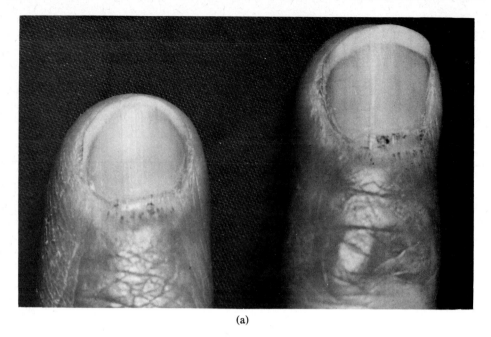

(a)

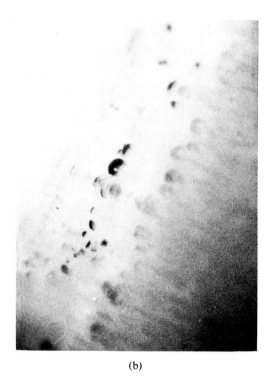

(b)

Figure 3.11. Nail-fold capillaries in a patient affected by severe Raynaud's syndrome (a). The dark blobs are extravasated blood and should be compared to the non-haemorrhagic thrombosed vessel in Figure 3.12. (b) Higher magnification.

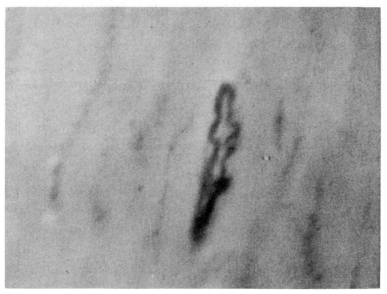

Figure 3.12. Nail-bed capillary, thrombosed and in the process of extrusion — clinically diagnosed as a 'splinter haemorrhage' but clearly there is no haemorrhage. ×50.

The skin lesions resulting from arterial necrosis are of several types. Clearcut, relatively small, deep ulcers are characteristic of complete obstruction of arteries (Figure 3.13). When arterioles are involved, the smallest mid-dermal lesions which result may not ulcerate but can heal with white atrophy — the porcelain scar of Degos' malignant atrophic papulosis. Much commoner is the infarction with ulceration of the skin in the centre of a rather more diffuse, irregular plaque of capillary-venular pathology. The typical purpuric lesion of Henoch's purpura, in which there is considerable capillary and venular damage in the upper dermis, may eventually proceed to central necrosis because flow through the artery supplying the area ceases (Figure 3.14). Rupture of arteries as a result of ischaemic necrosis produces a painful swelling with eventual tracking of blood to the surface as a bruise or ecchymosis.

When the microvasculature is the main site of injury, the morphology of the resulting skin lesion is determined by the distribution of the affected vessel. In this respect there are two types of pattern of rash — punctate or reticulate (Copeman and Ryan, 1971) — both of which result from the candelabra array of vessels supplying the epidermis (Figure 3.15). Figure 3.16 represents the anatomy of the papillary vessels and shows how they drain into the superficial horizontal venous plexus. Figure 3.17 shows the clinical counterpart of this diagram; the dot-like pattern making up the lesion is explained by bleeding and blockage in the papillary system. The disposition of the central arteriole and central venous drainage of the candelabra is such that blood flows not only upwards from the central vessel to the surface but also laterally to the periphery of the system and thence into the horizontal vessels. Flow through this candelabra is uneven, being faster through the central arteriole and slower through the capillaries and veins.

Cooling of the blood at the surface and variation in the metabolism of the epidermis and upper dermis cause still further variation in flow, which is, moreover, slower at the periphery than at the centre. The effect of this uneven flow is to cause vascular dilatation in some areas, short-circuiting of some channels and sometimes, where flow is slowest, atrophy of the vessels. These secondary changes in vascular morphology and distortion

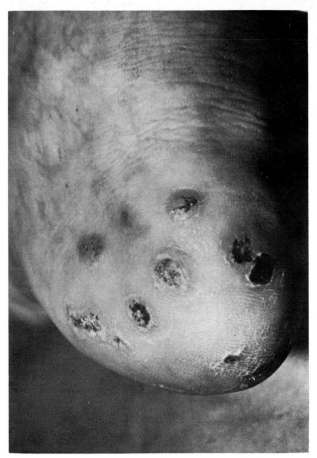

Figure 3.13. Truly arterial lesions are deep and well-defined, and they are often more localised than venous lesions. Elbow in suspected polyarteritis nodosa.

of flow patterns give rise to the reticular patterns of skin (Figure 3.18). In them, the central white area has normal-looking papillary vessels with little variation in flow, and is usually warmer than the surrounding blue area which represents a more dilated system with a slower flow. The latter is preferentially affected by pathology induced by circulating immune complexes, bacterial toxins, and the like. Following infarction due to arteriole occlusion the central pale area develops a different character: it becomes cooler than the surrounding tissue and may assume a slate-blue hue with a slightly depressed centre. Copeman and Ryan (1971) have discussed the interaction of blood flow and vascular patterns, and Table 3.2 summarises some aspects of their discourse.

ULCERATION AND NECROSIS

A break in the surface continuity of epithelium as a manifestation of vascular pathology is usually caused by ischaemic necrosis. It occurs in minute form when papillary vessels bleed or extrude white cells to such a degree that the epidermis becomes

Table 3.2. Interrelationship of some non-immunological factors that affect blood flow in skin vessels.

1. Vessel outflow blocking by:
   Red cell aggregates
   Platelet aggregates $\rightarrow$ small punctate (capillary) or larger livedo reticularis patterns.
2. Viscosity of blood
3. Fluidity of blood
4. Pressure:
   Internal, e.g. haemodynamic back-pressure from dependency.
   External on vessels.
5. Anatomical:
   Arrangement of deeper vessels, e.g. small punctate and larger reticular patterns; shunts; 'thoroughfare channels'

Aggregation of red blood cells depends on
A. Nature of fluid suspension
    Velocity of flow: Plasma (axial flow, marginal zone, turbulence)
                  RBC (rouleaux, collision aggregates)
    Viscosity: Rate of flow; surface cooling; back pressure
                  Haematocrit; properties (including internal viscosity) of RBC
                  Fluidity of blood
                  Plasma proteins (cold precipitable, fibrinogen)
    Platelet adhesiveness (enhanced by contact with damaged cells, collagen)
B. Nature of vessel
    Size; shape; elasticity, distensibility and tone of wall; bifurcation; response to surface temperature, trauma, vasoactive substances — capillary-venule particularly vulnerable

Platelet aggregation and adhesion depend on
A. ADP from platelets themselves stimulated by collagen or by injury to any cell (e.g. RBC, endothelial)
B. Collision: opportunity altered by flow rate and turbulence
C. Catecholamines, fibrin and its degradation products, prostaglandins, and other hormones and chemicals

Fluidity of blood depends on
    Velocity of flow (e.g. slowed by RBC aggregates, cold)
    Plasma: Coagulation-fibrinolysis
            Proteins (cold precipitable, fibrinogen concentration)
    Platelet: Adhesion and aggregation
    Endothelial integrity

Fibrinolytic system   Inhibitors (origin ? epithelium)
                                                   ↙ ↙
                        Plasminogen activators
                        (endothelial origin)
Plasminogen (β-globulin in plasma)————————————→ Plasmin
                                          ↑ ↑
                                Plasmin inhibitors

Coagulation mechanisms depend on
  Intrinsic system: blood
    (Factors V, VIII, IX, X, XI, XII, platelet phospholipid)

    Extrinsic system: tissues
                  (tissue factor, factors V, VII, X)
↓Ca^{++} ↓ Ca^{++} Prothrombin
Thromboplastin (blood or tissue)————————————→ ↓
                                  Thrombin
             Fibrinogen————————————————→ Fibrin

isolated from its blood supply by a wall of cellular material. This is most likely to occur when the papillary vessel is a gigantic coil and there are few vessels in the surrounding area, as in the case of the telangiectasic vessel of gravitational stasis with atrophie blanche.

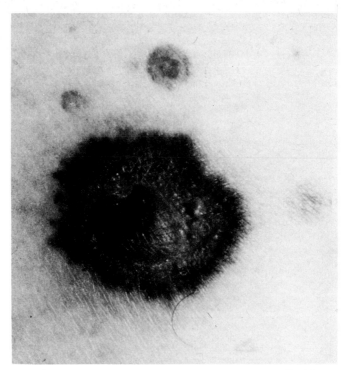

Figure 3.14. The type of lesion 3 cm in diameter that was initiated as a capillaritis—venulitis and then progressed as a result of arterial infarction. The adjacent smaller lesion remains a pure capillaritis.

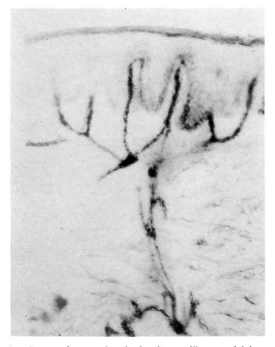

Figure 3.15. Alkaline phosphatase of upper dermis showing capillary candelabra.

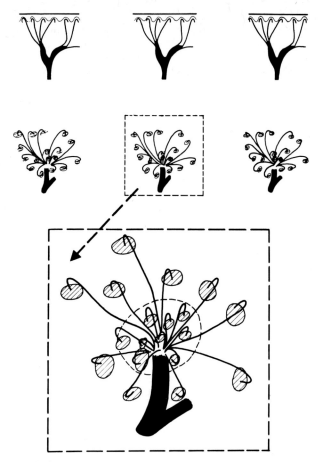

Figure 3.16. The venular drainage system when superimposed on the arterial candelabra explains the pattern of many of the lesions illustrated in Figure 3.17.

Arterial block occurs most commonly in the elderly and is then usually caused by microemboli or ischaemic necrosis of the wall. The latter occurs in hypertension and its site of predilection lies proximal to arteriovenous shunts of the minor kind so commonly seen in association with venous stasis of the lower leg. Ischaemic necrosis of the wall of an artery also occurs when all its branches become blocked as in a capillary vasculitis. Arterial block produces a well-defined punched-out ulcer which tends to remain the same size and takes a long time to heal (Figure 3.13).

Venous gangrene, by contrast, produces an ulcer which appears less suddenly and often enlarges slowly. The distribution of the venules in the skin is such that lateral spread and involvement of deeper tissues by a coagulation necrosis and neutrophil abscesses is to be expected. This is often preceded by a lesion resembling those of erythema nodosum or nodular vasculitis, and the necrosis is frequently multifocal (Figure 3.19). The edge of the ulcer usually merges into a slightly swollen reddish blue periphery which is commonly undermined. Because spread of venous pathology is downwards as well as radially, deep dermal and subcutaneous tissues are often involved, and the dividing line between affected and uninvolved tissues is less well defined than in the case of arteriolar lesions, the territory of which is clearly determined by the

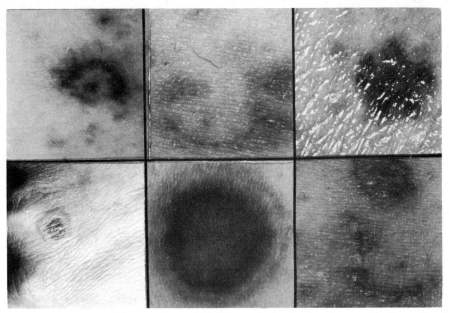

Figure 3.17. Six lesions from different patients which illustrate the localisation of purpura in the venules of the upper dermis as in Figure 3.16.

anatomical disposition of the vessel. Venous gangrene of the type described as pyoderma gangrenosum often involves sites with a large fat component, such as the buttocks, breasts and thighs (see Chapter 13).

REGIONAL VARIATION

Regional variation has been one of the main excuses for subclassification and separation of certain patterns of disease. It accounts for such terms as temporal arteritis, erythrocyanosis crurum frigidarum puellarum, acrocyanosis and midline granuloma.

The legs are affected more often than any other part of the body in most forms of vasculitis, particularly in those at the purpuric and infarctive end of the spectrum; this is less obviously so in urticarial forms which are rarely confined to the legs. The most likely reason for this is the effect of the upright posture on the vasculature. The long-term effect of gravity on the vasculature of the lower legs is to dilate the deeper arteriovenous anastomoses through which blood is short-circuited; this leads to stasis in the capillaries even when supine.

The legs, like the arms, face and ears, are influenced also by the effects of exposure to ultraviolet radiation and to cold. The acrocyanotic circulation is usually blamed on cold; but large pads of fat around the lower leg, particularly in women, often insulate the skin from the heat in the core of the limb and predispose it to the acrocyanotic picture (Figure 3.20).

Limited patterns of disease such as erythema nodosum on the shins, erythema induratum on the calves, Wegener's granulomatosis affecting the respiratory tract or Behçet's disease affecting the mouth, genitalia and eyes, have been over-emphasised. As

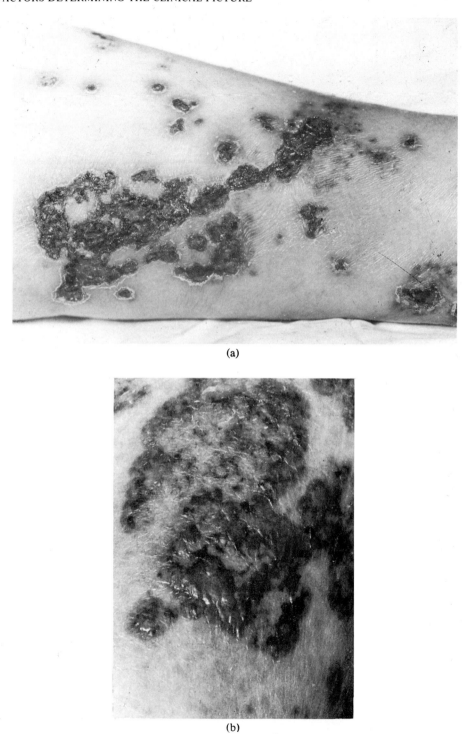

(a)

(b)

Figure 3.18. (a) and (b) Two areas of infarction illustrating the reticulate pattern of vascular disease in the skin.

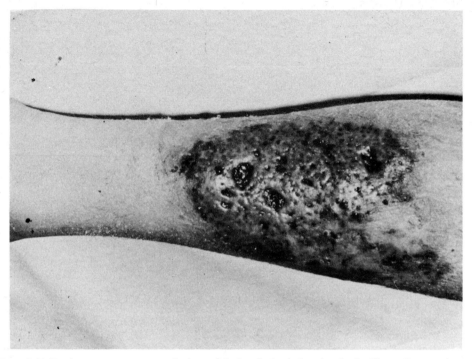

Figure 3.19. Pyoderma gangrenosum on the front of the leg. Such a lesion often begins like erythema nodosum before developing its violaceous hue and multifocal necrosis due to venous infarction.

a result it is sometimes difficult to name a disease in which erythema nodosum-like lesions affect areas other than the shins, or in which the less common associations of Behçet's syndrome, such as thrombophlebitis, superior vena caval obstruction or a papulo-necrotic reaction to needle punctures, occur in the absence of or precede the classic triad.

Vasculitis sometimes seems to favour areas that have a large fat component; this obviously applies to the deeper and more persistent varieties, or to the deep necrotic forms, and to the gangrene sometimes caused by the coumarin drugs. Temporal arteritis has been renamed giant-cell arteritis and this is an example of a successful lobby against naming diseases according to site. It has yet to be renamed according to mechanism.

In Chapter 9 some of the factors localising vasculitis to the nose are discussed. Many of these are applicable to other areas of the body. The observations by Cherry in Chapter 5 are also relevant. Skin flaps formed by the surgeon's knife develop a severe interference of their blood supply and this vascular insult is responsible for the resulting histological evidence of vasculitis. The skin is sometimes blue, warm and swollen and at other times white. Kanan and Ryan describe some differences in histology in such grafts in Chapter 4.

AGE VARIATION

Age is responsible for considerable variation in morphology because of changes in the vascular anatomy.

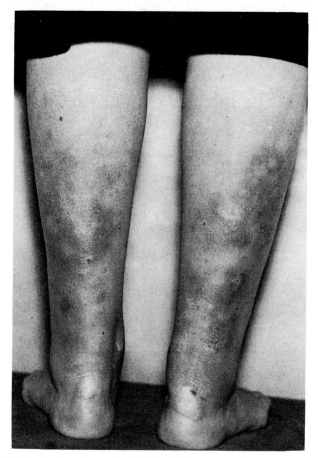

Figure 3.20. Typical fat legs that predispose to chilblains. Such areas are always cold and the superficial skin blood flow is very sluggish.

At birth there is no papillary system as the candelabra pattern has not yet formed. The dermis is relatively oedematous and wealing is lost in this hyperpermeable environment. The cardinal signs of Celsus, too, are much less obvious in the newborn, and the distribution of rashes does not particularly favour the legs compared to the arms and face. Eruptions are much more completely and rapidly resolved and even severe gangrene may leave relatively little scarring.

In children and teenagers, however, the urticarial component of rashes is more obvious than in adults, and punctate eruptions are a feature of the exanthemata. Necrosis is not a common feature of vasculitis in this age group.

A main consequence of old age is vascular atrophy and a wider range and frequency of abnormal anatomical vascular patterns. The urticarial and punctate component of rashes is less obvious partly because the upper dermis is atrophic and, on the lower leg, the papillary vessels are fewer in number per unit area. Haemorrhage, when it occurs, spreads more widely and irregularly in the tissues and is more slowly removed by the macrophage system. Purpuric lesions, too, are often larger, irregular in shape and long-lasting. Atrophy of capillaries and venules and an increasing number of arterio-venous shunts account for a *relatively* larger arterial component in the atrophic skin.

Local or systemic hypertension in this age group contributes to changes in the vessel wall and commonly leads to sudden total occlusion of a vessel. Infarction with punched-out ulcers is a feature particularly of elderly skin and is seen most commonly on the lower legs (Figure 3.21).

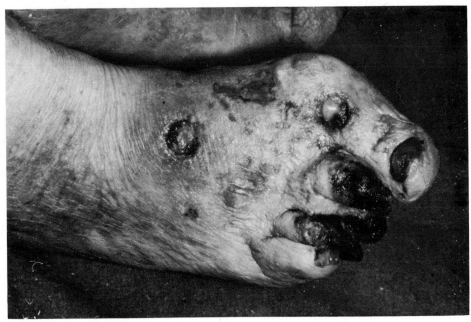

Figure 3.21. Typical ischaemia in foot of elderly patient. Hypertension and arteriosclerosis complicate venous stasis particularly in the elderly.

THE OVERLAP OF URTICARIA AND VASCULITIS

Urticaria was extensively reviewed by Warin and Champion (1974) in their volume in this series. That urticaria overlaps with normal physiological responses can hardly be doubted when dermographism and cholinergic urticaria are considered. Dermographism is an exaggerated form of the triple response and is found in approximately five per cent of the population, the exact figure depending on the intensity of the scratch. Cholinergic urticaria has been likened to an exaggerated blush, and in so far as blushing is associated with an increased permeability of the skin's microvasculature and is triggered by emotion, exercise or overheating, the similarities are obvious. But urticaria also overlaps with vasculitis, which in turn overlaps with intravascular coagulation. The exudative process can therefore be understood only as a spectrum and not as a group of disorders each with its own distinct pathological boundaries. The suggested spectrum is: normal permeability—urticaria—vasculitis—intravascular coagulation.

The overlap between urticaria and vasculitis is accepted in the literature on Schönlein—Henoch purpura. Thus Ansell (1970) observed urticarial lesions, some of which were followed by purpura, in 30 per cent of her patients with that disease.

Moreover, 45 per cent of her series had localised oedema which sometimes affected the face, hands, arms, feet and scrotum. Most texts on Schönlein—Henoch purpura emphasise the initial urticarial nature of the purpuric lesion.

Studies of urticaria have shown that the delayed pressure variety and vasculitis overlap. Ryan, Shim-Young and Turk (1968) described a relatively pure form of delayed pressure urticaria but Ryan has subsequently observed some 50 patients with this complaint which, in most, was associated with ordinary chronic urticaria; four had been classified by others as vasculitis. Wealing can be elicited in cases of delayed pressure urticaria by applying a weight to the skin — 10 lb for five to ten minutes — or by injecting histamine into the skin. Between two and six hours after applying the weight, the patient develops a deep tender weal which lasts for several hours, and the histamine inoculation, which in normal persons produces a weal lasting several hours, produces in these cases a weal which, after an initial period of two hours or so, increases in size. Inoculation of saline may sometimes have the same effect in such patients.

This type of urticaria is painful and may ultimately lead to bruising; it occurs in those patients who have long-lasting lesions and it is delayed in onset. In Chapter 10 it is pointed out that the delayed element has been much emphasised even though its mediators have not been identified. The kinins, complement, fibrinolysins and prostaglandins are contenders for this role. The histology of the delayed lesion is similar to that sometimes seen in vasculitis, namely a swollen endothelium and a mainly neutrophilic population of white cells. In addition Soter, Austen and Gigli (1974) also referred to urticaria and arthralgia as manifestations of vasculitis in a study from Boston.

Forms of vasculitis that have a prominent urticarial element (MacDuffie et al, 1973) are less likely to show infarction. Such lesions are usually widespread rather than confined to the legs and they develop rapidly in the course of a few minutes just like urticarial weals or an erythema. Some disappear within an hour or two, but others become purpuric and persist for several days. The urticarial process not only promotes the diffusion of activators of fibrinolysis but also is initiated by histamine released from mast cells in the company of heparin. These factors make urticaria more or less incompatible with the ischaemic and thrombotic state; by and large, therefore, less infarction is seen in vasculitis when urticaria is present. Handel et al (1975) have suggested that severe activation of coagulation, as occurs in disseminated intravascular coagulation, precludes the development of the acute necrotising lesions. This may be due to a reduction in the recruitment of neutrophils from the bloodstream when the vessels are totally occluded. The chronicity of this urticarial form of vasculitis is remarkable; it can persist for more than ten years — three such patients being known to the author. Urticaria has been described also in the vasculitis of lupus erythematosus (Williams, 1967).

The urticaria of Schönlein, emphasised by some authors as morphologically pure, is less commonly seen in the adult than in children (Cream, Gumpel and Peachey, 1970). Another urticarial form of vasculitis has recently been recognized and is associated with hypocomplementaemia, but rarely shows frank purpura and almost never necroses. One such patient was investigated by the author and found to have positive tests for delayed pressure urticaria; she was referred for further investigation when she was found to have a low serum complement, and she has been reported by Sissons (1974). The delayed pressure type of urticaria responds to aspirin, though any associated ordinary urticaria may be aggravated. Ryan, Shim-Young and Turk (1968) reported that these patients react to their own leucocytes, an observation confirmed by Dilorenzo and Peterka (1968) in a similar group of patients; in this respect the condition overlaps with psychogenic purpura (see Chapter 10 on the painful bruising syndrome). Perhaps it is significant that the painful bruising syndrome is a disease of women while delayed pressure urticaria is much commoner in men.

References

Ansell, B. M. (1970) Henoch—Schönlein purpura with particular reference to the prognosis of the renal lesions. *British Journal of Dermatology,* **82,** 811.

Audry, C. (1898) Étude de la lésion de l'érythème induré. *Annals de Dermatologie et de Syphiligraphie,* **3,** 209.

Bazin, E. (1861) *Extrait des Leçons Théoriques et Cliniques sur la Scrofule.* p. 146.

Copeman, P. W. M. & Ryan, T. J. (1970) The problems of cutaneous angiitis with reference to histopathology and pathogenesis. *British Journal of Dermatology,* **82,** 2.

Copeman, P. W. M. & Ryan, T. J. (1971) Cutaneous angiitis patterns of rashes explained by 1) flow properties of blood, 2) anatomical disposition of vessels. *British Journal of Dermatology,* **85,** 205.

Cream, J. J., Gumpel, J. M. & Peachey, R. D. G. (1970) Schönlein—Henoch purpura in the adult. A study of 77 adults with anaphylactoid or Schönlein—Henoch purpura. *Quarterly Journal of Medicine,* **34,** 461.

Cunliffe, W. J. & Menon, I. S. (1969) Blood fibrinolytic activity in diseases of small blood vessels and the effect of low molecular weight dextran. *British Journal of Dermatology,* **81,** 220.

Dilorenzo, P. A. & Peterka, E. S. (1968) Auto-leucocyte sensitivity. *Acta Dermato-venereologica,* **48,** 397.

Handel, D. W., Roenigk, H. H., Shainoff, J. & Deodhar, S. (1975) Necrotizing vasculitis. *Archives of Dermatology,* **111,** 847.

MacDuffie, F. C., Mitchell-Sams, W., Maldonado, J. E., Andreini, R. H., Conn, D. L. & Samayoa, E. A. (1973) Hypocomplementaemia with cutaneous vasculitis and arthritis. Possible immune complex syndrome. *Mayo Clinic Proceedings,* **48,** 340.

Malak, J. A. & Kurban, A. K. (1971) "Catharsis". An excretory function of the epidermis. *British Journal of Dermatology,* **84,** 516.

Osler, W. (1914) The visceral lesions of purpura and allied conditions. *British Medical Journal,* **i,** 517.

Ryan, T. J. (1973) In *Physiology and Pathophysiology of the Skin* (Ed.) Jarrett, A. New York: Academic Press.

Ryan, T. J., Shim-Young, N. & Turk, J. L. (1968) Delayed pressure urticaria. *British Journal of Dermatology,* **80,** 485.

Schneider, W. & Undeutsch, W. (1965) Vasculitiden des subcutanen Fettgewebes. *Archiv für klinische und experimentelle Dermatologie,* **221,** 600.

Siemens, H. W. (1958) *General Diagnosis and Therapy of Skin Diseases.* Chicago: University of Chicago Press. London: Cambridge University Press.

Sissons, J. G. P. (1974) Cutaneous vasculitis and hypocomplementaemia. *Proceedings of the Royal Society of Medicine,* **67,** 654.

Soter, N. A., Austen, F. & Gigli, I. (1974) Urticaria and arthralgias as manifestations of necrotising angiitis (vasculitis). *Journal of Investigative Dermatology,* **63,** 485.

Warin, R. P. & Champion, R. H. (1974) *Urticaria. Major Problems in Dermatology,* Volume 1. London, Philadelphia, Toronto: W. B. Saunders.

Wilhelm, D. L. (1971) Increased vascular permeability in acute inflammation. *Revue Canadienne de Biologie,* **30, 153.**

Williams, D. I. (1967) Systemic lupus erythematosus. *Proceedings of the Royal Society of Medicine,* **60,** 299.

4. The Pathology of Ischaemia, Stasis and Vasculitis

T. J. RYAN, M. W. KANAN AND G. W. CHERRY

Ischaemia and stasis form an integral part of vasculitis. They usually cause necrosis of the skin when they cut off its blood supply, unless they do so slowly enough to allow a collateral circulation to be established. Wilkinson (1972) reviewed the clinical causes of obstruction to the arterial blood flow, of which there were three principal varieties: extramural compression or strangulation of vessels; disease of the vessel wall; or changes in the composition or coagulability of the blood leading to occlusion by thrombosis or embolism. Rarely, necrosis is caused by a failure of the blood supply to meet increased metabolic demands, as can occur in tumours.

ISCHAEMIA

In the past, research on ischaemia of the skin has been limited, but from recent studies certain important observations and conclusions on the cause and effects of ischaemia have emerged. Fundamental to the understanding of the mechanisms involved is the realisation that ischaemia means more than hypoxia or anoxia, however crucial these may be to the survival of the tissue concerned.

The final outcome of restriction of blood flow to an organ has been shown to depend on several factors:

1. *The resistance of the component cells to the effects of obstructed blood flow.* The epidermis and dermis, for example, seem to be more resistant to an ischaemic insult than the muscles and hypodermal fat, and the brain cells show almost no resistance at all (Willms-Kretschmer and Majno, 1969).

2. *The ability of blood vessels and supporting tissues to recover when the cause of ischaemia ceases to exist* (Hills, 1964; Ames et al, 1968; Chiang et al, 1968; Kowada et

al, 1968). For instance, the so-called 'no-flow' phenomenon in brain ischaemia is due to compression of the small blood vessels by swollen perivascular glial cells (Ames et al, 1968).

3. *The length of the ischaemic period.* As explained by Cherry in Chapter 5, the revival time varies with the specific tissue susceptibility and with the type of vessel occluded. In their study in the rat and the rabbit, Wilms-Kretschmer and Majno (1969) found that compression ischaemia for four to six hours produced no skin damage but that ischaemia for eight hours caused complete necrosis a few days later. An exception was the ischaemic skin of the rabbit's ear which suffered no significant damage after eight hours of compression. However, growth of hair in the ischaemic area of the ear was impaired and this they ascribed to the fact that hair follicles depend completely on the deep dermal vessels supplying their papillae. The epidermis, on the other hand, can, in the early hours of ischaemia, be oxygenated in part by surface diffusion from the atmospheric air (Bullough, 1952).

4. *The type of occluded vessel.* Experimental studies on skin flaps have shown that the most important cause of flap necrosis is combined arterial and venous insufficiency, the arterial component being the crucial one (Myers and Cherry, 1967).

5. *States of stress.* Selye (1967) showed that the resistance of rat skin to ischaemia could be increased by subjecting the animal to some form of stress such as starvation for 48 hours, hypothermia, spinal cord transection or parenteral adrenaline. On the other hand, Palmer (1972) found in the rat that the survival of freshly raised flaps was reduced when the animal was subjected to the stress of restraint. Cherry in Chapter 5 attributes this difference to the fact that all the nerves supplying the vessel were severed in Palmer's experiments, whereas in Selye's experiment they were not.

6. *Delay phenomenon.* As described by Cherry in Chapter 5, delay is a surgical technique using staged operations to improve the blood supply of a skin flap before it is transplanted to a new site (Myers and Cherry, 1967; Milton, 1969). However, Milton (1972) was surprised to find that delayed flaps could withstand only four hours of ischaemia, whereas freshly raised (non-delayed) island skin flaps could tolerate on average eight hours of ischaemia.

In collaboration with Cherry the authors studied the morphological changes in delayed and non-delayed pig skin flaps subjected to six hours of ischaemia followed by reperfusion. The following is an outline of their findings:

Light microscopy

Biopsies taken from the centre of ischaemic, freshly raised island flaps six hours after clamping their main artery and vein and before reperfusion differed little from normal control skin.

Biopsies taken from identical flaps 18 hours after reperfusion revealed minimal focal oedema in the dermis but moderate changes in and around the deep vessels in the hypodermis and panniculus carnosus. Oedema, congestion and leakage of polymorpho-nuclear leucocytes through some veins and venules were noted in the adipose tissue (Figure 4.1). The striated muscle fibres of the panniculus showed cloudy swelling and interfascicular oedema (Figure 4.2).

In contrast, biopsies obtained from the centre of *delayed* island flaps 18 hours after reperfusion showed marked oedema of the dermis with prominent lymphatics (Figure

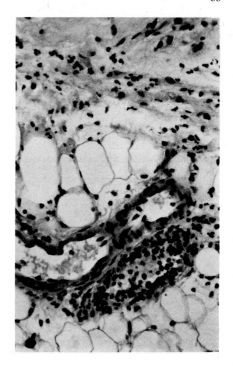

Figure 4.1. Oedema and predominantly neutrophilic infiltrates are seen in and around veins and venules in the septa of the hypodermal fat. Ischaemia and reperfusion in freshly raised island flaps. H. & E. × 150.

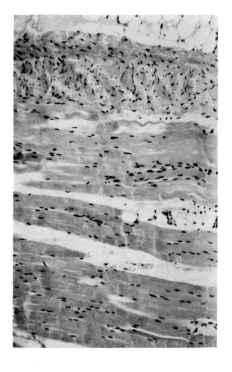

Figure 4.2. Moderate oedema separating the muscle bundles of panniculus carnosus. Cloudy swelling and crowding of the sarcolemmal nuclei from same flap as in Figure 4.1. H. & E. × 60.

4.3). In the hypodermis, the connective tissue septa were remarkably thickened, presumably due to severe transudation of fluid and plasma proteins (Figure 4.4). The blood vessels, mainly the venules and veins, were engorged with polymorphs which leaked into the extravascular spaces, especially in the deep fat (Figure 4.5). Many of the fat cells had burst and the rest were separated by intercellular oedema. The muscle fibres in the panniculus showed severe cloudy swelling, loss of their striations and prominent interstitial oedema (Figure 4.6).

Further biopsies obtained from identical flaps, one and two weeks after reperfusion, revealed remarkable morphological signs of repair. The epidermis and dermis were hypertrophic and showed residual oedema and prominent lymphatics (Figure 4.7). A moderate perivascular polymorphonuclear infiltrate was still to be seen in these sections. The connective tissue septa of the hypodermis and the panniculus carnosus showed obvious hypertrophy (Figure 4.8) and there was massive necrosis of the muscle fibres in the panniculus associated with fibrous tissue replacement (Figure 4.9). Deep to the panniculus lay a thick inflamed area of granulation tissue composed mainly of endothelial sprouts, new vessel formation and actively proliferating fibroblasts (Figure 4.10).

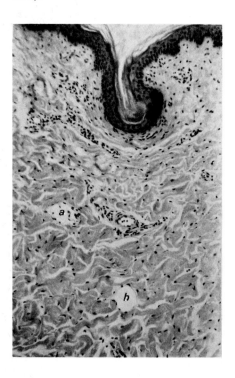

Figure 4.3. Dermal oedema and wide separation of collagen fibres. Dilated lymphatics (a & b) seen in mid and deep dermal levels. Effect of ischaemia and reperfusion in delayed island flaps. H. & E. × 80.

Electron microscopy

A few of the flaps were studied in the electron microscope. In the delayed flaps, upwards of 18 hours after reperfusion, focal changes were present mainly in the deep venules of the dermis and hypodermis. The endothelial cytoplasm was often swollen and narrowed the vascular lumen. Intracellular oedema of the endothelial cells caused multiple discrete bulges in their peripheral cytoplasm resulting in the so-called blebbing phenomenon (Figure 4.11) described by Chiang et al (1968) and by Wilms-Kretschmer and Majno (1969).

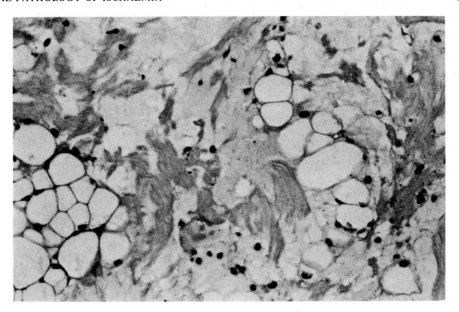

Figure 4.4. Marked thickening of interlobular fat septa with oedema fluid and plasma proteins. Ischaemia and reperfusion in delayed island flap. H. & E. × 150.

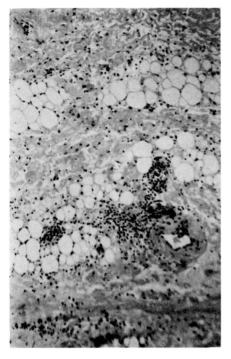

Figure 4.5. Deep hypodermal venules engorged with blood cells and extravascular neutrophil infiltrates. H. & E. × 60.

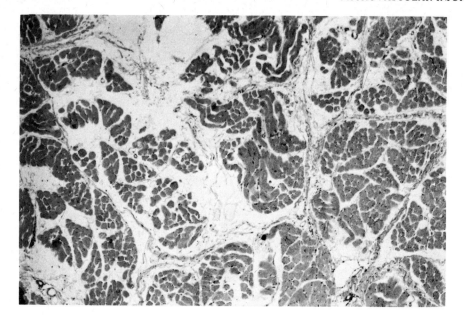

(a)

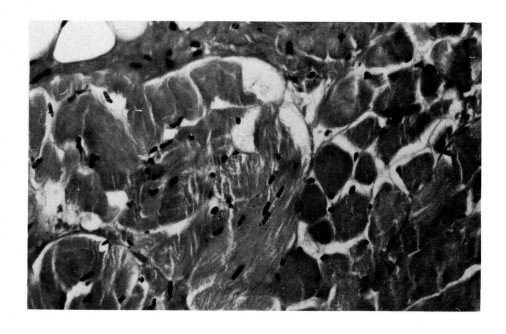

(b)

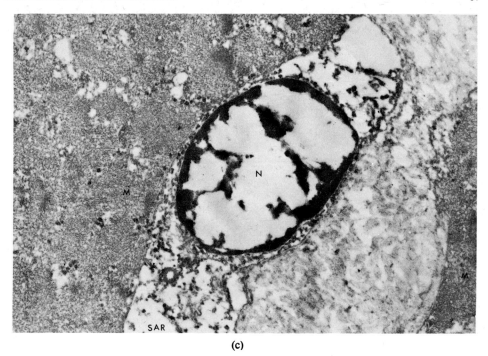

(c)

Figure 4.6. (a) Marked swelling of the panniculus carnosus with oedema widely separating the muscle bundles. Same flap as in Figure 4.5. H. & E. × 32.
(b) Cloudy swelling and necrosis of some muscle fibres. H. & E. × 200.
(c) Electron micrography of panniculus carnosus. Muscle fibres (M) show oedema, necrotic changes and loss of bands (striations). Nucleus (N) of sarcolemma (SAR) shows oedema and degeneration. Magnification × 19 800.

Another ultrastructural feature in these vessels was swelling of the rough endoplasmic reticulum in the endothelial cells and in the pericytes nursing them. In both these types of cell, collections of glycogen granules were present and were reminiscent of a similar finding in the cardiac muscle of rats exposed to chronic hypoxia, as described by Sulkin and Sulkin (1965). In areas of advanced tissue damage in the hypodermis and panniculus carnosus, extravasation of neutrophils and red cells and deposits of fibrin were encountered.

The increased vulnerability of a delayed flap to a second ischaemic insult, in contradistinction to that of a freshly raised island flap, is still a mystery. However, a study of fibrinolysis in these flaps (Cherry, Ryan and Ellis, 1974) suggested that, because damage to the endothelium of the blood vessels in the flap occurs 18 hours after reperfusion, depression of fibrinolytic activity must occur even later. But this does not explain why the new vessel formation in the delayed flap should be accompanied by a lowering of its resistance to an ischaemic insult. On the other hand, ultrastructural studies showed that newly formed capillaries in healing wounds were more permeable and fragile as a result of their loose inter-endothelial junctions, thin endothelium and incomplete basement membrane (Majno, 1965). It is tempting to compare the delay phenomenon, produced intentionally by plastic surgeons to improve the survival length of the skin flaps, to the phenomenon of 'preparation', or to the so-called 'locus minores resistentiae' caused by repeated minor ischaemic insults in certain cutaneous and endonasal sites (referred to in Chapters 5 to 9). By doing so, the propensity of such sites to succumb to a new insult of acute onset becomes more understandable.

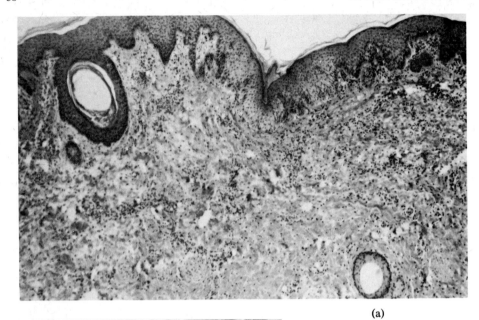

(a)

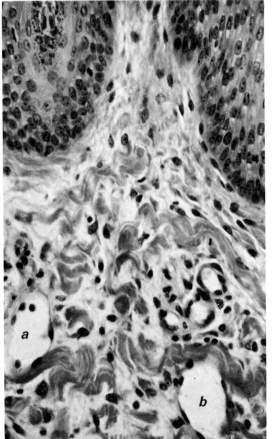

(b)

Figure 4.7. (a) Marked hypertrophy of the epidermis and dermis two weeks after reperfusion of ischaemic delayed flap. H. & E. × 32.
(b) High power of Figure 4.7a showing residual dermal oedema and dilated lymphatics (a and b). H. & E. × 200.

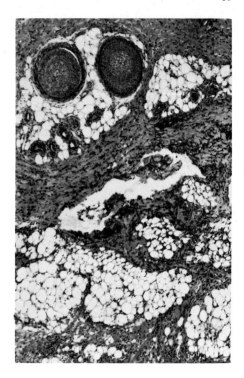

Figure 4.8. Obvious hypertrophy of interlobular fat connective tissue septa. H. & E. × 24. Same flap as Figure 4.7.

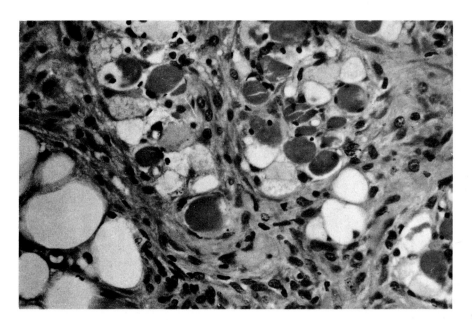

Figure 4.9. Marked necrosis of muscle fibres of panniculus carnosus with fibrous tissue replacement. Same flap as Figure 4.7. H. & E. × 200.

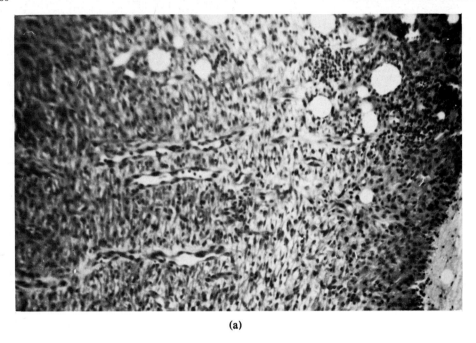

(a)

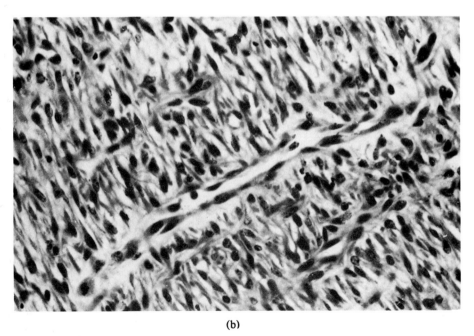

(b)

Figure 4.10. (a) Thick inflamed granulation tissue deep to the panniculus carnosus. H. & E. × 80.
(b) High power of central area of Figure 4.10a showing new capillary sprouts with hyperplasia of endothelial cells and fibroblasts. Same flap as in Figure 4.7. H. & E. × 200.

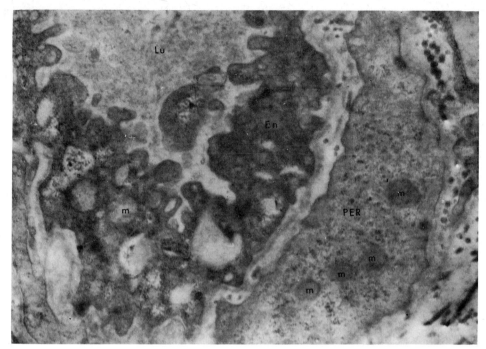

Figure 4.11. Electron-micrograph of dermal venule showing endothelial swelling with intraluminal polypoid projections or blebbing phenomenon. En = endothelium; Lu = lumen of venule. Pericyte (PER) with damaged mitochondria (m). Magnification × 27 300.

STASIS

The histopathology of venous stasis depends on the rate and degree of obstruction to the venous outflow in a particular tissue. According to Farber and Batts (1954) chronic venous insufficiency results in cutaneous oedema, dilatation of the venules and lymphatics and separation of the collagen fibres. Later, raised pressure in the capillaries makes them congested, dilated and tortuous with extravasation of erythrocytes and some monocytic cells into the interstitial tissue. Haemosiderin granules usually take the place of erythrocytes in the later stages of the stasis syndrome, and this picture is often replaced by features of a nonspecific dermatitis. Endothelial proliferation and thrombosis of the vessels may follow and interference with the nutrition of the overlying epidermis may end in ulcer formation. In the more dramatic post-thrombotic syndrome the protein-rich oedema fluid stimulates fibroblastic activity with the result that the blood vessels and lymphatics become entangled in a fibrous tissue mass with increasing lymphoedema and hypertrophy of the skin and subcutaneous tissues. In some cases of chronic stasis ulcers the end-organ hypertrophy of the epidermis in the margin of the ulcer may become pseudoepitheliomatous. In cases complicated by lymphoedema the lymphatic vessels are numerous, tortuous and dilated.

In a recent experiment in the pig in which tubed skin flaps were used as a model, Cherry compared the changes in such flaps raised vertically, perpendicular to the long axis of the animal, with those in similar flaps kept in a dependent position for periods of one to seven days. In cooperation with Cherry the authors studied morphological changes in these two groups of tubed flaps, with the following results:

Microscopic findings

In the erect flaps

Sections prepared from the skin near the distal end of the tubed flaps showed a moderate degree of oedema in the dermis and clogging of the superficial and deep capillaries and venules with red blood cells (Figure 4.12). Diapedesis into the dermal connective tissue of erythrocytes, but of very few leucocytes, was a prominent feature in these sections. Examination of the hypodermis showed that, in the septa of the adipose tissue, the venules and veins were distended and that, on rupture, they spilled their contents (Figure 4.13) to form an extravasated mass consisting mainly of red blood cells, monocytic cells, a few neutrophils and serum proteins. In several sections many lipocytes were also found to have ruptured.

It was thought that these findings were due to congestion of the venular tree, caused probably by twisting and obstruction of the deep veins when the proximal end of the tubed flap was raised. The clogging of the dermal capillaries with red cells seems to leave no space for polymorphs and other white cells to escape into the surrounding connective tissue. This sequence of events is similar to that seen in the disseminated intravascular coagulation syndrome where severe endothelial damage is one cause of early intravascular clotting and cessation of blood flow, and as a result no neutrophils or eosinophils have a chance to participate in the inflammatory response.

In the dependent flaps

Microscopic examination of biopsies obtained from the skin near the distal end of these flaps demonstrated features of dependency stasis. In the dermis there was diffuse oedema of the connective tissue, swelling and wide separation of the collagen fibres and dilatation of the lymphatics (Figure 4.14). This resulted in compression of the capillaries and venules, some of which contained erythrocytes. A few leucocytes seemed to have

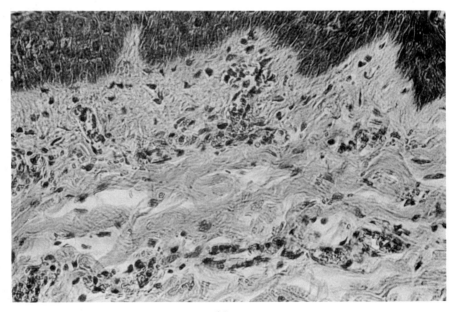

(a)

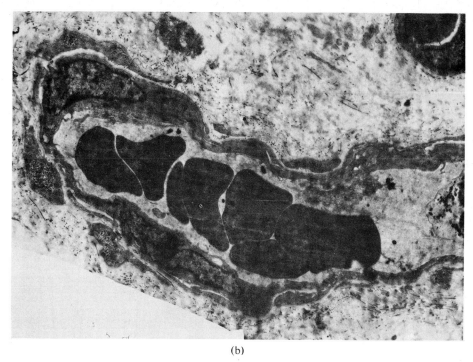

(b)

Figure 4.12. Dermal capillaries and venules show clogging of their lumina with red blood cells (a) H. & E. ×
200.
(b) An electron-micrograph with red cells and one neutrophil impeded by projections of the endothelial wall.
Blood flow from left to right. × 5700.

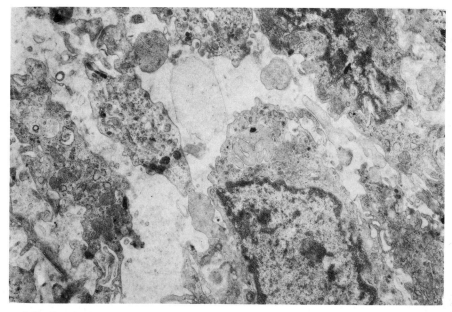

Figure 4.13. Hypodermal venules and veins with considerable disruption of the endothelial cells. Electron
micrograph × 13 500.

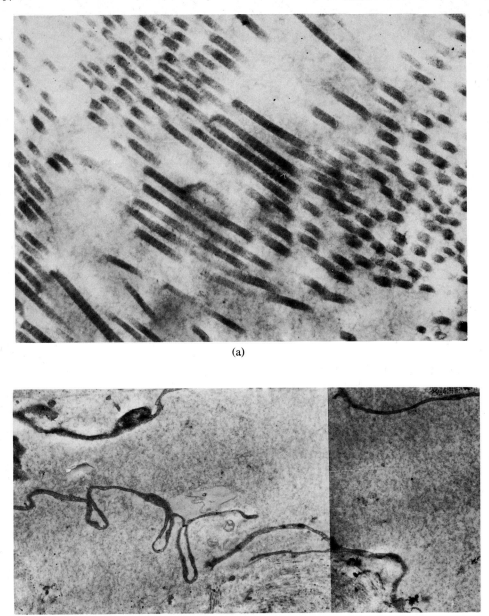

(a)

(b)

Figure 4.14. (a) Marked dermal oedema widely separating the collagen fibres. $\times$ 31 500.
(b) Dilatation of the lymphatics in a dependent skin flap. $\times$ 6825.

leaked earlier on through the vascular walls. Deeper down, the panniculus carnosus was the site of severe oedema, widely separating the muscle bundles which showed minimal focal degenerative changes (Figure 4.15). In the veins of the panniculus there was early damage to the endothelial cells which appeared to exfoliate and to stick to the blood cells in the lumen (Figure 4.16).

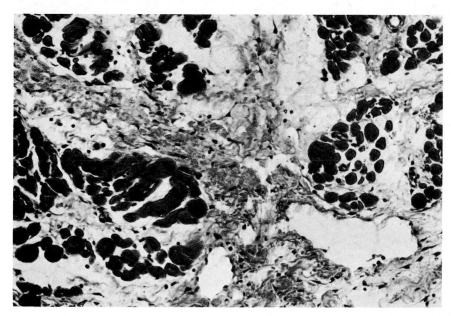

Figure 4.15. Severe oedema of panniculus carnosus with widely separated muscle bundles and dilated lymphatics. H. & E. × 80.

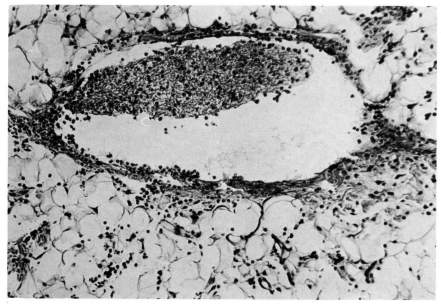

Figure 4.16. Venules of the hypodermis showing endothelial damage and stickiness of the blood cells in the lumen. H. & E. × 200.

References

Ames, A. III, Wright, R. W., Kowada, M., Thurston, J. M. & Majno, G. (1968) Cerebral ischemia II. The no-reflow phenomenon. *American Journal of Pathology*, **52**, 437.

Bullough, W. S. (1952) The energy relations of mitotic activity. *Biological Review*, **27**, 133.

Cherry, G. W., Ryan, T. J. & Ellis, J. P. (1974) Decreased fibrinolysis in reperfused ischaemic tissue. *Thrombosis et Diathesis Haemorrhagica*, **32**, 659.

Chiang, J., Kowada, M., Ames, A. III, Wright, L. & Majno, G. (1968) Cerebral ischaemia III. Vascular changes. *American Journal of Pathology*, **52**, 455.

Farber, E. M. & Batts, E. E. (1954) Pathologic physiology of stasis syndrome. *Archives of Dermatology and Syphilology*, **70**, 653.

Hills, C. P. (1964) Ultrastructural changes in the capillary bed of the rat cerebral cortex in anoxic-ischaemic brain lesions. *American Journal of Pathology*, **44**, 531.

Kowada, M., Ames, A. III, Majno, G. & Wright, R. L. (1968) Cerebral ischemia. An improved experimental method for study: cardiovascular effects and demonstration of an early vascular lesion in the rabbit. *Journal of Neurosurgery*, **28**, 150.

Majno, G. (1965) In *Handbook of Physiology*, Volume 3. Chapter 64. Washington: American Physiological Society.

Milton, S. H. (1969) The effects of 'delay' on the survival of experimental pedicled skin flaps. *British Journal of Plastic Surgery*, **22**, 244.

Milton, S. H. (1972) Experimental studies on island flaps. II. Ischaemia and delay. *Plastic and Reconstructive Surgery*, **49**, 444.

Myers, M. B. & Cherry, G. (1967) Design of skin flaps to study vascular insufficiency. *Journal of Surgical Research*, **7**, 399.

Palmer, B. (1972) The influence of stress on the survival of experimental skin flaps. *Scandinavian Journal of Plastic and Reconstructive Surgery*, **6**, 110.

Selye, H. (1967) Ischemic necrosis: prevention by stress. *Science*, **156**, 1262.

Sulkin, N. M. & Sulkin, D. F. (1965) An electron microscopic study of the effects of chronic hypoxia on cardiac muscle, hepatic and autonomic ganglion cells. *Laboratory Investigation*, **14**, 1523.

Wilkinson, D. S. (1972) Ischaemic (arterial) ulceration of the leg. In *Textbook of Dermatology* (Ed.) Rook, A., Wilkinson, D. S. & Ebling, F. J. G. Volume 1, 2nd edition. Oxford: Blackwell.

Wilms-Kretschmer, K. & Majno, G. (1969) Ischaemia of the skin. *American Journal of Pathology*, **54**, 3327.

VASCULITIS

A study of the histopathology of vasculitis supplements clinical observation but adds problems of interpretation. No single histopathological pattern is a regular feature of any one clinical picture. It could not be otherwise, for the section under the microscope represents only a moment in the life history of the lesion. Moreover, vasculitis expresses a reaction pattern to vascular injury, for which there is only a limited repertoire including a variable degree of endothelial disintegration and repair, exudation, which may be slow or fast, and a variable cellular component involving other components of the vessel wall or the adjacent tissues. Coagulation, platelet aggregation and ischaemic necrosis are further features. Neither capillary, venule, arteriole nor artery is the sole site of the pathology in any variety of vasculitis. Where the injured part of the vascular tree is situated determines which other tissues, such as the epidermis or fat, are affected; in fact, they often become the most prominently inflamed. The histopathological features seem to depend not only on the intensity of the injury but also on the timing of the biopsy — necrosis, for instance, is a late feature.

The attitude of the 'lumper' (see page 1) usually stems from an attempt to find pathogenetic mechanisms common to many forms of vasculitis. The 'splitter' on the other hand (see page 1) is fond of classifications, subclassifications and definitions based on subtle differences among basically similar morphological patterns. His activities often lead to unwarranted confusion of the whole issue of vasculitis. To regard as a separate entity a newly recognised variant of an accepted pathological pattern should be welcomed only if it adds to the understanding of the mechanisms involved in its pathogenesis, or if it promotes prophylaxis or control of the disease. The 'splitting' attitude is sometimes helpful if a newly described variant is shown to have a more favourable prognosis than that already recorded for the main disease entity.

All authors writing on vasculitis would agree that inflammation does produce some sort of change in the blood vessels of the inflamed area irrespective of whether the noxious agent reaches the skin from without or from within the bloodstream. Pinkus and Mehregan (1969) argued that vasculitis must not be diagnosed unless there is evidence of organic damage to the vessel wall in the form of necrosis, hyalinisation, fibrinoid change or granulomatous involvement. To them the changes in pityriasis lichenoides acuta and certain lymphocytic drug eruptions represent perivascular infiltration rather than a true lymphocytic vasculitis. Lever (1968), on the other hand, included the latter conditions under inflammatory purpura or vasculitis. An intriguing facet of this argument is the difficulty in demonstrating in every case, either by light or by electron microscopy, that there is organic damage to the vessel wall. However, neutrophils, nuclear dust and fibrin deposits have been shown to occur in some cases of pityriasis lichenoides acuta (Kruger and Weise, 1959; Ritzenfeld, 1963).

More often than not the difference between two variants of a lesion lies in the degree rather than in the nature of the underlying pathological change. Therefore, to emphasise the mechanisms involved in the pathogenesis of vasculitis and paravasculitis is more fruitful than to argue about definitions, classifications and subclassifications. Morphology (Chapter 3), in fact, is rarely a reliable clue to the nature of the initial cause of vasculitis. For although both urticaria and vasculitis are manifestations of the same wide spectrum embracing altered permeability, blood flow and integrity of the vessel wall, the usual type of common urticaria is a transient local disturbance, while vasculitis is a more persistent reaction due to vascular occlusion or necrosis. However, the delayed deep type of urticaria may be purpuric, often having features characteristic of vasculitis, including deposition of fibrin and release of activators of fibrinolysis and of fibrinogen degradation products (FDP).

Micro-anatomical considerations

The angio-architecture of the skin is determined by the nutritional needs of the epidermis and its adnexae and the acquired ability to divert blood to sweat glands or through shunts in response to changes in temperature.

In the fetus and neonate, where the nutritional needs are considerable, the vasculature is a rather primitive network of capillaries and venules. Shunting of blood is a frequent response to stasis in and to clogging of one part of the network, but fully-formed glomus-type anastomoses do not develop until the skin has experienced cooling and its resultant effects on blood flow. Arteries supply the skin at fairly regular intervals, piercing its undersurface, and initially — at least in the fetus — veins have a more or less similar distribution. Subsequently, differential rates of growth, variation in nutritional requirements and the effects of gravitational stasis and of cooling all combine to produce differentiation, stretching and redistribution of skin vasculature.

In the skin of the adult, the upper dermis, sweat glands, dermal papillae and the peripheries of the fat lobules are very well endowed with capillaries and venules, arranged in a kind of network through which blood can take a variety of channels. These are the main areas of normal transudation and they easily become the places where exudation occurs and where noxious agents silt out; they are thus the commonest sites for vasculitis. Arteries feature only in the deeper dermis, at single points of entry into fat lobules (Figure 4.17) and as relatively sparse vessels crossing the subcutaneous tissues to reach the tissues they supply; these, then, are the sites where arteritis is met.

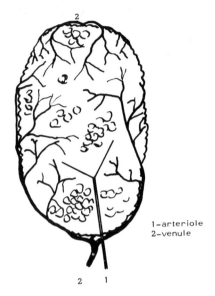

1–arteriole
2–venule

Figure 4.17. Diagram of blood supply to fat lobule. Capillaries and venules are peripheral.

Ultramicroscopic features of capillaries

In general, normal dermal capillaries are of the closed type and have no gaps between their endothelial cells (Figure 4.18). They show relatively little pinocytosis and have rather fewer microfibrils in their cytoplasm than the endothelial cells of the venules. The nuclei of the capillary endothelial cells do not show the marked indentations seen in the venules. In the legs, the vascular basement membrane has been shown to be much thicker than that in the upper half of the body (Figure 4.19); this was illustrated in a comparative study of the human and giraffe vascular basement membrane by Williamson, Vogler and Kilo (1971). A sleeve of pericytes surrounds the endothelial tube.

In any condition, or at any site, where increased transport of metabolites from the bloodstream to the tissue and vice versa is a feature, there is some adaptation of the microcirculation. Such sites are usually relatively hypoxic and the blood flow relatively static.

The minor state of 'prevasculitis' of normal skin

Any interpretation of vessel injury must take into account the normal appearance of that vessel, bearing in mind that several variations in 'normal' morphology exist, and that there are a number of sites which cannot be considered representative because the vessels they contain are exposed to repeated micro-injuries. This applies particularly to sites of blood stasis such as the lower leg, the anterior mucosa of the nasal septum and turbinates or the habitually cold skin of perniosis; it also applies to scarred tissues and virtually any vessels that have been injured in the past.

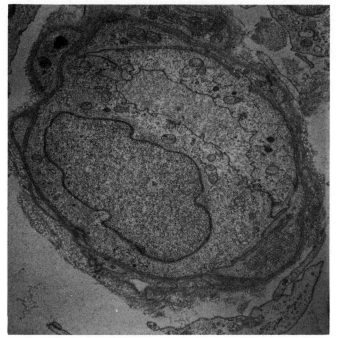

Figure 4.18. Dermal capillary with characteristic tight junctions and absence of fenestrations.

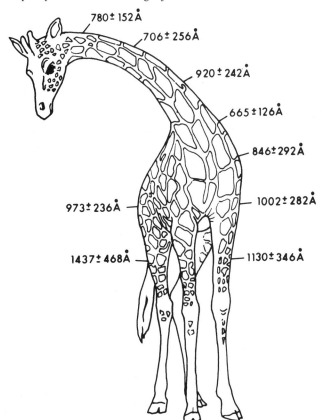

780 ± 152 Å

706 ± 256 Å

920 ± 242 Å

665 ± 126 Å

846 ± 292 Å

973 ± 236 Å

1002 ± 282 Å

1437 ± 468 Å

1130 ± 346 Å

Figure 4.19. Capillary basement membrane thickness in a study of giraffe and man by Williamson et al (1971).

In later chapters, such vessels will be described in various contexts, such as 'prepared', 'pathergic', 'locus minores resistentiae', altered reactivity, altered constitution, skin 'memory', and the vasculature of 'delay'. As bacteria or immune complexes are preferentially lodged in areas of stasis and of increased permeability, it is not surprising that the problem of vasculitis tended to be concerned with gaps between endothelial cells and fenestrations in or increased porosity of the endothelial cell itself. Some of these features are a direct consequence of injury, but probably the vessels also harbour a change prior to overt vasculitis which makes them a preferred site for subsequent pathology. Studies of the preferential localisation of particulate matter in certain sites in the nose tend to confirm this (see Chapter 9).

Much more needs to be known about those factors in skin which alter endothelium so that it develops fenestrae or endothelial gaps. Interesting examples of the results of these features are Campbell de Morgan spots, perniosis and pustular psoriasis. These factors are discussed in more detail in another monograph (Ryan, 1973) but the effects of epidermal metabolism or injury, of cooling and of sex hormones are important aspects covered elsewhere in this monograph.

References

Kruger, H. & Weise, H. J. (1959) Uber klinische und histologische Beziehungen bestimmter Formen der Parapsoriasis guttata zur allergischen Vaskulitis (Ruiter). *Dermatologische Wochenschrift,* **140,** 813.
Lever, W. F. (1968) In *Histopathology of the Skin,* 4th edition. Philadelphia: J. B. Lippincott.
Pinkus, H. & Mehregan, A. H. (1969) Dermal vasculitides. In *A Guide to Dermatohistopathology.* New York: Meredith Corporation.
Ritzenfeld, P. (1963) Uber das Verhaltnis der Parapsoriasis guttata zur Vasculitis allergica. *Dermatologische Wochenschrift,* **147,** 8.
Ryan, T. J. (1972) The pathogenesis of vasculitis. *Eighth Symposium of Advanced Medicine* (Ed.) Neale, G. p. 319. London: Pitman Medical.
Ryan, T. J. (1973) In *Physiology and Pathophysiology* (Ed.) Jarratt, A. Volume 2. London, New York: Academic Press.
Ryan, T. J. (1974) In *Physiology and Pathophysiology of the Skin* (Ed.) Jarratt, A. Volume 3. London, New York: Academic Press.
Williamson, J. R., Vogler, N. J. & Kilo, C. (1971) Regional variations in the width of the basement membrane of muscle capillaries in man and giraffe. *American Journal of Pathology,* **63,** 359.

The basic features of vasculitis

In interpreting the histopathology of vasculitis one should remember that injury to the vessel wall brings about a complex of effects illustrated in Figure 4.20.
1. Coagulation, fibrinolysis, kinins and the complement system are activated and may be exhausted.
2. Endothelial cells alter their contour, swell and are often fragmented, and by separating they are exfoliated (Table 4.1). Usually they migrate and proliferate in response to injury.
3. Platelets and leucocytes stick to the vessel wall, infiltrate it and migrate through it, particularly between endothelial cells, but some phagocytosis by endothelium also occurs. Within 12 hours many of the neutrophils disintegrate.
4. The contractile elements in the vessel wall become more or less activated.
5. Adjacent tissues react to interference with their blood supply and, in responding, effect a further stimulus or injury to the vessels.
6. Local stasis occurs and blood is diverted through alternative channels, many of which are capillaries that rapidly enlarge to become significant pathways.

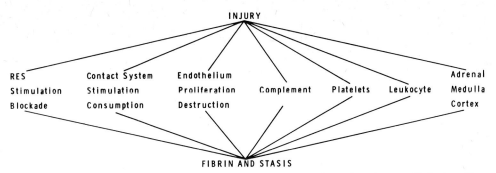

Figure 4.20. Changes in microvascular system in response to injury which ultimately cause fibrin deposition and stasis.

Leucocytoclastic vasculitis

The basic pathological changes in allergic vasculitis are deposition of fibrinoid within and around the walls of the small cutaneous vessels and a perivascular infiltrate composed predominantly of neutrophils whose nuclei fragment into nuclear dust (Figure 4.21).

At the ultrastructural level swelling of the endothelial cells of the superficial dermal venules is in part due to increased pinocytotic activity, swelling of the rough endoplasmic reticulum, increased numbers of ribosomal granules and folding up of the nucleus. The contractility of the venular endothelium leads to separation of the cells and opening of the inter-endothelial spaces (Figure 4.22). Many polymorphonuclear leucocytes are found both in the lumen of these vessels and in the extravascular spaces and they exhibit fragmentation of their nuclei and rupture of their plasma membranes with release of their lysosomal granules into the surrounding matrix (Figure 4.23). Similar findings were described by Ruiter and Molenaar (1970), who also noted deposits of an amorphous material infiltrating the vessels and coating almost everything; this was believed to be fibrin-like. Perrot et al (1971) reported similar findings. The granular floccular precipitate of fibrin similar to that described by McKay et al (1967) in eclampsia probably represents partially polymerised fibrin. However, although fibrin and fibrin degradation products are a common feature of the more infarctive and necrotising forms of vasculitis, they are not an invariable accompaniment of leucocytoclasis and they rarely feature in the most urticarial forms of vasculitis. The fibrin deposits illustrated in Figures 10.2 and 10.3 were seen in so-called necrotising angiitis.

Endothelial contraction seems to have a definite topography for, while it can be induced in the venules of certain tissues, e.g. muscle, skin, peritoneum and bronchial vessels, it cannot be induced in others, such as the brain, testis or pulmonary vessels (Gabbiani, Badonnel and Majno, 1970; Gabbiani et al, 1972); capillaries, on the other hand, do not react anywhere (Majno et al, 1961). Attempts to explain this may be helped by Becker's immunofluorescence studies (Becker and Murphy, 1969; Becker, 1972) which showed that venular endothelium contains more smooth muscle actomyosin than is found in capillaries in the liver and kidney. Majno et al (1972) assume that the contractile system of the endothelial cells corresponds to the microfilaments which have so often been described (Majno, Shea and Leventhal, 1969). In the author's experience this has also been the case in vasculitis (Figure 4.24) and it is conceivable that the capillaries of the skin are more vunerable in this respect. Recently, Hammersen (personal communication, 1975) has attributed vascular leakage to the ultrastructural necrotic changes in the interdigitating processes of opposed endothelial plasma membranes.

Table 4.1. Cell responses to injury.

Changes in leucocytes	Platelet aggregation and changes in endothelial cells
Stage 1. The formation of blebs, granules and minor changes in the size of the nucleus and cytoplasm.	Stage 1. Oedema of the endothelial cells with the cytoplasm staining less intensely.
Stage 2. Mitochondria decrease in number and increase in size.	Stage 2. Bleb formation of the endothelial cytoplasm greater than twice the normal thickness of neighbouring endothelial cells. This was often associated with loss of contact of the anchoring regions of the cell to the underlying basement membrane.
Stage 3. At a central point in a rather narrow range the cell bursts releasing part of its contents, resulting in diminution in the size of the cell though a protein framework remains within the cytoplasm and the nucleus remains intact. Although rupture of the cell occurs the nuclear substance is substantially intact within its membrane and the cytoplasmic organelles are still grouped in a perinuclear fashion.	Stage 3. Stripping of the endothelial cells from the basement membrane results in the cells lying free within the lumina of the vessels. In these most severely damaged vessels endothelial cells are usually in contact with aggregated platelets which still possess their granules.
Stage 4. The terminal phase in which a few irregularly stained nuclei are embedded in precipitated protein.	Stage 4. Peripheral margination of chromatin in endothelial nuclei is noted at a late stage together with other features indicative of a pyknotic type of necrosis.

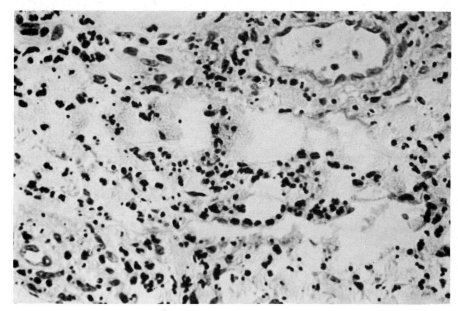

Figure 4.21. Leucocytoclastic angiitis. There are numerous neutrophils and many are disintegrated.

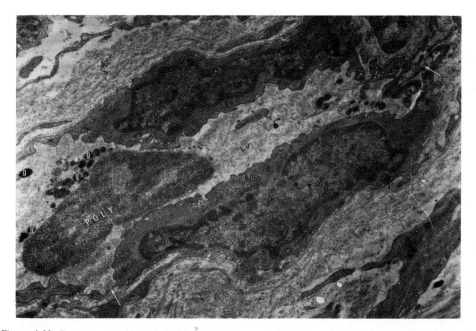

Figure 4.22. Dermal venule from an early case of leucocytoclastic vasculitis showing separation of inter-endothelial junctions (white arrows). Granules (g) of polymorphonuclear leucocyte (POLY) seen free in the lumen (Lu). En = endothelium. $\times$ 11 500.

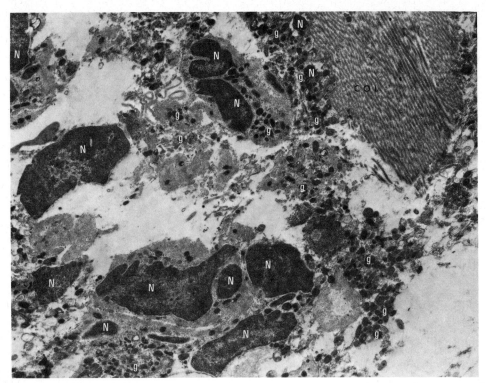

Figure 4.23. Electron-micrograph of polymorphs showing fragmentation of their nuclei (N) and rupture of their lysosomal granules (g) floating in connective tissue matrix outside a dermal venule from same case of vasculitis in Figures 4.21 and 4.22. COL = collagen. × 9900.

The term leucocytoclasis is popular and neatly describes one of the most common phases of vessel injury. It may perhaps be most characteristic of the Arthus reaction, in which lysis of leucocytes by complement is an important mediator. Nevertheless, complement should not be regarded as a purely immunological factor, for it plays a significant part in nonspecific injury (Ratnoff and Lepow, 1963; Willoughby, Coote and Turk, 1969; Spector and Willoughby, 1972). Intracapillary leucocytoclasis in an early lesion of vasculitis (Figure 4.23) of the skin suggests that severe injury to the neutrophil occurs within seconds of its arrival via the bloodstream.

The relationship between vascular permeability, accumulation of neutrophils, blood flow and haemoconcentration has been the subject of extensive investigation by Steele and Wilhelm (1966, 1967, 1970) and was reviewed by Wilhelm (1971). Leucocytoclastic angiitis is equivalent to a mixture of 'the delayed-onset prolonged-duration response' and 'the early-onset strong-intensity moderate-duration response' that they found so often in their experiments on guinea-pigs, rabbits and rats. The first of these responses was induced with short-wave ultraviolet radiation, and by applying xylene, chloroform or benzene to the surface of the skin, or after injecting various salts into the skin. It was also evoked by tuberculin, bacterial toxins and dinitrochlorobenzene (DNCB). They showed that intravenously injected carbon collected within the capillary and venular walls after entry through large inter-endothelial gaps; the venules affected were the small and medium-sized ones throughout the dermis and subcutaneous tissue. The second response was induced by strong heating, immune complexes, surgical incision, crush injury and chemical injury. Venules, capillaries and arterioles were all involved, and

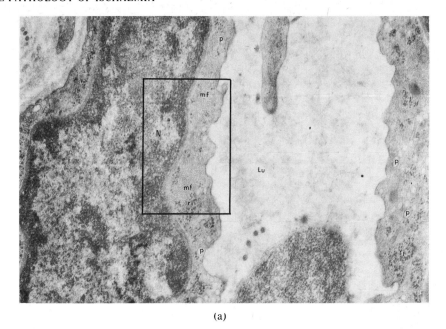

(a)

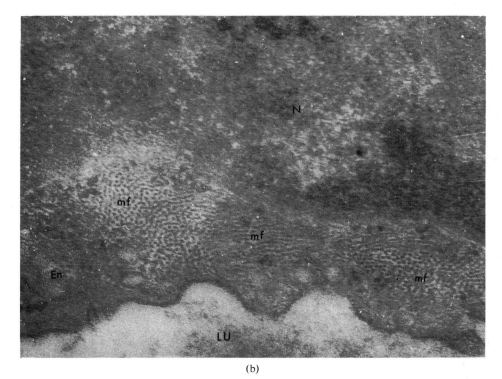

(b)

Figure 4.24. (a) Showing venular endothelium from same case of vasculitis as in Figures 4.21 and 4.23, exhibiting obvious micropinocytosis (p), rich ribosomal aggregates (ri) and contractile protein microfilaments (mf). Lu = lumen; N = nucleus of endothelial cell. × 30 000.
(b) High power of rectangular section indicated by frame in Figure 4.25a. Lu = lumen of venule; En = endothelium; N = nucleus.

electron microscopy revealed damage to endothelium and pericytes with fragmentation and even sloughing of endothelial cells. Occlusion with fibrin, platelets and carbon was common. In this type of response circulation is maintained through deeper vessels and also, to a significant extent, through alternative channels and arteriovenous anastomoses.

Surface application of acids and alkalis of different strengths has been used to show that the response to injury depends on its intensity. Steele and Wilhelm (1970), for instance, recorded that the stronger a superficial injury, the greater was the accumulation of neutrophils, even in the case of deep dermal vessels. The escape of neutrophils reached a peak at two to three hours after injury and the majority were degenerate by 12 to 24 hours.

Leucocytoclasis is characteristic of vasculitis but represents a relatively early phase. In the spectrum ranging from urticaria to ischaemia illustrated on page 28, it must be regarded as central, although it certainly is a feature of some forms of urticaria, particularly the prolonged painful lesions (see Chapter 6). It is sometimes followed by necrosis but is not a consequence of acute infarction. This is understandable because once blood flow has ceased, neutrophils no longer reach the area and, as those already there tend to disintegrate after a few hours, the presence of many neutrophils in a section implies that blood flow is maintained or has only just ceased. It follows, therefore, that neutrophils are not a feature of tissues whose blood supply has been obstructed for many hours by disseminated coagulation. On the other hand, mononuclear cells tend to proliferate locally and extravascularly in such circumstances and many granulomas maintain their own cellularity without necessarily recruiting via the bloodstream.

Fibrin also is important in the histogenesis of vasculitis. Boyd (1970), emphasising that neutrophils must have a framework on which to crawl out of vessels, stated: "It is fibrin which provides the interfacing pathways that bridge across the fluid in distended spaces on which the leucocytes can move". It is also the fabric in which reparative connective tissue is laid down (Astrup, 1968).

The timing of cell arrival in infiltrates has been studied recently and it appears that monocytes and neutrophils begin to emigrate from blood vessels into the wound simultaneously (Simpson and Ross, 1972). The predominance of the neutrophil early on after injury has been ascribed to its relatively greater rate of movement as measured in vitro (Snyderman, Gewurz and Mergenhagen, 1968; Snyderman and Mergenhagen, 1972). In this context, it is relevant that contractile protein has been extracted from neutrophils (Senda et al, 1969) and that cytochalasin B affects their chemotactic movements (Becker et al, 1972).

References

Astrup, T. (1968) Blood coagulation and fibrinolysis in tissue culture and tissue repair. *Biochemical Pharmacology*, **241**, 257.
Becker, C. G. (1972) Demonstration of actomyosin in mesangial cells of the renal glomerulus. *American Journal of Pathology*, **66**, 97.
Becker, C. G. & Murphy, G. E. (1968) Demonstration of actomyosin in cells of heart valve endothelium, intima, the arteriosclerotic plaque and endocardial and myocardial Aschoff bodies. *American Journal of Pathology*, **52**, 22a.
Becker, C. G. & Murphy, G. E. (1969) Demonstration of contractile protein in endothelium and cells of the heart valves, endocardium, intima, arteriosclerotic plaques and Aschoff bodies of rheumatic heart disease. *American Journal of Pathology*, **55**, 1.
Becker, E. L., Davis, A. T., Estensen, R. D. & Quie, P. G. (1972) Cytochalasin B. IV. Inhibition and stimulation of chemotaxis of rabbit and human polymorphonuclear leucocytes. *Journal of Immunology*, **108**, 396.
Boyd, W. (1970) *Textbook of Pathology*, 8th Edition. London: Henry Kimpton.
Gabbiani, G., Badonnel, M. C. & Majno, G. (1970) Intra-arterial injections of histamine, serotonin or bradykinin; a topographic study of vascular leakage. *Proceedings of the Society for Experimental Biology and Medicine*, **135**, 447.

Gabbiani, G., Badonnel, M. C., Gervasoni, C., Portmann, B. & Majno, G. (1972) Carbon deposition in bronchial and pulmonary vessels in response to vasoactive compounds. *Proceedings of the Society for Experimental Biology and Medicine,* **140,** 958.

Majno, G., Palade, G. E. & Schoefl, G. I. (1961) Studies on inflammation. II. The site of action of histamine and serotonin along the vascular tree: A topographic study. *Journal of Biophysical and Biochemical Cytology,* **11,** 607.

Majno, G., Shea, S. M. & Leventhal, M. (1969) Endothelial contraction induced by histamine-type mediators: an electron microscopic study. *Journal of Cell Biology,* **42,** 647.

Majno, G., Ryan, G. B., Gabbiani, G., Hirschel, B. J., Irle, C. & Joris, I. (1972) Contractile events in inflammation and repair. In *Inflammation, Mechanisms and Control* (Ed.) Lepow, I. H. & Ward, P. A. New York, London: Academic Press.

McKay, D. G., Goldenberg, V., Kaunitz, H. & Csavossy, I. (1967) Experimental eclampsia. An electron microscope study and review. *Archives of Pathology,* **84,** 557.

Perrot, H., Leung, T. K., Schmitt, D. & Thivolet, J. (1971) Étude ultrastructurale des lésions vasculaires dermiques du trisyndrôme de Gougerot vasculite leucocytoclasique. *Archiv für Dermatologische Forschrift,* **241,** 44.

Ratnoff, O. D. & Lepow, I. H. (1963) Complement as a mediator of inflammation. *Journal of Experimental Medicine,* **118,** 681.

Ruiter, M. & Molenaar, J. (1970) Ultrastructural changes in arteriolitis. *British Journal of Dermatology,* **83,** 14.

Senda, N., Shibata, N., Tatsumi, N., Kondo, K. & Hamada, K. (1969) A contractile protein from leucocytes. Its extraction and some of its properties. *Biochimica et Biophysica Acta,* **181,** 191.

Simpson, D. M. & Ross, R. (1972) The neutrophilic leucocyte in wound repair: a study with antineutrophilic serum. *Journal of Clinical Investigation,* **51,** 2009.

Snyderman, R. & Mergenhagen, S. E. (1972) Characterization of polymorphonuclear leukocyte chemotactic activity in serums activated by various inflammatory agents. In *Proceedings of the Canadian Immunology Society Fifth International Symposium on the Biological Activities of Complement, Guelph, 1970.* Basel: S. Karger.

Snyderman, R., Gerwurz, H. & Mergenhagen, S. E. (1968) Interactions of the complement system with endotoxic lipopolysaccharide. Generation of a factor chemotactic for polymorphonuclear leukocytes. *Journal of Experimental Medicine,* **128,** 259.

Spector, W. G. & Willoughby, D. A. (1972) Evaluation of the role of individual mediators in inflammation. In *Methods in Microcirculation Studies* (Ed.) Ryan, T. J., Jolles, B. & Holli, G. p. 4. London: H. K. Lewis.

Steele, R. H. & Wilhelm, D. L. (1966) The inflammatory reaction in chemical injury. Increased vascular permeability and erythema induced by various chemicals. *British Journal of Experimental Pathology,* **47,** 612.

Steele, R. H. & Wilhelm, D. L. (1967) The inflammatory reaction in chemical injury. Vascular permeability changes and necrosis induced by intracutaneous injection of various chemicals. *British Journal of Experimental Pathology,* **48,** 592.

Steele, R. H. & Wilhelm, D. L. (1970) Leucocytosis and other histological changes induced by superficial injury. *British Journal of Experimental Pathology,* **51,** 265.

Wilhelm, D. L. (1971) Increased vascular permeability in acute permeability. *Revue Canadienne de Biologie,* **30,** 153.

Willoughby, D. A., Coote, E. & Turk, J. L. (1969) Complement in acute inflammation. *Journal of Pathology,* **97,** 295.

The role of the eosinophil

This mysterious cell features prominently in some types of vasculitis. Parish (1970) summarised the functions ascribed to it as follows:

1. Eosinophils are attracted by histamine into the tissues where they inactivate excess histamine, serotonin and bradykinin (Archer, 1963).
2. Eosinophils are attracted by antigen—antibody complexes which they ingest and destroy (Litt, 1964).
3. Eosinophils have the same function as neutrophils and other phagocytic cells and may have no specific function of their own (Archer and Hirsch, 1963).

4. Eosinophils participate in antibody synthesis, ingesting antigen and modifying it before it is taken up by those mononuclear cells that eventually transform into plasma cells (Speirs, 1958a, b).

Parish's own experiments suggested that eosinophils turn up in situations that also attract mast cells but that histamine and immune complexes are no more attractive to eosinophils than they are to neutrophils. In reporting that eosinophils are mobilised during disseminated intravascular coagulation, myocardial infarction and strokes, Riddle and Barnhart (1969) also stressed the relevant point that these cells are attracted by fibrin degradation products and that they have a special feature in being well endowed with materials which enhance fibrinolysis (Honsinger, Silverstein and Van Arsdel, 1972). It is unlikely that a cell would show such a feature unless it were to have some affinity for fibrin. In the authors' view, any explanation of the behaviour of the eosinophil must take into account not only the heavy infiltrate of these cells in injured human neonatal skin (Harris and Schick, 1956; Bret, Duperrat and Dubois, 1961) but also the prominence of eosinophils in conditions such as angiolymphoid hyperplasia.

There is a group of disorders in which a local eosinophilia accompanies changes in the vessels of the skin, and it includes this subcutaneous angiolymphoid hyperplasia with eosinophilia (Wells and Whimster, 1969) as well as pseudopyogenic granuloma (Wilson Jones and Bleehen, 1969). However, other workers, describing similar cases, have considered the two conditions to be a single entity (Mehregan and Shapiro, 1971; Reed and Terazakis, 1972) and thought them to be similar to the eosinophilic lymphofolliculosis of the skin described in the Japanese literature (Kawada, Takashashi and Anzai, 1966; Ofuji et al, 1970).

When the site of a previous delayed hypersensitivity skin reaction is *injected* with the relevant allergen — the re-test situation — the resulting infiltrate is characteristically composed of eosinophils (Arnason and Waksman, 1963) and when DNCB is the relevant allergen and is applied *topically* to such a site, it produces at one hour, a mononuclear infiltrate which, at two hours, infiltrates the epidermis (Dolby, Williamson and Adams, 1969). In the delayed hypersensitivity reaction itself, however, mononuclear cells appear at five hours and infiltrate the epidermis at five hours. The re-test situation, therefore, produces an accelerated response. Vasodilatation and oedema were obvious at two hours in the re-test site, and although eosinophils were significantly increased in number, this occurred only at a later stage, from one to 24 hours onwards, implying that eosinophilia is not part of the initial response (Rebuck, Sweet and Barth, 1967).

Eosinophils have also been seen to line the endothelium of graft capillaries in lung transplants (Warren and de Bono, 1969).

Pastinsky and Kovacs (1965) made the interesting observation that blood within the vessels of haemangiomata shows an eosinophilia. In a study of 23 patients they found a decreased platelet count and an eosinophilia (40 per cent in the peripheral blood); they believed that the changes were due to intravascular coagulation and were important for the protection of newly formed vessels. They discussed similar findings in granulation tissue.

It is of interest that, whereas there is no eosinophilia in hereditary angio-oedema (Sheffer et al, 1971), a disorder which is well controlled by inhibitors of fibrinolysis and in which fibrin deposition and inflammatory cells are absent, there is an eosinophilia in anaphylaxis, in which consumption of coagulation factors has been demonstrated. Prostaglandins E_1 and F_{1a} do not incite an eosinophil response (Sondergaard and Wolf Jurgenson, 1972).

Of further interest is the role of iodides, for eosinophilia occurs not only in iododerma (Jacobs et al, 1964; Nelson, 1972) (Figure 4.25) but also in the iodide patch test in dermatitis herpetiformis; in both these reactions fibrin is plentiful.

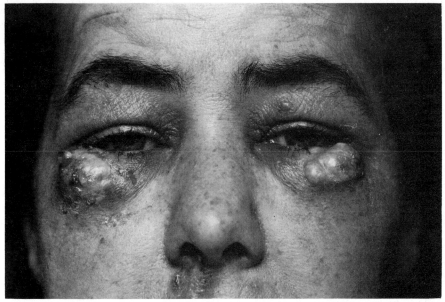

Figure 4.25. Clinical appearance of iododerma in which eosinophilia was a feature.

The presence of mast cells

It is notable that mast cells are prominent in all these conditions and that blood flow is vigorously maintained. Moreover, no matter how proliferative or inflammatory the lesion may be, thrombosis and ischaemic necrosis are unusual and it is the tissues with a heavy infiltrate of mast cells and eosinophils which do not necrose (Figure 4.26).

Despite an adequate protective code of mast cells in the anterior nasal septum, its low Po_2 (see Chapter 9) often renders it prone to ulceration and perforation from micro-vascular injury.

Mast cell infiltration is a late development in vasculitis and is a feature particularly of chronic pathology (Kulaga, Talovskaya and Supowitsky, 1971). These authors empha-sised the close relationship of the mast cells to endothelium which they may even penetrate to reach the lumen; in the process endothelial cells phagocytose the mast cell granules.

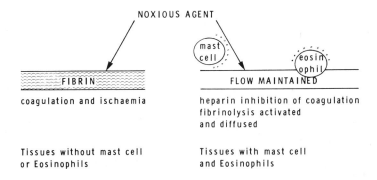

Figure 4.26. A suggested role of the mast cell and eosinophil in vasculitis.

Dolowitz and Dougherty (1965) have argued that as heparin binds histamine it is in many senses protective in inflammatory states. It is significant, too, that mast cells are a feature not only of pigmented purpuric eruptions, in which infarction is rare, but also of non-infarctive forms of livedo reticularis. They accumulate also in venous stasis (Témine, 1956). They are particularly well-marked in non-ulcerative lesions such as elephantiasis nostras, in tissues after ligation of their venous drainage (Asboe-Hansen, 1964), and in certain areas such as the septum of the nose (Figure 4.27) and perniotic skin.

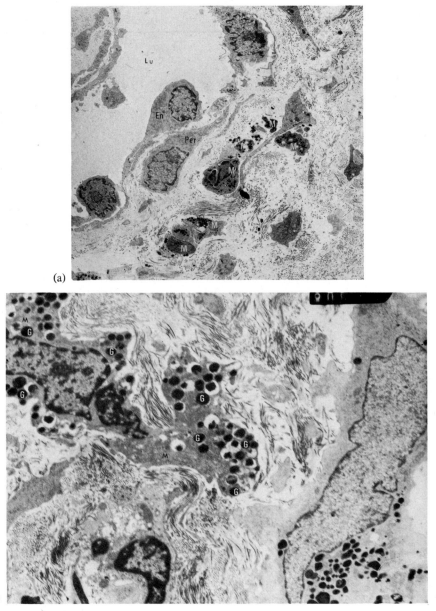

(a)

(b)

Figure 4.27. Perivascular mast cells are numerous in the nasal mucosa at sites of maximum vulnerability. G = granules; M = mast cell; En = endothelium; Per = pericyte. (a) × 3900. (b) × 9300.

'Sleeving' by cellular infiltrate

'Sleeving' of vessels by a cellular infiltrate is a common feature in pathology. White cells leave the bloodstream by first sticking to the vessel wall and then migrating through any gaps that they can find. Although they can migrate upstream, most will be carried downstream; consequently an inflammatory exudate will form mainly at or distal to the site of injury. The mediators of inflammation are commonly produced extracellularly and extravascularly. But when there is damage to tissue such as epidermis or fat supplied by the vessel, it will release such agents, and these will, to some extent, diffuse through the tissues unevenly; but some will be carried along the venules to produce their effects downstream. Thus it is common for epidermal injury to be associated with a perivascular infiltrate extending along the venules to the level of the lower dermis. The interpretation of such an appearance must of course take into account the effects of damage to the tissues supplied. Therefore, much of the infiltrate that one observes in vasculitis is secondary to ischaemic injury, especially to fat cells and smooth muscle cells which are the most vulnerable. However, there is a far greater degree of cellular response to injury when the skin is hypertrophic, and therefore more metabolically demanding, than when it is atrophic. Some of the sparsest and most feeble inflammatory responses are, in fact, observed in very atrophic skin.

Venules are more permeable to particulate matter than other vessels; they are sites of stasis, and the preferred location for neovascularisation. In these and many other ways they differ from the arterial tree. Because of these features and because they lie downstream from the area where injury is most severe, they are responsible for the anatomical pattern of the response to injury. Waksman (1960 a,b) has emphasised this point in several studies of injury to the tissues. He was interested at first in the localisation of demyelinisation in neurological diseases, which he observed was mainly perivenular. Later, in a study of autoradiographs and of the skin's reaction to agents such as Old Tuberculin, he was able to show that the vascular reaction pattern was determined by the anatomical distribution of venules. He found that skin well endowed with dermal vessels developed dermal reactions, while that with sparse dermal vessels draining almost directly into deeper fatty layers responded with panniculitis similar to erythema nodosum.

References

Archer, R. K. (1963) *The Eosinophil Leucocytes*. Oxford: Blackwell.

Archer, R. K. & Hirsch, J. G. (1963) Motion picture studies on degranulation of horse eosinophils during phagocytosis. *Journal of Experimental Medicine*, **118**, 287.

Arnason, B. & Waksman, B. H. (1963) The re-test reaction in delayed sensitivity. *Laboratory Investigation*, **12**, 737.

Asboe-Hansen, G. (1964) Connective tissue response to injury. In *Injury, Inflammation and Immunity* (Ed.) Thomas, L., Uhr, J. W. & Grant, L. p. 22. Baltimore: Williams and Wilkins.

Bret, A. J., Duperrat, B. & Dubois, J. P. (1961) Dermite allergique de nouveau-né. Erythema allergican de Mayerhofer. *Archiv für Pediatrica*, **18**, 109.

Dolby, A. E., Williamson, J. J. & Adams, D. (1969) The re-test contact hypersensitivity reaction in guinea pig skin and oral mucosa. *British Journal of Experimental Pathology*, **50**, 343.

Dolowitz, D. A. & Dougherty, T. P. (1965) The use of heparin in the control of allergies. *Annals of Allergy*, **23**, 309.

Duperrat, B. & Bret, A. J. (1961) Erythema neonatorum allergicum. *British Journal of Dermatology*, **73**, 300.

Harris, J. R. & Schick, B. (1956) Erythema neonatorum. *American Journal of Diseases of Children*, **92**, 27.

Honsinger, R. W. Jr, Silverstein, D. & Van Arsdel, P. P. G. (1972) The eosinophil and allergy, why? *Journal of Allergy and Clinical Immunology*, **49**, 142.

Jacobs, H. S., Sidd, J. J., Greenberg, B. H. & Lingley, J. F. (1964) Extreme eosinophilia with iodide hyper-sensitivity. *New England Journal of Medicine*, **271**, 1138.

Kawada, A., Takashashi, H. & Anzai, T. (1966) Eosinophilic lymph folliculosis of the skin (Kimura's disease). *Japanese Journal of Dermatology,* **76,** 61.

Kulaga, V. V., Talovskaya, Z. S. & Supowitsky, V. Y. (1971) On the study of morphology of mast cells in allergic vasculitis of the skin. *Vestnik Dermatologii i Venerologii,* **45,** 26.

Litt, M. (1964) Eosinophils and antigen—antibody reactions. *Annals of the New York Academy of Sciences,* **116,** 964.

Mehregan, A. H. & Shapiro, L. (1971) Angiolymphoid hyperplasia with eosinophilia. *Archives of Dermatology,* **103,** 50.

Nelson, C. T. (1972) Iododerma. *Archives of Dermatology,* **105,** 448.

Ofuji, S., Ogiwo, A., Horio, T., Ohseko, T. & Uehara, M. (1970) Eosinophilic pustular folliculitis. *Acta Dermato-venereologica,* **50,** 195.

Parish, W. E. (1970) Investigations on eosinophilia. The influence of histamine, antigen—antibody complexes containing γ1 or γ2 globulins, foreign bodies (phagocytosis) and disrupted mast cells. *British Journal of Dermatology,* **82,** 42.

Pastinsky, I. & Kovacs, M. (1965) Untersuchungen uber den lokalen Blutstatus der vaskalaren Haut tumoren. *Dermatologische Wochenschrift,* **151,** 514.

Rebuck, J. W., Sweet, L. C. & Barth, C. L. (1967) Increased fibrin deposition in allergic inflammation in relation to eosinophil migration. *Federation Proceedings,* **26,** 745.

Reed, R. J. & Terazakis, N. (1972) Subcutaneous angioblastic lymphoid hyperplasia with eosinophilia (Kimura's disease). *Cancer,* **19,** 489.

Riddle, J. M. & Barnhart, M. I. (1969) Eosinophil mobilization during intravascular coagulation. *Thrombosis et Diathesis Haemorrhagica,* **36,** 99.

Sheffer, A. L., Craig, J. M., Wilms-Kretschmer, K., Austen, K. F. & Rosen, F. S. (1971) Histopathological and ultrastructural observations on tissues from patients with hereditary angioneurotic oedema. *Journal of Allergy,* **41,** 292.

Sondergaard, J. & Wolf Jurgenson, P. (1972) The cellular exudate of human cutaneous inflammation induced by prostaglandins E_1 and F_{1a}. *Acta Dermato-venereologica,* **52,** 361.

Speirs, R. S. (1958a) A theory of antibody formation involving eosinophils and reticuloendothelial cells. *Nature,* **181,** 681.

Speirs, R. S. (1958b) Advances in the knowledge of the eosinophil in relation to antibody formation. *Annals of the New York Academy of Sciences,* **59,** 706.

Témine, M. (1956) *Les Troubles Trophiques des Membres Inférieurs d'Origine Veineuse* (Ed.) Charpy, P. J. p. 263. Paris: Masson et Cie.

Waksman, B. H. (1960a) The pattern of rejection in rat skin homografts and its relation to the vascular network. *Laboratory Investigation,* **12,** 46.

Waksman, B. H. (1960b) The distribution of experimental autoallergic lesions. Its relation to the distribution of small veins. *American Journal of Pathology,* **37,** 673.

Warren, B. A. & de Bono, A. H. B. (1969) The ultrastructure of early rejection phenomena in lung homografts in dogs. *British Journal of Experimental Pathology,* **50,** 593.

Wells, G. C. & Whimster, I. W. (1969) Subcutaneous angiolymphoid hyperplasia with eosinophilia. *British Journal of Dermatology,* **81,** 1.

Wilson Jones, E. & Bleehen, S. S. (1969) Inflammatory angiomatous nodules with abnormal blood vessels occurring about the ears and scalp (pseudo atypical pyogenic granuloma). *British Journal of Dermatology,* **81,** 804.

The epidermis

The participation of the epidermis in vasculitis is variable. Mostly it is affected by ischaemia which, if acute, causes necrosis and, if chronic, causes atrophy. But in some conditions, such as the pigmented purpuric eruptions, one observes elongation and coiling of the capillary vessels with prominent extravasation of red cells, in which case there may be an associated elongation of the rete pegs, often with increased numbers of mast cells.

In all patterns of response in the skin of the legs there tends to be an overall reduction in the number of papillary vessels per surface area. In some patients one observes a simple hypertrophy of the epidermis and elongation of the papillae, but in the more atrophic forms the epidermis is somewhat thinned and there is usually an associated

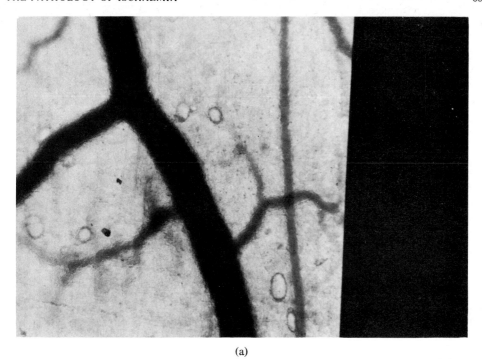

(a)

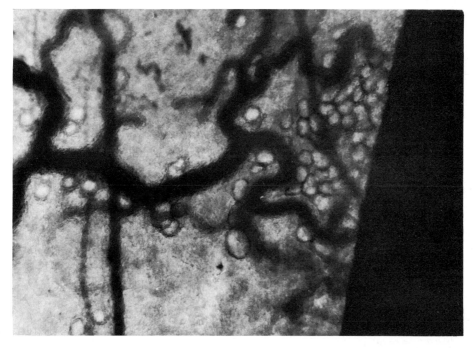

(b)

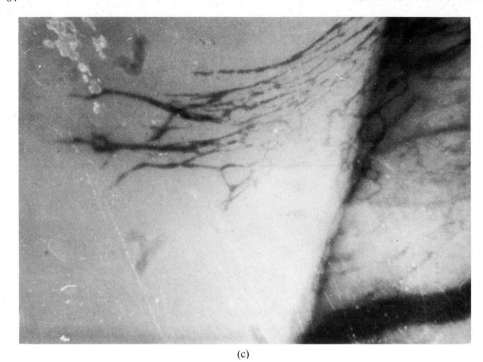

(c)

Figure 4.28. Studies of an epidermal angiogenic factor (Nishioka and Ryan, 1972): (a) hamster cheek pouch normal vasculature showing no tortuosity a few minutes after insertion of epidermal graft embedded in millepore filter paper (Rt). (b) Tortuosity of vessels in response to graft some 24 hours later. (c) New vessel growth over the graft at six days.

atrophy of the upper dermis with poor structural support for the vessels which consequently dilate to produce telangiectases as described by Majocchi (1896). All such areas tend to be warm; they usually have some shunting with associated venous hypertension and these probably account for the hypertrophy of the walls of deeper vessels. In the lichenoid forms of pigmented purpuric eruptions a greater degree of liquefaction degeneration of the epidermis is associated inevitably with a heavy perivascular infiltrate in the dermis.

The epidermis can be shown to possess angiogenic factors (Figure 4.28) some of which appear to act by encouraging fibrin deposition and therefore a scaffold for vessel growth (Nishioka and Ryan, 1972; Wolf and Harrison, 1973). The role of epidermal inhibitors of fibrinolysis (Nishioka and Ryan, 1971) could also be important.

References

Majocchi, D. (1896) Sopra una telangiectode non ancora descritta "purpura annularis". *Giornale Italia Medica di Venezia,* **31,** 263-264.
Nishioka, K. & Ryan, T. J. (1971) Inhibitors and proactivators of fibrinolysis in human epidermis. *British Journal of Dermatology,* **85,** 561.
Nishioka, K. & Ryan, T. J. (1972) The influence of the epidermis and other tissues on blood vessel growth in the hamster cheek pouch. *Journal of Investigative Dermatology,* **58,** 33.
Wolf, J. & Harrison, R. G. (1973) Demonstration and characterization of an epidermal angiogenic factor. *Journal of Investigative Dermatology,* **61,** 130.

Deep dermal and subcutaneous vasculitis

Injury to the vessels of the deep dermis and subcutaneous tissues is associated with endothelial and vessel wall changes which differ very little from those seen in the upper dermis (see above). However, it is in these tissues that the larger veins and arteries lie and fat necrosis as a complication occurs.

One of the commonest forms of vasculitis at this level is erythema nodosum. Montgomery (1967) doubted whether this is a specific entity, but most observers agree that it is an inflammatory process affecting the deep dermis and subcutaneous tissues and that it stops short of necrosis. It is a reasonable assumption, therefore, that the blood flow is never completely interrupted, in which case it is hardly surprising that thrombosis is not a feature of erythema nodosum, and that, as Vesey and Wilkinson (1959) pointed out, bruising is a common characteristic. The present author has noted on several occasions that erythema nodosum is one form of vasculitis in which local fibrinolysis is sometimes unimpaired. The tissues in this disorder are initially infiltrated by neutrophils and there may be considerable proliferation of the endothelium, particularly intraluminally. Sometimes there is little inflammation in the surrounding tissues, possibly because neutrophils have relatively less fibrin scaffolding to climb on.

Vasculitis in the deep dermis and subcutaneous tissue shows a greater degree of fibrin deposition, is liable to last much longer and tends to be associated with still greater capillary proliferation and with some degree of granuloma formation. This is true not only of the sub-acute nodular migratory panniculitis of Vilanova and Aguade (1959) but also of Behçet's disease, nodular vasculitis and thrombophlebitis migrans. One suspects that, in these conditions, impairment of blood flow, ischaemia and — as has been mentioned above — resulting damage to fat may all be greater. Fat is, in fact, particularly susceptible to ischaemia and may well be damaged by chronic stasis.

References

Montgomery, H. (1967) *Dermatopathology,* Volume II, p. 677. New York: Hoebner Medical Division, Harper and Row.
Vesey, C. M. R. & Wilkinson, D. S. (1959) Erythema nodosum, a study of seventy cases. *British Journal of Dermatology,* **71,** 139.
Vilanova, X. & Aguade, J. P. (1959) Subacute nodular migratory panniculitis. *British Journal of Dermatology,* **71,** 45.

Factors contributing to granulomata

Antigen—antibody complexes produce a severe local inflammatory response, as was shown by Opie (1924) and Cochrane and Weigle (1958). The latter observed an acute polymorphonuclear leucocytic response in the skin of rabbits following injection of both bovine serum albumin (BSA) and anti-BSA rabbit serum; the reaction was transient and cleared in two to three days.

The matter was studied further by Spector and Heesom (1969) to see under what circumstances a more persistent granuloma could be produced. They found that immune complexes prepared with BSA and anti-BSA serum in the region of antigen—antibody equivalence caused granulomata after being injected into rat skin; rat or rabbit antibodies were equally effective. By contrast, complexes prepared at moderate antigen excess had little activity in spite of inducing severe acute inflammatory reactions. But by labelling either the antigen or the antibody with ^{125}I it was shown that granuloma formation was associated with persistence within macrophages of both constituents of the immune complex. It was also found that granulomata occurred in association with the local persistence of antigen when rats were actively sensitised with antigen in complete Freund's adjuvant.

The conclusion was that deposition of immune complexes may cause granulomatous disease provided an excess of antibody is available to render the complex indigestible. Support for this interpretation was already available, as Sorkin and Boyden (1959) had found that an excess of antibody delayed the intracellular degradation of antigen and Cohn (1963) had demonstrated that it also delayed the breakdown of phagocytosed bacteria.

Ischaemia and granuloma formation

Another mechanism suspected of contributing to granuloma formation is ischaemia. Tissues adjacent to vasculitis with impaired blood flow may be rendered ischaemic and in this way large extravascular necrobiotic granulomata may be formed in the vicinity of large vessels. Such granulomata may or may not be centred on capillaries and venules in the adventitiae; if they are, these vessels maintain a supply of white cells for a while before they themselves necrose.

Wegener's granulomatosis is an example of a granuloma that frequently is extra-vascular and which usually occurs adjacent to the severest necrotising vasculitis. The earliest lesion is leucocytoclastic, and it is significant that eosinophils are rarely a feature. In contradistinction, allergic granulomatosis (Churg and Strauss, 1951) exhibits a heavy infiltrate of eosinophils in its central core where a small necrotic vessel is frequently found (Churg and Strauss, 1951; Zeek, 1952).

Ischaemia is most harmful to fat cells which can survive only a few hours of anoxia (Willms-Kretschmer and Majno, 1969), but the histopathology it produces depends on whether or not the tissues have previously experienced ischaemia. In the experiments described in Chapter 5, tissues that had suffered ischaemia in the past were more vascular but, perhaps because of more cells with hypermetabolism, they were nevertheless more vulnerable. There is an interesting parallel here with the effects of chronic stasis on smooth muscle and fat.

Repetitive ischaemia could explain many of the features both of subcutaneous vasculitis and of necrotising vasculitis when smooth muscle of the media of the vessel is involved, for smooth muscle can survive only limited ischaemia. However, the brunt of subcutaneous vasculitis falls on the capillaries in the periphery of the fat lobule lying within the border of the fibrous septa. These show many features of an ischaemic granuloma with increased vascularity and a somewhat variable infiltrate of white cells.

Foreign body giant cells

Foreign body giant cells accompany vasculitis and Montgomery (1967) has described their presence in the walls of vessels in, for example, thrombo-angiitis obliterans and temporal arteritis, or in association with the chronic panniculitis in perniosis, livedo reticularis, erythema nodosum, sub-acute nodular migratory panniculitis, nodular vasculitis and allergic granulomatosis.

Multinucleate giant cells have long been recognised as a characteristic component of many granulomatous infiltrates, where they are formed most probably by fusion of non-proliferating macrophages. Their lifespan is only a few days (Papadimitrio,

Sforsina and Papaelias, 1973) during which time they are capable of phagocytosis. Most granulomata are now believed to be dynamic collections of dividing cells with some recruitment from the circulation (Mariano and Spector, 1974).

Even experimental granulomata show a direct relationship to vascular injury, and when Ebert, Ahern and Bloch (1948) inoculated mycobacteria into the rabbit's ear chamber, considerable new vessel formation was initiated. Then between the 10th and 24th day leucocytes quite suddenly began to stick to the vessel walls and this was followed by haemoconcentration, stasis and thrombosis. Until this had occurred no avascular tubercles with necrotic centres were formed. After undertaking similar experiments, Florey (1970) suggested that the vascular injury is always secondary to trauma to the adjacent tissue. A further point, made by Boyd (1970), was that when individual macrophages are unable to deal with particles which have to be removed, they fuse to form multinucleate giant cells, and that such behaviour is not due to the indigestibility of the particles but may be due rather to some change in the environment such as anoxia. In fact, one giant cell well known to be a consequence of anoxia is the osteoclast (Payling Wright, 1958).

Granulomata have the effect of partially walling off areas of necrobiosis or necrosis, thereby modifying the gradients of supply and demand to the walled-off area. Indeed, when there is a heavy infiltrate, blood vessels supplying a tissue often cease to provide an effective nutritional supply; when this happens they may atrophy or new compensatory patterns may develop.

References

Boyd, W. (1970) *Textbook of Pathology*, 8th edition. London: Henry Kimpton.
Churg, J. & Strauss, L. (1951) Allergic granulomatosis, allergic angiitis and periarteritis nodosa. *American Journal of Pathology*, **27**, 277.
Cochrane, C. G. & Weigle, W. O. (1958) The cutaneous reaction to soluble antigen—antibody complexes. *Journal of Experimental Medicine*, **108**, 591.
Cohn, Z. A. (1963) The fate of bacteria within phagocytic cells. The modification of intracellular degradation. *Journal of Experimental Medicine*, **117**, 43.
Ebert, R. H., Ahern, J. J. & Bloch, R. G. (1948) Development of tuberculous infection, in vivo observations in rabbit ear chamber. *Proceedings of the Society for Experimental Biology*, **68**, 625.
Florey, L. (1970) *General Pathology*, 4th edition, p. 1203. London: Lloyd-Luke Medical Books.
Mariano, M. & Spector, W. G. (1974) The formation and properties of macrophage polykaryons (inflammatory giant cells). *Journal of Pathology*, **113**, 1.
Montgomery, H. (1967) *Dermatopathology*. Volume II, p. 677. New York: Hoebner Medical Division, Harper and Row.
Opie, E. L. (1924) Pathogenesis of specific inflammatory reaction of immunized animals (Arthus phenomenon); relation of local sensitization to immunity. *Journal of Immunology*, **9**, 259.
Papadimitriou, J. M., Sforsina, D. & Papaelias, L. (1973) Kinetics of multinucleate giant cell formation and their modification by various agents in foreign body reactions. *American Journal of Pathology*, **73**, 349.
Payling Wright, G. (1958) *An Introduction to Pathology*. London: Longman Green.
Sorkin, E. & Boyden, S. V. (1959) Studies on the fate of antigens in vitro. I. The effect of specific antibody on the fate of I[131] trace labelled human serum albumin in vitro in the presence of guinea pig monocytes. *Journal of Immunology*, **82**, 332.
Spector, W. G. & Heesom, N. (1969) The production of granulomata by antigen—antibody complexes. *Journal of Pathology*, **98**, 31.
Willms-Kretschmer, K. & Majno, G. (1969) Ischaemia of the skin. *American Journal of Pathology*, **54**, 3327.
Zeek, P. M. (1952) Periarteritis nodosa. A critical review. *American Journal of Clinical Pathology*, **22**, 777.

Endothelial proliferation

Endothelial proliferation is a common feature of vasculitis. This is inevitable because injury to endothelium must be repaired, and the proliferation occurs mainly to fill gaps and spaces in the vessel wall. Migration of adjacent endothelial cells is a prominent initial phenomenon, and being particularly encouraged by fibrin, it is an automatic accompaniment of disseminated intravascular coagulation; in extent it is sometimes bizarre (Figure 4.29, a and b). This proliferation is a feature of the complete spectrum of vasculitis including perniosis, erythema nodosum, sub-acute nodular migrating panniculitis and endocarditis lenta (Ruiter and Mandema, 1965). Tappeiner and Pfleger (1963) described a systematised angio-endotheliomatosis proliferans, which is similar to that observed in patients with bacterial endocarditis by Gottran and Nikolarski (1958) and later by Ruiter and Mandema (1965). Lever (1967) believed it to be merely a variant of vasculitis. There is always occlusion of small vessels with fibrin and plump hyperchromatic endothelial cells. The latter are almost certainly the effect of shedding of endothelial cells into the bloodstream and their consequent enmeshment and destruction as they are torn apart while flowing between and over strands of fibrin (Stalker, Brown and Hall, 1969).

Three patients were described by Scott, Silvers and Helwig (1975). Some of these patients had bizarre neurological manifestations and a histological picture suggestive of sarcoma. Whether the condition is a true sarcoma is in fact very doubtful.

Endothelial proliferation in the reticuloses is a usual feature and has been blamed on a failure of the mononuclear phagocytic system to remove the debris that stimulates new vessel growth (Ryan, 1973). Ashton (1957) suggested that anaerobic metabolism in areas of profound venous stasis is responsible for the accumulation of vasoformative factors. Ditzel (1975) uses the same explanation to account for the new vessels in diabetes mellitus.

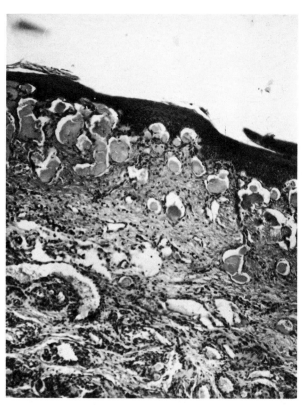

(a)

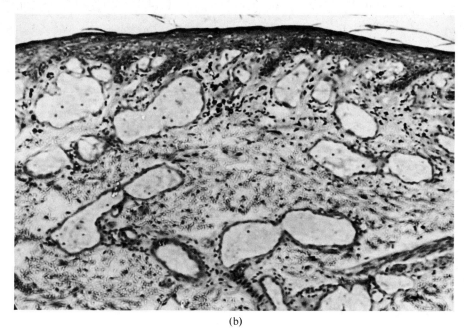

(b)

Figure 4.29. Tortuosity, dilatation and probable angiogenesis of upper dermal vessels in disseminated intra-vascular coagulation in (a) patient described by Brödthagen et al (1968) (See also Figures 9.7 and 9.8). (b) Patient with pancreatic tumour and hepatic failure.

In Cherry's experiments (Chapter 5) new vessel formation with shunts occurred in response to temporary ischaemia. The role of fibrin and impaired fibrinolysis is emphasised both in these studies and elsewhere (Ryan, 1973). New vessel formation and shunts are features of all hypermetabolic and ischaemic tissues such as psoriasis or cancer, and they are also the feature of angiolymphoid hyperplasia wherever it occurs. Dermatological examples are pseudopyogenic granuloma, mycosis fungoides (tumour stage) and Kaposi's sarcoma.

Valdes et al (1975) and Frizzara, Moran and Rappaport (1974) have also drawn attention to the proliferation of endothelium in lymphomas (see also Chapter 6). Lymphocyte-induced angiogenesis has been described in graft versus host reactions (Sidky and Auerbach, 1975). However, all these conditions have a similar degree of nonspecific injury, hypoxia, coagulation and a failure to clear debris and accumulated angiogenic stimuli. In these respects they differ little from the ischaemic skin flaps described in Chapter 5. Accumulation of nonspecific vaso-formative factors is a consequence of stasis or of macrophage paralysis. Often these occur together.

References

Ashton, N. (1957) Retinal vascularization in health and disease. *American Journal of Ophthalmology*, **44**, 7.
Ditzel, J. (1975) The problems of tissue oxygenization in diabetes mellitus. *Acta Medica Scandinavica*, **578**, 69.
Frizzera, G., Moran, E. M. & Rappaport, H. (1974) Proliferation and swelling of endothelial cells in lymphomas. *Lancet*, **i**, 1070.
Gottran, H. A. & Nikolarski, W. (1958) Extrarenal lohlein herdnephritis der haut bei endocarditis. *Archiv für klinische und experimentelle Dermatologie*, **20**, 156.

Lever, W. F. (1967) *Histopathology of the Skin*. Philadelphia: J. B. Lippincott.
Ruiter, M. & Mandema, E. (1965) Hochgradige mit ungewohnlichen haut manifestationen einhergehende gefassendothelwucherung bei subakuter bacterieller endokarditis. *Hautarzt*, **16**, 205.
Ryan, T. J. (1973) *Physiology and Pathophysiology of the Skin* (Ed.) Jarrett, A. London, New York: Academic Press.
Scott, P. W., Silvers, D. N. & Helwig, E. B. (1975) Proliferating angio-endotheliomatosis. *Archives of Pathology*, **99**, 323.
Sidky, Y. A. & Auerbach, R. J. (1975) Lymphocyte induced angiogenesis. *Journal of Experimental Medicine*, **141**, 1084.
Stalker, A. L., Brown, L. J. & Hall, J. (1969) Microcirculatory and histological observations on experimental defibrination. *Bibliotheca Anatomica*, **10**, 366.
Tappeiner, J. & Pfleger, L. (1963) Angioendotheliomatosis proliferans systeminata. *Hautarzt*, **14**, 67.
Valdes, E. F., Herrero, M., De Las, V. & Calb, I. (1975) Skin microvascular lesions in lymphomas. *Lancet*, **i**, 855.

Hyaline and fibrinoid deposition

Chronic, insidious and minimal leakage of cholesterol, triglycerides, phospholipid and fibrinogen explain hyalinisation (Baker and Selikoff, 1952; Adams, 1967). Initially there is minor leakage through gaps in the endothelium, and subsequently subendothelial deposition occurs particularly in arterioles where the higher intravascular pressure may play a part. The vessel is converted into a homogeneous hyaline tube with considerable narrowing of the lumen.

Fibrinoid necrosis is a stage in which leakage is more acute and fibrin, its precursors and split products are deposited. At one time many authors were reluctant to accept fibrinoid as having much to do with fibrin but most would now agree that it has (see discussion in Chapter 10). There is an interesting relationship between ischaemia and fibrinoid: according to Ashton (1972) and his co-workers, prolonged vasoconstriction of arterioles is responsible for ischaemia, and in malignant hypertension one consequence of this is smooth muscle necrosis. The necrosed wall dilates and gaps in the endothelium allow plasma to exude into the wall and to coagulate.

When Rossmann and Vavra (1969) produced acute disturbances of blood pressure and respiration in experimental animals, they observed that, within seconds of apnoea, mesenteric muscular arteries became strongly vasoconstricted. Ischaemic necrosis of the vessel wall could result from such vasoconstriction, although thrombosis, or merely prolonged stasis — such as occurs in shock, local inflammation or capillary sludging — could have the same effect (Figure 13.1). Patterns of reaction such as polyarteritis nodosa are thus ascribable to hypertension, intravascular coagulation or leucocytoclastic angiitis (see Chapter 13).

References

Adams, C. W. M. (1967) *Vascular Histochemistry*. London: Lloyd-Luke (Medical Books). p. 270.
Ashton, N. (1972) The eye in malignant hypertension. *Transactions of the American Academy of Ophthalmology and Otology*, **76**, 17.
Baker, R. D. & Selikoff, E. (1952) The cholesterol of hyaline arteriosclerosis. *American Journal of Pathology*, **28**, 573.
Rossmann, P. & Vavra, I. (1969) Morphology of freeze dried muscular arteries in acute experimental disturbance of blood pressure and respiration. *Angiologica*, **6**, 326.

Arterialisation

Many of the most distinguished authors seem to give the name artery to any inflamed thick-walled vessel, and several textbooks provide illustrations of vasculitis in the upper dermis over a caption of necrotising arteritis or polyarteritis nodosa. But arteries and even arterioles are not part of the upper dermal vasculature, and it is noteworthy in this respect that, in the skin, veins are more like arteries than they are in other tissues (Darier et al, 1936). The veins in the skin of the foot, for example, have twice as much muscle in their walls as those in the forearm (Kugelgen, 1951, 1955). Furthermore, Kulwin and Hines (1950), in studies on the dermatohistopathology of chronic venous insufficiency, made the important observation that blood vessels smaller than those at the junction of the dermis with the subcutis cannot always be identified as arterioles or venules. They described thickening of the media in 84 per cent of the arterioles and fragmentation or reduplication of the internal elastic lamina in 30 per cent. Six out of 30 (20 per cent) venules showed intimal proliferation and 13 out of 30 (43 per cent) had broadening of their media. The most characteristic difference between the venous and arterial vasculature is a direct result of pulsatile flow; this causes elastic tissue to be deposited as a thick lamina just deep to the intima and, of course, occurs only in arteries.

With ageing, as in solar or senile elastosis, altered collagen in the vessel wall stains like elastic tissue (Jackson, Puchtler and Sweat, 1968); this is also a feature of hypertension.

Other changes in the arterioles of the skin in essential hypertension were studied by Farber et al (1947). They found the wall to lumen ratio to be 1:1.57 compared to the control ratio of 1:2.4, and they recorded endothelial proliferation, thickening of the internal elastic lamina, periarteriolar fibrosis and occasional thrombotic occlusion.

Inflamed veins, especially when also thrombosed, are very difficult to distinguish from arteries. Walker et al (1973), for instance, studied 55 long saphenous veins selected from legs that had no evidence of varicosity or thrombosis; these were from patients ranging in age from three to 88 years. Only three veins were 'normal'. The others showed subendothelial fibrosis and a prominent internal elastic lamina.

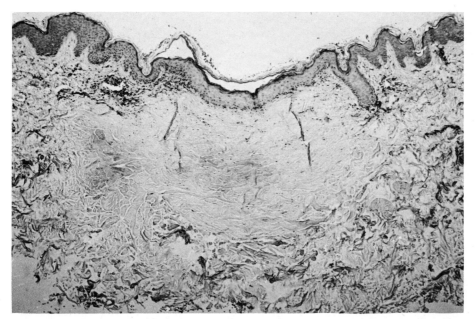

Figure 4.30. Atrophic malignant papulosis. Note relative acellularity and avascularity of the affected area.

Gradual absorption of capillaries and venules is a feature of ageing (Strobel, 1948; Ryan, 1973), is associated with hypertension and is more marked in diseases such as scleroderma or rheumatoid arthritis. It is a particular feature of those patterns of vasculitis of the lower leg presenting with atrophie blanche and described under a variety of names including livedoid vasculitis. A more acute reduction in dermal vasculature producing atrophy and acellularity of the dermis is seen in atrophic malignant papulosis (Figure 4.30).

Atherosclerosis is associated with an increase in 'shunting' in the lower leg as measured by increased oxygenation of venous blood and decreased circulation time (reviewed by Ryan, 1973). A consequence of such shunting is venous hypertension, and whether there is a true diversion from existing vascular channels or whether a virtually complete absorption of the capillary system has left only these alternative channels to carry the arterial blood supply, the end-result is the same. There is a rapid-flowing, sometimes pulsatile, column of blood impinging on arterioles and venules, causing arterialisation of both and making interpretation of the histology all the more difficult. Old skin, shunted skin, and scarred skin are the most difficult to analyse.

References

Darier, J., Civatte, A., Flandin, C. & Tsanck, A. (1936) Anatomie de la peau. In *Nouvelle Pratique Dermatologique* (Ed.) Darier, J., Darier, J. S., Abouraud, R., Gougerot, H., Milian, G., Pautrier, L. M., Ravaut, P., Sezary, A. & Simon, C. Paris: Masson and Cie.

Farber, E. M., Hines, E. A. Jr, Montgomery, H. & Craig, W. M. K. (1947) Arterioles of skin in essential hypertension. *Journal of Investigative Dermatology*, **9**, 285.

Jackson, J. G., Puchtler, H. & Sweat, F. (1968) Investigation of staining, polarization and fluorescence microscopic properties of pseudo-elastic fibres in the renal arterial system. *Journal of the Royal Microscopical Society*, **88**, 473.

Kugelgen, A. V. (1951) Uber den wandbau der groben venen. *Morphologisches Jahrbuch*, **91**, 447.

Kugelgen, A. V. (1955) Uber das verhaltnis ron Ringmuskulatur und snnendruck in menschlichen groben venen. *Zeitschrift für Zellforschung*, **43**, 168.

Kulwin, M. H. & Hines, E. A. (1950) Blood vessels of the skin in chronic venous insufficiency. Clinical and pathological study. *Archives of Dermatology and Syphilology*, **62**, 293.

Ryan, T. J. (1973) In *Physiology and Pathophysiology of the Skin* (Ed.) Jarrett, A. London, New York: Academic Press.

Strobel, H. (1948) Die Gewetsveranderungen der Haut im Verlaufe des Lebens. *Archiv für Dermatologie und Syphilologie*, **186**, 636.

Walker, F., Dhall, D. P., Walker, M. G. & Mavor, G. E. (1973) The normal and arterialised human saphenous vein. 7th European Conference on Microcirculation, Aberdeen 1972. *Bibliotheca Anatomica*, **11**, 495.

5. The Effect of Ischaemia and Reperfusion on Tissue Survival

G. W. CHERRY AND T. J. RYAN

There are few greater disasters for the surgeon than complete necrosis of skin flaps, as for instance in the closure of the wound following a radical mastectomy. Myers and his colleagues in a series of studies on skin flaps concluded that the amount of surviving skin was dependent solely on the inherent blood supply, and that the most common cause of flap necrosis was combined arterial and venous insufficiency, with the arterial component being the more important. Thus they managed to produce necrosis in flaps by venous occlusion but only if every visible vein in the dermal and subdermal plexus also was occluded; even then 60 per cent of the flaps survived.

Tissue survival can be increased by lowering its metabolism either by cooling (Kiehn and Desprez, 1960; Brooks, 1973) or by giving appropriate drugs (Vasko, DeWall and Riley, 1972). Clinically atrophic skin, too, often survives a vascular insult better than normal skin.

It has been known for years that raising a skin flap in two or more stages encourages its survival, partly because the staging causes increased vascularity (Myers and Cherry, 1967, 1968) and partly because the skin is conditioned to ischaemia, the flap surviving when it is relatively starved of blood (McFarlane et al, 1965). However, a switch to a greatly increased anaerobic metabolism may have the opposite effect. Reinisch (1974) believed that sympathetic denervation of arteriovenous shunts, and subsequent denervation hypersensitivity, contribute to this skin flap behaviour, a view determined largely by his finding that ischaemic flaps often are warm and that chromium-labelled red cells are present in high proportions in the ischaemic flaps. Strontium 85-labelled microspheres 15 μm in diameter have been used to confirm that in these flaps the blood flows mostly through large vessels, not small nutrient capillaries.

The experiments described in this chapter reveal a relationship between blood flow, ischaemia, coagulation and new vessel formation and shunts. In vasculitis, whether leucocytoclastic, atrophie blanche or granulomatous, this is important.

The relationship between ischaemia, followed by reperfusion, and subsequent tissue viability has been studied in most organs. One of the clinical objectives of such research is to determine the 'revival time', meaning the length of time between the onset of

93

ischaemia and the occurrence of irreversible tissue damage (Table 5.1). Establishing exactly when vascular obstruction starts is almost impossible in most pathological conditions such as vasculitis, but it can usually be determined in devascularisation caused by trauma or surgery. This is especially true in plastic surgery where skin is

Table 5.1. The effect of temporary ischaemia time on reflow and tissue survival in different organs.

Organ	Animal	Maximum ischaemia time before no reflow	Maximum ischaemia time before maximum tissue death	Author
Brain	Rabbit	15 min		Ames, Wright and Kowanola (1968)
Heart	Dog	5 hours	60 min	Jennings and Wartmann (1957) Bresnahan et al (1974)
Heart	Cat	120 min		Krug and Du Mesnil de Rochemont (1966)
Kidney	Rabbit	120 min		Sheehan and Davis (1959)
Kidney	Rat	230 min	230 min	Milton, Craddock and Brennan (1972)
Adrenal gland	Rat	120 min	120 min	Kovacs, Carroll and Tapp (1966)
Intestine	Dog		7 hours 15 min	Glotzer et al (1962)
Intestine	Dog		10 hours	Carter, Cherry and Myers (1970)
Skin	Pig	21 hours	9 hours 16 hours	Milton (1972)

devascularised intentionally for free grafts, or unintentionally should a full thickness skin flap be raised on a vascular pedicle too small to supply the whole flap (Figure 5.1). Much information about the 'revival time' for different organs has been obtained in the

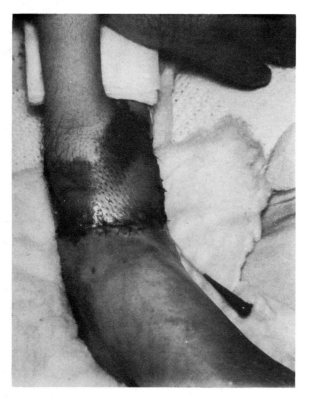

Figure 5.1. Demonstrating the effect of total ischaemia caused by surgical devascularisation of a transplanted tube pedicle. The transplanted end is becoming necrotic, the extent of devascularisation at the time of surgery could have been determined with a vital dye.

field of transplantation, especially for the kidney and heart. For instance, it is well established in this field that temperature and perfusion can affect an organ's tolerance of ischaemia. However, the studies reviewed and presented in this chapter are concerned mainly with the effect of total ischaemia (no flow with hypoxia) on tissue at normothermic conditions.

Another problem associated with an organ's ability to withstand ischaemia concerns the consequences of re-establishing its blood supply. The blood vessels in the organ devoid of blood supply experience hypoxic injury, and this is thought to be more detrimental to its survival than are the direct effects of ischaemia on the tissues.

The failure of blood to reach an ischaemic organ once the occlusion is removed has been termed the 'no reflow phenomenon' (Ames, Wright and Kowanola, 1968). Unquestionably integrity of the endothelium following ischaemia and reperfusion is a major consideration here, and this aspect seems particularly relevant to the problem of vasculitis.

ISCHAEMIA AND PRESSURE IN THE AETIOLOGY OF EXPERIMENTAL DECUBITUS ULCERS

Surprisingly little work has been done on the effect of ischaemia on tissue survival in skin. Most studies undertaken on skin have been concerned with the pathogenesis of decubitus ulcers, more attention having been paid to the effect of pressure on underlying muscle degeneration. Husain's (1953) much quoted study on rats showed that a pressure of 100 mm Hg for two hours was necessary to produce histological changes in the muscles of the hind limb. When, however, the same pressure was applied for six hours, complete muscle degeneration occurred. Husain noted that localised pressure obliterated more vessels in the skin and subcutaneous tissue than in the muscle. This study appears to be the only one which has investigated what effect a previous injury to the vasculature of a tissue, such as a wound or trauma, has on its survival. A second episode of ischaemia applied to a limb three days after ligation of the femoral artery was shown to produce degeneration of muscle fibres, as little pressure as 50 mm Hg for only one hour being sufficient. In other words the threshold tolerance to pressure and to duration of ischaemia had been considerably reduced by the previous vascular insult, which had originally caused no necrosis.

This is an important consideration in clinical vascular pathology where most occlusions leading to total ischaemia occur in tissue where chronic vascular occlusion has produced a sublethal amount of ischaemia in the past. In vasculitis, too, as will be described in the section on the Shwartzman phenomenon, the vessel injury that eventuates in gross pathology is often preceded by some form of 'preparation' of that vessel. In particular, many organs such as the skin of the lower leg or the mucosa of the nasal septum habitually display venous stasis prior to the final occlusive episode. Most experimental studies on ischaemia and tissue survival are performed on healthy organs spared previous vascular insults. However, the authors' experiments described later in this chapter were designed to circumvent this objection.

Kosiak (1961) applied a pressure of 100 to 550 mm Hg to the skin of dogs for periods of one to twelve hours and he found that the higher the pressure the more rapid the skin ulceration, i.e. there is an inverse time—pressure relationship which follows a parabolic curve. Kosiak's article also presents a thorough review of previous experimental work on decubitus ulcers.

In rabbits, Lindan (1961) found that a special pressure clip applied to the ear for seven hours at a pressure of 100 mm Hg did not lead to any ulceration of the skin surface within 12 days. However, healing of the skin was retarded and hair failed to grow in the area subjected to pressure. When pressure was applied for as long as 13 to 15 hours, necrosis occurred. It is interesting to note that when the pressure was less than 100 mm Hg (20, 40, 60 mm Hg), but its duration was the same, no ulceration occurred. In other words a pressure less than systolic did not result in necrosis. This is not surprising as it has been shown in experimental skin flaps that venous obstruction by itself seldom causes necrosis (Myers and Cherry, 1968).

Recently, a study on normal and paraplegic swine by Dinsdale (1973) demonstrated that when an external pressure in excess of 150 mm Hg in conjunction with friction was applied to the skin for 3.5 hours, superficial epidermal necrosis resulted seven days later. With light microscopy, fibrin thrombus was seen in the venules in specimens that had epidermal necrosis and ulceration. Electron microscopy revealed that the venular endothelial cells often had swollen mitochondria with fragmented cristae and blebs projected into the lumen. Skin from paraplegic and control pigs did not differ in their reactions to this trauma. Although Dinsdale stated that friction in conjunction with ischaemia was necessary to produce ulceration, he did not explain the mechanism involved. It may be relevant, however, that Turner, Kurban and Ryan (1969) demonstrated in patients that stripping the epidermis with cellophane tape leads to a decrease in the fibrinolytic activity of skin, and that Cherry, Ryan and Ellis (1974) showed ischaemia coupled with reperfusion to have the same effect. It is conceivable, therefore, that by adding friction the period of ischaemia necessary to produce necrosis is shortened by accelerated depletion of the local fibrinolytic system in the dermis.

SKIN SURVIVAL FOLLOWING ISCHAEMIA AND REPERFUSION

Two recent studies have demonstrated that skin can withstand ischaemia for up to eight hours in situ in normothermic conditions before irreversible damage takes place (Selye, 1967; Willms-Kretschmer and Majno, 1969). Selye's experiment showed that the resistance of rat skin to ischaemia could be increased if the animals were subjected to a form of stress before the blood supply was occluded. In control animals, a fold of skin occluded by an umbilical clamp for nine hours underwent necrosis after reperfusion. It is interesting to note in passing that no thrombus formation was seen until there had been at least six hours of reperfusion. There is, in fact, considerable controversy about the sequence and timing of tissue death and thrombus formation, especially in myocardial infarction, for although there have been many studies on the development of thrombi following vascular injuries, little is known about the true role of ischaemia in this process. In other words, what comes first, ischaemia or thrombus?

Returning to Selye's experiment, the occluded skin fold in animals pretreated with stress (starvation for 48 hours, hypothermia, spinal cord transection or epinephrine) underwent little or no necrosis when reperfused after nine hours of ischaemia. However, when the rats were pretreated with cortisol acetate and cortisol succinate the same amount of necrosis occurred as in the controls. Selye postulated that underlying this protective mechanism there might be a chemical, possibly liberated by systemic endogenous catecholamines released during stress.

Palmer (1972), on the other hand, found that the survival of freshly raised skin flaps in rats was reduced if the animals had been stressed by restraint. The clinical implication of this is important in plastic surgery where the patient often has to be immobilised.

When Palmer pretreated rats with an adrenergic alpha receptor blocking agent, skin flap survival was prolonged. He had also demonstrated previously that the vessels in skin flaps in the rat become denervated within 18 to 30 hours of surgery (Palmer, 1970). Myers and Cherry (1968) too had shown that skin flap survival could be increased with phenoxybenzamine, an adrenergic alpha receptor blocking drug. Such denervation has been shown by several investigators to increase the sensitivity of vessels to circulating catecholamines (Trendelenberg, 1963; Malmors and Sachs, 1965) and this state of affairs may account for the different results and conclusions reached by Selye who worked with normally innervated skin. Of course, the effect of innervation on coagulation and fibrinolysis must be taken into account; this is discussed in Chapters 10 and 11.

Willms-Kretschmer and Majno's (1969) study dealt in greater detail with the histological changes that occur during the period of ischaemia preceding necrosis. They occluded a fold of skin on the backs of rats with a pressure device for varying periods. Skin rendered ischaemic for two hours and then reperfused for 24 hours showed no abnormalities, but after ischaemia for four to six hours, muscle and fat necrosis could be seen. Eight hours of occlusion resulted in complete necrosis of the compressed skin. In the same study a similar experiment was performed on the ears of rabbits and, unlike the rats, their skin underwent no significant necrosis after eight hours of ischaemia. The authors offered no explanation for this species difference, but pointed out that, compared with rat skin, rabbit's ear contains relatively little fat and muscle and these are known to be more susceptible to ischaemia than is skin.

Neither of the above studies attempted to quantify the amount of tissue surviving after periods of temporary ischaemia. The studies by Milton (1972) on delayed* and undelayed island skin flaps were the first to do this. He found that freshly raised island flaps could tolerate on average eight hours of ischaemia (Figure 5.2). This is surprisingly similar to the findings of Selye (1967) and Willms-Kretschmer and Majno (1969).

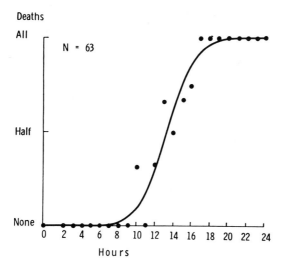

Figure 5.2. Survival curves of delayed and undelayed skin flaps (island) after ischaemia obtained by Milton (1972).

---

*The terms *island flap* and *delay* have special meanings in plastic surgery. An island flap is a skin flap (subcutaneous tissue included) that has a vascular pedicle consisting of blood vessels only. Delay is a term used to describe the surgical technique of improving the blood supply to the skin flap by staged operations before transplanting the skin to a new site.

Delayed island flaps, however, were found to withstand on average only four hours of ischaemia. This was unexpected, because delaying the raising of a skin flap in stages is known to increase the vascularity of the skin and to increase the amount of tissue surviving by up to 100 per cent (Myers and Cherry, 1967; Milton, 1969).

One of the mechanisms thought to promote increased vascularity of a skin flap with delay is conditioning of the tissues to withstand hypoxia, while the flap is raised in stages (McFarlane et al, 1965). If this is so one would expect delayed flaps to withstand ischaemia better than freshly raised skin flaps. Milton's results failed to support this theory. Angiograms of the delayed flaps (Figure 5.3) showed that the vessels had increased in size, and this led Milton to conclude that there was a complete disassociation

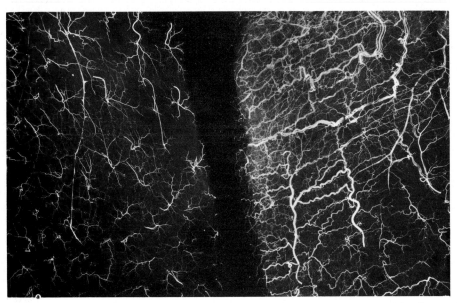

Figure 5.3. Angiogram of pig skin injected with 35 per cent micropaque. Delayed and undelayed seven-day skin flaps. The skin flap on the right shows marked increased vascularity with increased number and calibre of vessels. The flap on the left is from the other side of the pig and represents the normal vascular pattern of pig skin.

between vessel calibre and the ability of the skin to withstand ischaemia. This discrepancy between the increased vascularity and the survival time in skin has been noted by other investigators. De Haan and Stark (1958, 1961), for example, showed that histamine iontopheresis increased the vascularity of pedicled skin flaps. This was demonstrated indirectly by an increased pulse wave on plethysmography and an increased vascular tree by vinyl casts. However, when tissue survival was used to determine the effectiveness of the treatment the results were disappointing. The distal ends of the skin pedicles that had been raised in an area of histamine-pretreated skin not only failed to survive but showed a more rapid and progressive slough than those raised in the normal or less vascular skin of the controls.

McEwan and Ledingham (1971) found that patients with ischaemic feet due to advanced arteriosclerotic disease have an increased blood supply but poor tissue nutrition. The blood flow in their feet was five times greater than in patients with normal feet. They also found the temperature of the ischaemic feet to be significantly higher than that of normal feet, suggesting an increase in blood flow. The authors postulated that the lesions in ischaemic feet might be due to abnormal perfusion at the cellular level.

Burton (1961), in a review article on special aspects of the circulation of the skin, has also pointed to this dissociation of blood flow from tissue nutrition: "It is of the greatest importance for those concerned with the health of the skin itself to realise that this increase of total blood flow through shunts does not supply oxygen and nutrition to the skin cells as in the case of capillary flow. Thus ointments, etc., applied to the skin to increase its circulation may do so without comparable improvement in the oxygenation of the skin, if they merely open these shunts rather than the metarterioles supplying the capillaries."

Experiments to demonstrate skin survival following ischaemia and reperfusion

The experimental model used by Milton (1969, 1972) to study skin survival following ischaemia and reperfusion was the island flap, in which the cutaneous and lymphatic vessels are completely severed and the only blood supply is from a few segmental arteries and veins that perforate from the deep fascia. However, the cutaneous vessels and the lymphatic system undoubtedly play a role in the ability of normal intact skin to withstand ischaemia. Another criticism of Milton's original work is that the animals were under anaesthesia during the ischaemic periods which in some cases lasted for 24 hours. The difference in the maximum survival times — nine hours when the animals were anaesthetised during the ischaemic period, and 16 hours when they were awake — was thought by Milton to be due to this variable. Experiments were designed to mitigate or to counter these criticisms.

Four proposed skin flaps were outlined on the flanks of 14 pigs. Two of these flaps were randomly chosen to be delayed. This was done by making parallel incisions through the full thickness of the skin to the deep fascia and then undermining the centre of the skin flap. After two weeks the animals were re-anaesthetised and the wounds of the delayed flaps re-opened and extended. Once this had been done the dorsal end of the bipedicle delayed skin flap was cut, leaving its vascular supply at the ventral end. This consisted of branches of the internal mammary artery and veins, cutaneous vessels and lymphatics. Two fresh or control flaps were raised at the same time and of the same dimensions. To estimate the blood supply to the skin flaps before ischaemia a vital dye, disulphine blue, was given intravenously and the extent of its penetration into the skin was measured after 30 minutes. The pedicles of the skin flaps were then clamped with vascular clips for two, four, six, eight, ten, 12, 14, 16 or 18 hours. The animals were then placed in a special restrainer cage after being allowed to regain consciousness. At the end of the chosen ischaemic period another vital dye, fluorescein, was given intravenously to the awakened animals to verify that the clips were still securely closed and that reperfusion occurred. Seven days later the survival of the skin flaps was measured.

The average blood supply of the skin flaps before ischaemia in terms of disulphine blue penetration was 19 cm compared with 10 cm for the control flaps. In other words alteration of the blood supply by delaying a flap led to a 190 per cent increase in its survival. Angiograms of the delayed flaps revealed an increase in calibre and number of small vessels. Because the flaps were in different positions on the flanks it was necessary to correct for the inevitably differential initial blood supply in each flap. This was done by subtracting the ultimate survival obtained seven days after the ischaemia from the distance of dye penetration before the flaps were rendered ischaemic. All of the analyses were carried out on the following transformed observations:

$$Y \text{ (corrected survival time)} = \text{survival} - \text{dye}$$

Figure 5.4. shows how this measurement relates to ischaemia time for both delayed and undelayed skin flaps. Straight lines were fitted to the data by the method of regression analysis. The amount of survival and the duration of ischaemia show a linear relationship for both undelayed and delayed flaps. Were there no difference in the response of the, delayed and the undelayed skin flaps to ischaemia, these lines would remain parallel, but this can be seen not to be the case. In fact there was a significant difference between the two in their response to ischaemia; in the delayed flaps and in skin with increased vascularity, survival was more profoundly reduced by ischaemia.

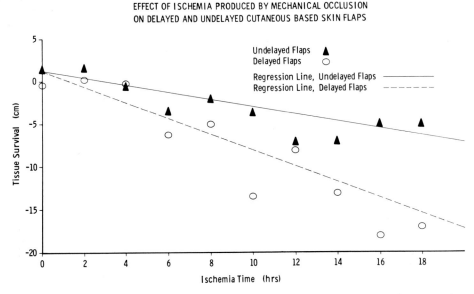

Figure 5.4. Graph of survival following ischaemia and reperfusion of delayed and undelayed cutaneous based flaps, showing an increased susceptibility to ischaemia by delayed flaps.

One of the criticisms rightly levelled against the above experiment is that clamping the base of pedicles with surgical instruments is highly unphysiological. To circumvent this criticism the authors did a similar experiment in which the skin and blood supply were occluded by constricting the vessels with tissue. This was achieved by designing a skin flap of such a width that when it was tubed the vessels in the skin and subcutaneous tissue would become obstructed. After a specified time the skin flap was untubed and reperfusion occurred. The blood supply both before ischaemia and after reperfusion was assessed as above with vital dyes, but this time the effect of position was eliminated by having the delayed and undelayed flaps on the same location on the pig.

The results of this experiment and of the previous one were similar, and because there was no position factor, survival was expressed in terms of eventual tissue survival (Figure 5.5).

Experiments to demonstrate metabolic changes following ischaemia and reperfusion

The results of the experiments just described confirmed Milton's original conclusion that skin with an increased vascularity fails to tolerate ischaemia as well as normal skin.

The next problem was to elucidate the mechanisms that might be responsible for this difference in survival. One such mechanism could be an increased vasculature leading to an elevated anaerobic metabolic rate which it was thought might be reflected in changes in tissue Po_2, Pco_2, pH and water accumulation following ischaemia. Experiments were designed to measure these variables in ischaemic and reperfused, delayed and undelayed skin flaps.

Tissue gas tensions in the flaps were measured using a silastic coil technique. Briefly, this consists of making a small wound in the subcutaneous tissue and inserting a length of silastic tube shaped in the form of a coil. After implantation, the wound is closed and

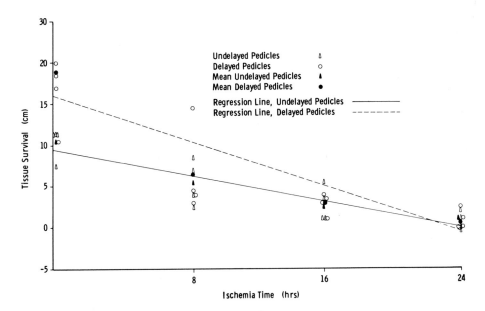

Figure 5.5. Graph of tissue survival of delayed and undelayed tube pedicles made ischaemic by tissue occlusion of the vessels in the base instead of surgical instrument occlusion.

the tube is filled with saline. After a time, the gas tension in the saline equilibrates with that in the surrounding tissue. Silastic is a silicon rubber highly permeable to gas, and previous work has shown that full equilibration occurs within an hour (Cherry and Myers, 1970). The vascular pedicles of the skin flaps were occluded for six hours, after which they were reperfused. Saline was extracted from the coil at hourly intervals during the ischaemic period and up to three hours after reperfusion. Specimens were also taken the next day, 16, 17 and 18 hours after reperfusion. The partial pressures of the gases in the saline were measured in a standard clinical gas analysis machine. In a similar experiment on four pigs, the surface pH of a wound made in the skin flaps was also measured.

The results of the gas tension studies showed a linear fall in Po_2 coupled with a linear rise in Pco_2 (Figure 5.6). There was, however, a significant decline in pH with ischaemia in the delayed flaps. After restoration of the blood supply, all of these values returned to normal. These was also a significant difference in the amount of water that accumulated in the delayed island flaps (Figure 5.7). Such a difference was not evident in cutaneous flaps with intact lymphatic and cutaneous vessels. It would appear, therefore, that these vessels are probably more important in relieving oedema formation following ischaemia than in influencing survival.

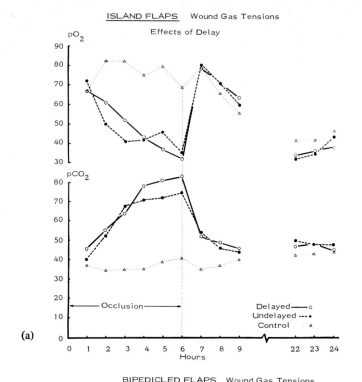

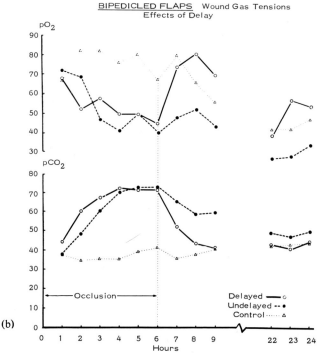

Figure 5.6. (a) Wound gas tensions in delayed and undelayed island skin flaps following ischaemia and reperfusion. (b) Wound gas tensions in bipedicle delayed and undelayed skin flaps following ischaemia and reperfusion.

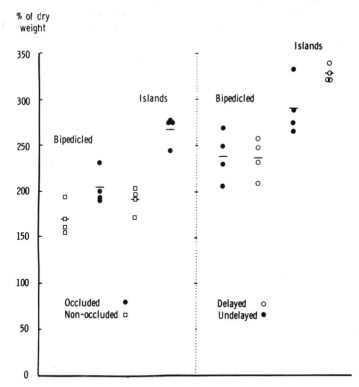

Figure 5.7. Water content of delayed and undelayed bipedicle and island skin flaps following ischaemia and reperfusion.

Experiments to demonstrate fibrinolysis and skin survival following ischaemia and reperfusion

One of the major events in inflammation is fibrin deposition. The role of this phenomenon in inflammation following injury to the skin and the effect of interfering with fibrinolysis have been investigated by Ryan, Nishioka and Dawber (1971). They demonstrated that fibrin deposition was related to the phase or time of inflammation (see Chapter 10). Previous investigations on the mediators of inflammation have, in fact, led several investigators to separate such inflammatory response to injury into two phases, early and late (Cotran and Majno, 1964; Steele and Wilhelm, 1966, 1970). Ryan and colleagues found that in the early phase there was increased fibrinolysis while in the late phase fibrinolytic activity was definitely reduced or lost and fibrin was deposited.

The injury involved in delaying a skin flap surgically to increase its vascularity results in inflammation. This led to the belief that by the time the skin flap is finally raised (i.e. after one to two weeks) its tissues will be in the late phase of inflammation; it will then be more susceptible to thrombus formation because local fibrinolytic activity is reduced. Experiments were designed to test this hypothesis as follows:

A skin flap was delayed on one side of each of five pigs by making parallel incisions 10 cm apart and 20 cm long. The skin and subcutaneous tissue between the two wounds were separated from the deep fascia. The wounds were closed and one week later re-opened. Fresh incisions were made at the cephalic and caudal end of the flap to isolate completely a rectangular section of skin. At the caudal end of the flap one artery accompanied by two veins was left intact to provide a blood supply to the isolated segment of skin. After the skin flap had been raised it was replaced in its bed and partially sutured to the surrounding skin. Vital dyes were given intravenously before ischaemia and after reperfusion to assess the blood supply of the skin. Immediately after the initial injection of the vital dye, approximately 100 μCi/ml of ^{125}I human fibrinogen was given intravenously. The thyroid had been saturated with non-radioactive iodine 24 hours previously. After a 30-minute control period, the extent of the blue dye on this flap was measured and biopsies were taken from the stained areas and from an adjacent unmolested control area of skin. The biopsies were then divided into three sections for measurement of fibrinolytic activity and isotope activity and for routine histological analysis. The specimens were taken at the end of the six-hour ischaemic period, and two hours, 18 hours, seven days, and 14 days after reperfusion. The same protocol was followed on a skin flap on the other side of the pig, which was not delayed but was raised in one stage. To eliminate time-operative factors, the choice of treatment (delayed or control) was randomly chosen. Fibrinolytic activity was measured by Todd's (1959) technique of fibrinolytic autography and by the assessment method of Dodman et al (1972).

Normal and non-delayed skin. Fibrinolysis was normal in control skin and in skin rendered ischaemic for up to 18 hours but not reperfused. It was slightly reduced in skin which had been ischaemic for 24 hours and which later necrosed. The activity was unchanged two hours after reperfusion, but it was essentially absent by 18 hours, although the tissue was still viable (Figure 5.8 a, b, c).

Delayed flap. There was an inconsistent reduction in fibrinolytic activity in delayed flaps before ischaemia. Table 5.2 summarises the results of one experiment representative of the others:

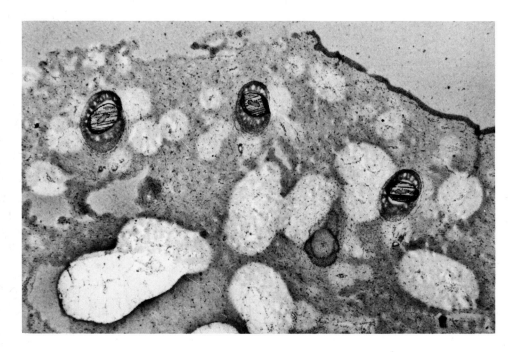

(a)

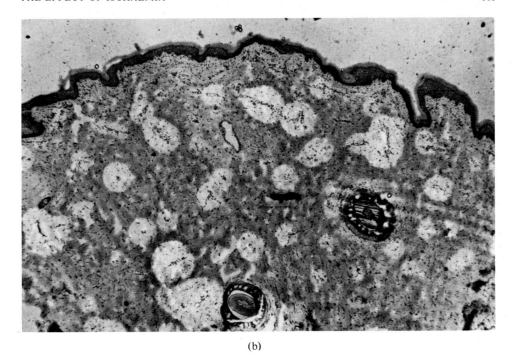

(b)

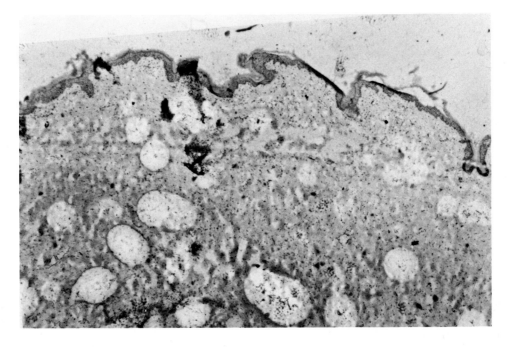

(c)

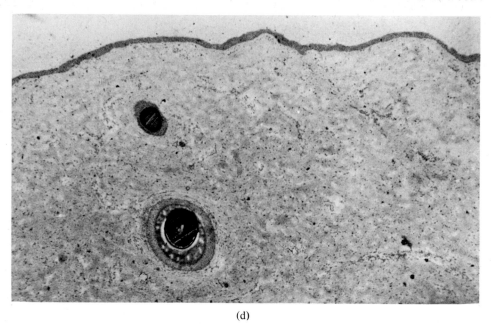

(d)

Figure 5.8.
(a) Skin; control normal fibrinolytic activity, clear areas represent lysed fibrin.
(b) Skin; six hours of ischaemia demonstrating no alteration in fibrinolytic activity.
(c) Skin; six hours of ischaemia and two hours of reperfusion showing slight decrease in fibrinolytic activity.
(d) Skin; six hours of ischaemia and 18 hours of reperfusion with absence of fibrinolytic activity.

In this case fibrinolysis in the delayed flap showing increased vascularity was somewhat reduced at 30 per cent, but this was not a consistent finding. (The dye penetration in the control flap before ischaemia was 13 cm whilst that in the delayed flap was 25 cm — nearly double, demonstrating the increased vascularity.) After the ischaemic period there was no further change in lysis. Two hours of reperfusion did not produce any changes in fibrinolysis, though there was a slight increase in ^{125}I-fibrinogen activity. After 18 hours of reperfusion, that is 24 hours from the beginning of the

Table 5.2. Showing fibrinolysis, ^{125}I-fibrinogen activity and the blood supply of a control flap and the delayed flap on the same pig before and after ischaemia and followed by reperfusion.

	Control flap (normal vascularity)				Delayed flap (increased vascularity)			
	% Lysis		^{125}I-fibrinogen activity counts/g	Vital dye (cm)	% Lysis		^{125}I-fibrinogen activity counts/g	Vital dye (cm)
Time	Flap	Skin			Flap	Skin		
0	58	51	3338	13.0	30	51	4100	25.0
6 h ischaemic (reperfused)	55	58	3035		39	38	4890	
8 h	46	63	4500	10.0	43	38	5450	19.0
24 h	14	59	8565	11.0	6	42	9400	12.0
7 days	—	—	—	10.0	10	47	6332	11.0

ischaemia, the fibrinolytic activity in both skin flaps was greatly reduced, figures of 14 per cent and six per cent being obtained in the delayed flap. The fibrinolytic activity of control skin taken at this time was essentially unchanged, indicating that the systemic effect of surgery was not responsible for the decline in fibrinolytic activity in the skin flaps. At the same time its fibrinogen activity was greatly elevated. The blood supply of the control flap 24 hours later had been reduced to 11.0 cm as compared to 13.0 cm before the ischaemia. The reduction in survival following ischaemia and reperfusion was 15 per cent for the control flap and 56 per cent for the delayed flap. In two cases the delayed flaps were completely cyanotic and swollen the day after ischaemia, but part of the flap managed to survive (Figure 5.9a, b).

An additional experiment was performed to determine whether fibrinolytic activity is reduced in the presence of ischaemia without reperfusion. In this experiment the skin was not reperfused but biopsies were taken at the same time as those in the previous experiment with 10 and 24 hours of ischaemia followed by reperfusion. Skin which had not been reperfused showed no reduction in fibrinolytic activity with the exception of one skin flap, and this was a delayed flap.

Experiments to demonstrate fibrinolysis in blood vessels following ischaemia and reperfusion

Plasminogen activators have been shown to be present in the endothelium of vessels (Warren, 1964) and around the vessels in the vasa vasorum (Kwaan, 1969). Interference with the blood supply by venous occlusion has produced changes in fibrinolytic activity, consisting of an increased amount of lysis coupled with a change in its location (Constantini et al, 1969). These workers demonstrated in veins from apparently healthy patients that the location of this activity shifts from the adventitia to the vessel lumen after venous occlusion. In most investigations only short-term interference with the blood flow has been studied using a sphygmomanometer to occlude the blood supply and then estimating the fibrinolytic activity in the blood rather than in tissues (Nilsson and Robertson, 1968). In this way the plasminogen activator of sclerotic arteries has been shown by Constantini (1972) to be reduced in patients with chronic occlusive arterial disease.

The effect of ischaemia and reperfusion on blood vessel fibrinolysis was assessed in two pigs by clipping a 4-cm segment of the femoral vein and artery to make it ischaemic for six hours (Cherry, Ryan and Ellis, 1974). The vessels in the opposite leg were subjected to a sham operation. Twenty-four hours later, that is 18 hours after reperfusion, the vessels were removed and sections were taken from the centre of the clipped segment of vessel. The fibrinolytic activity was assessed as previously described. In a portion of the vessel wall the endothelium was examined by a stripping technique described by Pugatch and Sanders (1968).

Fibrinolytic activity was easily demonstrated in the control vessels mainly around the adventitia, whereas the clipped arteries showed no activity 18 hours after removal of the occlusion. The activity in the veins was markedly reduced (Figure 5.10). The endothelial stripping technique demonstrated very few intact endothelial cells, the artery being completely denuded of endothelium (Figure 5.11). The changes in fibrinolysis found in pig arteries subjected to ischaemia and reperfusion were remarkably similar to those found by Constantini in the sclerotic arteries of patients. In renal allograft rejection the sequence of events is very similar. Svalander (1971), for example, described separation of endothelial cells and simultaneous aggregation of platelets followed by precipitation of fibrin and accumulation of polymorphonuclear leucocytes.

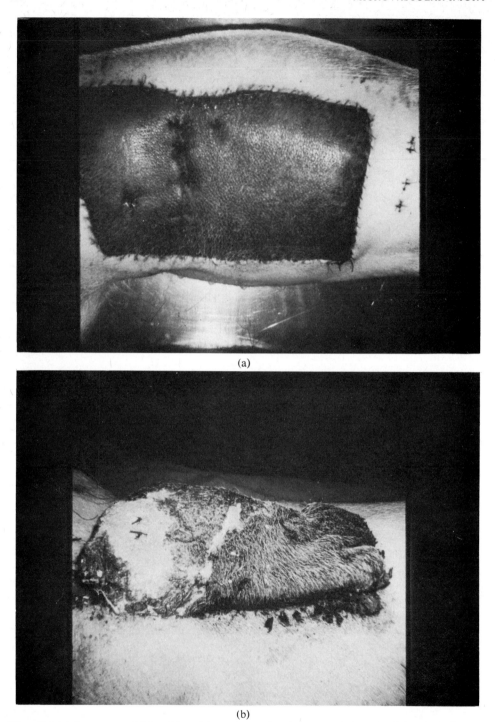

(a)

(b)

Figure 5.9. (a) Appearance of delayed flap eighteen hours after six hours of ischaemia. Although the flap was extremely oedematous and cyanotic at this time, after the administration of fluorescein dye spotty staining occurred. The fibrinolytic activity of the skin from the flap was markedly depressed. (b) The same skin flap seven days later showing that some tissue survived.

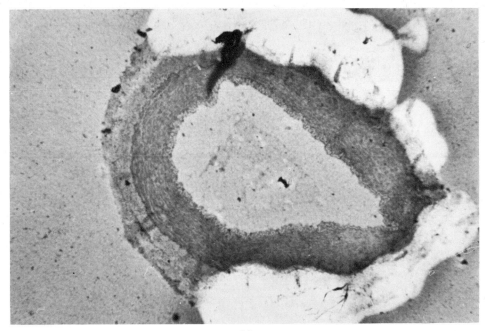

(a)

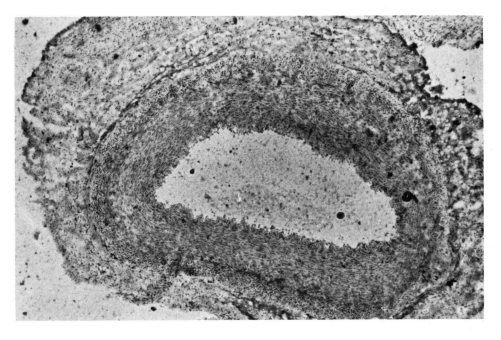

(b)

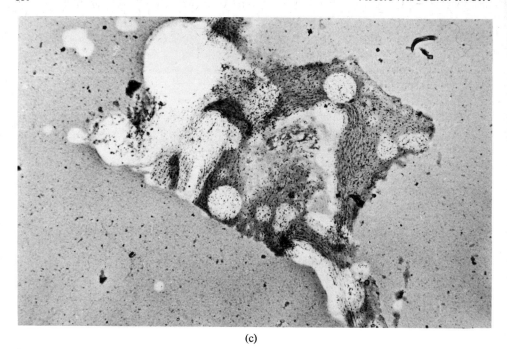

(c)

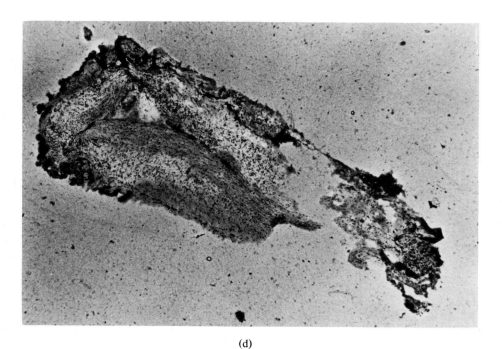

(d)

Figure 5.10.
(a) Control pig artery (femoral) — clear area around adventitia represents lysed fibrin.
(b) Ischaemic reperfused artery demonstrating absence of fibrinolytic activity.
(c) Control pig vein (femoral) — clear areas are lysed fibrin.
(d) Ischaemic and reperfused vein demonstrating reduction in fibrinolytic activity.

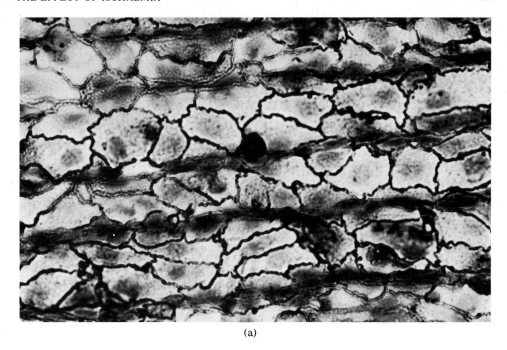

(a)

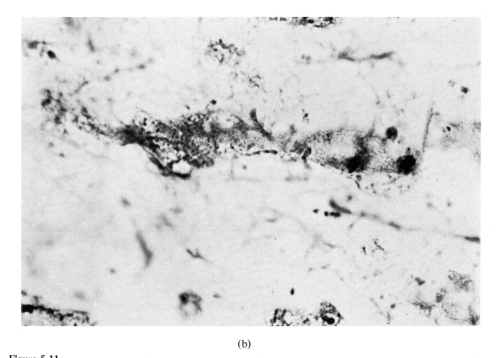

(b)

Figure 5.11.
(a) Hautchen demonstrating mosaic pattern of endothelium in the pig femoral artery.
(b) Hautchen of pig femoral vessel after six hours of ischaemia and reperfused for eighteen hours. Endothelium completely denuded.

Experiments to demonstrate fibrinolytic activity in reperfused myocardial infarcts

Several clinical investigations have demonstrated a decrease in the fibrinolytic activity of patients with myocardial infarction (Chakrabarti, Hocking and Fearnley, 1968). This deficiency in the fibrinolytic system has been implicated as an aetiological factor. Much controversy continues as to the actual role of thrombus in the pathogenesis of myocardial infarction, and it has not even been resolved whether thrombosis precedes or follows infarction. But a recent investigation by Erhardt, Lundman and Mellstedt (1973) has shed some light on this problem. They administered ^{125}I-fibrinogen to patients shortly after admission to hospital for acute infarction, and found at necropsy that labelled

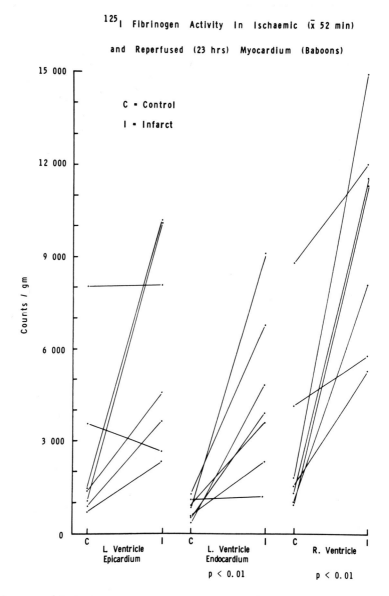

Figure 5.12. Graph of ^{125}I fibrinogen activity in reperfused myocardial infarcts.

fibrinogen was present in most of the thrombi formed in the coronary vessels of six of the seven patients studied. This suggests that thrombus formation continues after the initial ischaemic episode.

In a study designed to determine if temporary ischaemia affects the fibrinolytic system in the heart as it does in the skin and large vessels, temporary myocardial ischaemia was produced in baboons. This was done by temporarily occluding the anterior descending coronary artery at a point halfway from its origin. The time chosen for ischaemia was 30 minutes, an interval of ischaemia shown to produce partial irreversible myocardial cellular death (Jennings and Wartmann, 1957) and alteration of the endothelium (Gavin, Wheeler and Hardson, 1973).

After occlusion, a distinct area of avascular tissue was demonstrated by injecting the vital dye disulphine blue into the blocked anterior descending artery (Cherry and Myers, 1968). Reperfusion of the infarct was shown by the dye test to be complete. Thirty minutes after reperfusion ^{125}I-fibrinogen was injected intravenously and the animals were allowed to survive for 24 hours. Biopsies taken the next day for fibrinolytic activity and fibrinogen content showed a definite increase in fibrin deposition in the ischaemic and reperfused infarcts in comparison with control animals that had sham operations (Figure 5.12). Fibrinolytic activity in the ischaemic and reperfused myocardium also was reduced (Table 5.3) (Cherry and Opie, 1975).

Table 5.3. Mean myocardial fibrinolytic activity (% area of lysis) in baboon myocardium following ischaemia (52 min) and reperfusion (23 hours 8 min).

No.	Condition	Epicardium	Endocardium
(7)	Control	82.5 ($\pm$ 13.3)	99.5 ($\pm$ 13.5)
(7)	Ischaemic reperfused	52.6 ($\pm$ 7.5)	45.3 ($\pm$ 11.9)
	x̄ *Difference*	—29.9 ($\pm$ 13.0)	—54.2 ($\pm$ 12.5)
	P	N.S.	<0.005

x̄ = mean.
P = level of significance.
N.S. = not significant.

Fibrinolytic activity has been thought to be relevant to atheroma, arteriosclerosis, deep vein thrombosis, dermatoses and hyperperfusion of the lung in newborns, all of which are influenced by blood flow. In the above studies ischaemia alone has little effect on fibrinolytic activity for at least 24 hours. In contrast, re-establishment of blood flow in ischaemic tissue resulted in severe depression of activity coupled with fibrin deposition. The author believes that this may be due to endothelial injury caused by the re-establishment of blood flow in the ischaemic tissues. In other studies (Chapter 4) electron-microscopic examination of skin capillaries subjected to similar ischaemia and reperfusion has revealed severe damage to the endothelium; the relevance of this to vasculitis is discussed in Chapter 10. It is probable that injury of any kind, sufficient to produce changes in endothelium such as those observed in this experiment, prepares the vessel so that subsequent changes in flow cause endothelial shedding and consequent fibrin and platelet deposition.

References

Ames, A. zd., Wright, R. L. & Kowanola, M. (1968) Cerebral ischemia II. The no-flow phenomenon. *American Journal of Pathology*, **52**, 437.
Bresnahen, G. F., Roberts, R., Shell, W. E., Ross, J. & Sobel, B. E. (1974) After myocardial reperfusion. *American Journal of Cardiology*, **33**, 82.

Brooks, H. W. (1973) Controlled hypothermia to pedicle flaps. *Medical Exhibition at the American Society of Plastic and Reconstructive Surgery, 1973.*

Burton, A. (1961) Special features of the circulation of the skin in blood vessels and circulation. In *Advances in Biology of the Skin* (Ed.) Montagna, W. & Ellis, R. A. p. 117. Oxford: Pergamon Press.

Carter, K., Cherry, G. & Myers, M. B. (1970) Determination of the viability of ischemic intestine. *Archives of Surgery,* **100,** 695.

Chakrabarti, R., Hocking, E. D. & Fearnley, G. R. (1968) Fibrinolytic activity and coronary-artery disease. *Lancet,* **i,** 987.

Cherry, G. & Myers, M. B. (1968) The use of vital dyes to predict survival after experimental coronary artery ligation. *Surgery,* **63,** 929.

Cherry, G. & Myers, M. B. (1970) A new method to measure tissue pO_2 and CO_2 with results in normal and ischaemic skin. *Federation Proceedings,* **29,** 317 (abstract).

Cherry, G. & Opie, L. H. (1975) Decreased myocardial fibrinolytic activity following ischaemia and re-perfusion. *Thrombosis et Diathesis Haemorrhagica,* **34,** 210.

Cherry, G. W., Ryan, T. J. & Ellis, J. P. (1974) Decreased fibrinolysis in reperfused ischaemic tissue. *Thrombosis et Diathesis Haemorrhagica,* **32,** 659.

Constantini, R., Spottl, E., Holzknecht, F. & Braunstein, H. (1969) The role of the stable plasminogen activator of the venous wall in occlusion induced fibrinolytic state. *Thrombosis et Diathesis Haemorrhagica,* **22,** 544.

Cotran, R. S. & Majno, G. (1964) A light and electron microscopic analysis of vascular injury. *Annals of the New York Academy of Sciences,* **116,** 750.

De Haan, C. R. & Stark, R. B. (1958) Vascular reinforcement of pedicled tissues: quantitation by arteriography of increase in circulation obtained using histamine iontophoresis. *Surgical Forum,* **8,** 578.

De Haan, C. R. & Stark, R. B. (1961) Changes in efferent circulation of tubed pedicles and in the trans-plantability of large composite grafts produced by histamine iontophoresis. *Plastic and Reconstructive Surgery,* **28,** 577.

Dinsdale, S. M. (1973) Decubitus ulcers in swine: light and electron microscopy study of pathogenesis. *Archives of Physical Medicine and Rehabilitation,* **54,** 51.

Dodman, B. A., Cunliffe, W. J., Dodman, E. A. & Webster, J. A. (1972) A method of measuring well-defined areas within sections applied to the assessment of tissue fibrinolysis. In *Methods in Microcirculation Studies* (Ed.) Ryan, T. J., Jolles, B. & Holti, G. p. 104. London: H. K. Lewis.

Erhardt, L. R., Lundman, T. & Mellstedt, H. (1973) Incorporation of ^{125}I-labelled fibrinogen into coronary arterial thrombi in acute myocardial infarction in man. *Lancet,* **i,** 387.

Gavin, J. B., Wheeler, E. E. & Hardson, P. B. (1973) Scanning electron microscopy of the endocardial endothelium overlying early myocardial infarcts. *Pathology,* **5,** 145.

Glotzer, D. J., Villegas, A. H., Anekamaya, S. & Shaw, R. S. (1962) Healing of the intestine in experimental bowel infarction. *Annals of Surgery,* **155,** 183-190.

Husain, T. (1953) An experimental study of some pressure effects on tissues, with reference to the bed-sore problem. *Journal of Pathology and Bacteriology,* **66,** 347.

Jennings, R. B. & Wartmann, W. B. (1957) Production of an area of homogenous myocardial infarction in the dog. *Archives of Pathology,* **63,** 580.

Kiehn, C. L. & Desprez, J. D. (1960) Effects of local hypothermia on pedicle flap tissue. *Plastic and Reconstructive Surgery,* **25,** 349.

Kosiak, M. (1961) Etiology of decubitus ulcers. *Archives of Physical Medicine,* **42,** 19-29.

Kovacs, K., Carroll, R. & Tapp, E. (1966) Temporary ischaemia of the rat adrenal gland. *Journal of Pathology and Bacteriology,* **91,** 235.

Krug, A. & Du Mesnil de Rochemont, K. G. (1966) Blood supply of myocardium after temporary coronary occlusion. *Circulation Research,* **19,** 57.

Kwaan, H. (1969) Endothelial fibrinolytic activity in the prevention and resolution of thrombosis. In *Dynamics of Thrombosis Formation.* Philadelphia: J. B. Lippincott.

Lindan, O. (1961) Etiology of decubitus ulcers: an experimental study. *Archives of Physical Medicine and Rehabilitation,* **42,** 774-783.

Malmors, T. & Sachs, C. (1965) Direct studies on the disappearance of the transmitter and the changes in the uptake storage mechanisms of degenerating adrenergic nerves. *Acta Physiologica Scandinavica,* **64,** 211.

McEwan, A. J. & Ledingham, I. McA. (1971) Blood flow characteristics and tissue nutrition in apparently ischaemic feet. *British Medical Journal,* **iii,** 220.

McFarlane, R. M., Heagy, F. C., Radin, S., Aust, J. C. & Wermuth, R. E. (1965) Experimental pedicle flaps. *Plastic and Reconstructive Surgery,* **35,** 245.

Milton, S. (1969) The effects of 'delay' on the survival of experimental pedicled skin flaps. *British Journal of Plastic Surgery,* **22,** 244.

Milton, S. H. (1972) Experimental studies on island flaps. II. Ischaemia and delay. *Plastic and Reconstructive Surgery,* **49,** 444.

Milton, S. H., Craddock, G. N. & Brennan, J. M. (1972) Detrimental effects of removal of the renal capsule following acute ischaemia. *Archives of Surgery,* **104,** 90.

Myers, M. B. & Cherry, G. (1967) Augmentation of tissue survival by delay. *Plastic and Reconstructive Surgery,* **39,** 245.

Myers, M. B. & Cherry, G. (1968) Enhancement of survival in devascularised pedicles by the use of phenoxy-benzamine. *Plastic and Reconstructive Surgery,* **41,** 254.

Nilsson, I. M. & Robertson, B. (1968) Effect of venous occlusion on coagulation and fibrinolytic components in normal subjects. *Thrombosis et Diathesis Haemorrhagica,* **20,** 397.

Palmer, B. (1970) Sympathetic denervation and reinervation of cutaneous blood vessels following surgery. *Scandinavian Journal of Plastic and Reconstructive Surgery,* **4,** 93.

Palmer, B. (1972) The influence on the survival of experimental skin flaps. *Scandinavian Journal of Plastic and Reconstructive Surgery,* **6,** 110-113.

Pugatch, E. M. J. & Saunders, A. M. (1968) A new technique for making Häutchen preparations of unfixed aortic endothelium. *Journal of Atherosclerosis Research,* **8,** 735.

Reinisch, J. (1974) The pathophysiology of skin flap circulation. *Plastic and Reconstructive Surgery,* **54,** 585.

Ryan, T. J., Nishioka, K. & Dawber, R. P. R. (1971) Control of inflammation through fibrinolysis. *British Journal of Dermatology,* **84,** 501.

Selye, H. (1967) Ischemic necrosis: prevention by stress. *Science,* **156,** 1262.

Sheehan, H. L. & Davis, J. C. (1959) Renal ischemia with failed reflow. *Journal of Pathology and Bacteriology,* **78,** 105.

Stark, R. (1956) Vascular reinforcement of pedicled tissue: a preliminary report. *Plastic and Reconstructive Surgery,* **18,** 329.

Steele, R. H. & Wilhelm, D. L. (1966) The inflammatory reaction in chemical injury. I Increased vascular permeability and erythema induced by various chemicals. *British Journal of Experimental Pathology,* **47,** 612.

Steele, R. H. & Wilhelm, D. L. (1970) The inflammatory reaction in chemical injury. III Leucocytosis and other histological changes induced by superficial injury. *British Journal of Experimental Pathology,* **51,** 265.

Svalander, C. (1971) Microthrombolic occlusions in renal allografts. In *Microcirculatory Approaches to Current Therapeutic Problems; 6th European Conference on Microcirculation, Aalborg, 1970* (Ed.) Ditzel, J. & Lewis, D. H. p. 79. Basel: S. Karger.

Todd, A. S. (1959) The histological localisation of fibrinolysin activator. *Journal of Pathology and Bacteriology,* **78,** 281.

Trendelenburg, U. (1963) Supersensitivity and subsensitivity to sympathomimetic amines. *Pharmacological Review,* **15,** 225.

Turner, R. H., Kurban, A. K. & Ryan, T. J. (1969) Fibrinolytic activity in human skin following epidermal injury. *Journal of Investigative Dermatology,* **53,** 458.

Vasko, N. A., DeWall, R. A. & Riley, A. M. (1972) Effect of allopurinol in renal ischaemia. *Surgery,* **71,** 787.

Warren, B. (1964) Fibrinolytic activity of vascular endothelium. *British Medical Bulletin,* **20,** 213.

Willms-Kretschmer, K. & Majno, G. (1969) Ischaemia of the skin. *American Journal of Pathology,* **54,** 327-343.

6. The Triggers and the Chemical and Cellular Contribution of the Tissues to Altered Reactivity

When Copeman and Ryan (1970) introduced their mechanistic classification of vasculitis, they based it on fibrin (Table 6.1). They viewed vasculitis as an expression of vessel damage triggered by various agencies, such as immune complexes or bacterial endotoxin which, in the presence of constitutional factors, tend to enhance fibrin production and platelet aggregation. A third set of mechanisms was thought to play a complicating and perpetuating role once fibrin had been deposited in or around the vessel. It is acknowledged that other agents, such as complement or leucocytes, can be included in a mechanistic classification, but compared to fibrin none seems quite so invariable a feature of the injured vessel.

Fibrin and platelet interaction are difficult to separate from endothelial injury, and any one of these three may initiate the chain of events leading to vasculitis. However, fibrin is the most likely agent to determine progression of the inflammation, so that factors controlling its removal are important therapeutically. The breakdown products of fibrin elicit inflammation by potentiating mediators such as histamine and kinins and because they are chemotactic. But intact fibrin acts as a scaffold, blocks small vessels, and encourages migration of leucocytes, macrophages and fibroblasts into the vessel wall and surrounding tissues.

TRIGGERS

Important triggers of endothelial injury, platelet aggregation and fibrin deposition in vasculitis include direct trauma to the vessel wall by physical agents, immune complexes, bacterial endotoxin and various biochemical or metabolic disorders.

Physical agents

Direct trauma by the application of various noxious materials through micro-needles has been used experimentally to injure endothelium and to study fibrin and platelet deposition and leucocyte migration. The end-result of such experiments is a reaction pattern indistinguishable from clinical vasculitis. However, the role of trauma as such is not easy to define in clinical disease or in experiments of this type. Injury, especially to the leg, commonly precedes the usual clinical pattern of vasculitis, and in some of the more peculiar forms such as pyoderma gangrenosum or Behçet's disease, inflammatory lesions at the site of venepunctures are a well-known feature.

Table 6.1. Cutaneous angiitis: classifications of mechanisms.

1. Initiation of fibrin and platelet deposition
   - (a) immune complexes
   - (b) bacterial endotoxin
   - (c) ischaemic, pharmacological and biochemical damage to vessel wall.

2. Enhancement of fibrin and platelet deposition
   - (a) fibrinolysis and its impairment
   - (b) coagulopathies
   - (c) blood viscosity
   - (d) blood flow
     - (i) central venous and gravitational pressure
     - (ii) anatomical distribution of vessels in upper dermis
     - (iii) changes (e.g. anatomical) in papillary capillaries.

3. Modification of pathology that results from fibrin and platelet deposition
   - (a) red cell extravasation
   - (b) white cell extravasation
   - (c) alteration of macrophage activity
   - (d) vasoactive substances
   - (e) secondary involvement of the environment: epidermis, fat, etc.

The experiments described by Cherry in Chapter 5 illustrate trauma from the surgeon's knife and from biochemical injury, as in ischaemia. The final clinical pattern, be it purpura or necrotic skin, is determined by the surgical approach, but the pathology is always vasculitis.

In the experiments described by Kanan in Chapter 9, the clumps of platelets around injected particulate carbon and other agents also exemplify physical injury that can progress to vasculitis.

Immune complexes

Immunological injury will be described in Chapter 7. As in the Arthus reaction, such injury may be due to circulating immune complexes, or, as in the vasculitis of erythema nodosum leprosum, to the antibody probably combining with the antigen already present in the tissues to form a complex that produces only a local response. Cytotoxic antibody and delayed hypersensitivity mechanisms may also produce vasculitis at specific sites in this way.

Infection

Infective agents will be described in Chapter 8. They can be viral, bacterial, fungal or parasitic, and can act as toxins, as particulate matter or as antigens. No matter how they act, the triad of endothelial injury, platelet aggregation and fibrin deposition is a usual consequence.

Food and drugs

Of all the factors causing vasculitis these are the least understood and are described in Chapter 8. Their action as antigens is probably rarer than their activity as pharmacological agents. Penicillin allergy, aspirin enhancement of urticaria and vasculitis, similar rashes from food additives such as tartrazine, and the earlier work of Ackroyd on Sedormid purpura (see page 183) are probably the most fully investigated effects of food and drugs and supply examples from the whole field of the immunology and pharmacology of blood vessels. Some foods may be regarded as direct triggers; others probably act indirectly via the constitutional background that controls tissue reactivity.

Constitution

As emphasised by Copeman and Ryan (1970), endothelial injury, platelet aggregation and fibrin deposition can be very transient, and at times almost physiological. Certainly micro-injury must be occurring all the time due to the metabolism of living, feeding and dying cells. Such transience is mostly due to quick repair.

Many factors can, however, enhance injury. For example, transient ischaemia may make endothelial cells more susceptible to the trauma of high perfusion rates (see Chapter 5), or a lack of certain serum factors may interfere with local phagocytosis (see page 126).

Fibrin deposition may be either enhanced by coagulation factors or prevented by fibrinolysis, and so the individual's constitution or make-up may determine whether or not fibrin is deposited in amounts sufficient to block a vessel.

There are marked individual differences in the proteolytic capacity of human plasma which are genetically determined (Jacobson, 1968). As Ygge (1969) has pointed out, each normal individual has a specific and distinctive pattern of biological values, and it is to be expected that small but significant differences will be concealed in figures for normal values obtained by averaging a sample of normal persons.

The studies of the Shwartzman phenomenon discussed in Chapter 10 provide a good example of triggers interacting with constitution. Injury from bacterial toxin triggers coagulation, but vessel damage results only if the fibrinolytic mechanisms are impaired or if the removal of fibrin by the phagocytic system is paralysed. Ischaemia, a fall in pH, and various other metabolic factors enhance the Shwartzman phenomenon. Vasoconstriction and stasis make a further contribution and may be modified by circulating noradrenaline or adrenal steroids. It is factors such as these which make up the constitution.

Once it is accepted that micro-injury is occurring all the time, it becomes conceivable that constitutional defects could, on their own, enhance it into the realms of pathology to produce vasculitis. Superimpose a far more virulent trigger such as *E. coli* or immune complexes — which occasionally circulate in anyone — and one must be thankful that one's constitution is for the most part effective in dealing with them. Thus vasculitis, which is usually explained by triggers, can equally be due to constitutional disturbances, and these require much more careful analysis if a fuller understanding is to be obtained and correct treatment given.

One important response to injury is vessel leakiness. Gaps between endothelial cells are a feature of vasculitis, and increased capillary permeability is accepted as a general phenomenon in all inflammatory states. Marks, Birkett and Shuster (1972) detected increased capillary permeability to serum albumin in several patients with collagen vascular diseases and in erythroderma from eczema and psoriasis (Marks and Shuster, 1966). Such leakiness must increase the escape of haematogenous agents. The importance of such leakiness is emphasised in Chapter 9 in Kanan's studies of the nose, in Chapter 7 in descriptions of the localisation of circulating immune complexes and in Chapter 13 in the discussion of the escape of protein and fibrinogen into the vessel wall as a result of high blood pressure or ischaemic injury.

Kanan refers in Chapter 9 to the roles of pregnancy, endocrine status and cold exposure. These modify the constitution in many ways, for example by affecting the fibrinolytic system or mononuclear phagocytosis. Kanan who studies localisation using the nose as his model, considers that a theme common to the many pathological states affecting the anterior septum seems to be vascular reactivity, influenced by local and systemic events. Furthermore, some of these events are developmental, occurring in the fetus or in the period immediately after birth.

The systemic or local constitution develops and adapts throughout life, and its reactivity at any one time is determined by a complex balance between oscillating and opposing systems of chemical and physical agents. The coagulation cascade in opposition to the fibrinolytic mechanism, on the one hand, and its interaction with the kinin and complement cascade, on the other, form but one example of the complexity of the balance underlying our constitution.

Both Kanan's and Cherry's experiments illustrate clearly how the local constitution can be changed by previous exposure, in the one case to the environment, and in the other to ischaemic injury. The vasculature of the anterior nasal septum may be modified by exposure to cold (and its reactivity to circulating carbon or colloidal gold is clearly affected by such exposure) or by an endocrine disturbance such as ovariectomy or pregnancy. The survival of a skin flap, when made ischaemic, is greatly influenced by previous interference with its blood supply and by the pathology of previous inflammation and repair. A corollary of this is that an area of vasculitis in previously unaffected skin may require very different management compared with recurrence in that site as, for example, in an area of stasis of the lower leg.

Winkelmann and Ditto (1964), in their discussion of the pathogenesis of necrotising vasculitis, wrote of aggravating factors such as stasis, menstruation, emotional upsets and exposure to cold. These phenomena alter the constitution and localise circulating triggers; the mechanisms whereby such alteration and localisation are achieved are becoming clearer. The term locus minoris resistentiae is often used to describe the altered behaviour of a local area which predisposes it to disease.

Pathology, however minor, predisposes the tissue to further pathology and there is no better example of this than the Shwartzman phenomenon. In Chapter 12 are described various stasis syndromes; some are gravitational, others are perniotic. The legs act as a locus minoris resistentiae for vasculitis because of the effects of gravitational stasis. Similarly, as was beautifully emphasised by Haxthausen (1930) in a monograph on cold, perniosis is a locus for much pathology. Probably stasis is the common denominator and is the most frequent cause of changes in vascular reactivity to circulating triggers.

The isomorphic response

When tissue injury causes pathology identical to that already featured at several other sites, the phenomenon is called the isomorphic response. It is common in psoriasis (Figure 6.1) and lichen planus, in which it is termed the Koebner phenomenon, but it also occurs in vasculitis and related disorders and in eczema. It can be induced by a whole range of agents or physical phenomena including scratching the skin, stripping it with cellotape, exposing it to ultraviolet radiation, the intradermal injection of bacterial antigen, or the topical application of tetrahydrofurfuryl ester of nicotinic acid (Trafuril). In psoriasis it is known to be dependent on an intact blood supply (Ryan, 1969).

Traumatised skin in patients with vasculitis, erythema multiforme, Behçet's disease, or pyoderma gangrenosum will develop lesions identical to the primary disorder (Juhlin and Michaelsson, 1971). It is assumed that the whole constitution or system is in some way altered so that the tissues — usually the skin — react in an altered fashion that is nevertheless predictable on the basis of responses already observed. The tendency to develop the isomorphic response fluctuates, being more acute at the height of the illness, and possibly no longer reproducible after recovery from the primary disease. In the case of pyoderma gangrenosum or psoriasis, it is easier to produce an isomorphic response near an existing lesion than at a more distant site.

The fault lies with the constitution; it is more disturbed near existing pathology, and triggers such as trauma, bacterial antigen or immune complexes can detect the underlying fault. When Michaelsson, Pettersson and Juhlin (1974) used Trafuril to reveal a purpuric tendency in the presence of a leucocytoclastic histology in persons sensitive to food additives, it is probable that they were inducing the isomorphic response locally in people whose constitution was temporarily altered by the ingested agents.

THE PHARMACOLOGICAL CONSTITUTION

Tissue behaviour in inflammation depends on the availability, concentration and rate of activation, inhibition or removal of mediators. Wilhelm (1971) has described six patterns of permeability response in inflammation, and most of these show an approximate division into the early and late phases of inflammation, a fact emphasised by most writers in this field. These patterns are illustrated in Figure 6.2.

The peaks of permeability occurring within the first two hours are mediated mainly by histamine and 5-hydroxytryptamine. The mediators of the delayed and prolonged phases are of uncertain nature. Kinins, plasmin, prostaglandins and complement are important factors. They are often released in the early phase and are partly responsible for the changes in coagulation and cellular infiltration that contribute to altered structure and organisation — the more persistent features of inflammation. As many of the activators, substrates and inhibitors of the mediators of inflammation are carried to the tissues by the bloodstream, blood stasis, induced by inflammation, is a controlling factor. But ischaemia, when a consequence of stasis, is a complicating factor.

Once a tissue has been inflamed, it carries a memory of the event, probably in the form of microscarring, altered vascularity, or an infiltrate by, for example, mast cells. The nervous system also retains a memory of the event and 'conditioning' may be an important influence of the central nervous system (see Chapter 11). Evidence of skin memory is provided by Holti's experiments discussed on page 268; these showed that reflex vasodilatation is greatest at sites of previous inflammation and that this persists for many months after histamine release, ultraviolet radiation or the Mantoux reaction.

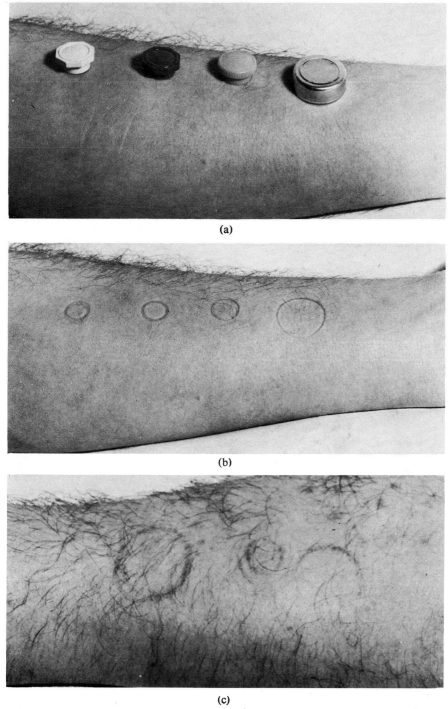

(a)

(b)

(c)

Figure 6.1. Isomorphic response. Injury to the skin produces a response in the skin which is morphologically identical to whatever skin lesions are most in evidence at that time. Indentation marks from the caps of tubes of ointments applied for only 24 hours were the site of psoriasis 10 days later: (a) caps, (b) marks at 24 hours, (c) psoriasis.

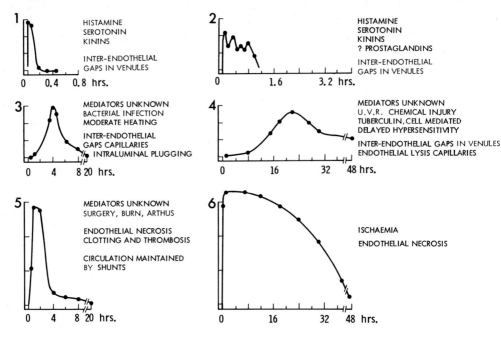

Figure 6.2. Six different types of permeability response. 1 and 2 early inflammatory response equivalent to acute urticaria; 3 and 4 delayed urticaria; 4, 5 and 6 vasculitis.

Factitious wealing at the site of previous injury to the skin is another example (James and Warin, 1970).

Only these examples of the complexity of the local pharmacological constitution will be discussed — histamine and mast cells, prostaglandins and complement.

Histamine and mast cells

Histamine is generated in the tissues by the action of histidine decarboxylase on histidine (Schayer, 1962, 1964), a reaction enhanced by stasis and hypoxia. It is liberated from mast cells either by the release reaction of secretion (Størmorken, 1969), or by toxic changes causing irreversible disruption of the cell. Mast cells also release hyaluronidase and heparin. This combination of factors not only produces an immediate increase in vascular permeability but also prevents the more deleterious effects of coagulation and ischaemia.

Fibrin is not likely to be deposited in the presence of heparin, and if histamine is present too, it will attract profibrinolysin-containing eosinophils (Archer, 1963). These agents also greatly encourage the diffusion of fibrinolytic enzymes throughout the tissues (Ryan et al, 1968).

Prolonged or acute experimental stasis (Asboe-Hansen, 1964) encourages not only the generation of histamine but also mast cell infiltration, hence it is not surprising that these cells are increased in number in the legs of patients with venous stasis disorders (Témine, 1956). A tissue well endowed with mast cells and eosinophils for long periods rarely shows thrombosis or ischaemic necrosis. This is illustrated by patients with proliferative or warty hyperkeratosis and lymphoedema in whom the grossest of congestive changes rarely proceed to ulceration (Figure 6.3).

Histamine is destroyed by diamine oxidase and imidazole N-methyl-transferase, but there is species as well as tissue variation (Kowalewski, Russel and Koheil, 1969).

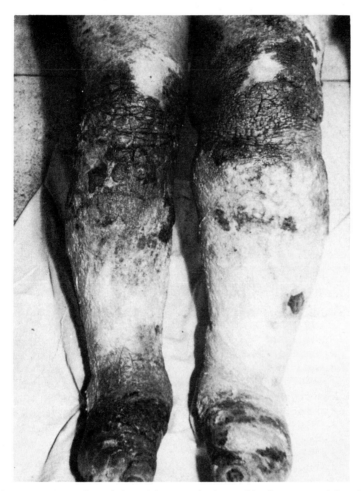

Figure 6.3. Gross hyperkeratosis and dermal hypertrophy in combined venous and lymphatic stasis, a condition in which mast cells are very plentiful and skin necrosis rare.

Prostaglandins

The evidence that prostaglandins are mediators of inflammation includes the following:
1. Increased levels of prostaglandins have been found in inflamed skin.
2. Intradermal injection of small amounts of prostaglandins (PGE_1) produces erythema that lasts for 10 to 12 hours. Accompanying wealing is in part due to histamine release (Sondergaard and Greaves, 1971).

3. Prostaglandin lowers the threshold to itching and pain and, in a variety of experimental situations, appears to potentiate the activity of other mediators such as histamine and kinins.

Injury to the tissues results in the release of arachidonic acid from cell membranes, which in all probability becomes freely available at most sites of inflammation. This acid is the substrate for prostaglandin synthetase, an enzyme present in the neutrophils, which is responsible for prostaglandin biosynthesis. If excessive amounts of readily available enzyme are present locally, they may lead to increased tissue levels of prostaglandins. Such a situation may well be operative in skin memory.

Complement

Complement as part of immune complexes has long been regarded as a significant factor in vasculitis. In recent years the pathways of complement activation and the role of complement in inflammation have become better understood, though no less complex.

Rather in the same way that cleavage by thrombin converts fibrinogen into the more electron-dense fibrin, so cleavage of the complement component converts it into the more electron-dense C_3b. This material coats particles and causes them to adhere to and injure platelets or endothelium.

There are two important ways in which this cleavage into C_3b comes about. In the first, the so-called classical pathway, C_1 and C_2 are activated — usually by immune complexes in vasculitis. In the second, the alternate pathway, properdin is activated usually by endotoxin and by plasmin, but in dermatitis herpetiformis it is probably activated by IgA (Seah et al, 1973).

It is probable that intravascular coagulation induced by endotoxin is mediated by C_3b (Figure 6.4), which becomes fixed to endotoxin and attracts neutrophils, eosinophils, monocytes, macrophages and platelets. Activation of complement in this way releases peptides that cause increased vascular permeability and make platelets and polymorphs sticky to endothelium. Other components of complement may be formed in the process and cause lysis of lipid-containing membranes, and the release of platelet factor 3 and anti-heparin factor all of which contribute to coagulation (Figure 6.4). At the same time vasoactive amines and endogenous ADP are discharged from the platelet (Henson, 1969; Siraganian, 1972). The consumption of complement has also been described in the disseminated intravascular coagulation met in *Plasmodium falciparum* malaria (Srichaikul et al, 1975).

Baart de la Faille Kuyper, Van der Meer and Baart de la Faille (1974) found C_3b, C_3c, C_3d and C_5 in the basement membrane zone in a study of 23 biopsies of skin from normal people. The walls of capillaries frequently contained C_3d and sometimes C_4, C_3c and C_5. Presumably these are synthesised by skin macrophages as was indicated by Lai et al (1974). Baart de la Faille Kuyper, Van der Meer and Baart de la Faille (1974) suggested that the vessel deposits represent "residual products of the activities of the 'daily' immunological defence", a physiological rather than a pathological phenomenon. The presence of such material in normal skin provides yet another aspect of the local constitution, the recruitment of which may eventuate in pathology.

Hypocomplementaemia has been reported (MacDuffie et al, 1973) in patients with a persistent low-grade urticarial type of vasculitis due to immune complex disease. In one such patient, referred to and reported by Sissons (1974), a positive pressure test suggested some overlap with delayed pressure urticaria. This result probably can be explained by the localisation of immune complexes. The histology of these morphologically pure urticarial lesions is leucocytoclastic as in the Arthus reaction. The amount of cryoglobulin detectable in these patients is usually very small, and it is suggested that a defect in complement itself rather than immune complex formation is responsible for this disease.

Ballow et al (1975) studying complement activator pathways in 152 patients with urticaria found four with low serum levels of the third component of complement. There was nothing clinically distinctive about these patients, their C_1 inhibitor levels were normal and there was no evidence of immune complexes.

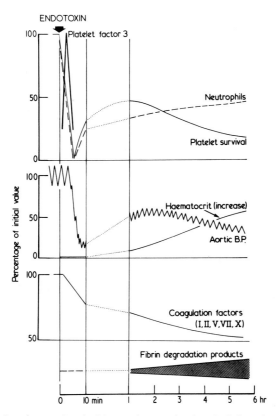

Figure 6.4. Effects of endotoxin complexed with complement showing depletion of neutrophils, release of platelet factor 3, fall in blood pressure and eventual coagulation.

THE MONONUCLEAR PHAGOCYTIC SYSTEM

The term mononuclear phagocytic system is gradually replacing that of the reticulo-endothelial system. Phagocytosis is now recognised as a feature of virtually all cells given the appropriate environment for such a process. It is a process that is influenced by a number of pharmacological agents, and it cannot take place in the absence of certain other factors, some of which are provided from the bloodstream and are therefore in short supply at sites of blood stasis.

In 1903 Wright and Douglas showed that normal human serum contains a substance which they called 'opsonin'. This coats bacteria making them more susceptible to phagocytic ingestion.

In Chapter 9 Kanan describes his experiments on intravascular phagocytosis and stresses the considerable influence of stasis. This feature has been reviewed by Saba (1970) and he referred to the marked depression of the reticuloendothelial system in circulatory failure. Much, however, depends on how the function of this system is measured. If it is assessed by the clearance of materials from the bloodstream, as in Kanan's experiments, then local permeability and chance contact of particulate matter with phagocytic cells at sites of stasis should be taken into account. Certainly activation of the clearance system may be modified by factors influencing permeability and stasis. Moreover, the way blood flow affects the phagocytosis of particulate matter is determined in part by the blood volume and the velocity at which the particulate matter flows past the phagocytic cells, and in part by the availability of metabolites and opsonins in the serum. There is thus an optimum degree of stasis below which, no matter how much contact there is between cells and particulate matter, lack of oxygen and opsonins prevents phagocytosis.

Factors which concentrate particulate matter at a particular site, and at the same time maintain flow, may well enhance phagocytosis. The balance between the coagulation and the fibrinolytic systems is important in this respect. Congested haemoconcentrated blood may nevertheless be kept free-moving by an effective fibrinolytic system. The role of oestrogens here could be significant since they appear to enhance fibrinolysis and phagocytic potential and at the same time increase permeability. This localised increase in permeability is a factor turning up in almost every aspect of vasculitis. It is a feature of gravitational eczema and ulcers (see Chapter 12), and it is prominent in collagen vascular disease (Marks, Birkett and Shuster, 1972). The localisation of immune complexes extravascularly, where they often do most damage, is discussed in Chapter 7. Anything that increases local permeability may allow harmful circulating material to become lodged extravascularly where the mononuclear phagocytic system may or may not be able to deal with it.

The factor stimulating phagocytic activity in Kupffer cells is dependent more on heparin availability than on complement (Saba, 1970). Saba argued that heparin, by altering the dynamics of the coagulation process, probably encourages larger amounts of altered fibrinogen to be locally available and that this affects chemotaxis, clotting, particle charge and slippage. A variety of plasma proteins participate in opsonic activity; many of them acting as antibody impart specificity to the system.

The phagocytic mononuclear system is important in vasculitis, stasis and ischaemia because of its role in removing noxious agents and the by-products of inflammation and repair. Its local performance contributes significantly to the constitution and is, in turn, influenced by age, organ size, weight, blood flow, temperature, cellular metabolism, hormone levels and cell population dynamics (Saba, 1970).

References

Archer, R. K. (1963) *The Eosinophil Leucocytes.* Oxford: Blackwell.
Asboe-Hansen, G. (1964) Connective tissue response to injury. In *Injury, Inflammation and Immunity* (Ed.) Thomas, L., Uhr, J. W. & Grant, L. p. 22. Baltimore: Williams and Wilkins.
Baart de la Faille Kuyper, E. H., Van der Meer, J. B. & Baart de la Faille, H. (1974) An immunohistochemical study of the skin of healthy individuals. *Acta Dermato-venereologica,* **54,** 271.
Ballow, M., Ward, G. W., Gershwin, M. E. & Day, N. K. (1975) C_1 by pass complement-activation pathway in patients with chronic urticaria and angio-oedema. *Lancet,* **ii,** 248.
Copeman, P. W. M. & Ryan, T. J. (1970) The problems of cutaneous angiitis with reference to histopathology and pathogenesis. *British Journal of Dermatology,* **82,** Supplement 5, 2.
Haxthausen, H. (1930) *Cold in Relation to Skin Diseases.* Copenhagen: Levin & Munksgaard.
Henson, P. M. (1969) Role of complement and leukocytes in immunologic release of vasoactive amines in platelets. *Federation Proceedings,* **28,** 1721.

Jacobson, C. D. (1968) *Studies on the Plasminogen Plasmin System of Human Plasma with Special Reference to Methodology and Genetics.* Thesis, University of Oslo.

James, J. & Warin, R. P. (1969) Factitious wealing at the site of previous cutaneous response. *British Journal of Dermatology,* **81,** 882.

James, J. & Warin, R. P. (1970) Chronic urticaria. The effect of aspirin. Letter. *British Journal of Dermatology,* **32,** 204.

Juhlin, L. & Michaelsson, G. (1971) Abnormal cutaneous reactions to a nicotinic acid ester. *Acta Dermatovenereologica,* **51,** 448.

Kowalewski, K., Russel, J. C. & Koheil, A. (1969) Blood and tissue histamine in mice, rats, hamsters and guinea pigs. *Proceedings of the Society for the Comparative Study of Experimental Biology and Medicine,* **132,** 443.

Lai A. Fat, R. F. M., Cormane, R. H. & Van Furth, R. (1974) An immunohistopathological study and the synthesis of immunoglobulins and complement in normal and pathological skin and the adjacent mucous membrane. *British Journal of Dermatology,* **90,** 123.

MacDuffie, F. C., Mitchell-Sams, W., Maldonado, J. E., Andreini, P. H., Conn, D. L. & Samayoa, E. A. (1973) Hypocomplementaemia with cutaneous vasculitis and arthritis. Possible immune complex syndrome. *Mayo Clinic Proceedings,* **48,** 340.

Marks, J. & Shuster, S. (1966) Method for measuring capillary permeability and its use in patients with skin diseases. *British Medical Journal,* **ii,** 88.

Marks, J., Birkett, D. A. & Shuster, S. (1972) "Capillary permeability" in patients with collagen vascular diseases. *British Medical Journal,* **i,** 782.

Michaelsson, G., Pettersson, L. & Juhlin, L. (1974) Purpura caused by food and drug additives. *Archives of Dermatology,* **109,** 49.

Ryan, T. J. (1969) A study of the epidermal capillary unit in psoriasis. *Dermatologica,* **138,** 459.

Ryan, T. J., Nishioka, K. & Dawber, R. P. R. (1971) Epithelial—endothelial interactions in the control of inflammation through fibrinolysis. *British Journal of Dermatology,* **84,** 501.

Saba, T. M. (1970) Physiology and physiopathology of the reticuloendothelial system. *Archives of Internal Medicine,* **126,** 1031.

Schayer, R. W. (1962) Evidence that induced histamine is an intrinsic regulator of the microcirculatory system. *American Journal of Physiology,* **202,** 66.

Schayer, R. W. (1964) Histamine and the autonomous responses of the microcirculation relationship to glucocorticoid action. *Annals of the New York Academy of Sciences,* **116,** 891.

Seah, P. P., Fry, L., Mazaheri, M. R. & Mowbray, J. F. (1973) Alternate pathway complement fixation by IgA in the skin in dermatitis herpetiformis. *Lancet,* **ii,** 175.

Siraganian, R. P. (1972) Platelet requirement in the interaction of the complement and clotting systems. *Nature,* **239,** 208.

Sissons, J. G. P. (1974) Cutaneous vasculitis and hypocomplementaemia. *Proceedings of the Royal Society of Medicine,* **67,** 654.

Sondergaard, J. & Greaves, M. W. (1971) Prostaglandin E1, effect on human cutaneous vasculature and skin histamine. *British Journal of Dermatology,* **84,** 424.

Srichaikul, T., Puwasatien, P., Puwasatien, P., Karnjanjetanee, J. & Bokisch, V. A. (1975) Complement changes and disseminated intravascular coagulation in plasmodium falciparum malaria. *Lancet,* **i,** 770.

Størmorken, H. (1969) The release reaction of secretion. *Scandinavian Journal of Haematology,* Supplement **9,** 1.

Témine, M. (1956) In *Les Troubles Trophiques des Membres Inférieur d'Origine Veineuse* (Ed.) Charpy, P. T. p. 263. Paris: Masson et Cie.

Wilhelm, D. L. (1971) Increased vascular permeability in acute inflammation. *Revue Canadienne de Biologie,* **30,** 153.

Winkelmann, R. K. & Ditto, W. B. (1964) Cutaneous and visceral syndromes of necrotising or allergic angiitis. A study of thirty-eight cases. *Medicine* (Baltimore), **43,** 59.

Wright, A. E. & Douglas, S. R. (1903) An experimental investigation of the role of the blood fluids in connection with phagocytosis. *Proceedings of the Royal Society,* **72,** 357.

Ygge, J. (1969) Variation in the individual subject of some parameters in blood coagulation and fibrinolysis. A longitudinal study in young healthy women. *Scandinavian Journal of Haematology,* **6,** 343.

MALIGNANCY

Lethal reticuloendothelial diseases predispose to necrotising vasculitis (Sams, Harville and Winkelmann, 1968) and Ryan (1968) has described vascular proliferation and necrosis in skin reticuloses where there probably is a failure to clear the products of a metabolically active skin. Bard and Winklemann (1967) described vasculitis in sarcoidosis and in Hodgkin's disease and other reticuloses. Perreau et al (1971) described polyarteritis nodosa in association with lymphoma, and Perry and Winkelmann (1972) reported pyoderma gangrenosum in three cases of leukaemia.

The role of malignancy in determining why and when vasculitis develops in some patients but not others has been insufficiently studied, considering the frequency of the association. There have in fact been many relevant reports, for instance: erythema nodosum has been described in Hodgkin's disease, leukaemia (Pinski and Stanisfer, 1964; Sams and Winklemann, 1968), and after radiotherapy for pelvic malignancy (Ryan and Wilkinson, 1972) (see page 237); Copeman (1970) too has emphasised this relationship, and McCombs (1965) described five cases of vasculitis in association with lymphoproliferative disorders. Figure 6.5 illustrates the vasculitis which was the presenting sign in one fulminant case of Hodgkin's disease. Urticaria, anaphylactoid

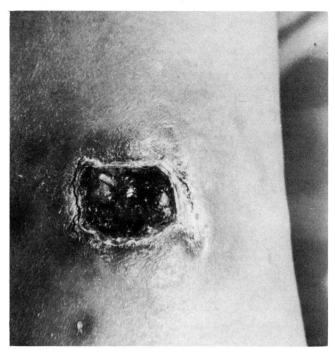

Figure 6.5. Infarct localised to the calf as the presenting sign of Hodgkin's disease from which the patient died a few months later.

purpura and angioneurotic oedema were reported by Kamenetskii and Reiderman (1965) to be present in a case of hypernephroma and in two cases of cancer of the stomach. In these cases the skin manifestations were the presenting sign, and in a patient with carcinoma of the breast, they heralded widespread metastasisation.

Several manifestations of this association are noteworthy, thus nodular vasculitis in the subcutaneous tissues is a not infrequent complication of cancer of the pancreas (De Graciansky et al, 1965), and arteritis in association with malignant reticuloses was described by Scheuer-Karpin and d'Heureuse-Gerhardt (1965). Palmer and Vedi (1974) described digital vascular disease in one case of reticulum cell sarcoma and in two cases of abdominal cancer, and gangrene of the fingers in malignant disease was described by

Hawley, Johnston and Rankin (1967) (Table 6.2, Figure 6.6). The underlying mechanism is not known in these cases. Palmer and Vedi (1974) suggested that immune complexes might be responsible on the basis of evidence from case 6 of Hawley, Johnston and Rankin (1967) and from the vasculitis described in a case reported by Friedman, Bienenstock and Richter (1969).

Table 6.2. Malignancies reported in association with digital ischaemia.

No.	Age	Sex	Neoplasm	Severity of changes	Authors
1	59	F	Carcinoma of maxillary antrum	Gangrene	
2	54	F	Hypernephroma	Gangrene	
3	45	F	Carcinoma ovary, colon and uterus	Raynaud's phenomenon Splinter haemorrhages	Hawley, Johnston and Rankin (1967)
4	45	F	Carcinoma ovary	Gangrene	
5	58	F	Carcinoma stomach or pancreas	Raynaud's phenomenon	
6	42	F	Hodgkin's disease Cryoglobulinaemia	Gangrene	
7	32	F	Carcinoma cervix	Gangrene	
					Friedman, Bienenstock and Richter, 1969
8	57	F	Carcinoma breast	Gangrene (toes and fingers)	
9	7	M	Acute lymphatic leukaemia	Gangrene	Powell, 1973
10	62	F	Reticulum-cell sarcoma	Pre-gangrene	
11	74	F	Carcinoma stomach or pancreas	Splinter haemorrhages Pulp atrophy	Palmer and Vedi, 1974
12	66	F	Carcinoma stomach	Splinter haemorrhages Pulp atrophy	

Another reaction pattern consists of symmetrical violaceous plaques of the extremities with a histological picture that includes coagulation necrosis; this is seen in elderly men with monocytosis and neutropenia. The differential diagnosis of the clinical lesions in such cases includes perniosis or sarcoidosis (Marks, Lim and Borrie, 1969), and when first described they were recorded as showing a 'low-grade arteritis with mild fibrinoid necrosis' and were named chilblain lupus erythematosus (Marks, 1967).

The effect of malignancy on the coagulation system is described in Chapter 10. Patients with malignant disease produce thrombi very much earlier in the postoperative period than do patients treated regularly for other diseases (Roberts et al, 1972). Hills et al (1972) used intermittent compression of the calf to reduce postoperative venous thrombosis in non-malignant disease but found that it gave no such protection in malignancy. However, Roberts and Cotton (1974) introduced an improved method of maintaining venous blood flow and managed to reduce the frequency of deep vein thrombosis even in malignant disease. In an endeavour to find an explanation Sun et al (1974) studied 61 patients with various malignancies associated with intravascular coagulation with fibrinolysis. They suggested that chronic depletion of coagulation factors followed by a compensatory increase in their production may be the reason.

The phagocytic system is more active in some neoplastic diseases (Salky et al, 1967); however, opsonic activity is decreased in others (Pisano, Di Luzio and Salky, 1970) and cytotoxic factors inhibiting lymphocyte transformation were found in the sera of patients with lymphoma by Langner, Pawinska-Proniewska and Glinski (1971).

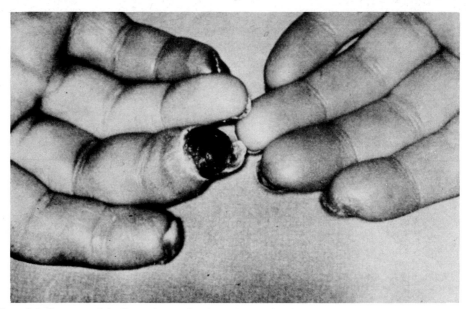

Figure 6.6. Gangrene of the finger tip associated with internal malignancy.

The skin reactivity in patients with cancer was studied by Johnson, Maibach and Salmon (1971) and they found that delayed hypersensitivity to 2,4-dinitrochlorobenzene was impaired. Perhaps even more significant was their observation that the skin of such patients also failed to react to the nonspecific inflammatory stimulus of 10 per cent croton oil solution. Judged by a study of allergy in patients with malignant lymphoma and chronic lymphocytic leukaemia (McCormick et al, 1971), such a depression of reactivity cannot be blamed entirely on therapy but could be related to circulating IgE levels. Thus, patients with hyporeactive skin may have lower serum levels of IgE, whereas the hyper-reactivity in the atopic diathesis is related to high levels of IgE. Dermographism, which is present in at least five per cent of the general population, has also been explained by IgE levels (Aoyama, 1971). Such impairment of the early phases of the inflammatory response in malignancy may be associated with an exhausted or inhibited fibrinolytic system and hence an enhanced deposition of fibrin is to be expected (see Chapter 10).

References

Aoyama, H. (1971) IgE as a dermographism—inducing principle of urticaria factitia. *Japanese Journal of Dermatology,* **81B,** 266.
Bard, J. W. & Winkelmann, R. K. (1967) Livedo reticularis, segmental hyalinizing vasculitis of the dermis. *Archives of Dermatology,* **96,** 489.
Copeman, P. W. M. (1970) Investigations into the pathogenesis of acute cutaneous angiitis. *British Journal of Dermatology,* **82,** Supplement 5, 51.
De Graciansky, P., Paraf, A., Rautureau, J. & Texier, J. (1965) Panniculite nodulaire ague fébrile récidivante au course d'un cancer 'acineux' de pancreas. Le problème de la maladie de Weber—Christian. *Bulletin de la Société Médicale des Hôpitaux de Paris,* **116,** 261.
Friedman, S. A., Bienenstock, H. & Richter, I. H. (1969) Malignancy and arteriopathy. *Angiology,* **20,** 136.
Hawley, P. R., Johnston, A. W. & Rankin, J. T. (1967) Association between digital ischaemia and malignant disease. *British Medical Journal,* **iii,** 208.

Hills, N. H., Pflug, J. J., Jeyasingh, K., Boardman. L. & Calnan, J. S. (1972) Prevention of deep vein thrombosis by intermittent pneumatic compression of calf. *British Medical Journal*, **i**, 131.

Johnson, M. W., Maibach, H. I. & Salmon, S. E. (1971) Skin reactivity in patient with cancer: impaired delayed hypersensitivity or faulty inflammatory response. *New England Journal of Medicine*, **284**, 1255.

Kamenetskii, S. I. & Reiderman, M. L. (1965) Athrombopenic anaphylactoid purpura and similar conditions: malignant neoplasms. *Klinicheskaya Meditsina* (Moskva), **43**, 117.

Langner, A., Pawinska-Proniewska, M. & Glinski, W. (1971) Cytotoxic factors in inhibitions of lymphocyte transformation in lymphomata. *British Journal of Dermatology*, **85**, 7.

McCombs, R. P. (1965) Systemic 'allergic' vasculitis; clinical and pathological relationships. *Journal of the American Medical Association*, **194**, 1059.

McCormick, D. P., Ammann, A. J., Ishizaka, K., Miller, D. G. & Hong, R. (1971) Study of allergy in patients with malignant lymphoma and chronic lymphocytic leukaemia. *Cancer*, **27**, 93.

Marks, R. (1967) Chilblain lupus erythematosus as a manifestation of lymphoma. *Proceedings of the Royal Society of Medicine*, **60**, 12.

Marks, R., Lim, C. C. & Borrie, P. F. (1969) Aperniotic syndrome with monocytosis and neutropenia. A possible association with a pre-leukaemic state. *British Journal of Dermatology*, **81**, 327.

Palmer, H. M. & Vedi, K. K. (1974) Digital ischaemia and malignant disease. *Practitioner*, **213**, 819.

Perreau, P., Bertrand, G., Gardias, J. & Pithon, G. (1971) Periartèrite noueuse et lymphôme malin. *Archives Médicales de l'Ouest*, **3**, 489.

Perry, H. O. & Winkelmann, R. K. (1972) Bullous pyoderma gangrenosum and leukaemia. *Archives of Dermatology*, **106**, 901.

Pinski, J. B. & Stanisfer, P. D. (1964) Erythema nodosum as the initial manifestation of leukaemia. *Archives of Dermatology*, **89**, 339.

Pisano, J. C., Di Luzio, N. R. & Salky, N. K. (1970) Depletion of serum opsonic activity in humans with neoplastic disease. *Journal of the Reticuloendothelial Society*, **7**, 633.

Powell, K. R. (1973) Raynaud's phenomenon preceding acute lymphatic leukaemia. *Journal of Pediatrics*, **82**, 539.

Roberts, V. C. & Cotton, L. T. (1974) Prevention of postoperative deep vein thrombosis in patients with malignant disease. *British Medical Journal*, **i**, 358.

Roberts, V. C., Berguer, R., Clark, A. W. & Cotton, L. T. (1972) Prevention of deep vein thrombosis. *British Medical Journal*, **i**, 628.

Ryan, T. J. (1968) The blood supply of the epidermis in the reticuloses. *British Journal of Dermatology*, **80**, 298.

Ryan, T. J. & Wilkinson, D. S. (1972) Cutaneous vasculitis angiitis. In *Textbook of Dermatology* (Ed.) Rook, A., Wilkinson, D. S. & Ebling, F. P. G. 2nd edition, p. 920. Oxford: Blackwell.

Salky, N. K., Di Luzio, N. R., Levin, A. G. & Goldsmith, H. S. (1967) Phagocytic activity of the reticuloendothelial system in neoplastic disease. *Laboratory and Clinical Medicine*, **70**, 393.

Sams, W. M. & Winkelmann, R. K. (1968) The association of erythema nodosum with ulcerative colitis. *Southern Medical Journal*, **61**, 676.

Sams, W. M. Jr, Harville, D. D. & Winkelmann, R. K. (1968) Necrotising vasculitis associated with lethal reticuloendothelial diseases. *British Journal of Dermatology*, **80**, 555.

Scheuer-Karpin, R. & d'Heureuse-Gerhardt, R. (1965) Proceedings of the Third Congress of the Asian and Pacific Society of Haematology. *Israel Journal of Medical Sciences*, **1**, 819.

Sun, N. C. J., Bowie, E. J. W., Kazmier, F. J., Elveback, L. R. & Owen, C. A. (1974) Blood coagulation studies in patients with cancer. *Mayo Clinic Proceedings*, **49**, 636.

THE INFLUENCE OF SEX HORMONES

During the first half of the menstrual cycle the ovary secretes increasing amounts of 17β-oestradiol under the influence of the pituitary. The oestrogen, in its turn, causes a burst of pituitary activity at mid-cycle, which can be inhibited by stress. This is followed by progesterone secretion by the ovary and then the second rise and subsequent fall of oestrogen and progesterone prior to menstruation. In some animals oestrogen and progesterone stimulate prostaglandin F_2 production by the endometrium. These hormones, particularly the oestrogen—progesterone combination in the second half of the cycle, prepare the endometrium to receive the fertilised ovum and are also responsible for secondary sexual development.

Menstruation is due to profound instability and spasm of the vascular tree following withdrawal of oestrogen.

At the menopause, gradually decreasing levels of oestrogen and increasing secretion of pituitary hormones are indicative of a loss of feedback control. Endometrial growth is reduced and the secretory phase normally encouraged by progesterone is lacking. Secondary sexual characteristics tend to be reduced.

Oral contraceptives provide a steady level both of oestrogen, that suppresses pituitary activity, and of progesterone, which prevents endometrial hyperplasia. The interpretation of some of the side-effects of oral contraceptives, as compared to pregnancy or the menopause, must take into account their being synthetic agents. Natural oestrogens, for instance, seem to have little effect on coagulation and fibrinolysis (Notelovitz and Greig, 1974), whereas synthetic analogues are associated with a 'hypercoagulable' state in which the "blood forms thrombi more readily in vivo than other blood when subjected to the same stimulus" (Kim et al, 1963; Leader, *Lancet,* December 14th, 1974). Nevertheless, the platelet count falls shortly before menstruation and the prothrombin time is at the same time prolonged (Catel and Schotola, 1940).

The influence of the menstrual cycle, pregnancy and oral contraceptives on vasculitis is an important but still much debated issue. There also is a significant sex difference in the incidence of diseases affecting the vasculature. Pregnancy is one of the main preparatory states for the Shwartzman phenomenon in rabbits (McKay, 1963) and there is a slow state of intravascular coagulation and reduced fibrinolysis in toxaemia of pregnancy (Wardle and Menon, 1969); in addition, cryofibrinogen levels are raised even in normal pregnancy (McKay and Corey, 1964).

Many diseases have a premenstrual exacerbation and these tend to improve during pregnancy. Premenstrual changes in vascular permeability and in tissue fluid may explain exacerbations of such non-dermatological disorders as epilepsy, vertigo or the carpal-tunnel syndrome.

During menstruation engorgement of the nasal mucosa is a well recognised feature (Mortimer, Wright and Collip, 1936; Dalton, 1964, 1969); varicose veins (Rivlin, 1955) and spontaneous bruising are more troublesome (Billig and Spaulding, 1947); and purpura and epistaxis are well-known (Weiner, 1947) as is a menstrual vasculitis of the erythema multiforme type (Figure 6.7). In the fourth week of the cycle there is increased capillary fragility and permeability (Brewer, 1938; Clemetson, Blair and Brown, 1962) with stasis and arteriolar narrowing in the nail-fold vessels (Hagen, 1922). Premenstrual prominence of naevi (Bean, 1958) and increased skin temperature, probably due to shunting, may be observed (Edwards and Duntley, 1949; Dintenfass, Julian and Miller, 1966).

Oestrogen tends to loosen the vascular support to vessels and encourages vasodilatation, whereas progesterone reduces vascular smooth muscle tone. Increased numbers of endothelial pores were noted in rabbit vessels under the influence of oestrogen (Wolff and Merker, 1966; Wolff, Schwartz and Merker, 1967). Taylor (1961) recorded an increase in the size of vessel lumina in the nose of the rabbit and rat after the administration of oestrogens and, in the rabbit, during pregnancy; he referred to a large pre-World War II literature on the subject. Bicknell (1971) described vascular proliferation in the nasal mucosa during the fifth month of pregnancy, and bleeding from this site was thought to be due to thrombocytopenia and hypothrombinaemia.

Oestrogens and possibly prolactin are the strongest of agents stimulating carbon clearance from the circulatory system, and they possibly constitute the principal natural stimulant of the body defences (Nicol and Bilbey, 1960; Nicol et al, 1964). The technique of carbon clearance may, however, merely indicate two phases of increased vascular permeability which facilitate the escape of cells of the macrophage system from the bloodstream into the tissues, particularly those in the endometrium. While women may be more efficient at 'leaking' immune complexes into the tissues, they are consequently more likely to develop immune complex disease.

Erythema nodosum has been related to the ingestion of oral contraceptives (Holcomb, 1965; Matz, 1967; Baden and Holcomb, 1968; Savel, Madison and Meeker, 1970; Darlington, 1974); oral ulceration (Dalton, 1955) and Behçet's syndrome are worse premenstrually; and Shelley, Preucel and Spoont (1964) reported a case of Behçet's syndrome which always became worse with menstruation and was suppressed by progesterone. Furthermore, many patterns of vasculitis, particularly the chronic intermittent non-infarctive forms, have premenstrual exacerbations.

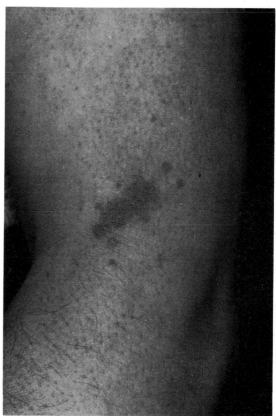

Figure 6.7. Vasculitis appearing monthly at time of menstruation.

Lupus erythematosus in the reproductive years is a disease predominantly of women but it affects the sexes equally in childhood and old age (Dubois and Tuffanelli, 1964). The effect of pregnancy on systemic lupus erythematosus is very variable, although post-partum exacerbation is common.

On the other hand, oestrogens appear to protect women from the cardiovascular disease so commonly encountered in men, and their withdrawal coincides with an increasing incidence of osteoporosis.

The menstrual period was at one time considered to be a bad time to apply patch tests or to perform the Dick test for scarlet fever (Hansen-Pruss and Raymond, 1942). The reactivity to allergens was said to be highest on the last day of menstruation, and to be lowest on the day before the onset of menstruation. In other words, the greatest reactivity coincides with the period of oestrogen deprivation. By contrast, oestrogen given parenterally to mice, at the same time that the animals were infected with *Escherichia coli*, caused more animals to develop pyelonephritis (Hurle, Bullen and Thomson, 1975).

References

Baden, H. P. & Holcomb, F. D. (1968) Erythema nodosum from oral contraceptives. *Archives of Dermatology*, **98**, 634.

Bean, W. B. (1958) *Vascular Spiders and Related Lesions of the Skin.* Springfield, Illinois; Charles C. Thomas.

Bicknell, P. G. (1971) Granulomata arising in the nasal mucosa during pregnancy. *Journal of Laryngology and Otology*, **85**, 515.

Billig, H. E. & Spaulding, C. A. (1947) Hyperinsulinism of menses. *Industrial Medicine*, **16**, 336.

Brewer, J. I. (1938) Rhythmic changes in the skin capillaries and their relation to menstruation. *American Journal of Obstetrics and Gynecology*, **36**, 597.

Catel, W. & Schotola, H. (1940) Über beziehungen zwischen hrombozyten menstruation und corpusluteum-hormon. *Medizinische Klinik*, **36**, 973.

Clemetson, C. A., Blair, L. & Brown, A. B. (1962) Capillary strength and the menstrual cycle. *Annals of the New York Academy of Sciences*, **116**, 990.

Dalton, K. (1955) Discussion on the premenstrual syndrome. *Proceedings of the Royal Society of Medicine*, **48**, 337.

Dalton, K. (1964) *The Premenstrual Syndrome.* London: William Heinemann Medical Books.

Dalton, K. (1969) *The Menstrual Cycle.* London: Penguin.

Darlington, L. G. (1974) Erythema nodosum and oral contraceptives. *British Journal of Dermatology*, **90**, 209.

Dintenfass, L., Julian, D. G. & Miller, G. (1966) Viscosity of blood in healthy young women. *Lancet*, **i**, 234.

Dubois, E. L. & Tuffanelli, D. L. (1964) Clinical manifestations of systemic lupus erythematosus. Computer analysis of 520 cases. *Journal of the American Medical Association*, **190**, 104.

Edwards, E. A. & Duntley, S. Q. (1949) Cutaneous vascular changes in women in reference to the menstrual cycle and ovariectomy. *American Journal of Obstetrics and Gynecology*, **57**, 501.

Hagen, W. (1922) Periodische, konstitutionelle und pathologische schwankungen im verhalten der Blut-capillaren. *Archiv für Pathologische anatomie und Physiologie*, **239**, 504.

Hansen-Pruss, O. C. & Raymond, R. (1942) Skin reactivity during the menstrual cycle. *Journal of Clinical Endocrinology*, **2**, 161.

Holcomb, F. D. (1965) Erythema nodosum associated with the use of an oral contraceptive. Report of a case. *Obstetrics and Gynecology*, **25**, 156.

Hurle, E. M. J., Bullen, J. J. & Thomson, D. A. (1975) Influence of oestrogens on experimental pyelonephritis caused by Escherichia coli. *Lancet*, **ii**, 283.

Kim, D. N., Lee, K. T., Kiokarn, Y. & Thomas, W. A. (1963) Dietary lipids and thrombosis; studies of the role of surface factors in the production of the 'hypercoagulable states'. *Experimental Molecular Pathology*, **2**, Supplement 1, 62.

McKay, D. G. (1963) A partial synthesis of generalized Shwartzman reaction. *Federation Proceedings*, **22**, 1373.

McKay, D. G. & Corey, A. E. (1964) Cryofibrinogenemia in toxemia of pregnancy. *Obstetrics and Gynecology*, **23**, 508.

Matz, M. H. (1967) Erythema nodosum and contraceptive medication. *New England Journal of Medicine*, **278**, 351.

Mortimer, H., Wright, R. P. & Collip, J. B. (1936) Effect of administration of oestrogenic hormones on nasal mucosa; their role in naso sexual relationship; and their significance in clinical rhinology. *Canadian Medical Association Journal*, **35**, 503, 615.

Nicol, T. & Bilbey, B. L. J. (1960) The effect of various steroids on the phagocytic activity of the R.E.S. In *Reticulo-endothelial Structure and Function* (Ed.) Heller, J. H. p. 301. New York: Ronald Press.

Nicol, T., Bilbey, B. L. J., Charles, L. M., Dingley, J. L. & Vernon-Roberts, B. (1964) Oestrogen: the natural stimulant of body defence. *Journal of Endocrinology*, **30**, 27.

Notelovitz, M. & Greig, H. B. W. (1974) Effect of natural oestrogens on coagulation. *British Medical Journal*, **iii**, 171.

Savel, H., Madison, J. F. & Meeker, C. I. (1970) Cutaneous eruptions and in vitro lymphocyte hypersensitivity with oral contraceptives and mestranol. *Archives of Dermatology*, **101**, 187.

Shelley, W. B., Preucel, R. W. & Spoont, S. S. (1964) Autoimmune progesterone dermatitis; cure by oophorectomy. *Journal of the American Medical Association*, **190**, 35.

Taylor, M. (1961) An experimental study of the influence of the endocrine system on the nasal respiratory mucosa. *Journal of Laryngology and Otology*, **75**, 521.

Wardle, E. N. & Menon, I. S. (1969) Slow state of intravascular coagulations and reduced fibrinolysis in toxaemia. *British Medical Journal*, **ii**, 625.

Weiner, K. (1947) *Skin Manifestations of Internal Disorders.* p. 351. London: Henry Kimpton.

Wolff, J. & Merker, H. J. (1966) Ultrastruktur und Bildung von Poren im endothel von Porosen und geschlossenen Kapillaren. *Zeitschrift für Zellforschung und Mikroskopische Anatomie*, **73**, 174.

Wolff, J., Schwarz, W. & Merker, H. J. (1967) Influence of hormones on the ultrastructure of capillaries. *Bibliography of Anatomy*, **9**, 334.

7. Immunological Aspects of Vasculitis

In recent years the immunological basis of vasculitis has received intense and detailed analysis, aimed chiefly at the role of triggers, such as immune complexes, and at cellular immunity, particularly with respect to the vascular injury in transplanted tissues. Readers of the vast literature on this subject can easily become confused by the finer points, most of which are still debated. To avoid such side issues one should remember that in vasculitis it is endothelial damage that matters most, and one should not lose sight of the relationship of the immunological reaction to this (Figure 7.1).

Immunological injury to endothelium occurs at three levels:

1. Primary and specific injury occurs when the antibody formed is directed specifically against the endothelial cell or when the endothelial cell is 'attacked' by lymphocytes.
2. Primary and nonspecific injury results from contact with circulating immune complexes which have no special affinity for the endothelial cell.
3. Secondary injury occurs when an immune reaction: (a) acts against neighbouring tissues such as basement membrane, smooth muscle, mast cells or adjacent epithelium, (b) is directed against foreign material such as mycobacteria or transplanted tissue, or (c) deposits nonspecific immune complexes in adjacent tissues, usually because of an increase in permeability which may or may not be the result of an earlier specific immunological reaction in the tissues, e.g. an IgE and mast cell interaction.

The endothelial cell responds to graded injury like any other cell. Irritation may merely make it more motile, phagocytic and secretory, or it may destroy it. If the injury is mild, then features such as increased permeability, stickiness to leucocytes, and release of activators of fibrinolysis will be the consequences. If the stimulus persists and the cell becomes exhausted, permeability will continue to be a feature but fibrinolysis will decrease and fibrin and platelet deposition will be enhanced. If the endothelial cell is killed it is shed and the blood passes more freely into the vessel wall unless a substantial thrombus prevents it.

None of this behaviour should be regarded as an inevitable consequence of a particular type of immunological injury. The intensity of action and the amount of a

135

noxious agent and the degree and rate of repair of the injury are dependent on numerous other variables. The response of endothelium to injury can be compared to the behaviour of the mast cell. This cell can be made to secrete its granules by a number of different immunological processes which, when very aggressive, will kill it. The rate of recovery also has to be taken into account. The urticarial or 'anaphylactic' behaviour of endothelium cannot be separated easily from its behaviour in more prolonged or delayed inflammatory states. This is why a spectral view has been taken in Chapters 3 and 4, and why, in this chapter, a strict adherence to a classification of immunological reactions such as that of Gell and Coombs (1963) is avoided.

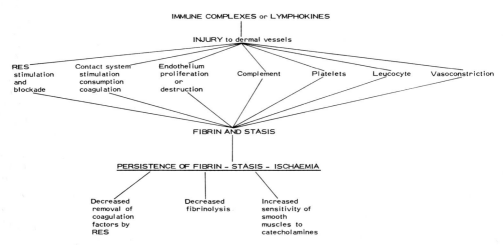

Figure 7.1. Injury to dermal vessels by immune complexes, the consequences of which are dependent on the effectiveness of the removal of fibrin and on the sensitivity of smooth muscle to catecholamines. RES = reticuloendothelial system.

One cannot look at a rash or at a histological section and be certain that it represents a particular type of immunological response, but one can assess the degree of vascular injury, permeability, ischaemia and leucocyte emigration. Thus it is wrong to regard every example of a leucocytoclastic angiitis as an Arthus reaction, for the same picture is produced by the Shwartzman phenomenon or by an acute reaction to physical injury.

The patterns of vascular response in inflammation as described by Wilhelm (1971) were divided into six phases or types, which are not specific in an immunological sense (Figure 6.2). In Wilhelm's classification the Arthus responses do not differ from those caused by surgical incision or by crush, chemical or thermal injury, and the response in cellular immunity can be mimicked by reactions to toxins or by ultraviolet radiation. It is because most responses are nonspecific that an immunological classification of vasculitis serves only as a partial explanation of the rash. Immune complexes, for instance, can produce all grades of vessel damage from urticaria and necrotising angiitis to granulomata (Cream and Turk, 1971).

ANTIBODY AND CELLULAR IMMUNITY AIMED AT ENDOTHELIAL CELLS

Stefanini and Mednicoff (1954), studying two cases of acute idiopathic thrombocytopenic purpura associated with Schönlein—Henoch anaphylactoid purpura, obtained a precipitin from the serum of these patients which acted against a saline-soluble antigen obtained from newborn aortic intima. This precipitin fixed complement and was a gamma-globulin. They followed this up by making a preparation of aortic antigen, and they found that it gave a positive precipitation reaction with sera from six out of eight cases of anaphylactoid purpura, and from three out of four cases of polyarteritis nodosa.

The fact that Katsura (1923) had produced purpura in guinea-pigs stimulated the study by Clark and Jacobs (1950) who were able to produce purpura in dogs with serum containing antibodies to vascular endothelium. Winkelmann, Kim and Wells (1964), however, were unable to reproduce this result in guinea-pigs, and Fabius (1959) had similar difficulty in 47 patients with vasculitis. These early experiments were updated with better control by Stefanini and his colleagues (Piomelli, Stefanini and Mele, 1959) in their studies on a specific antibody to endothelium. Their results led them to suggest that the precipitins referred to above are entirely nonspecific and that most cases of vasculitis are due to nonspecific damage by immune complexes. Paronetto and Strauss (1962) also failed to demonstrate any specific antibody to endothelium in a case of vasculitis. On the other hand, White and Grollman (1964) managed to produce a polyarteritis in the rat with an endothelial antibody, and Seaman, Marsical and Moffat (1971) caused multiple arterial emboli by injecting antivessel antibodies intra-arterially. However, circulating heart binding antibody has been demonstrated by Ellis, Lillehei and Zabriskie (1970a) and Goldman (1970) on sarcolemmal membrane but only rarely on endothelial elements (Ellis, Lillehei and Zabriskie, 1970b).

CIRCULATING IMMUNE COMPLEXES DAMAGING ENDOTHELIAL CELLS

Maurice Arthus (1903) sensitised a rabbit to human serum albumin and then injected the same material intradermally and produced erythema purpura and necrosis. It is now realised that circulating IgG antibody reacting with antigen and fixing complement is responsible for this inflammation. The sensitising material initially is not toxic but becomes so once it is complexed with the antibody and complement. Various studies by Opie (1924) and by other workers in subsequent years have demonstrated a close correlation between the intensity of the Arthus reaction and the amount of circulating antibody. Immunofluorescence techniques were used by Cochrane and Weigle (1958) and by many subsequent workers to show deposition of antigen, antibody and complement in vessel walls in the experimental Arthus reaction (Levenson and Cochrane, 1964).

It was postulated that circulating complexes were responsible for serum sickness (Germuth, 1953; Dixon et al, 1958), and in allergic vasculitis, the pronounced neutrophilic infiltrate which accompanies heavy deposition of immunoglobulin and complement led Stringa et al (1967) to compare the clinical picture to the Arthus phenomenon. Also, the belief, if true, that complement-fixing complexes attract polymorphonuclear leucocytes which then disintegrate and destroy the vessel (Cochrane, 1967) would explain the leucocytoclastic angiitis seen so commonly in vasculitis. The use of immune complexes to study leucocyte stickiness under direct vision in rabbit ear chambers (Cliff, 1966) has given the clearest possible evidence of the injury sustained by endothelium. Other such evidence has been derived from studies on intravascular coagulation induced by immune complexes or antigen in which shedding and subsequent circulation of endothelial cells indicates the damage done to the vessel wall (Wright and Giacometti, 1972; Evensen, Elgjo and Shepro, 1973). Circulating injured endothelial cells are also found in the Shwartzman phenomenon induced by circulating immune complexes (see Chapter 10). The large volume of work done in this field is reviewed by Cream and Turk (1971).

ANTIBODY DIRECTED AGAINST MAST CELLS AND BASOPHILS

This reaction depends on reaginic antibody, known as IgE. In the serum IgE is present in much lower concentrations than IgG, but its level tends to be increased in atopic states and parasitic infections. Its particular role is related to its affinity for the mast cell and the basophil. It attaches itself to these in such a way that the antigen-binding area of its molecule is exposed. Combination with allergen results in the release of cell contents to which there is an immediate but short-lasting reaction consisting predominantly of a marked increase in the permeability of capillaries and venules. This helps to rid mucosal surfaces of harmful antigen but it can, at the same time, cause circulating immune complexes to lodge in the tissues where they incite further activity.

Hypersensitivity reactions can be induced by a wide range of allergens which may either be 'complete', e.g. pollens, fungal products, the saliva and venom of insects and other animals, ingested food and applied cosmetics, or be 'haptens', e.g. penicillin and other allergenic drugs or simple industrial chemicals (Cruickshank, 1969). Such allergens may also induce IgG antibody formation but exactly which type of response occurs depends on the duration of the effect and constitutional factors such as the atopic diathesis. An important consequence of this IgE response is an increase in permeability that allows IgG complexes to settle deep in the tissues.

ANTIBODY TO BASEMENT MEMBRANE AND OTHER TISSUES

Studies of specific immunological attack on renal tissue in glomerulonephritis have been intense and productive. In particular the role of the streptococcus in the induction of glomerulonephritis has been analysed. Soluble fractions obtained from pooled human glomeruli have been shown to cross-react immunologically with similar fractions of cell membranes of streptococci type 12, known to be capable of inducing nephritis (Markowitz and Lange, 1964). The antigen is contained in the glomerular basement membrane. The renal response to streptococcal infection has been usefully reviewed by Freedman et al (1970) following their study of 1246 patients suffering from a beta haemolytic streptococcal upper respiratory tract infection. Damage to the kidney by the streptococcus was thought to be common and to lead to disturbances of structure and function. Occasionally there is a secondary immunological phase in which excess antibody is deposited in the renal tissue.

Administration of antiglomerular basement membrane antibody to animals causes nephritis. When the antibody and the basement membrane combine they form a product which is antigenic, and to this the host forms autoantibody. It is the combination of this autoantibody with the enjoined antibody and glomerular basement membrane that produces the immune complexes injurious to endothelium. The best known example of anti-basement membrane antibody occurs in Goodpasture's syndrome in which both renal and lung tissue are affected.

Studies such as those of Lai a Fat, Cormane and Furth (1974) have shown that immunoglobulins are often synthesised in the skin and mucosae by plasma cells and lymphocytes. The scattering of these cells suggests that they may reach the skin by the bloodstream rather than by proliferation locally in the tissues. As Kanan points out in Chapter 9, using the nose as a model, the presence of such cells in a tissue predisposes it to persistent localised flare-up reactions in response to circulating antigens.

ANTIBODY DIRECTED AT LOCALISED FOREIGN ANTIGEN

Good examples of immune complexes forming in situ are found in the mycobacterial diseases leprosy and tuberculosis. In erythema nodosa leprosum degenerating bacteria are found in the lesions and high levels of precipitating antibody are found in the serum (Turk, 1970). Immunoglobulin and complement are found in these lesions (Wemambu et al, 1969). Pepys (1972) has demonstrated similar Arthus-type lesions arising from circulating antibody directed at *Thermopolyspora polyspora* localised in the lung, and it is reasonable to suppose that gluten localised in the gut could be another form of local antigen to which antibody and complement combine to produce irritating complexes.

Polak, Frey and Turk (1970) used divalent chrome as an allergen to demonstrate that guinea-pigs sensitive to an inorganic metal experience a flare-up reaction when the antigen is injected intravenously. They blamed the formation of local immune complexes with antibody fixed in the skin as the cause of the reaction. Cream, Levene and Calnan (1971) studied a case of erythema elevatum diutinum and concluded that the persistent localisation and the recurrence of the vasculitis could have been due to fixed antibody to streptococcal antigen. Kanan in Chapter 9 draws attention to Cormane's observations on immunoglobulin-producing cells in the nose. These afford a persistent form of antibody and may thus account for persistent local pathology, should there be a circulating allergen; and one possible example akin to the studies of Polak, Frey and Turk (1970) is the recurrent inflammation in the nasal septum that used to be so common in chrome workers. Persistent recurrent injury of this kind explains the usually nonspecific Shwartzman phenomenon (see Chapter 10).

Prolonged active synthesis of immunoglobulins occurs locally in the synovial tissue and explains the persistence of chronic inflammatory reactions to antigen in the synovium in rheumatoid arthritis (Cooke and Jasin, 1972). It may even account for antigen remaining localised instead of being rapidly eliminated. These authors suggested that high levels of pre-existing circulating antibody result in the formation of antigen—antibody complexes that are more likely to persist for a prolonged period in the tissues.

VASCULAR DAMAGE IN TRANSPLANTATION

Several mechanisms for vascular injury in transplanted tissue may be postulated. The close association of lymphocyte blast cells with the cells of a foreign graft at the time of rejection contributes to the release of a number of directly injurious agents, and also attracts macrophages and polymorphs. Circulating antibodies induced by previous antigenic stimulus cause a more immediate hyper-acute response, namely vaso constriction of interlobular arteries (Klassen and Milgrom, 1971) or intravascular coagulation (Starzl et al, 1970).

Slowly progressive obliterative lesions occur in blood vessels of patients on immuno-suppressive drugs, and immunoglobulins and complement can be demonstrated in the vessel walls. Several groups of workers doubt the role of cellular immunity in such changes. But antibody to graft tissue has been eluted from damaged kidneys of these cases (Melzgar et al, 1972), and interest now lies in whether such antibodies, by shielding graft antigen, can be protective rather than cytotoxic. It is also conceivable that such protection could block the stimulus from the epidermis which is necessary for new vessel formation. In this way a wall of leucocytes or immunoglobulin lying between the epithelium and the blood vessels could provide an explanation of the vascular atrophy seen in several autoimmune diseases (Ryan, 1973).

BIOLOGICAL PROPERTIES OF IMMUNOGLOBULINS AND THE ROLE OF IMMUNE COMPLEXES

There are five types of immunoglobulins: IgD, IgE, IgA, IgM and IgG. *IgD* is the least understood; it does not fix complement but it is an antibody. Cormane and Giannetti (1971) believed it to have a role in contact dermatitis. *IgE* is a reaginic antibody; it fixes to basophil leucocytes and mast cells and when it then combines with antigen histamine is released. *IgA* is found predominantly in secretions such as milk, saliva, nasal mucus and gastrointestinal fluid, and it is formed locally in these tissues. It does not fix complement, and may therefore be less irritant when combined with antigen in the gut. It is not easily digested by trypsin and may protect the antigen to which it adheres. It forms non-absorbable stable complexes in the gut. Persons deficient in IgA have raised levels of anti-food antibodies in their blood (Ammann and Hong, 1970), and they are also more prone to autoimmune diseases. *IgM*, which is a large molecule with several binding sites is found mainly in serum. It combines with antigenic proteins and it also fixes complement. *IgG,* the main immunoglobulin class in man, is widely distributed in all tissues and in blood and unlike other immunoglobulins, even crosses the placenta. As it binds readily to the surface of macrophages, those immune complexes containing IgG are the more readily ingested. A subclass, IgG_3, forms cross-links when in excess or when cooled and accounts for increased blood viscosity in some cases of myelomatosis.

IgM, IgG, IgG_2 and IgG_3 are complement-fixing, whereas IgA, IgG_4 and IgE are not. Complement fixation leads to histamine release, chemotaxis of neutrophils and platelet clumping and lysis. As indicated above, the amount of damage done by immune complexes depends not only on their concentration and rate of removal but also on their site of activity, whether in the bloodstream, in the vessel wall or in the tissues. One important factor is the ratio of antibody to antigen in the complex. When antigen and antibody are combined in equivalent proportions, the aggregate is insoluble and is associated particularly with persistence in the tissues and with granuloma formation (Spector and Heesom, 1969). On the other hand, when antigen is in excess, the complex is smaller and is less easily phagocytosed by circulating macrophages. It therefore persists in the circulation and it can be shown to be more irritating when isolated and injected into the skin (Ishizaka and Campbell, 1958). Degradation of phagocytosed antigen is somewhat impaired when antibody is in excess; this is commonly the case when small amounts of antigen released from foci of infection or damaged tissues react with large numbers of antibody-producing cells located in other sites.

A single large dose of antigen often produces an acute and overwhelming immune complex disease in which complement is depleted and the brunt of the damage is borne by renal tissues, synovia and the small vessels throughout the body (Dixon et al,

1958; Dixon, Feldman and Vasquez, 1961). Repeated small doses of antigen are more likely to cause isolated glomerulonephritis. In skin disease, by analogy, a single acute episode is more likely to result from overwhelming single infection, whereas persistent or recurrent episodes of vasculitis require the presence of small foci of infection, persistently high levels of antibody and perhaps some additional localising factors in the skin. Also involved is a non-immunological hyper-reactivity of the tissues, equivalent to the prepared state observed in the Shwartzman phenomenon and a consequence of blockade of the monocyte—phagocytic system, of impaired fibrinolysis, or of both (see Chapter 10).

TIMING OF ARRIVAL AND CLEARANCE

Figure 7.2 illustrates the effect at five hours of suction applied to the skin for eight minutes in a patient with circulating immune complexes. The timing of the arrival and

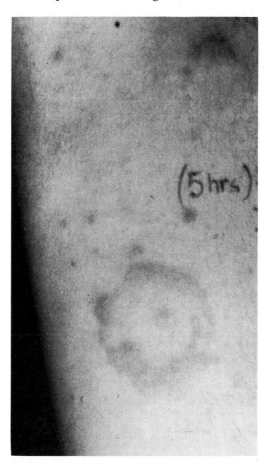

Figure 7.2. Reaction in the skin due to the localisation of immune complexes by suction for eight minutes, five hours earlier. A biopsy from this site showed immuno-fluorescence for IgG and complement as well as absence of fibrino-lysis.

disappearance of globulin and other agents in lesions is not known in most studies. However, Cream, Bryceson and Ryder (1971), studying the Arthus phenomenon in guinea-pigs, observed deposits of complement and gamma-globulin from 20 minutes onwards, coinciding with margination of polymorphs which seemingly ingested the deposits. By 30 minutes the vessel wall was outlined as a continuous ring of fluorescence. Cells began to migrate through the vessel wall at one hour and had spread widely in the tissues at four hours, by which time the vessels were already necrotic. From 8 to 18 hours all immunofluorescent globulin and complement had been cleared from the lesion.

Cochrane, Weigle and Dixon (1959) showed, by an immunofluorescence technique in the rabbit, that antigen had been largely removed from an Arthus reaction by 24 hours and was no longer detectable at 48 hours, whereas Eisen (1969), using autoradiography in the guinea-pig, noted that the antigen gradually disappeared after eight hours. Cream, Bryceson and Ryder (1971) made the point that immune complexes usually are no longer visible once haemorrhage is a feature.

Bianchi et al (1967), using the Rebuck skin window technique, found IgG and C'3 in polymorphonuclear leucocytes at the surface of experimentally scarified lesions in patients with vasculitis.

SPECIFICITY AND PATHOGENICITY

In the experimental animal it is certain that immune complexes, whether circulating or formed in situ, are capable of causing considerable injury. However, it is more difficult to be certain that they are the cause of injury in patients presenting with vasculitis. The presence of immune complexes in the circulation is not evidence of their pathogenicity, even though some authors feel strongly that there is a direct relationship between an abnormal complement-fixing antigen—antibody immune reaction and the pathogenesis of vasculitis (Heitmann and Kluken, 1970, 1971).

Increased capillary and venular permeability are responsible for trapping immuno-globulin in the tissues, and are the most likely explanation of heavy deposits in the vessels in diabetes mellitus, porphyria cutanea tarda, erythropoietic protoporphyria and amyloidosis (Baart de la Faille Kuyper and Cormane, 1968). Thus the mere presence of immunoglobulins or complement or both in the tissues does not mean that they are playing a primary pathogenic role, and even when antigen is demonstrable, its localisation in the tissues does not imply pathogenicity. Nevertheless, inflammation can be caused by such materials and undue protection by immunoglobulin can prevent their adequate removal, and this too can give rise to pathology.

Doubts about the significance of immunoglobulins in the tissues are partly due to technical problems such as whether small amounts of materials are pathogenic but are not detectable by present techniques. Masking can also prevent detection by immuno-fluorescence techniques. Other doubts arise because of lack of correlation between materials known to be circulating and those revealed in the tissues. Cream (1971), for instance, described IgG, IgA and IgM in the tissues but no IgA in the circulating complexes. Yet other doubts arise in cryoglobulinaemia for the clinical picture is not related to the amount of cryoglobulin present but to the constitutional response to it (Meltzer and Franklin, 1966). In one study (Cream, 1971) cryoglobulin components were found in the vessels of four patients, but in two of these non-cryoglobulin immunoglobulins were also present. In another two, no significant deposits were found. Cream offered three explanations for failure to show cryoglobulins at the site of vasculitis: (a) rapid removal, (b) masking and (c) insufficient amounts.

Concern that the detection of immune complexes in situ may be a nonspecific finding is enhanced by the presence of complement in pustulosis palmaris et plantaris and in generalised pustular psoriasis (Husky, Rajka and Larsen, 1973), as well as in ordinary psoriasis (Fierz, 1971) and in normal skin (Baart de la Faille Kuyper, Van der Meer and Baart de la Faille, 1974). The lack of correlation between levels of antibody and disease has been discussed both in relation to bullous disorders (Mitchell-Sams and Jordon, 1971) and in several studies of probands in whom levels of complement, antinuclear factor and rheumatoid factor were high yet overt disease was absent (Pollack, 1964; Svec and Viet, 1965; Whittingham et al, 1969; McDuffie, 1970; Bole and Ledger, 1971).

The question of specificity of immunofluorescence findings in lupus erythematosus has been discussed by Jablonska and Chorzelski (1974). Using these techniques the distinction can be made between (a) peripheral staining of nuclei by antinuclear antibodies, (b) diffuse homogenous staining of nuclei by antibodies against DNA—histone nucleoprotein, (c) speckled staining of nuclear ribonucleoprotein, and (d) nucleolar staining. These authors discussed overlap between lupus erythematosus, dermatomyositis and scleroderma. But even nucleolar antibody, which is more characteristic of scleroderma, was described in a titre of 1:5120 in the healthy mother of a patient with systemic lupus erythematosus (SLE). These authors believed that the titre of antinuclear factor reflects the dynamics of the disease in SLE but reveals nothing about the clinical activity of scleroderma. The difficulties of interpreting immunofluorescent staining of basement membrane are considerable because of the positive results in rosacea, lichen planus, polymorphic light eruption and porphyria, and these serve to emphasise therefore the value of a positive result in non-lesional skin in lupus erythematosus.

In very few cases the antigen has been isolated from tissues. In recent years examples receiving most interest have been Australia antigen (Gocke et al, 1970) and those listed in Table 7.1. Viruses are implicated also in the much-studied NZB/W mice and in Aleutian mink disease (see Chapter 8, page 167 in which the important observations of Parish on bacterial antigen are discussed).

IgG, attached to infective agents, tumours and the like, often incites the production of autoantibody. This is the basis of the rheumatoid factor and occurs in a number of autoimmune diseases (Torrigiani and Roitt, 1967; Klein et al, 1968; Barnett et al, 1970).

Table 7.1. Diseases in which isolation of antigen has been reported.

Systemic lupus erythematosus — DNA/anti-DNA (Tan et al, 1966; Koffler, Schur and Kunkel, 1967)
Nephrotic syndrome — *Plasmodium malariae* (Ward and Kibukamusoke, 1969)
Post-streptococcal nephritis (Treser et al, 1970)
Shunt nephritis, subacute bacterial endocarditis (Black, Challacombe and Ockenden, 1965; Stickler et al, 1968; Williams and Kunkel, 1962)
Glomerulonephritis — Australia antigen (Coombes et al, 1971)
Nephrotic syndrome — penicillamine (Lachmann, 1968)
Tumour-associated nephrotic syndrome (Loughridge and Lewis, 1971)
Proliferative glomerulonephritis — triple antigen (Sissons et al, 1974)

References

Ammann, A. J. & Hong, R. (1970) A selective IgA deficiency and autoimmunity. *Clinical and Experimental Immunology,* **7,** 833.
Arthus, M. (1903) Injections répétées de sérum de cheval chez le lapin. *Compte Rendu des Séances de la Société de Biologie,* **55,** 817.
Baart de la Faille Kuyper, E. H. & Cormane, R. H. (1968) The occurrence of certain serum factors in the dermal—epidermal junction and vessel walls of the skin in lupus erythematosus and other (skin) diseases. *Acta Dermato-venereologica,* **48,** 578.
Baart de la Faille Kuyper, E. H., Van der Meer, J. B. & Baart de la Faille, H. (1974) An immunohistochemical study of the skin of healthy individuals. *Acta Dermato-venereologica,* **54,** 271.

Barnett, E. V., Bluestone, R., Cracchiolo, A., Goldberg, L. S., Kantor, G. L. & McIntosh, R. M. (1970) Cryoglobulinemia and disease. *Annals of Internal Medicine,* **73,** 95.

Bianchi, C., Stringa, S., Casalá, A., Inglesini, C., Sanchez Avalos, J. C. & Vidal Pich, E. (1967) Allergic vasculitis: an immunofluorescence study of the cellular infiltrates obtained by the skin window method. *Dermatologica Ibero Latino-Americana,* **9,** 331.

Chakrabarti, R., Hocking, E. D. & Fearnley, G. R. (1969) Reaction pattern to three stresses — electropexy, surgery and myocardial infarction of fibrinolysis and plasma fibrinogen. *Journal of Clinical Pathology,* **22,** 659.

Clark, W. G. & Jacobs, E. (1950) Experimental non-thrombocytopenic vascular purpura: a review of the Japanese literature with preliminary confirmatory report. *Blood,* **5,** 320.

Cliff, W. J. (1966) The acute inflammatory reaction in the rabbit ear chamber with particular reference to the phenomenon of leukocyte migration. *Journal of Experimental Medicine,* **124,** 543.

Cochrane, C. G. (1967) Mediators of the Arthus and related reactions. *Progress in Allergy,* **11,** 1.

Cochrane, C. G. & Weigle, W. O. (1958) The cutaneous reaction to soluble antigen—antibody complexes. *Journal of Experimental Medicine,* **108,** 591.

Cochrane, C. G., Weigle, W. O. & Dixon, F. J. (1959) The role of polymorphonuclear leukocytes in the initiation and cessation of the Arthus vasculitis. *Journal of Experimental Medicine,* **110,** 480.

Cooke, T. D. & Jasin, H. E. (1972) The pathogenesis of chronic inflammation in experimental antigen induced arthritis. 1. The role of antigen on the local immune response. *Arthritis and Rheumatism,* **15,** 327.

Cormane, R. H. & Giannetti, A. (1971) IgD in various dermatoses; immunofluorescence studies. *British Journal of Dermatology,* **84,** 523.

Cream, J. J. (1971) Immunofluorescent studies of the skin in cryoglobulinaemic vasculitis. *British Journal of Dermatology,* **84,** 48.

Cream, J. J. (1972) Cryoglobulins in vasculitis. *Clinical and Experimental Immunology,* **10,** 117.

Cream, J. J. & Turk, J. L. (1971) A review of the evidence for immune complex deposition as a cause of skin disease in man. *Clinical Allergy,* **1,** 235.

Cream, J. J., Bryceson, A. D. M. & Ryder, G. (1971) Disappearance of immunoglobulin and complement from the Arthus reaction and its relevance to studies of vasculitis in man. *British Journal of Dermatology,* **84,** 106.

Cream, J. J., Levene, G. M. & Calnan, C. D. (1971) Erythema elevatum diutinum: an unusual reaction to streptococcal antigen and response to dapsone. *British Journal of Dermatology,* **84,** 393.

Cruickshank, C. N. D. (1969) Type I hypersensitivity and the skin. *British Journal of Dermatology,* **81,** 7.

Dixon, F. J., Feldman, J. D. & Vasquez, J. J. (1961) Experimental glomerulonephritis, the pathogenesis of a laboratory model resembling the spectrum of human glomerulonephritis. *Journal of Experimental Medicine,* **113,** 899.

Dixon, F. J., Vazquez, J. J., Weigle, W. D. & Cochrane, C. G. (1958) Pathogenesis of serum sickness. *Archives of Pathology,* **65,** 18.

Eisen, A. H. (1969) Fate of antigen in delayed hypersensitivity and Arthus reactions. *Journal of Immunology,* **103,** 1395.

Ellis, R. J., Lillehei, C. W. & Zabriskie, J. B. (1970a) Detection of circulating heart-reactive antibody in human heart transplants. *Journal of the American Medical Association,* **211,** 1505.

Ellis, R. J., Lillehei, C. W. & Zabriskie, J. B. (1970b) The significance of heart-binding antibody in human cardiac rejections. *Annals of Thoracic Surgery,* **10,** 432.

Evensen, S. A., Elgjo, R. F. & Shepro, D. (1973) Platelets, endothelium and the triggering mechanisms of intravascular coagulation. *Thrombosis et Diathesis Haemorrhagica,* Supplement **54,** 207.

Fabius, A. J. (1959) Failure to demonstrate precipitating antibodies against vessel extracts in patients with vascular disorders. *Vox Sanguinis,* **4,** 247.

Fierz, U. (1971) Ungereimtes der immunfluoresanz. *Dermatologica,* **142,** 274.

Freedman, P., Meister, H. P., Lee, H. J., Smith, E. A., Co, B. S. & Nidus, B. D. (1970) The renal response to streptococcal infections. *Medicine* (Baltimore), **49,** 433.

Fyrand, O. (1974) Heparin-precipitable fraction (HPF) in an unselected material of dermatological inpatients. *Acta Dermato-venereologica,* **54,** 293.

Gell, P. G. H. & Coombs, R. R. A. (1963) *Clinical Aspects of Immunology.* Oxford: Blackwell.

Germuth, F. G. Jr (1953) Comparative histologic and immunologic study in rabbits of induced hypersensitivity of the serum sickness type. *Journal of Experimental Medicine,* **97,** 257.

Gocke, D. J., Hsu, K., Morgan, C., Bombardieri, S., Lockshin, M. & Christian, C. L. (1970) Association between polyarteritis and Australia antigen. *Lancet,* **ii,** 1149.

Goldman, B. S. (1970) Discussion of the significance of heart binding antibody in human cardiac rejection. *Annals of Thoracic Surgery,* **10,** 441.

Gutman, R. A., Striker, G. E., Gilliland, B. C. & Cutler, R. E. (1972) The immune complex glomerulo-nephritis of bacterial endocarditis. *Medicine* (Baltimore), **51,** 1.

Heitmann, H. J. & Kluken, N. (1970) Immunofluorescenz-serologische Untersuchungen bei der vasculitis Ruiter. *Archiv für klinische und experimentelle Dermatologie,* **237,** 59.

Heitmann, H. J. & Kluken, N. (1971) Immunofluorescent serological studies in vasculitis superficialis "Ruiter". *British Journal of Dermatology*, **85**, 397.

Husky, G., Rajka, G. & Larsen, T. E. (1973) Immunofluorescence studies in pustular palmoplantaris. *Acta Dermato-venereologica*, **53**, 123.

Ishizaka, K. & Campbell, D. H. (1958) Biological activity of soluble antigen—antibody complexes. I. Skin reactive properties. *Proceedings of the Society for Experimental Biology and Medicine*, **97**, 635.

Jablonska, S. & Chorzelski, T. P. (1974) Lupus erythematosus. In *Immunological Aspects of Skin Diseases* (Ed.) Fry, L. & Seah, P. P. pp. 66-152. Lancaster England: Medical and Technical Publishing Company Ltd.

Katsura, H. (1923) Experimental study on purpura of guinea pigs. Purpura by the anti-haemangio endothelial cell serum. *Journal of Osaka Medical Association*, **22**, 373.

Kay, D. R., Bole, G. G. & Ledger, W. J. (1971) Antinuclear antibodies, rheumatoid factor and C reactive protein and serum of normal women using oral contraceptives. *Arthritis and Rheumatism*, **14**, 239.

Klassen, J. & Milgrom, F. (1971) Studies on cortical necrosis in rabbit renal transplants. *Transplantation*, **11**, 35.

Klein, F., Van Rood, J. J., Van Furth, R. & Radema, H. (1968) IgM and IgG cryoglobulinaemia with IgM paraprotein component. *Clinical and Experimental Immunology*, **3**, 703.

Lai a Fat, R. F. M., Cormane, R. H. & Furth, R. Van (1974) An immunohistopathological study on the synthesis of immunoglobulins and complement in normal and pathological skin and the adjacent mucous membranes. *British Journal of Dermatology*, **90**, 123.

Levenson, H. & Cochrane, C. G. (1964) Non-precipitatory antibody in the Arthus vasculitis. *Journal of Immunology*, **92**, 118.

Markowitz, A. S. & Lange, C. F. Jr (1964) Streptococcal related glomerulonephritis. *Journal of Immunology*, **92**, 565.

McDuffie, F. C. (1970) Serum complement levels in cutaneous diseases. *British Journal of Dermatology*, **82**, 20.

Meltzer, M. & Franklin, E. C. (1966) Cryoglobulinemia — A study of 29 patients. IgG and IgM cryo-globulins and factors affecting cryoprecipitability. *American Journal of Medicine*, **40**, 828.

Metzgar, R. S., Siegler, H. F., Ward, F. E. & Rowlands, D. T. (1972) Immunological studies on eluates from human renal allografts. *Transplantation*, **13**, 131.

Mitchell-Sams, W. & Jordon, R. E. (1971) Correlation of pemphigoid and pemphigus antibody titres with activity of disease. *British Journal of Dermatology*, **84**, 7.

Opie, E. L. (1924) Pathogenesis of specific inflammatory reaction of immunized animals (Arthus phenomenon); relation of local sensitisation to immunity. *Journal of Immunology*, **9**, 259.

Paronetto, F. & Strauss, L. (1962) Immunocytochemical observations in nodosa. *Annals of Internal Medicine*, **56**, 289.

Pepys, J. (1972) Immunopathology of allergic lung disease. *Clinical Allergy*, **3**, 1.

Pinski, J. B. & Stanisfer, P. D. (1964) Erythema nodosum as the initial manifestation of leukaemia. *Archives of Dermatology*, **89**, 339.

Piomelli, S., Stefanini, M. & Mele, R. H. (1959) Antigenicity of human vascular endothelium. Lack of relationship to the pathogenesis of vasculitis. *Journal of Laboratory and Clinical Medicine*, **54**, 241.

Polak, L., Frey, J. R. & Turk, J. L. (1970) Studies on the effect of systemic administration of sensitisers to guinea pigs with contact sensitivity to inorganic metal compounds. IV. Studies on the mechanism of the "flare up" reaction. *Clinical and Experimental Immunology*, **7**, 739.

Pollak, V. E. (1964) Antinuclear antibodies in families of patients with systemic lupus erythematosus. *New England Journal of Medicine*, **271**, 165.

Seaman, A. J., Marsical, I. & Moffat, Ch. (1971) Intravascular observations of fibrinolysis in an isolated organ. *Thrombosis et Diathesis Haemorrhagica*, Supplement **XLVI**, 263.

Spector, W. G. & Heesom, N. (1969) The production of granulomata by antigen—antibody complexes. *Journal of Pathology*, **98**, 31.

Starzl, T. E., Boehmig, H. J., Amemiya, H., Wilson, C. B., Dixon, F. J., Giles, G. R., Simpson, K. M. & Halgrimson, C. G. (1970) Clotting changes, including disseminated intravascular coagulation during rapid renal homograft rejection. *New England Journal of Medicine*, **283**, 383.

Stefanini, M. & Mednicoff, I. B. (1954) Demonstration of antivessel agents in serum of patients with anaphylactoid purpura and periarteritis nodosa. *Journal of Clinical Investigation*, **33**, 967.

Stringa, S. G., Bianchi, C., Casala, A. M. & Bianchi, O. (1967) Allergic vasculitis. Gougerot—Ruiter syndrome. Immunofluorescent study. *Archives of Dermatology*, **95**, 23.

Svec, K. H. & Viet, C. (1965) Age related antinuclear factors. Immunologic characteristics and associated clinical aspects. *Arthritis and Rheumatism*, **8**, 457.

Torrigiani, G. & Roitt, I. M. (1967) Antiglobulin factor in sera from patients with rheumatoid arthritis and normal subjects. *Annals of the Rheumatic Diseases*, **26**, 334.

Turk, J. L. (1970) Contribution of modern immunological concepts to an understanding of diseases of the skin. *British Medical Journal*, **iii**, 363.

Wemambu, S. N. C., Turk, J. L., Waters, M. F. R. & Rees, R. J. W. (1969) Erythema nodosum leprosum: a clinical manifestation of the Arthus phenomenon. *Lancet, ii,* 933.

White, F. N. & Grollman, A. (1964) Experimental periarteritis nodosa in the rat. *Archives of Pathology,* **78,** 31.

Whittingham, S., Irwin, J., Mackay, I. R., Marsh, S. & Cowling, D. C. (1969) Autoantibodies in healthy subjects. *Australian Annals of Medicine,* **18,** 130.

Wilhelm, D. L. (1971) Increased vascular permeability in acute inflammation. *Revue Canadienne de Biologie,* **30,** 153.

Winkelmann, R. K., Kim, R. & Wells, D. (1964) Unpublished data.

Wright, H. P. & Giacometti, N. J. (1972) Circulating endothelial cells and arterial endothelial mitosis in anaphylactic shock. *British Journal of Experimental Pathology,* **53,** 1.

Table 7.2. Fibrinolysis and immunofluorescence studies in various forms of vasculitis.

| Case no. | Diagnosis | Biopsy | Fibrinolysis | Immunofluorescence vessel deposits Ig | | | | | | |
				F	G	A	M	C'_3	T	Mac
1	Vasculitis	Purpura	Loss	+++	+	+	+	+	±	—
2	Vasculitis	Urticaria	No loss	+++	+	+	+	+	±	—
2	Vasculitis	Purpura	Loss	+++	+	+	+	+	±	—
3	Vasculitis	Livedo	Loss	+++	+	+	±	+	±	±
3	Vasculitis	Purpura	Loss	+++	+	—	—	+	—	—
4	Vasculitis	Purpura	Loss	+++	+	—	—	—	—	—
4	Vasculitis	Normal	No loss	—	+	+	+	+	±	—
5	Vasculitis	Purpura	Loss	+++	—	—	—	+	—	—
6	Vasculitis	Urticaria	Slightly reduced	+	+	+	+	+	+	—
7	Polyarteritis nodosa	48 hour Mantoux	Loss	±	—	..	..	—	—	—
7	Polyarteritis nodosa	Polyarteritis nodosa	Loss	++	+	+	+	+	+	+
8	Cold urticaria	Urticaria	No loss	—	—	—	—	—	—	—
9	Lichen amyloidosis	Amyloid	No loss	±	+	+	+	+	+	+
10	Vasculitis	Purpura	Loss	+	—	—	—	—	—	—
11	Erythema multiforme	Erythema multiforme	No loss	—	—	—	—	—	—	—
12	Pityriasis lichenoides chronica	Pityriasis lichenoides chronica	No loss	±	diffuse staining					
13	Platinum sensitivity	Arthus	Loss	+	+	+	—	+	—	—
14	Schönlein— Henoch purpura	Purpura	Loss	+++	+	—	—	—	±	—
15	Erythema elevatum diutinum	Plaque	Loss	+	+	+	+	+	+	+
15	Erythema elevatum diutinum	Bacterial antigen reaction	Loss	+++	+	±	—	—	—	+
16	Vasculitis	Purpura	Loss	+++	±	—	—	—	—	—
17	Vasculitis		No loss	++	+	..	..	+	—	—
18	Condylomata	Condylomata	Loss	+++	+	..	..	—	+	..
19	Cryoglobulin- aemia	Early purpura	Loss	+	+	+	+	—	—	—
20	Cryoglobulin- aemia	Late purpura	Loss	+++	—	—	+	—	—	—

F = Fibrinogen; T = Transferrin; Mac = a_2-macroglobulin. +++ = large amount present; — = none detected; .. = not done.

IMMUNOFLUORESCENCE IN VASCULITIS

Mellors and Ortega (1956) were the first to demonstrate gamma-globulin in the lesions of clinical vasculitis caused by a reaction to penicillin. Freedman, Peters and Kark (1960) also demonstrated gamma-globulin in renal blood vessels in vasculitis, but Paronetto and Strauss (1962) suggested its nonspecificity by showing gamma-globulin as well as fibrinogen and albumin in lesions of vasculitis and of human malignant hypertension. Strauss herself had seen such material in early experimental studies on necrotising arteritis induced by hypertension in the rat (Ohta, Cohen and Singer, 1959).

Lesions of human vasculitis were shown to contain complement by Lachmann et al (1962). A larger study of human cutaneous vasculitis by Scott and Rowell (1965) began the vogue for immunofluorescence analysis by dermatologists. However, these latter workers did not record any involvement of venules and thereby may have unwittingly contributed to the mistaken impression that most vasculitis involves arteries. A larger more detailed immunofluorescence study by Schroeter et al (1971) demonstrated IgG, IgM and complement in the lesions of various types of vasculitis. The absence of IgA was of particular interest as it very rarely forms a part of immune complexes. Scott and Rowell (1965) emphasised that globulins reflected neither the severity nor even the existence of the pathological change. Proof that the immune material is anything but a chance accumulation is usually lacking because antigen, the third component of the immune complex, is usually not demonstrable. Parish and Rhodes (1967) were able to identify antigenic components of Group A streptococci in the lesions of one patient and also to demonstrate the presence of mycobacteria and tuberculosis antigen in the lesions of two other patients. In such instances it is not known whether the immune complex is formed in situ or is a circulating complex. Sams et al (1975) studying 13 patients with necrotising vasculitis found complement and immunoglobulin in clinically normal skin. Other antigens that have been identified in the tissues are illustrated in Table 7.1. One immunofluorescence study (Ryan, Nishioka and Dawber, 1971) on the role of immuno-globulins and fibrin in fibrinolysis is illustrated in Table 7.2.

References

Freedman, P., Peters, J. H. & Kark, R. M. (1960) Localisation of gammaglobulin in the diseased kidney. *Archives of Internal Medicine,* **105,** 524.

Lachmann, P. J., Muller-Borhaad, H. J., Kunkel, H. G. & Paronetto, F. (1962) The localisation of in vivo bound complement in tissue sections. *Journal of Experimental Medicine,* **115,** 63.

Mellors, R. C. & Ortega, L. G. (1956) Analytical pathology. III. New observations on the pathogenesis of glomerulonephritis, lipid nephrosis, periarteritis nodosa and secondary amyloidosis in man. *American Journal of Pathology,* **32,** 455.

Ohta, G., Cohen, S. & Singer, E. (1959) Demonstration of gamma-globulin in vascular lesions of experimental necrotising arteritis in the rat. *Proceedings of the Society for Experimental Biology and Medicine,* **102,** 187.

Parish, W. E. & Rhodes, E. L. (1967) Bacterial antigens and aggregated gamma globulin in the lesions of nodular vasculitis. *British Journal of Dermatology,* **79,** 131.

Paronetto, F. & Strauss, L. (1962) Immunocytochemical observations in periarteritis nodosa. *Annals of Internal Medicine,* **56,** 289.

Ryan, T. J., Nishioka, K. & Dawber, R. P. R. (1971) Epithelial—endothelial interactions in the control of fibrinolysis. *British Journal of Dermatology,* **84,** 501.

Sams, W. M., Claman, H. N., Kohler, P. F., McIntosh, R. M., Small, P. & Mass, M. F. (1975) Human necrotising vasculitis: immunoglobulins and complement in vessel walls of cutaneous lesions and normal skin. *Journal of Investigative Dermatology,* **64,** 441.

Schroeter, A. L., Copeman, P. W. M. & Jordon, R. E. (1971) Immunofluorescence of cutaneous vasculitis associated with systemic disease. *Archives of Dermatology,* **104,** 254.

Scott, D. G. & Rowell, N. R. (1965) Preliminary investigations of arteritic lesions using fluorescent antibody techniques. *British Journal of Dermatology,* **77,** 211.

CIRCULATING IMMUNE COMPLEXES

The modern era of immunology, as it concerns vasculitis, began with experiments by Dixon et al (1959). They injected bovine serum albumin intravenously into the rabbit daily and found that rabbit precipitating antibody gradually rose but that, at the eighth to twelfth day, there was enough to precipitate all the inoculated albumin, at which time a widespread vasculitis developed. Thus was demonstrated the role of antigen—antibody complexes and the effect of such complexes when antibody is in excess. The injury is nonspecific in the sense that the complexes are noxious to all cells and not just to endothelium. Only rarely do immune complexes show any special affinity, as is the case with stibophen—IgM when the antibody is fixed to red cells, and with quinine—IgG when the antibody is fixed to platelets (Shulman, 1958). In the absence of such affinity, localisation of immune complexes depends on blood stasis more than any other factor, and the disease patterns being determined by localising factors (see Chapter 6) affect the legs and feet particularly (Figures 7.3 and 7.4). Unless demonstrated in the

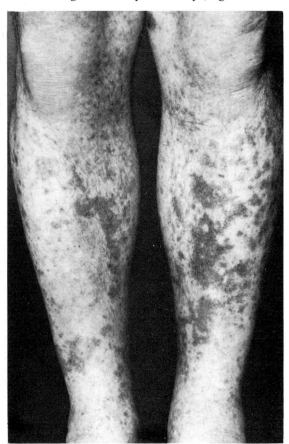

Figure 7.3. Purpura of the skin in a patient presenting with herpes zoster and cryoglobulinaemia illustrating localising role of gravitational stasis.

blood it is difficult to be certain whether complexes in the tissues are formed in situ or arrive there by way of the bloodstream.

Complexes in the bloodstream are not difficult to demonstrate in rheumatoid arthritis and Waldenström's benign hypergammaglobulinaemic purpura. A mixture of two immunoglobulins, the one being the antibody to the other, usually precipitates in vitro in

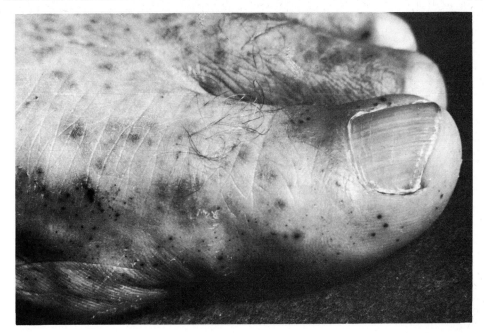

Figure 7.4. Punctate lesions of the toes in patient (as in Figure 7.3) with cryoglobulinaemia.

the cold as cryoglobulins and can also be precipitated by the first component of complement, C1q. Because many complexes fix complement, a drop in the complement level in the serum is often a feature of immune complex disease.

The diversity of reactions induced by immune complexes was once well illustrated by serum sickness but this has largely been superseded by allergy to drugs, such as penicillin, and to infections (see Chapter 8). Systemic lupus erythematosus is an example of widespread vascular damage due to immune complexes composed of DNA and antibody (see below).

The role of immune complexes in human allergic vasculitis has been emphasised by the presence of cryoglobulins in some 30 per cent of patients (Cream, 1971). Moreover, the inoculation of cryoprecipitates into the skin reproduces the pathology, but it is not species-specific (McIntosh, Kulvinskas and Kaufman, 1971; Whitsed and Penny, 1971).

A list of conditions in which circulating immune complexes have been identified as cryoglobulins is given in Table 7.3. That such cryoglobulins are noxious has been demonstrated by vasculitis resulting from their inoculation into the skin (Whitsed and Penny, 1971; Cream, 1971; Penny et al, 1971).

Table 7.3. List of conditions associated with cryoglobulinaemia.

Monoclonal cryoglobulinaemia	Kala-azar
Multiple myeloma	Lymphosarcoma
Waldenström's macroglobulinaemia	Acute haemolytic anaemia
Essential mixed cryoglobulinaemia	Cold urticaria
(Meltzer and Franklin, 1966)	Chronic hepatitis
Secondary cryoglobulinaemia	Chronic lymphatic leukaemia
Infectious mononucleosis	Acute glomerulonephritis
Cytomegalovirus infection	Systemic lupus erythematosus
Secondary syphilis	Rheumatoid arthritis
Lymphogranuloma venereum	Sjögren's syndrome
Leprosy	

Some cryoglobulins include an autoantibody, usually IgM, formed against and complexed with an IgG antibody which has acted as an antigen. This happens when antibody is complexed with foreign antigen such as an infectious agent, or in an autoimmune disease, and occasionally in neoplasia. Autoantibody is also known as rheumatoid factor (Barnett et al, 1970). Autoimmunity should always be considered as a possible cause in any case of vasculitis. The collagen diseases have long been viewed in this light, but other disorders such as Hashimoto's thyroiditis should be approached in the same way. Calder et al (1974), for example, found small immune complexes circulating in 59 per cent of patients with Hashimoto's disease; this is also a common finding in sub-acute bacterial endocarditis. In addition, Winkelmann and Ditto (1964) detected a circulating rheumatoid factor in 50 per cent of their cases of vasculitis at the Mayo Clinic.

The reason why rheumatoid factor features so prominently in the pathogenesis of immune complex disease is gradually becoming clearer. Rheumatoid factor activity is a particular pattern of response to antigenic stimuli and special clones of cells may be involved in its production. This possibility is suggested by the high incidence of IgM proteins with rheumatoid factor activity found in Waldenström's macroglobulinaemia.

In rabbits a cryoglobulinaemia has been produced experimentally in response to pneumococcal vaccine (Askonas, Farthing and Humphrey, 1960; Catsoulis, Franklin and Rothschild, 1965) and to streptococcal vaccine (Bokisch and Bernstein, 1972). The prominent rheumatoid factor activity of such cryoglobulins seemed to depend on genetic factors since it was present in only certain strains of animals and could be produced by only certain types of vaccine. This led to the suggestion that there is a complex relationship between the host's genetic background and the type of antigen, and that this determines whether or not rheumatoid factor is formed. There may be some advantage in producing rheumatoid factor because the large complexes to which it contributes are readily eliminated. It may also enhance the ingestion of antigen by plasma cell precursors and hence speed up antibody formation.

The association between distinctive nodular types of radiographic opacities in the lungs of coal miners and rheumatoid arthritis was described by Caplan (1953) and confirmed in a larger study by Miall et al (1953) (Figure 7.5). The association can also occur if the miners have a high level of rheumatoid factor but no joint disease (Caplan, Payne and Withey, 1962). Moreover, as pointed out by Soutar, Turner-Warwick and Raymond-Parkes (1974), many diseases characterised by fibrosis of the lung have high titres both of antinuclear factor and of rheumatoid factor; examples include asbestosis, silicosis and pneumoconiosis.

ENDOTHELIAL SPECIFICITY FOR THE TISSUE IT SERVES

There are reasons for believing that endothelial growth is stimulated by byproducts of growth and metabolism of the tissue supplied by the vessel (Ryan, 1973). It is conceivable that endothelium growing in a particular chemical environment could develop some features specific to that environment and that it would thereafter react specifically to the products of that environment. Thus, upper dermal vessels would learn to react to agents diffusing from the epidermis, and the venules in lymph glands would learn to react in like fashion to the material from the periphery in which they are habitually bathed.

There is in fact some evidence that the lymphocyte cell membrane has receptor sites which are antigenic and react with specific antibody such as antibasement membrane or

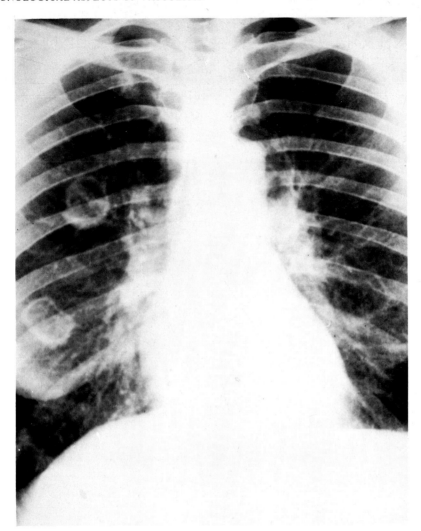

Figure 7.5. Cavity in the lungs of a coal miner suffering from rheumatoid arthritis: Caplan's syndrome.

anti-intracellular antibody (Cormane, Hammerlick and Husz, 1974). Lymphocytes which have such antigenic properties in common with the epidermis might be expected to affect endothelium that is reactive to such antigen or antibody. Ryan (1973) has suggested that some features of vasculitis are to be found in the vasculature supplying areas of skin reticulosis and that this can be explained by failure of control by lymphoid and mononuclear phagocytic tissue, which normally monitors the material diffusing from the epidermis to its vasculature.

References

Askonas, B. H., Farthing, C. P. & Humphrey, J. H. (1960) The significance of multiple antibody components in serum of immunized rabbits. *Immunology*, **3,** 336.
Barnett, E. V., Bluestone, R., Cracchiolo, A., Goldberg, L. S., Kantor, G. L. & McIntosh, R. M. (1970) Cryoglobulinemia and disease. *Annals of Internal Medicine*, **73,** 95.

Bokisch, V. A. & Bernstein, D. (1972) 19S and 7S anti IgG in rabbits immunised with streptococcal vaccines. *Arthritis and Rheumatism,* **15,** 104.

Calder, E. A., Penhale, W. J., Barnes, E. W. & Irvine, W. J. (1974) Evidence for circulating immune complexes in thyroid disease. *British Medical Journal,* **ii,** 30.

Caplan, A. (1953) Certain unusual radiological appearances in the chest of coal miners suffering from rheumatoid arthritis. *Thorax,* **8,** 29.

Caplan, A., Payne, R. B. & Withey, J. L. (1962) A broader concept of Caplan's syndrome related to rheumatoid factors. *Thorax,* **17,** 205.

Catsoulis, E. A., Franklin, E. C. & Rothschild, M. A. (1965) Cryoglobulinaemia in rabbits hyperimmunised with a polyvalent pneumococcal vaccine. *Immunology,* **9,** 327.

Cormane, R. H., Hammerlick, N. & Husz, S. (1974) Elution of antibodies from the lymphocyte membrane in certain dermatoses. *British Journal of Dermatology,* **91,** 315.

Cream, J. J. (1971) Immune complex diseases. *British Journal of Dermatology,* **85,** 189.

Dixon, F. J., Vazquez, J. J., Weigle, W. O. & Cochrane, C. G. (1959) In *Immunopathology.* Basel, Stuttgart: Benno Schwabo.

Grey, H. M. & Kohler, P. F. (1973) Cryoglobulins. *Seminars in Hematology,* **10,** 87.

McIntosh, R. M., Kulvinskas, C. & Kaufman, D. B. (1971) Quoted by Cream, J. J. & Turk, J. L. (1971) in a review of the evidence for immune complex disease in man. *Clinical Allergy,* **1,** 255.

Meltzer, M. & Franklin, E. C. (1966) Cryoglobulinaemia, a study of twenty-one patients. I. IgG and IgM cryoglobulin and factors affecting cryoprecipitability. *American Journal of Medicine,* **40,** 828.

Miall, W. E., Caplan, A., Cochrane, A. L., Kilpatrick, G. S. & Oldham, P. D. (1953) An epidemiological study of rheumatoid arthritis associated with characteristic chest x-ray appearances in local workers. *British Medical Journal,* **ii,** 1231.

Penny, R., Fiddes, P. J., Whitsed, H. M. & Cooper, D. A. (1971) Skin testing in vasculitis. Personal communication, quoted by Whitsed, H. M. & Penny, R. (1971).

Ryan, T. J. (1973) In *Physiology and Pathophysiology of the Skin,* Volume 2 (Ed.) Jarratt, A. London: Academic Press.

Shulman, N. R. (1958) Immunoreactions involving platelets. I. Asteric and kinetic model for formation of a complex from a human antibody. Quinidine as a haptene; and platelets; and for fixation of complement by the complex. *Journal of Experimental Medicine,* **107,** 665.

Soutar, C. A., Turner-Warwick, M. & Raymond-Parkes, W. (1974) Circulating anti nuclear antibody and rheumatoid factor in coal pneumoconiosis. *British Medical Journal,* **iii,** 145.

Whitsed, H. M. & Penny, R. (1971) IgA/IgG cryoglobulinaemia with vasculitis. *Clinical and Experimental Immunology,* **9,** 183.

Winkelmann, R. K. & Ditto, W. B. (1964) Cutaneous and visceral syndromes of necrotising or "allergic angiitis". A study of 38 cases. *Medicine* (Baltimore), **43,** 59.

LUPUS ERYTHEMATOSUS

Lupus erythematosus is one of the most notable causes of the full spectrum of urticaria, vasculitis and ischaemia. It is not the intention in this monograph to try to do justice to its many facets; the aim is merely to refer, in this chapter, to the systemic form associated with immune complexes.

Table 7.4 lists the criteria of the American Rheumatism Association for its diagnosis (Cohen and Canoso, 1972). Features such as the cold sensitive state of Raynaud's phenomenon, the nasopharyngeal ulceration, and the joint and renal complications clearly warrant its inclusion in a text devoted to vasculitis. In fact Barnett's (1969) clinical criteria of rash, fever, arthritis, small vessel vasculitis, glomerulonephritis and central nervous system disease, together with circulating LE cells or antinuclear factors, were until recently used by many in diagnosis.

Table 7.5 lists clinical and laboratory criteria outlined by Jablonska and Chorzelski (1974). Of all the available criteria the complement level and the anti-DNA antibody titre are the best guides to management, particularly of the renal disease.

Table 7.4. American Rheumatism Association criteria for systemic lupus erythematosus.

1. Facial erythema (butterfly rash)
2. Discoid LE lesions
3. Raynaud's phenomenon
4. Alopecia
5. Photosensitivity
6. Oral or nasopharyngeal ulceration
7. Arthritis without deformity
8. LE cells
9. Chronic false positive serological tests for syphilis
10. Profuse proteinuria: above 3.5 g per day
11. Cellular casts
12. (a) Pleuritis or (b) pericarditis or (c) both
13. (a) Psychosis or (b) convulsions or (c) both
14. One or more of the following: (a) haemolytic anaemia; (b) leucopenia, W.B.C. under 4000/mm^3; (c) thrombocytopenia, platelet count under 100 000/mm^3

Circulating complexes composed of DNA combined with anti-DNA antibody have been demonstrated by Agnello, Winchester and Kunkel (1970). When the antibody is in excess they tend to form particles which are removed by the mononuclear phagocytic system. When, however, antigen is in excess, possibly as a result of widespread tissue damage from, for instance, a viral infection, complement is bound and the complex causes injury to the blood vessels or to any organ where it happens to be filtered out.

In 1972, Maas et al described 21 patients with a disease resembling systemic lupus erythematosus clinically but distinguishable from it serologically by the presence of mitochondrial antibodies and the absence of nuclear antibodies. The syndrome is characterised by recurrent fever, myalgia, arthralgia, pleuritis, pulmonary infiltrates, pericarditis and myocarditis. A current but relevant phenomenon is worth mentioning here. As many as 90 per cent of long-term users of a drug containing phenopyrozone — a horse-chestnut extract — and glycosides extracted from several plants were found to have such mitochondrial antibodies and 10 per cent developed the full syndrome (Grob et al, 1975). The drug is used regularly on the continent of Europe for venous disorders.

Yet another ill-defined syndrome related to lupus erythematosus is 'mixed connective tissue disease'. Sharp et al (1972) reported patients in whom features of systemic lupus erythematosus, polymyositis and scleroderma coexisted. They noted that, as distinct from systemic lupus erythematosus, high titres of antinuclear factor of the 'speckled' pattern persisted through periods of clinical remission. This led to the isolation of a

Table 7.5. Clinical and laboratory criteria for diagnosis of systemic lupus erythematosus.

Clinical	Laboratory
Arthritis, 90%	Elevated sedimentation rate
Erythema/telangiectasia, 75—80%	Hypergammaglobulinaemia
Sensitivity to u.v. radiation, 32.7%	Leucopenia
Alopecia	Thrombocytopenia
Oral and nasal lesions	Proteinuria and casts
Raynaud's phenomenon, 18.4%	Haemolytic anaemia
Vasculitis	False positive serological tests for syphilis
Fever, malaise and weight loss	Antinuclear (and anti-DNA) antibodies
Renal involvement	LE phenomenon
Panniculitis	Immunofluorescent band in the uninvolved skin
Pleurisy	Low serum complement
Hepatitis	
Myositis	
Lymphadenopathy, 58%	
Ocular or cerebral signs	

distinct extractable nuclear antigen, an RNA protein. Patients with so-called 'mixed connective tissue disease' showed extraordinarily high titres to this antigen and low or absent titres of anti-DNA antibodies and had no renal disease. The vascular involvement, manifest particularly as Raynaud's phenomenon, can be severe (Kitchener et al, 1975).

Another collagen disease related to an exogenous agent is the pseudoscleroderma caused by polyvinyl chloride in workers whose job includes cleaning out the vats used for its polymerisation. They develop scleroderma, extensive lytic bone changes, pulmonary fibrosis, Raynaud's phenomenon and altered serology. Cryoglobulins, cryofibrinogen, complement conversion, increased immunoglobulins and impaired T-cell function are part of the syndrome (Wilson et al, 1967; Dinman et al, 1971; Maricq, 1975).

References

Agnello, V., Winchester, R. J. & Kunkel, H. G. (1970) Precipitin reactions of the C1q component of complement with aggregated gamma-globulin and immune complexes in gel diffusion. *Immunology,* **19,** 909.

Barnett, E. V. (1969) Diagnostic aspects of lupus erythematosus cells and antinuclear factors in disease states. *Mayo Clinic Proceedings,* **44,** 645.

Cohen, A. S. & Canoso, J. J. (1972) Criteria for the classification of systemic lupus erythematosus. *Arthritis and Rheumatism,* **15,** 540.

Dinman, B. D., Cook, W. A., Whitehouse, W. M., Magnuson, H. J., Arbor, A. & Ditcheck, T. (1971) Occupational acroosteolysis 1) An epidemiological study. *Archives of Environmental Health,* **22,** 73.

Grob, P. J., Muller-Schoop, J. W., Hacki, M. A. & Joller-Jemelka, H. I. (1975) Drug induced pseudo lupus. *Lancet,* **ii,** 144.

Jablonska, S. & Chorzelski, T. P. (1974) Lupus erythematosus. In *Immunological Aspects of Skin Diseases* (Ed.) Fry, L. & Seah, P. P. pp. 66-152. Lancaster, England: Medical and Technical Publishing Company Ltd.

Kitchener, D., Edmonds, J., Bruneau, C. & Hughes, G. R. V. (1975) Mixed connective tissue disease with digital gangrene. *British Medical Journal,* **i,** 249.

Maas, D., Merz, K. P., Hahn, J. & Schubothe, H. (1972) Ein Lupus erythematodes ähnliches Syndrome mit antimitochondriahan Antikörpern. Bericht über zi fälle. *Verhandlungen der Deutschen Gesellschaft für innere Medizin,* **78,** 895.

Maricq, H. R., Johnson, M. N., Whetstone, C. L. & Leroy, E. C. (1975) In vivo skin capillary abnormalities in vinyl chloride workers. In *Proceedings of World Congress for Microcirculation* (Ed.) Grayson, J. & Zingg, W. New York: Plenum Publishing Corporation.

Sharp, G. C., Irvin, W. S., Tan, E. M., Gould, R. G. & Holman, H. R. (1972) Mixed connective tissue disease — an apparently distinct rheumatic disease syndrome associated with a specific antibody to an extractable nuclear antigen. *American Journal of Medicine,* **52,** 148.

Wilson, R. E., McCormick, W. E., Tatum, C. F. & Creech, J. L. (1967) Occupational acroosteolysis. Report of 31 cases. *Journal of the American Medical Association,* **202,** 577.

PARALLELS IN RENAL DISEASE

Many of the problems encountered in vasculitis of the skin are the same as those found in glomerulonephritis, malignant hypertension and renal transplantation. The renal diseases have received rather more detailed analysis and the mechanisms underlying them are becoming clearer. The following short review is written with these parallels in mind, the aim being to outline how the study of renal disease is relevant to skin diseases and experimental aspects of vasculitis discussed in other chapters of this book.

Glomerulonephritis

Cameron (1972) in his Goulstonian lecture drew attention to various aspects of glomerulonephritis in terms that seem equally applicable to the skin (Figure 7.6).

Clinical and pathological classifications often fail when clinical presentation and histological appearances are put together. The kidney, like the skin, can express damage only in a limited number of ways and these are not a good clue to aetiology, especially when it comes to identifying immunological, as opposed to non-immunological, mechanisms. Tissues 'trot' out the same response whatever stimulus is applied. Cameron (1972) believed that antibody-mediated assault on the kidney was important but

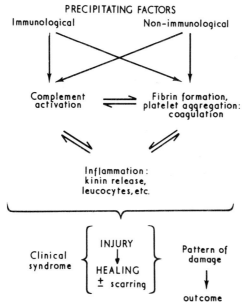

Figure 7.6. Levels of descriptive diagnosis in glomerulonephritis. This diagram illustrates how renal disease may be caused by immunologic and non-immunologic mechanisms acting through complement and fibrin formation.

probably not more so than injury to the surface of the endothelium and blood coagulation caused by other agents. He listed the following factors as determining the final overall response of the body to an antigen: inherited ability to mount a response; the balance between humoral and cellular immunity; the nature of the antigen, its route of presentation, mode of presentation and quantity, and the duration of exposure to it; and modifying factors such as coincident infection or inflammation. The antigen is rarely recognised in most cases of glomerulonephritis but has been identified in the diseases listed (Table 7.1).

Studies of experimental allergic glomerulonephritis reveal two main mechanisms of immunological injury to the glomerulus (Unanue and Dixon, 1967; Peters, 1974). In the first, circulating antibody reacts with antigen in the kidney, and in the second, the nonspecific circulating immune complex is filtered out by and hence is localised in the kidney. In 'one shot' serum sickness, the immune complexes are a transient phenomenon, whereas in chronic glomerulonephritis there is persistent formation of small amounts of immune complexes. Complement is generally regarded as one of the main causes of polymorphonuclear response in the tissues, and fibrin as the main stimulus to endothelial and epithelial cell proliferation. However, neither complement depletion (Henson and Cochrane, 1971) nor anticoagulants completely alleviate experimental glomerulonephritis.

There is good evidence that in serum sickness and in the experimental formation of soluble complexes in antigen excess, renal damage is caused by filtered 'toxic' material.

Animals producing little antibody may in consequence have persistent or recurrent renal injury in chronic infections. Because viruses are intracellular, long-lived and self-replicating, they are especially apt to produce a chronic antigen load; in fact the mouse, mink, horse and hog are all susceptible to viral diseases known to produce nephritis (Oldstone and Dixon, 1971).

New Zealand black mice crossed with New Zealand white mice develop an excess of anti-DNA antibody (Heyler and Howie, 1963), but their T lymphocytes are resistant to the induction of tolerance (Talal et al, 1971). Their production of anti-DNA antibody is enhanced by endemic gross virus infection, but lactic dehydrogenase virus affords protection (Dixon, Oldstone and Tonietti, 1971). Nephritis in these animals is common but depends not only on genetic factors and an imbalance between humoral and cellular defence mechanisms, but also on the type of virus to which they are exposed. Here it can be noted that Briggs et al (1972) suggested that the influenza virus precipitated renal transplant rejection in three patients.

Most of the viral diseases induce a somewhat inadequate antibody response so that elimination of virus is incomplete; it seems as if the various strains of animals thus infected have a genetically determined failure to produce effective antibody.

One pattern of renal disease not so far detected in animals is that in which IgA is the predominant tissue immunoglobulin (Berger, 1969). This is a focal proliferative glomerulonephritis sometimes associated with vasculitis of the skin (Evans et al, 1973), and it occurs usually at the height of a presumably viral upper respiratory tract infection. It has been suggested that mucosal injury by the viral infection evokes the IgA response, perhaps in the same way that coeliac disease may evoke IgA deposits in the skin in dermatitis herpetiformis. IgA does not activate the classic pathway of complement, but properdin is deposited in the tissues.

A new aspect of immunology is the observation that complement is low or defective in a number of patients suffering from a variety of renal diseases (reviewed by Peters, 1974). It is thought that complement deficiency, congenital or acquired, may lead to inadequate elimination of immune complexes by the mononuclear phagocytic system. It seems pertinent that vasculitis of the skin as in Schönlein—Henoch purpura has been described in association with C_2 deficiency (Jones et al, 1974, reported by Peters, 1974). This important association is discussed by Leddy et al (1975).

There is no doubt that in man chronic soluble immune complex deposition occurs in systemic lupus erythematosus (Christian, 1969; Koffler, Schur and Kunkel, 1967), in quartan malaria (Kibukamusoke, Hutt and Wilks, 1967; Houba et al, 1971), and occasionally also in disorders such as infection by Australia antigen, sub-acute bacterial endocarditis, malignancy and Hashimoto's disease (reviewed by Cream and Turk, 1971).

Cameron (1972) emphasised that complement, coagulation and kinins interact in renal disease at many levels and that investigative laboratory techniques have created an artificial separation of these factors. Excretion of fibrin degradation products in the urine is a feature of glomerulonephritis (Clarkson et al, 1971) and several studies have shown fibrin in the glomeruli (McCluskey et al, 1966; Urizar and Herdman, 1970) (the last report concerned the kidney in anaphylactoid purpura).

On the other hand, fibrin deposition in the mesangium of the glomerulus frequently is not associated with high titres of fibrin degradation products, and antibody deposition and complement in the basement membrane is often associated with fibrin deposition at a more distant site (Peters, 1974). A similar phenomenon in the skin can be explained by impaired fibrinolysis resulting from endothelial injury (see Chapter 10).

Boyd, Burden and Aber (1975) have drawn attention to the intrarenal vascular changes in patients receiving oestrogen-containing compounds. They emphasised the role of fibrin, stasis and shunting and recorded low serum complement in these patients. Microvascular thrombosis seemed to be the basic lesion.

References

Berger, J. (1969) IgA glomerular deposits in renal disease. *Transplantation Proceedings,* **1,** 939.

Black, J. D., Challacombe, D. N. & Ockenden, B. G. (1965) Nephrotic syndrome associated with bacteraemia after shunt operations for hydrocephalus. *Lancet,* **ii,** 921.

Boyd, W. N., Burden, R. P. & Aber, G. M. (1975) Intrarenal vascular changes in patients receiving oestrogen-containing compounds — a clinical, histological and angiographic study. *Quarterly Journal of Medicine,* **44,** 415.

Briggs, J. D., Timbury, M. C., Paton, A. M. & Bell, P. R. F. (1972) Viral infection and renal transplantation rejection. *British Medical Journal,* **iv,** 520.

Cameron, J. S. (1972) Bright's disease today: the pathogenesis and treatment of glomerulonephritis III. *British Medical Journal,* **iv,** 217.

Christian, C. L. (1969) Immune complex disease. *New England Journal of Medicine,* **280,** 878.

Clarkson, A. R., MacDonald, M. K., Petrie, J. J. B., Cash, J. D. & Robson, J. S. (1971) Serum and urinary fibrin/fibrinogen degradation products in glomerulonephritis. *British Medical Journal,* **iii,** 447.

Combes, B., Stasjny, P., Shorey, J., Bigenbrodt, E., Varrera, A., Hull, A. & Carter, N. (1971) Glomerulonephritis with deposition of Australia antigen—antibody complexes in glomerular basement membrane. *Lancet,* **ii,** 234.

Cream, J. J. & Turk, J. L. (1971) A review of the evidence for immune complex deposition as a cause of skin disease in man. *Clinical Allergy,* **1,** 235.

Dixon, F. J., Oldstone, M. B. & Tonietti, G. (1971) Pathogenesis of immune complex glomerulonephritis of New Zealand mice. *Journal of Experimental Medicine,* **134** (Supplement 65).

Evans, D. J., Williams, D. G., Peters, D. K., Sissons, J. G. P., Boulton-Jones, J. M., Ogg, C. S., Cameron, J. S. & Hoffbrand, B. I. (1973) Glomerular deposition of properdin in Henoch—Schönlein syndrome and idiopathic focal nephritis. *British Medical Journal,* **iii,** 326.

Henson, P. M. & Cochrane, C. G. (1971) Acute immune complex disease in rabbits. The role of complement and of leukocyte dependent release of vasoactive amines from platelets. *Journal of Experimental Medicine,* **133,** 554.

Heyler, B. J. & Howie, J. B. (1963) Renal disease associated with positive lupus erythematosus tests in a cross-bred strain of mice. *Nature,* **197,** 197.

Houba, V., Allison, A. C., Adeniyi, A. & Houba, J. E. (1971) Immunoglobulin classes and complement in biopsies of Nigerian children with nephrotic syndrome. *Clinical and Experimental Immunology,* **8,** 761.

Kibukamusoke, J. W., Hutt, M. S. R. & Wilks, N. E. (1967) The nephrotic syndrome in Uganda and its association with quartan malaria. *American Journal of Medicine,* **36,** 393.

Koffler, D., Schur, P. H. & Kunkel, H. G. (1967) Immunological studies concerning the nephritis of lupus erythematosus. *Journal of Experimental Medicine,* **126,** 607.

Koffler, D., Agnello, V., Thorburn, R. & Kunkel, H. G. (1971) Systemic lupus erythematosus; prototype of immune complex nephritis in man. *Journal of Experimental Medicine,* **36,** 393.

Lachmann, P. J. (1968) Nephrotic syndrome from penicillamine. *Postgraduate Medical Journal,* **44,** 23.

Leddy, J. P., Griggs, R. C., Klemperer, M. C. & Frank, M. M. (1975) Hereditary complement (C_2) deficiency with dermatomyositis. *American Journal of Medicine,* **58,** 83.

Loughridge, L. W. & Lewis, M. G. (1971) Nephrotic syndrome in malignant disease of non-renal origin. *Lancet,* **i,** 256.

McCluskey, R. T., Vassalli, P., Gallo, G. & Baldwin, D. S. (1966) An immunofluorescent study of pathogenic mechanisms in glomerular disease. *New England Journal of Medicine,* **274,** 695.

Oldstone, M. B. A. & Dixon, F. J. (1971) Chronic viral infection associated with immune complex disease. In *Progress in Immunology* (Ed.) Amos, B. p. 764. New York, London: Academic Press.

Peters, D. K. (1974) Symposium No. 14. The immunological basis of glomerulonephritis. *Proceedings of the Royal Society of Medicine,* **67,** 557.

Sissons, J. G. P., Evans, D. J., Peters, D. K., Eisinger, A. J., Boulton-Jones, J. M., Simpson, I. J. & Macanovic, M. (1974) Glomerulonephritis associated with antibody to glomerular basement membrane. *British Medical Journal,* **iv,** 11.

Stickler, G. B., Shin, M. H., Burke, E. C., Holley, K. E., Miller, R. H. & Segar, W. E. (1968) Diffuse glomerulonephritis associated with infected ventriculoatrial shunt. *New England Journal of Medicine,* **279,** 1027.

Talal, N., Steinberg, A. D., Jacobs, M. E., Chused, E. M. & Gazdar, A. F. (1971) Immune cell cooperation, viruses and antibodies to nucleic acids in New Zealand mice. *Journal of Experimental Medicine,* **134** (Supplement 52).

Tan, E. M., Schur, P. H., Carr, R. I. & Kunkel, H. F. (1966) Deoxyribonucleic acid (DNA) and antibodies to DNA in serum of patients with systemic lupus erythematosus. *Journal of Clinical Investigation,* **45,** 1732.

Treser, G., Semar, M., Ty, A., Sagei, I., Franklin, M. A. & Lange, K. (1970) Partial characterisation of antigenic streptococcal plasma membrane components in acute glomerulonephritis. *Journal of Clinical Investigation,* **49,** 762.

Unanue, E. R. & Dixon, F. J. (1967) In *Advances in Immunology* (Ed.) Humphrey, J. & Dixon, F. J. New York, London: Academic Press.
Urizar, R. E. & Herdman, R. C. (1970) Anaphylactoid purpura. III. Early morphologic glomerular changes. *American Journal of Clinical Pathology,* **53,** 258.
Ward, P. A. & Kibukamusoke, J. W. (1969) Evidence for soluble immune complexes in the pathogenesis of glomerulonephritis of quartan malaria. *Lancet,* **i,** 283.
Williams, R. C. & Kunkel, H. G. (1962) Rheumatoid factor, complement and conglutinin aberrations in patients with subacute bacterial endocarditis. *Journal of Clinical Investigation,* **41,** 666.

INTRAVASCULAR COAGULATION

In a series of 124 children with renal diseases Stiehm and Trygstad (1968) described three groups according to the level of serum fibrin degradation products:
1. The haemolytic uraemic syndrome or disseminated intravascular coagulation (DIC).
2. Localised intravascular coagulation or acute and chronic glomerulonephritis.
3. Those without coagulation, as in nephrosis or pyelonephritis.

The raised levels of fibrin degradation products in Group 2 may be a reflection of endothelial damage, the highest levels being found in patients with microangiopathic haemolytic anaemia. Malignant hypertension was chiefly responsible for the latter in one series (Briggs et al, 1972), and Wardle and Floyd (1973) postulated that the renal pathology observed in bacterial endocarditis is due to intravascular coagulation, because accelerated fibrinogen catabolism was found during the bacteriaemia and during the subsequent immunological phase of circulating immune complexes. In this latter phase, rheumatoid factors appear and serum complement is lowered (Cordeiro, Costa and Langinha, 1965).

Microangiopathic haemolytic anaemia, selective thrombocytopenia and renal impairment all are features of renal allografts (Pillay et al, 1973). The platelets which sequestrate in the kidney undergoing hyper-acute rejection probably result from the immunological injury (Myburg et al, 1969) and fibrin deposition (Starzl et al, 1970). Labelled platelets in fact disappear in transplanted kidneys (Mowbray, 1967).

It should be noted here that malignant nephrosclerosis can be produced by platelet embolisation from experimentally induced damage to the renal artery (Moore, 1976). Other features of transplant rejection were noted by Clark et al (1976) who studied microvascular thrombosis in particular. They showed that the earliest lesion occurs in the most venular compartment of the vascular tree, and that arteriolar—venular shunting and vascular disruptions were prominent findings. As in skin, stasis determines the site of the thrombosis in the kidney (Latour and Leger, 1976). The occurrence of glomerulonephritis in gammaglobulinaemia makes it probable that renal disease is due to primary intravascular coagulation and not always secondary to immune complexes (Avasthi, Avasthi and Tung, 1975).

Amery et al (1973) believe that the accelerated rejection of allografts which occurs when there is an excess of antibody to the graft may be delayed by heparin infusion. This prolongation of graft survival by heparin is probably due to its effect on platelets. The evidence presented in Chapters 4, 5 and 10 that endothelial cells may be shed after a period of ischaemia is relevant to the findings of endothelial disruption in peritubular capillaries (Porter, 1967), and of endothelial loss from larger vessels (Kosek et al, 1969). These authors attributed the vascular injury to hypoxia and noted that the pathology was similar to that seen in malignant hypertension. Sinclair (1972) showed that endothelial cells from the host could repopulate vessels of human renal allografts.

TRANSPLANTS

In the first large series of human renal homotransplants (Hume et al, 1955) severe arteriosclerotic changes in the vessels of the rejected kidneys were attributed to hypertension in rather the same way that Zeek (1952) explained some of the changes seen in polyarteritis nodosa. Porter et al (1963) described two phases or crises in similar patients; the first occurred at 15 to 19 days after transplantation, when the kidney became oedematous and infiltrated with lymphocytes and the patients developed a higher fever. The second febrile crisis occurred at 38 to 45 days and was associated with endothelial proliferation, marked splitting and necrosis of the internal elastic lamina, and partial obliteration of the blood vessels. By the 60th day several such patients showed patchy venous thrombosis. The first crisis was believed to be a cell-mediated immune response and the later change to be partly due to ischaemia. Simonson et al (1953) emphasised that there were histopathological similarities to polyarteritis nodosa with subsequent ischaemic changes, and Porter et al (1963) believed that an early immunological injury to the vessels caused impaired blood flow and eventually ischaemia. An initial ischaemic episode during surgery could account for some of the renal changes (Calne et al, 1963), and in this respect there are similarities to the observations Cherry describes in Chapter 5.

The intensity and rate of the rejection process, and its clinical and pathological picture, are variable (Dempster, Harrison and Shakman, 1964). Some kidneys are tense and oedematous, others are more purpuric; in some the changes resemble those of polyarteritis nodosa, and in others, scleroderma or thrombotic thrombocytopenic purpura. The gradually increasing emphasis on the underlying mechanisms, namely immunological processes, coagulation, thrombosis and ischaemia, is very similar to the changing views on vasculitis of the skin.

Darmady, Offer and Stranack (1964) observed that those patients who survived the shortest time showed more involvement of the smaller vessels, while those who survived for longer periods developed changes in the larger vessels. In skin diseases too the more acute processes involve more commonly the smaller vessels.

ISCHAEMIA

When the blood flow to the kidney is interrupted by pedicle clamping, it at first has a pale slate-blue colour. On releasing the clamp within about six hours, blood flow is quickly re-established and the kidney shows a pulsating redness. From about 10 to 30 seconds after re-establishing flow, the kidney develops a blotchy reticulate dark purple colour, but the red pulsation continues in intermediate areas for about two hours, after which flow through cortical vessels has apparently ceased. At this stage, examination of the renal vein shows an axial stream of bright red blood. Closer scrutiny shows that the smaller vessels of the kidney are filled with fibrin and that the blood seen in the renal vein is coming from shunts (Sheehan and Davis, 1959a, b).

The kidney has been extensively studied in experiments equivalent to those described for the skin in Chapter 5; the morphological and histological changes and the alteration in function have much in common with those found in the skin. The capillaries of both tissues show pyknotic nuclei followed by increased numbers of mitotic figures and evidence of considerable regeneration. Larger vessels show degeneration of the media.

The relationship of ischaemia to failed or good reflow and coagulation was clearly established by Sheehan and Davis (1959a, b). Ischaemia causes considerable necrosis of interstitial cells, an aspect that cannot be prevented by heparin infusion. Sheehan and Davis (1959) and Mathew et al (1974) also distinguished between the interstitial injury of cadaveric renal allograft that fails to respond to anticoagulants, and the glomerular and blood vessel injury that is greatly helped by a therapeutic regime aimed at preventing fibrin and platelet deposition in the vessels. Any assessment of ischaemic effects in the kidney, skin or other tissues must take into account the fact that some cell systems such as fat, smooth muscle or the interstitial cells of the kidney are particularly susceptible to deprivation of blood supply. Even if the blood vessels of the tissues survive an ischaemic insult, the surrounding tissue may not recover and will show a pattern of scarring that falls short of a typical infarction.

The inter-relationship of hypertension, coagulation and ischaemia so important in polyarteritis nodosa (see Chapter 13) has received much attention in the literature on pre-eclampsia (see Leader, *British Medical Journal,* 16th March, 1974). Hypertension may be a consequence of changes in renin and angiotensin (Gordon, Parsons and Simonds, 1969) and such changes may occur early in pregnancy. However, low-grade disseminated intravascular coagulation also occurs in pregnancy (McKay et al, 1953; McKay, De Bacalao and Sedlis, 1964; McKay, 1965; Bonnar, McNicol and Douglas, 1971; Howie, Prentice and McNicol, 1971; McCluskey, 1971; Brown and Stalker, 1969). Microangiopathic haemolytic anaemia occurs in severe pre-eclampsia (Brain, Kuah and Dixon, 1967) and this is suggestive of primary damage to endothelium and fibrin deposition. Some workers have drawn attention to similarities between this disease and renal allograft rejection and these have been reviewed by Petrucco et al (1974). It is probable that the behaviour of blood vessels during pregnancy differs from normal in respect to the localisation of immune complexes (Shirai and Sims, 1970), as is the case with colloidal gold (see Chapter 9, page 214). Injection of anti-kidney gamma-globulin in non-pregnant rats produces nephritis with the pre-eclampsia-type of lesion seen in the kidneys of pregnant rats. Also, Shirai and Sims (1970) and Petrucco et al (1974) found IgM, IgG and complement in the kidneys of eleven pre-eclamptic women.

Sophian (1972) and Speroff (1973) are the main proponents of the ischaemic theory of pre-eclampsia, and Sanerkin (1971) claimed that a period of ischaemia resulting from malignant hypertension leads to endothelial damage and that thrombosis follows this. Robertson (1958) stated that the lesions in the placenta in pre-eclampsia are like those seen in syphilis. Wardle (1973) also believed that the histology of pre-eclampsia is nonspecific and that intravascular coagulation is secondary to hypertension or placental damage. There is always abundant fibrin in the glomeruli (Morris et al, 1964).

References

Amery, A. H., Pegrum, G. D., Risdon, R. A. & Williams, G. (1973) Nature of hyperacute rejection in dog renal allographs and effect of heparin on rejection process. *British Medical Journal,* i, 455.

Avasthi, P. S., Avasthi, P. & Tung, K. S. K. (1975) Glomerulonephritis in agammaglobulinaemia. *British Medical Journal,* ii, 478.

Bonnar, J., McNicol, G. P. & Douglas, A. S. (1971) Coagulation and fibrinolytic systems in pre-eclampsia and eclampsia. *British Medical Journal,* ii, 12.

Brain, M. C., Kuah, K. B. & Dixon, H. G. (1967) Heparin treatment of haemolysis and thrombocytopenia in pre-eclampsia. Report of a case and review of the literature. *Journal of Obstetrics and Gynaecology of the British Commonwealth,* 74, 702.

Briggs, J. D., Timbury, M. C., Paton, A. M. & Bell, P. R. F. (1972) Viral infection of renal transplantation rejection. *British Medical Journal,* iv, 520.

Brown, L. J. & Stalker, A. L. (1969) Experimental defibrination. III. The maternal and foetal microcirculation following placental separation of trauma. *Microvascular Research,* 1, 403.

Calne, R. Y., Loughridge, L. W., MacGillivray, J. B., Zilva, J. F. & Levi, A. J. (1963) Renal transplantation in man. A report of five cases, using cadaveric donors. *British Medical Journal,* iii, 645.

Clark, R. L., Staab, E. V., Mandel, S. R. & Webster, W. P. (1976) Progressive microvascular obliteration during canine renal allograft rejection. In *Proceedings of the World Congress for Microcirculation* (Ed.) Grayson, J. & Zingg, W. London: Plenum.

Cordeiro, A., Costa, H. & Langinha, F. (1965) Immunologic phase of subacute bacterial endocarditis. A new concept and general considerations. *American Journal of Cardiology,* **16,** 477.

Darmady, E. M., Offer, J. M. & Stranack, F. (1964) Study of renal vessels by microdissection in human transplantation. *British Medical Journal,* **ii,** 976.

Dempster, W. J., Harrison, C. V. & Shackman, R. (1964) Rejection processes in human homotransplanted kidneys. *British Medical Journal,* **ii,** 969.

Gordon, R. D., Parsons, S. & Simonds, E. M. (1969) A prospective study of plasma serum activity in normal and toxaemic pregnancy. *Lancet,* **i,** 347.

Howie, P. W., Prentice, C. R. M. & McNicol, G. P. (1971) Coagulation fibrinolysis and platelet function in pre-eclampsia, essential hypertension and placental insufficiency. *Journal of Obstetrics and Gynaecology of the British Commonwealth,* **79,** 992.

Hume, D. M., Merrill, J. P., Miller, B. F. & Thorn, G. W. (1955) Experiences with renal homotransplantation in human: report of nine cases. *Journal of Clinical Investigation,* **34,** 327.

Kosek, J. C., Chartrand, C., Hurley, E. J. & Lower, R. R. (1969) Arteries in canine cardiac homografts, ultrastructure during acute rejection. *Laboratory Investigation,* **21,** 328.

Latour, J. G. & Leger, C. (1976) Production of glomerular capillary thrombosis by thrombin and vasoactive hormones. In *Proceedings of the World Congress for Microcirculation* (Ed.) Grayson, J. & Zingg, W. London: Plenum.

Leader (1974) *British Medical Journal,* **i,** 468.

Mathew, T. H., Clyne, D. H., Nanra, R. S., Kincaid-Smith, P., Saker, B. M. & Marshall, P. J. (1974) A controlled trial of oral anticoagulants and dipyridamole in cadaveric renal allografts. *Lancet,* **i,** 137.

McCluskey, R. T. (1971) The value of immunofluorescence in the study of human renal disease. *Journal of Experimental Medicine,* **134,** 242.

McKay, D. G. (1965) *Disseminated Intravascular Coagulation and Intermediary of Disease.* New York: Hoebner Medical Division, Harper & Row.

McKay, D. G., De Bacalao, E. B. & Sedlis, A. (1964) Platelet adhesiveness in toxaemia of pregnancy. *American Journal of Obstetrics and Gynecology,* **90,** 1315.

McKay, D. G., Merrill, S. J., Weiner, A. E., Hertig, A. T. & Reid, D. E. (1953) Pathologic anatomy of eclampsia, bilaterial renal cortical necrosis, pituitary necrosis and other acute fatal complications of pregnancy and its possible relationship to generalised Shwartzman phenomenon. *American Journal of Obstetrics and Gynecology,* **66,** 507.

Moore, S. (1976) Platelet aggregates in the microcirculation and human disease. In *Proceedings of the World Congress for Microcirculation* (Ed.) Grayson, J. & Zingg, W. London: Plenum.

Morris, R. H., Vassalli, P., Beller, F. K. & McCluskey, R. T. (1964) Immunofluorescent studies of renal biopsies in the diagnosis of toxemia of pregnancy. *Obstetrics and Gynecology,* **24,** 32.

Mowbray, J. F. (1967) Method of suppression of immune response. In *Integration in Internal Medicine, International Congress Series,* **137,** 106. Amsterdam: Excerpta Medica.

Myburg, J. A., Cohen, I., Gecelter, L., Meyers, A. M., Abrahams, C., Furman, K. I., Goldberg, B. & Van Bleck, P. J. P. (1969) Hyperacute rejection in human kidney allografts, Shwartzman or Arthrus phenomenon. *New England Journal of Medicine,* **281,** 131.

Papadimitriou, J. M., Sforsina, D. & Papaelias, L. (1973) Kinetics of multinucleate giant cell formation and their modification by various agents in foreign body reactions. *American Journal of Pathology,* **73,** 349.

Petrucco, O. M., Thompson, N. M., Lawrence, J. R. & Weldon, M. W. (1974) Immunofluorescent studies in renal biopsies in pre-eclampsia. *British Medical Journal,* **i,** 473.

Pillay, V. K. G., Kurtzman, N. A., Manaligod, J. R. & Jonasson, O. (1973) Selective thrombocytopenia due to localised microangiopathy of renal allografts. *Lancet,* **iv,** 988.

Porter, K. A. (1967) Rejection in treated renal allografts. *Journal of Clinical Pathology,* **20** (Supplement 2), 518.

Porter, K. A., Thompson, W. B., Owen, K., Kenyon, J. R., Mowbray J. F. & Peart, W. S. (1963) Obliterative vascular changes in four human kidney homotransplants. *British Medical Journal,* **iii,** 639.

Ryan, T. J. (1966) Periadenitis mucosae necroticans. *Proceedings of the Royal Society of Medicine,* **59,** 255.

Sanerkin, N. G. (1971) Vascular lesions of malignant essential hypertension. *Journal of Pathology,* **103,** 177.

Sheehan, H. L. & Davis, J. C. (1959a) Renal ischaemia with failed reflow. *Journal of Pathology and Bacteriology,* **78,** 105.

Sheehan, H. L. & Davis, J. C. (1959b) Renal ischaemia with good reflow. *Journal of Pathology and Bacteriology,* **78,** 351.

Shirai, T. & Sims, E. A. H. (1970) Pre-eclampsia and related complications of pregnancy, quoted by Sims, E. A. H. (1970) *American Journal of Obstetrics and Gynecology,* **107,** 154.

Simonson, M., Buemann, J., Gammel Toft, A., Jensen, F. & Jorgensen, K. (1953) Biological incompatibility in kidney transplantation in dogs; experimental and morphological investigations. *Acta Pathologica et Microbiologica Scandinavica,* **32,** 1.

Sinclair, R. A. (1972) Origin of endothelium in human renal allografts. *British Medical Journal,* **iv,** 15.

Sophian, J. (1972) *Pregnancy Nephropathy,* Vol. 2. London: Butterworths.

Speroff, L. (1973) Toxaemia of pregnancy; mechanism and therapeutic management. *American Journal of Cardiology,* **32,** 582.

Starzl, T. E., Boehmig, H. J., Amemiya, H., Wilson, C. B., Dixon, F. J., Giles, G. R., Simpson, K. M. & Halgrimson, C. G. (1970) Clotting changes, including disseminated intravascular coagulation, during rapid renal homograft rejection. *New England Journal of Medicine,* **283,** 383.

Stiehm, E. R. & Trygstad, C. W. (1968) Split products of fibrin in human renal disease. *American Journal of Medicine,* **46,** 774.

Wardle, E. N. (1973) Studies of animal models of toxaemia with respect to fibrinogen and platelet survival and selectivity of proteinuria. *Angiologica,* **10,** 173.

Wardle, E. N. & Floyd, M. (1973) Fibrinogen catabolism; study of three patients with bacterial endocarditis and renal disease. *British Medical Journal,* **iii,** 255.

Zeek, P. M. (1952) Periarteritis nodosa, a critical review. *American Journal of Clinical Pathology,* **22,** 777.

AUTOIMMUNE MECHANISMS IN HUMAN VASCULAR DISEASE—SKIN MEMORY

Mathews, Whittingham and Mackay (1974) supposed that many of the genetic and environmental causes of human vascular disease may act via immunological pathways. It was their thesis that ageing, genetic factors which determine autoimmune disease, diet, obesity, pregnancy, smoking, infection, tissue injury and breakdown, and stress all contribute to the production of autoantibodies and hence to the formation either of immune complexes or of specific antivessel antibodies. These, by repetitive injury to vessels, cause thrombosis, atherosclerosis and hypertension.

As reviewed by these authors and as referred to in various sections of this monograph, there can be little doubt that immune complexes do injure vessels and may thus contribute to their obliteration, thickening and infiltration by lipid or cells. Such effects are more common in diseases considered to be, at least in part, autoimmune — hypothyroidism or diabetes mellitus, for instance. A few would doubt that repetitive vascular injury and the response it produces in the vascular tree can ultimately contribute to hypertension and ageing. Mathews, Whittingham and Mackay (1974) argued that food and drugs not only provide additional material to which the immunological system may react but also provide the nourishment necessary for peak productiveness of this system.

It has been suggested by these authors that the immune system, unlike other physiological systems, is endowed with memory (Mathews, Whittingham and Mackay, 1974). However, although it is true that most tissues other than the immunological system, when injured, very often do return to their original state, this is not always so. Scarring and its associated changes in anatomical structure represent one form of memory. The 'prepared state' of the vascular tree in the Shwartzman phenomenon is memory in the short term. The accumulation of scars that occurs in the vascular tree is not confined to the immune system and it would be wrong to believe that obliteration of vessels or increase in their permeability are features especially of the immune system.

It is the vascular tree itself that provides the unifying concept. As Mathews, Whittingham and Mackay (1974) so rightly indicated, of all systems of the body the vascular tree may be exposed to the highest concentrations of immune complexes and autoantibodies but is also exposed to the highest concentrations of almost everything else. There is no simple 'all or none' response to such circulating agents, and whether or not a vessel becomes irreversibly damaged depends on many other factors such as fibrinolysis or the phagocytic mononuclear system. Success or failure to achieve restitution of the status quo with new vessel formation depends on yet other factors. In the skin, every component of the local environment of the vessel can be shown to exert an influence on vessel behaviour (Ryan, 1973). Within such a diverse system the role of immune complexes is but one factor and not such a big factor at that. They do contribute to vessel injury, they do 'prepare' the vessel and exhaust it of fibrinolytic and phagocytic potential, as in the Shwartzman phenomenon, but they have this effect mostly at prepared sites, at a locus minores resistentiae or where stasis is predominant. To understand human vascular disease it is necessary to understand the anatomy of stasis.

References

Mathews, J. D., Whittingham, S. & Mackay, I. R. (1974) Autoimmune mechanisms in human vascular disease. *Lancet,* **ii,** 1423.

Ryan, T. J. (1973) In *Physiology and Pathophysiology of the Skin* (Ed.) Jarrett, A. Volume 2. London: Academic Press.

8. Infection, Food and Drugs as Triggers of Vasculitis

Infection, food and drugs are exogenous agents frequently incriminated in vasculitis. They often act as triggers or provokers of vascular pathology (Figure 8.1.), but even more often they modify venular behaviour, contribute to the anatomy of stasis and 'prepare' the vessel so that subsequent injury has a greater effect.

Such a temporary state of altered reactivity is demonstrated in all of the following: the preparatory and provoking stages in the Shwartzman phenomenon, the aspirin and tartrazine provocation of vasculitis and its enhancement by trafuril, the isomorphic response to bacterial antigen or the strongly positive Mantoux reaction in some cases of nodular vasculitis, and the hyper-reactivity of the skin in Behçet's disease and in pyoderma gangrenosum.

As often as not this state has something to do with the biological effects of stasis, with the clotting and fibrinolytic mechanisms and with the complement cascade. It is a change in the behaviour of the vessel that not only makes it more susceptible to insults, including the effects of cold and to alterations in endocrine status or in the emotions, but also impairs its ability to repair itself and to rid itself of the insulting agent. It is not difficult to explain such a preparatory role since many data have been collected in studies of the Shwartzman phenomenon. It is merely a question of applying this information to the clinical manifestations of venulitis.

As indicated in Chapter 6 'preparation' of the vascular system, so that vasculitis develops when it is 'provoked', depends on the following factors:
1. Blockade of the reticuloendothelial system, also known as the mononuclear phagocytic system.
2. Decreased fibrinolysis.
3. Increased sensitivity of arteriolar smooth muscle to catecholamines.
The most significant of such provoking factors act by stimulating the coagulation system.

While food and drugs act chiefly as 'preparatory' agents, infections more commonly act both as 'preparatory' and as 'provoking' agents. Much of the confusion in the literature concerning the aetiology of vasculitis arises because it is difficult to demonstrate the actual presence of the preparatory agent at the time of provocation. However, it is not difficult to demonstrate the *hyper-reactivity* or *'preparedness'* of the tissues at the time of provocation since this is typified by the isomorphic response, the trafuril reaction in vasculitis, the hypersensitivity that is seen in Behçet's disease or pyoderma gangrenosum, and the enhanced Mantoux reaction in nodular vasculitis.

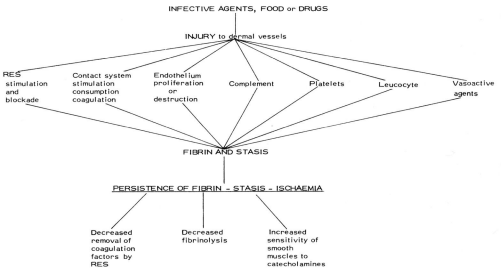

Figure 8.1. Diagram of effects of injury to dermal vessels by infective agents, food and drugs. Fibrin and stasis are a consequence of several associated phenomena.

The importance of the apparent specificity of invading organisms is now in doubt, not only in vasculitis but also in conditions such as progressive bacterial gangrene and necrotising fasciitis and in transplanted organs. Vicious circles of infection, local ischaemia, and reduced local and systemic host defence mechanisms need to be explored. Thus acute dermal gangrene following infection cannot be explained merely by the presence of a virulent organism (Ledingham and Tehrani, 1975). Moreover, to enable patients to live in symbiosis with foreign organs and yet remain free of the risk of infection requires much work on the biochemistry and pharmacology of the reticulo-endothelial cell system and on the microvascular system (Drivas, Uldall and Wardle, 1975). The influence of oestrogen on localisation of infection in the nose also is clearly in part a vascular effect (see Chapter 9), but the virulence of *E. coli* for the kidney in pregnancy seems to be specific for certain strains that are encouraged by oestrogens (Harle, Bullen and Thompson, 1975).

One other way in which bacteria can alter the constitution is through coagulation mechanisms by acting as a stimulus to fibrinogen formation by the liver (Ham and Curtis, 1938). The resulting high levels of fibrinogen increase blood viscosity which exaggerates stasis at sites of slow blood flow. This is but one example of how infection can perpetuate the mechanisms responsible for its own localisation.

THE ROLE OF INFECTIVE AGENTS

Rudzki et al (1964), reviewing the role of bacterial allergy in skin disease, gave some two dozen references to the concept of foci of infection. Several of these are sources of other references to what was at one time of major interest to the medical profession. These authors referred to 20 or so additional reports of remissions of disease following surgical removal or spontaneous clearance of foci of infection, or following a course of antibiotics.

This literature coincided with many other reports of the use of autologous vaccines and an associated increased incidence of fulminant vasculitis. Rudzki et al (1964) tested 1977 individuals with streptococcal antigens and 779 individuals with staphylococcal antigens. They were able to induce erythema nodosum-like lesions in 19 subjects, allergic vasculitis in 12 and urticaria in three. They emphasised that such reactions could be provoked only at the height of active disease and were rarely seen during remissions. These tests were more likely to be positive when there was gross infection, probably because the tissues were in some way altered or prepared by such infection. Vasculitis was the commonest disease pattern associated with positive skin tests, and it seemed that the vascular system is the locus minoris resistentiae for bacterial hypersensitivity. The ability of skin vessels to react to skin tests is transient and often expires after active disease has subsided. Rajka (1968) observed that atopic eczema subjects were less reactive than controls to both bacterial and viral allergens, and in another study (Rajka, 1969) he noted that the streptococcal antigen produced haemorrhagic leucocytoclastic reactions more commonly in the elderly.

Rostenberg (1953), in an article that drew the attention of dermatologists to a number of diseases that could be explained by the Shwartzman phenomenon, also referred to changes in reactivity at the height of the disease. He reported many examples of vasculitis induced by tuberculin, typhoid vaccine, and other vaccines prepared from staphylococci or E. coli. He emphasised that fulminant vasculitis provoked by bacterial vaccines occurred most commonly either when there was an excess of antigen at the height of the ragweed season or during a generalised infection.

A similar story is related by Winkelmann and Ditto (1964). Case 36 of their series of patients with allergic vasculitis had received bacterial antigen, and case 22 had received ragweed and dust antigens. Gougerot (1932) was one of the more influential exponents of the role of bacteria in vasculitis. At first he was concerned only with bacterial endocarditis but later he searched for septicaemia. It was only because the search was often fruitless that Gougerot became more interested in allergy (Gougerot and Duperrat, 1954). Focal sepsis continued to be recorded, however, and sinusitis, dental abscesses, gallstones, amoebic dysentery or hypersensitivity to tuberculin, to staphylococcal or to streptococcal antigen were reported. As indicated in Chapter 2, besides French authors, Ruiter, Storck and Miescher frequently wrote about infection and allergy in vasculitis (reviewed by Pevny and Metz, 1972).

The streptococcus and staphylococcus

Acute streptococcal sore throats have long been known to have an association with Schönlein—Henoch purpura (Gairdner, 1948), usually preceding the rash by one to three weeks. This association, however, is not an exact one, for no significantly increased incidence of streptococcal sore throat was found in one study of 45 children (Vernier et al, 1961), and the anti-streptolysin O titre was no higher than in the normal population in another study (Bywaters, Isdale and Kempton, 1957). Rudzki et al (1964) also found the anti-streptolysin O titre to be of little relevance. In another study, a history of sore throats in 70 per cent of 75 cases was associated only rarely with a positive throat swab, and less than half the patients had a raised anti-streptolysin O titre (Ansell, 1970). In her study, streptococcal infection seemed unimportant as a cause of renal changes presenting with haematuria. Others held the same view (Treser et al, 1970).

The majority of clinically important streptococcal infections are caused by beta haemolytic streptococci of Lancefield Group A. The cell wall carries a protein which includes an antigenic component M. Antigen M is responsible for virulence and inhibits phagocytosis by neutrophils and macrophages (Lancefield, 1962). Antibody to M coats the streptococcus and hence restores susceptibility to phagocytic activity. This antibody, however, also binds to heart muscle, to smooth muscle elements of arteries, arterioles and endocardium (Kaplan and Mayeserian, 1962; Kaplan and Svec, 1964), as well as to human fibroblasts and endothelium (Kingston and Glynn, 1971). Moreover, antigens from human glomeruli and from cell membranes of streptococci cross-react (Markowitz and Lange, 1964; Holm, Braun and Jönsson, 1968) and streptococcal antigen has been found in glomeruli by several workers (Andres et al, 1966; Michael et al, 1966; Lange et al, 1969). It is evident, therefore, that acute glomerulonephritis could arise from an immunological response aimed at the streptococcus but cross-reacting with the kidney (Zabriskie, 1971).

The streptococcus also has an adjuvant effect in the induction of autoimmune disease (Holborow, Schwab and Brown, 1969) and in the rejection of homografts (Chase and Rapaport, 1965).

In a review of vasculitis with widespread systemic vessel involvement, Rose and Spencer (1957) thought that an abnormal immune response to infection was a contributory factor, whereas Bartak (1970) and Rantz et al (1952), who studied other forms of vasculitis, found a high incidence of streptococcal infection in their cases.

Sensitivity to streptococcal skin tests has been described in a child with recurrent crops of tender nodules associated with livedo reticularis of the legs, feet and ankles (Orkin, 1970). Similarly, the particular role of streptococcal infection in nodular vasculitis, rheumatoid vasculitis and maladie trisymptôme has been demonstrated by the results of intradermal tests, passive transfer tests and lymphocyte transformation in 20 patients studied by Ky, Hazard and Laroche (1968).

Parish (1971a), studying vasculitis, found that the only definite correlation between a history of a febrile illness in the preceding three months and the presence of bacterial antigen in the vascular lesions was the occurrence either of streptococcal antigens in those lesions infiltrated by neutrophils, or (in two patients) of *Mycobacterium tuberculosis* antigen in lesions infiltrated predominantly by mononuclear cells. The bacterial antigen was usually intracellular and seemed to be in degraded rather than intact organisms. Parish concluded that his results reflect the harmless and fortuitous deposition of substances in damaged tissue containing active phagocytes.

In a second paper, Parish (1971b) stated "after infection, many persons form antibody to bacterial antigen capable of forming tissue-damaging complexes, but vasculitis may only occur in those in whom sufficient antigen is released into the blood to form complexes and whose tissues are 'prepared' for the penetration of the complexes into the vessel walls".

Parish also observed that patients with vasculitis had less circulating antibody to bacterial antigen, particularly to streptococcal protein and lipopolysaccharide cellular antigen, than did patients recovering from similar infections without vasculitis. Moreover, the complexes formed by the antibodies in the vasculitis patients were less harmful to the tissues than those formed by the patients without vasculitis. Such a finding may indicate that patients with vasculitis are forming harmful complexes in antigen excess of equivalence to antibody.

Parish and Rhodes (1967) were the first to detect streptococcal antigen in vasculitis of the skin. They found it in one of nine patients with nodular vasculitis of the legs; the serum of that patient contained antibody which, when complexed with streptococcal antigen, caused vasculitis in an experimental animal. Parish (1971c) later found streptococcal antigen in 14 of 80 cases of vasculitis and in four cases of erythema nodosum. By inoculating streptococcal antigen intradermally, Cream, Levene and Calnan (1971) produced haemorrhagic pustules with a massive neutrophil infiltrate and vasculitis in patients with erythema elevatum diutinum, a disease in which vasculitis has a particularly fibrotic and persistent healing phase. Both the skin test and the skin rash were suppressed by dapsone. It is interesting to recall that as long ago as 1929, Weidman and Besançon showed that in erythema elevatum diutinum, which is an example of a chronic low-grade form of vasculitis, reactions to skin testing with bacterial antigen are strongly positive and that the streptococcus was particularly implicated (Figures 8.2 and 8.3).

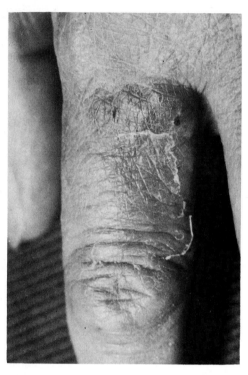

Figure 8.2. Erythema elevatum diutinum before response to dapsone in a middle-aged woman also suffering from interstitial fibrosis of the lung.

Parker (1969) in a review of glomerulonephritis following streptococcal skin infection referred to nephritogenic streptococci, the well-known type 12 and less familiar 49, which accounted for large epidemics of pyoderma among American Indians, often followed by nephritis. Type 49 also accounted for nephritis following skin infection in the Trinidad epidemics reported by Bassett (1972). Type 55 accounted for other epidemics probably spread by scabies (Poon-King et al, 1973).

The role of bacterial endocarditis was emphasised by Gougerot (1932) and later by Rowell (1968) and it has been suggested more recently by Hayward that in this disease the lesions previously ascribed to microemboli could in fact be due to immune complexes (Hayward, 1973). However, the proliferative glomerulonephritis seen in bacterial endocarditis would, according to Wardle and Floyd (1973), largely result from an intravascular coagulation, for they detected accelerated fibrinogen catabolism in three patients they studied. Further evidence that its genesis could be explained by an immune mechanism was provided by Boulton-Jones et al (1974), although in two of their cases the pathogenesis of the glomerulonephritis was attributable neither to emboli nor to immune complexes and was consequently unexplained. Other references to sub-acute bacterial endocarditis and shunt nephritis are available (Williams and Kunkel, 1962; Black,

Challacombe and Ockenden, 1965; Stickler et al, 1968; Gutman et al, 1972).

The problem was viewed from a different point of view by Freedman et al (1970) who studied 1246 patients with beta haemolytic streptococcal upper respiratory tract infection; they suggested that such infection produced a functional or even a morphological change in the tissues which was not, or was only weakly, immunological.

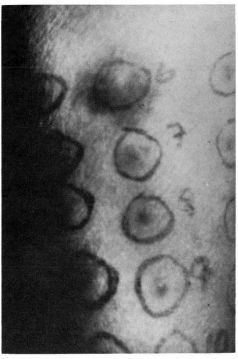

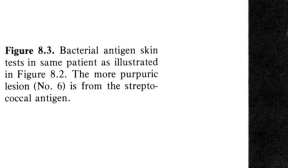

Figure 8.3. Bacterial antigen skin tests in same patient as illustrated in Figure 8.2. The more purpuric lesion (No. 6) is from the streptococcal antigen.

Little distinction has been made in the literature between the 'provoking' effect of a severe acute infection which was a feature in the cases of fulminant vasculitis described by Ruiter (1952, 1960, 1962), Wilkinson (1965) and Winkelmann and Ditto (1964), and the 'preparatory' effect of minor or concealed infection as is seen in the sub-acute or chronic forms of vasculitis. It is only in the latter that a close search for, and elimination of, foci of infection may be of value (Ruiter, 1952). For example, chronic *E. coli* infection was thought to be concerned in one closely followed and fully investigated case (Teilum, 1946) and others have been reported by Duperrat and Montfort (1958), Wilkinson (1954) and Vilanova (1951). Wilkinson (1954) found active infection in nine of 28 cases of nodular vasculitis; in three of these, resolution followed treatment of a streptococcal throat infection, and in four the vasculitis was related to a symptomless dental abscess and cleared after the tooth had been extracted. This situation was also emphasised by Duperrat and Montfort (1958) and Vilanova (1951).

Fedotov and Bazyka (1967) obtained serological evidence of sensitivity to staphylococci more often than to streptococci in 40 cases of deep vasculitis of the legs. As early as 1903, Loeb wrote of the influence of pathogenic coagulase-positive staphylococci on coagulation, and there is ample evidence that staphylococcal filtrates activate the production of a form of thrombosis which is not inhibited by heparin (Biggs and Macfarlane, 1962).

Martin, Crowder and White (1967) observed delayed necrosis in the skin of people with high blood levels of antibody to staphylococcal teichoic acids. They also reported that complexes of teichoic acid and antibody released lysosomes from neutrophils in vitro.

The staphylococcus and the streptococcus are probably the most significant human pathogens, but most bacteria have been incriminated at some time or other in disseminated intravascular coagulation, and it is the gram-negative organisms that have been most often blamed for the Shwartzman phenomenon (see Chapter 10). Cryoglobulinaemia and glomerulonephritis, as well as local inflammatory lesions, have been recorded in a nurse who repeatedly injected herself with diphtheria, pertussis and tetanus vaccine (Boulton-Jones, 1974a).

The control of gram-positive organisms has led to an increasing incidence of infections by gram-negative organisms which, in some respects, are more difficult to manage. Certain of these bacteria are fibrinolytically active, namely: *Pseudomonas fluorescens* (Adamis, 1961) and *Pseudomonas aeruginosa* (Bhagwat, 1962). They may initially stimulate fibrinolysis but in overwhelming infections fibrinolysis is presumably exhausted.

References

Adamis, D. M. (1961) A new fibrinolytic and anticoagulant enzyme. *Lancet*, **ii**, 1070.

Andres, G. A., Accinni, L., Hsu, K. C., Zabriskie, J. B. & Seegal, B. C. (1966) Electron microscope studies of human glomerulonephritis with ferritin conjugated antibody. Localisation of antigen antibody complexes in glomerular structures of patients with acute glomerulonephritis. *Journal of Experimental Medicine*, **123**, 399.

Ansell, B. M. (1970) Henoch—Schönlein purpura with particular reference to the prognosis of the renal lesion. *British Journal of Dermatology*, **82**, 211.

Bartak, P. (1970) Vascular patterns and the pathogenesis of nodular panniculitis of the legs. *British Journal of Dermatology*, **82** (Supplement 5), 15.

Bassett, D. C. J. (1972) Streptococcal pyoderma and acute nephritis in Trinidad. *British Journal of Dermatology*, **86** (Supplement 8), 55.

Beidleman, B. (1963) Wegener's granulomatosis; prolonged therapy with large doses of steroids. *Journal of the American Medical Association*, **186**, 827.

Bhagwat, A. G. (1962) New fibrinolytic and anticoagulant enzyme. *Lancet*, **i**, 487.

Biggs, R. & Macfarlane, R. G. (1962) *Human Blood Coagulation and its Disorders*, 3rd edition. Oxford: Blackwell.

Black, J. D., Challacombe, D. N. & Ockenden, B. G. (1965) Nephrotic syndrome associated with bacteraemia after shunt operations for hydrocephalus. *Lancet*, **ii**, 921.

Boulton-Jones, J. M., Sissons, J. G. P., Naish, P. F., Evans, D. J. & Peters, D. K. (1974a) Self induced glomerulonephritis. *British Medical Journal*, **ii**, 387.

Boulton-Jones, J. M., Sissons, J. G. P., Evans, D. J. & Peters, D. K. (1974b) Renal lesions of subacute infective endocarditis. *British Medical Journal*, **ii**, 11.

Bywaters, E. G. L., Isdale, I. & Kempton, J. J. (1957) Schönlein—Henoch purpura. *Quarterly Journal of Medicine*, **26**, 161.

Chase, R. M. & Rapaport, F. T. (1965) The bacterial induction of homograft sensitivity. I. Effects of sensitisation with Group A streptococci. *Journal of Experimental Medicine*, **122**, 721.

Cream, J. J., Levene, G. M. & Calnan, C. D. (1971) Erythema elevatum diutinum: an unusual reaction to streptococcal antigen and response to dapsone. *British Journal of Dermatology*, **84**, 393.

Drivas, G., Uldall, P. R. & Wardle, N. (1975) Reticulo-endothelial function in renal allograft recipients. *British Medical Journal*, **iii**, 743.

Duperrat, B. & Monfort, J. (1958) Les allergides vasculaires hypodermiques. *Annales de Dermatologie et de Syphiligraphie*, **85**, 385.

Fedotov, V. P. & Bazyka, A. P. (1967) Immunologic reactions in patients with allergic nodular dermohypodermal lesions. *Vestnik Dermatologii et Venerologii*, **22**.

Freedman, P., Meister, H. P., Lee H. J., Smith, E. A., Co, B. S. & Nidus, B. D. (1970) The renal response to streptococcal infection. *Medicine* (Baltimore), **49**, 433.

Gairdner, D. (1948) The Schönlein—Henoch syndrome and anaphylactoid purpura. *Quarterly Journal of Medicine*, **17**, 95.

Gougerot, H. (1932) Septicémie chronique indéterminée caractérisée par des petits nodules dermiques ("Dermatitis nodularis non necroticans") elements erythemato-papuleux purpura. *Bulletin de la Société Française de Dermatologie et de Syphiligraphie*, **39**, 1192.

Gougerot, H. & Duperrat, B. (1954) The nodular dermal allergides of Gougerot. *British Journal of Dermatology*, **66**, 283.

Gutman, R. A., Striker, G. E., Gilliland, B. C. & Cutler, R. E. (1972) The immune complex glomerulonephritis of bacterial endocarditis. *Medicine* (Baltimore), **51**, 1.

Ham, J. H. & Curtis, F. C. (1938) Plasma fibrinogen response in man, influence of nutritional state, induced hyperpyrexia, infectious disease and liver damage. *Medicine* (Baltimore), **17**, 413.

Harle, E. M. J., Bullen, J. J. & Thompson, D. A. (1975) Influence of oestrogen on experimental pyelonephritis caused by Escherichia coli. *Lancet*, **ii**, 283.

Hayward, G. W. (1973) Infective endocarditis, a changing disease. *British Medical Journal*, **ii**, 706.

Holborow, E. J., Schwab, J. H. & Brown, J. C. (1969) The capacity of isolated cell walls from Group A streptococci to induce auto-immune processes. *Folia Allergologica*, **16**, 287.

Holm, S. E., Braun, D. & Jönsson, J. (1968) Antigenic factors common to human kidney and nephritogenic and non-nephritogenic streptococcal strains. *International Archives of Allergy and Applied Immunology*, **33**, 127.

Houba, V., Allison, A. C., Adeniyi, A. & Houba, J. E. (1971) Immunoglobulin classes and complement in biopsies of Nigerian children with the nephrotic syndrome. *Clinical and Experimental Immunology*, **8**, 761.

Kaplan, M. H. & Mayeserian, M. (1962) Immunological studies of heart tissue. V. Antigens related to heart tissue revealed by cross-reaction of rabbit antisera to heterologous heart. *Journal of Immunology*, **88**, 450.

Kaplan, M. H. & Svec, K. H. (1964) Immunologic relation of streptococcal and tissue antigens. III. Presence in human sera of streptococcal antibody, cross reactive with heart tissue. Association with streptococcal infection, rheumatic fever and glomerulonephritis. *Journal of Experimental Medicine*, **119**, 651.

Kingston, D. & Glynn, L. E. (1971) A cross reaction between *S. pyogenes* and human fibroblasts, endothelial cells and astrocytes. *Immunology*, **21**, 1003.

Ky, N. T., Hazard, J. & Laroche, C. (1968) Allergies vasculaires cutanées d'origine streptococcus — a propos de vingt observations. *Presse Médicale*, **76**, 247.

Lancefield, R. C. (1962) Current knowledge of type and specific M antigens of Group A Streptococci. *Journal of Immunology*, **89**, 307.

Lange, K., Semar, M., Ty, A. & Treser, G. (1969) A specific antigen and antibody in acute post streptococcal glomerulonephritis. *Transactions of the Association of American Physicians*, **82**, 188.

Ledingham, I. McA. & Tehrani, M. A. (1975) Diagnosis, clinical course and treatment of acute dermal gangrene. *British Journal of Surgery*, **62**, 364.

Loeb, L. (1903) The influence of certain bacteria on the coagulation of the blood. *Journal of Medical Research* (Boston), **10**, 407.

Markowitz, A. S. & Lange, C. F. Jr (1964) Streptococcal related glomerulonephritis. *Journal of Immunology*, **92**, 565.

Martin, R. R., Crowder, J. G. & White, A. (1967) Human reactions to staphylococcal antigen. A possible role of leukocyte lysosomal enzymes. *Journal of Immunology*, **99**, 269.

Michael, A. F., Drummond, K. N., Good, R. A. & Vernier, R. L. (1966) Acute post-streptococcal glomerulonephritis: immune deposit disease. *Journal of Clinical Investigation*, **45**, 237.

Orkin, M. (1970) Cutaneous polyarteritis nodosa. *Archives of Dermatology*, **102**, 571.

Parish, W. E. (1971a) Studies in vasculitis. I. Immunoglobulins β1C, C-reactive protein and bacterial antigens in cutaneous vasculitis lesions. *Clinical Allergy*, **1**, 97.

Parish, W. E. (1971b) Studies on vasculitis. II. Some properties of complexes formed of antibacterial antibodies from persons with or without cutaneous vasculitis lesions. *Clinical Allergy*, **1**, 111.

Parish, W. E. (1971c) Studies on vasculitis. III. Decreased formation of antibody to M protein Group A, polysaccharide and to some exotoxins in persons with cutaneous vasculitis after streptococcal infection. *Clinical Allergy*, **1**, 295.

Parish, W. E. & Rhodes, E. L. (1967) Bacterial antigens and aggregated gamma globulin in the lesions of nodular vasculitis. *British Journal of Dermatology*, **79**, 131.

Parker, M. T. (1969) Streptococcal skin infection and acute glomerulonephritis. *British Journal of Dermatology*, **8**, (Supplement 1), 37.

Pevny, I. & Metz, J. (1972) Positiver Intracutantest, Fern- und Aufflammphanomen mit Streptokokken-antigen bei Vasculitis Allergica. *Hautarzt*, **23**, 350.

Poon-King, T., Porter, E., Svartman, M., Achong, J., Mohammed, I., Cox, R. & Earle, D. P. (1973) Epidemic acute nephritis with reappearance of M type 55 streptococci in Trinidad. *Lancet*, **i**, 475.

Rajka, G. (1968) Delayed dermal and epidermal reactivity in atopic dermatitis (Prurigo Besnier). III. Further studies with bacterial and viral allergens. *Acta Dermato-venereologica*, **48**, 186.

Rajka, G. (1969) Delayed reactivity to bacterial and viral extracts in the aged. *Acta Dermato-venereologica*, **49**, 503.

Rantz, L. A., Di Caprio, J. M. & Randall, E. (1952) Antistreptolysin O and anti-hyaluronidase titres in health and in various diseases. *American Journal of the Medical Sciences*, **224**, 194.

Rose, G. A. & Spencer, H. (1957) Polyarteritis nodosa. *Quarterly Journal of Medicine*, **26**, 43.

Rostenberg, A. (1953) The Shwartzman phenomenon: a review with consideration of some possible dermatological manifestations. *British Journal of Dermatology*, **65**, 389.

Rowell, N. R. (1968) Polyarteritis nodosa. In *Textbook of Dermatology* (Ed.) Rook, A., Wilkinson, D. S. & Ebling, F. J. G. p. 578. Oxford: Blackwell.

Rudzki, E., Moskalewska, K., Leszczynski, W., Maciejowska, E. & Blaszczyk, M. (1964) Bacterial allergy in the skin diseases. 1) The methods of evaluation. *Acta Dermato-venereologica,* **44,** 310.

Ruiter, M. (1952) Allergic cutaneous vasculitis. *Acta Dermato-venereologica,* **32,** 274.

Ruiter, M. (1960) Some histopathological aspects of vascular allergy. *International Archives of Allergy and Applied Immunology,* **17,** 157.

Ruiter, M. (1962) Vascular fibrinoid in cutaneous "allergic" arteriolitis. *Journal of Investigative Dermatology,* **38,** 85.

Stickler, G. B., Shin, M. H., Burke, E. C., Holley, K. E., Miller, R. H. & Segar, W. E. (1968) Diffuse glomerulonephritis associated with infected ventriculoatrial shunt. *New England Journal of Medicine,* **279,** 1027.

Teilum, G. (1946) Pathogenetic studies on lupus erythematosus disseminatus and related diseases. *Acta Medica Scandinavica,* **123,** 126.

Treser, G., Semar, M., Ty, A., Sagei, I., Franklin, M. A. & Lange, K. (1970) Partial characterization of antigenic streptococcal plasma membrane components in acute glomerulonephritis. *Journal of Clinical Investigation,* **49,** 762.

Vernier, R. L., Worthen, H. G., Peterson, R. D., Cole, E. & Good, R. A. (1961) Anaphylactoid purpura. I. Pathology of the skin and kidney and frequency of streptococcal infection. *Pediatrics,* **27,** 181.

Vilanova, Z. (1951) Vasculite nodulaire. *Semaine des Hôpitaux de Paris,* **27,** 2803.

Wardle, E. N. & Floyd, M. (1973) Fibrinogen catabolism study of three patients with bacterial endocarditis and renal disease. *British Medical Journal,* **iii,** 255.

Weidman, F. D. & Besançon, J. H. (1929) Erythema elevatum diutinum: role of streptococci and relationship to other rheumatic dermatoses. *Archives of Dermatology and Syphilology,* **20,** 593.

Wilkinson, D. S. (1954) The vascular basis of some nodular eruptions of the legs. *British Journal of Dermatology,* **66,** 201.

Wilkinson, D. S. (1965) Some clinical manifestations and associations of "allergic" vasculitis. *British Journal of Dermatology,* **77,** 186.

Williams, R. C. & Kunkel, H. G. (1962) Rheumatoid factor complement and conglutinin aberrations in patients with subacute bacterial endocarditis. *Journal of Clinical Investigation,* **41,** 666.

Winkelmann, R. K. & Ditto, W. B. (1964) Cutaneous and visceral syndromes of necrotising or "allergic" angiitis. A study of 38 cases. *Medicine* (Baltimore), **43,** 59.

Zabriskie, J. B. (1971) The role of streptococci in human glomerulonephritis. *Journal of Experimental Medicine,* **134,** (Supplement 180).

Mycobacterial infections

Subsequent to Bazin's (1861) description of deep indurated red areas on the lower legs of some female patients, the condition named erythema induratum was thought to be associated with tuberculosis. However, some distinguished authors such as Audry (1898), Whitfield (1901) and Galloway (1913) doubted this association, especially in older women in whom inflammation of the leg is often associated with thrombophlebitis, stasis and perniosis. Subsequently Montgomery, O'Leary and Barker (1945), after a process of exclusion of known causes, described the histological features of a doubtfully distinct entity which they called nodular vasculitis and which was supposedly a primary disease of the deep dermal or subcutaneous vessels.

Hewitt (1957) thought that some young women were subject to prolonged attacks of deep nodules, sometimes ulcerated which affected the legs (Figure 8.4), but were often painless and were worse in winter. Such nodules were often associated with tuberculosis and occasionally were even directly infected by mycobacteria. However, he also described a patient under the care of Degos, from whose lesions a streptococcus could be isolated, and emphasised the advisability of searching for other infections. He also referred to the role of ischaemia following obliteration of large veins and arteries. In his view, altered reactivity — 'allergy' — might be a consequence of tuberculosis or of other bacterial infections or even drugs; Hewitt came to the conclusion that nodular vasculitis is a polymorphic vascular disorder usually with painful lesions and often associated with strongly positive skin tests to tuberculin and to other bacterial allergens and perhaps less often associated with perniosis.

In a study of 42 patients with nodular eruptions of the legs Wilkinson (1954) found only three with associated tuberculosis. He believed that the mycobacterium was rarely the direct cause of the injury but that in some way it intensified nonspecific peripheral vascular reactivity.

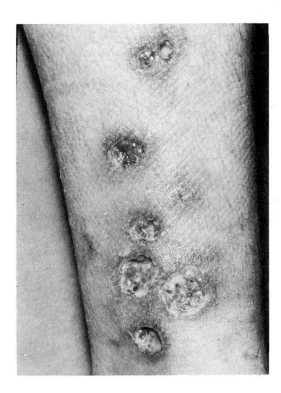

Figure 8.4. Ulceration of the leg in a patient with pulmonary tuberculosis.

Feiwel (1968) reviewed 30 patients in whom he considered that tuberculosis was the most likely cause of the skin nodules of their legs; this opinion was based on clinical or radiological evidence, or on a history of tuberculosis and a strongly positive Mantoux test. He began his review by describing a patient with ulceration and increased sensitivity of the fingers, an obvious case of papulonecrotic tuberculid. More recently, Findlay and Morrison (1973) have drawn attention to the tuberculous origin of acral gangrene in the African. It is relevant in this context that such cases of gangrene have been described in which gross defects in coagulation and fibrinolytic mechanisms have been present (Barr, Roy and Miller, 1972).

Papulonecrotic tuberculid is an extreme form of hypersensitivity to infection in which the tuberculin reaction is strongly positive and endarteritis and thrombosis of dermal vessels are characteristic features (Wilkinson, 1972) (Figure 8.5). Morrison and Fourie (1974) described 91 cases of papulonecrotic tuberculid; gangrene of the extremities due to arteritis was a feature in seven of them and erythema induratum was present in nine. The authors suggested that a high titre of precipitating antibody against *M. tuberculosis* alters the physical properties of the bacteria and that after they have settled out at sites of blood stasis, the antibody and complement are removed by neutrophils without reducing the viability of the bacilli.

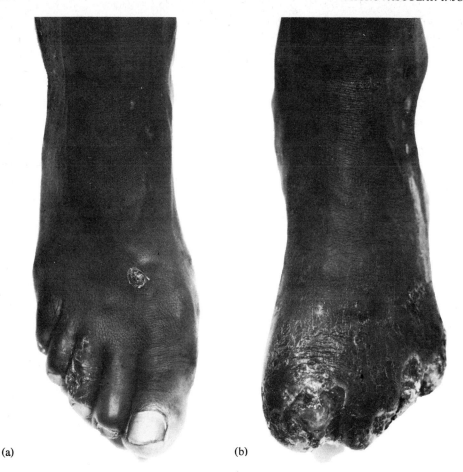

(a)   (b)

Figure 8.5. The feet of a patient affected by papulonecrotic tuberculid illustrating a pattern of gangrene still common in the African. Intravascular coagulation is often demonstrable.

References to the debate on the relationship of tuberculosis to redness and nodularity of the skin of the leg are given by Förström and Hannuksela (1970). These authors studied 72 such patients, nine men and 63 women. Antituberculous therapy was given to all patients and the nodules resolved in all but four, this being the case whether or not the patient had evidence of past or present tuberculosis.

The disappearance of disease in response to antibiotics is not absolute proof of a specific antibacterial effect. Thus Winkelmann and Ditto (1964) in discussing case 19 in their series, a patient with bullous, infarctive, necrotising vasculitis who was intensely sensitive to streptococcal antigen, pointed out that her response to sulphapyridine need be no more specific than the response to the same drug in ulcerative colitis and dermatitis herpetiformis. The suspicion that tetracycline may be of value in nodular vasculitis (Eberhartinger, 1963), because of a vascular rather than an antibacterial effect, is encouraged by Shelley's observations (1971) on the role of this drug in telangiectasia.

Förström, Hannuksela and Rauste (1973) performed lymphography on the legs of 90 patients, eight of whom had erythema nodosum, 44 had erythema induratum and 38 had other forms of panniculitis. Evidence of tuberculous pathology was found in the lymph glands in the pelvis of 1, 16 and 14 of the patients respectively; in 12 of 15 patients who had the lymphography repeated after antituberculous therapy, the affected lymph glands had diminished in size.

Erythema nodosum is associated with a variety of infective agents including streptococcus, tuberculosis, bedsoniae, lymphogranuloma venereum, cat-scratch disease, ornithosis, pasteurella and pseudotuberculosis, blastomycosis, coccidioidomycosis and kerion (Wilkinson, 1972). Many of these, as in tuberculosis, coccidioidomycosis and histoplasmosis, are associated with a high degree of sensitivity to antigen, thus suggesting good T-cell function. It is therefore difficult to understand why erythema nodosum is equally common in sarcoidosis and in lepromatous leprosy, both of which show depressed T-cell function. There is no proof that excessive humoral antibody accounts for this reaction in sarcoidosis. Leprosy is a mycobacterial infection that has received detailed immunological analysis during the past few years, especially the lepromatous form in which erythema nodosum is common (Figure 8.6). Cell-mediated immunity is depressed (Turk and Waters, 1969) and immunoglobulin and complement

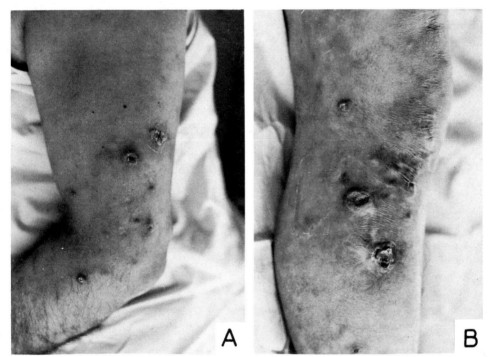

Figure 8.6. Ulcerating lepromatous leprosy in a Cypriot. McDougall and Rees (1973) reported the shedding from body ulcers into the environment of dapsone-resistant bacilli that could have been in excess of 20 million daily.

are deposited in the lesions (Wemambu et al, 1969) (see Figure 14.9). These lesions also show impaired fibrinolytic activity (Ryan, Nishioka and Dawber, 1969). Cryoglobulins are detected in some cases (Bonomo and Dammacco, 1971) and C1q precipitation has been reported (Moran et al, 1972; Rojas-Espinosa, Mendez-Navarrette and Estrada-Parra, 1972).

In Chapter 9, Kanan outlines some reasons for supposing that in certain sites in the body such as the nose, mycobacteria and other organisms tend to settle preferentially and to thrive. Such sites show stasis, hypoxia, impaired fibrinolysis and enhanced phagocytosis.

References

Audry, C. (1898) Étude de la lesion de l'érythème induré. *Annales de Dermatologie et de Syphiligraphie,* **3**, 209.

Barr, R. D., Roy, A. D. & Miller, J. R. M. (1972) Idiopathic gangrene in African adults. *British Medical Journal,* **iv**, 273.

Bazin, E. (1861) *Extrait des Leçons Théoriques et Cliniques sur la Scrofule.* p. 146.

Bonomo, L. & Dammacco, F. (1971) Immune complex cryoglobulinaemia in lepromatous leprosy — a pathogenic approach to some clinical features of leprosy. *Clinical and Experimental Immunology,* **9**, 175.

Eberhartinger, C. (1963) Das Problem des Erythema Induratum Bazin. *Archiv für klinische und experimentelle Dermatologie,* **217**, 196.

Feiwel, M. (1968) Erythema induratum Bazin. *Acta Dermato-venereologica,* **48**, 242.

Findlay, G. H. & Morrison, J. G. L. (1973) Idiopathic gangrene in African adults. *British Medical Journal,* **i**, 173.

Förström, L. & Hannuksela, M. (1970) Anti tuberculosis treatment of erythema induratum Bazin. *Acta Dermato-venereologica,* **50**, 143.

Förström, L., Hannuksela, M. & Rauste, J. (1973) Lymphographic investigation of panniculitis of the legs. *Acta Dermato-venereologica,* **53**, 347.

Galloway, J. (1913) Case of erythema induratum giving no evidence of tuberculosis. *British Journal of Dermatology,* **25**, 217.

Hewitt, J. (1957) Subacute hypodermic nodules of vascular origin. *British Journal of Dermatology,* **69**, 245.

Montgomery, H., O'Leary, P. A. & Barker, N. W. (1945) Nodular vascular diseases of legs; erythema induratum and allied conditions. *Journal of the American Medical Association,* **128**, 335.

Moran, C. J., Turk, J. L., Ryder, G. & Waters, M. F. R. (1972) Evidence for circulating immune complexes in lepromatous leprosy. *Lancet,* **ii**, 572.

Morrison, J. G. L. & Fourie, E. D. (1974) The papulonecrotic tuberculide. *British Journal of Dermatology,* **91**, 263.

Rojas-Espinosa, O., Mendez-Navarrette, I. & Estrada-Parra, S. (1972) Presence of C1q-reactive immune complexes in patients with leprosy. *Clinical and Experimental Immunology,* **12**, 215.

Ryan, T. J., Nishioka, K. & Dawber, R. P. R. (1971) Epithelial—endothelial interactions in the control of inflammation through fibrinolysis. *British Journal of Dermatology,* **84**, 501.

Shelley, W. B. (1971) Essential progressive telangiectasia — successful treatment with tetracycline. *Journal of the American Medical Association,* **216**, 1343.

Turk, J. L. & Waters, M. F. (1969) Cell mediated immunity in patients with leprosy. *Lancet,* **ii**, 243.

Wemambu, S. N. C., Turk, J. L., Waters, M. F. R. & Rees, R. J. W. (1969) Erythema nodosum leprosum, a clinical manifestation of the Arthus phenomenon. *Lancet,* **ii**, 933.

Whitfield, A. (1901) On the nature of disease known as erythema induratum scrofulosorum. *British Journal of Dermatology,* **13**, 323.

Wilkinson, D. S. (1954) The vascular basis of some nodular eruptions of the legs. *British Journal of Dermatology,* **66**, 201.

Wilkinson, D. S. (1972) Erythema nodosum. In *Textbook of Dermatology* (Ed.) Rook, A., Wilkinson, D. S. & Ebling, F. p. 953. Oxford: Blackwell.

Winkelmann, R. K. & Ditto, W. B. (1964) Cutaneous and visceral syndromes of necrotising or "allergic" angiitis. A study of 38 cases. *Medicine,* **43**, 59.

Miscellaneous infections

Vasculitis has also been recorded in association with fungus infections (Andriasian, 1967) and there is an unexplained relationship between chilblains and *Trychophyton rubrum* infections (Cremer, 1953). Halmy and Pintye (1968) described 12 patients with vasculitis in whom serum antibodies to *Trichophyton rubrum,* to *Candida albicans,* or to both were demonstrated by agar gel plates and intracutaneous tests were positive.

Erythema nodosum has been reported in 4.6 per cent of cases of coccidioidomycosis (Smith, 1940) and in blastomycosis (Smith et al, 1955; Medeiros et al, 1966). The association of kerion with erythema nodosum was reported by Sutter (1920), Bloch (1921), Ferguson-Smith (1963) and Warin (1963).

Older texts blamed vasculitis on syphilis, largely on circumstantial evidence, but in recent years an immunological basis for such vasculitis has become better documented.

Cryoprecipitates have been demonstrated in one series by Mustakallio, Lassus and Wager (1967) and in another large series of cases of vasculitis, Lassus et al (1969) found cryoglobulinaemia in 15 per cent. Rheumatoid factors were found in 13 per cent. Glomerulonephritis in congenital syphilis is also induced by immune complexes (Wiggelinkhuizen et al, 1973).

Chronic gonococcal sepsis has been responsible for a Shwartzman-like vasculitis of the skin and direct immunofluorescence for antigenic material of *Neisseria gonorrhoea* is helpful in such cases (Shapiro, Teisch and Brownstein, 1973; Danielsson, Norberg and Svanbom, 1975).

Rickettsial diseases, too, are relevant in vasculitis having been blamed for chronic purpuric eruptions with necrosis and a histological picture of microvascular thrombosis (Bazex et al, 1960). In fact a long time ago (Ash and Spitz, 1945; Allen, 1954) necrotising angiitis of typhus was compared to polyarteritis nodosa. Necrotic purpura lesions of the lower leg resembling stasis ulcers and infarcts were attributed to latent rickettsial infection by Nicolau, Noaghea and Bucur (1967). They established this relationship by using agglutination, complement fixation and skin tests as well as by the response to tetracycline; the organisms incriminated were *R. prowazekii*, *R. mooseri* and *R. conorii*. In Rocky Mountain spotted fever, Wolbach, Todd and Palfrey (1922) demonstrated intra-endothelial rickettsiae and necrotising angiitis. Thrombosis and symmetrical gangrene were reported by Snyder (1965) and livedo reticularis appeared in an illustration from a patient of Wolbach (Figure 8.7). A recent review of 50 cases (Torres, Humphreys and Bisno, 1973) confirmed the high incidence of disseminated intravascular coagulation.

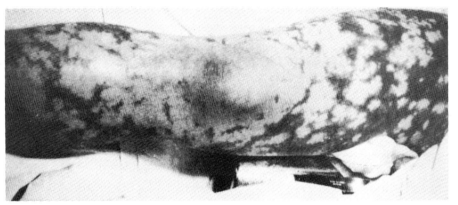

Figure 8.7. Reticulate pattern of vasculitis in a patient with Rocky Mountain spotted fever referred to by Snyder (1965).

Mycoplasmas

Like viruses, these are small and lack cell walls; unlike viruses they contain both DNA and RNA and possess independent metabolic systems. They are the smallest free-living organisms known and their role in skin disease is difficult to assess (Gordon and Lyell, 1970).

In erythema multiforme they have been isolated from the respiratory tract at the same time as raised titres of complement fixing antibody have been detected in the serum (Ludlam, Bridges and Benn, 1964; Katz et al, 1967; Cannell, Churcher and Milton-Thompson, 1969). They were not isolated from the skin according to these reports. Lyell et al (1967) isolated *M. pneumoniae* from the skin of two cases at a time when the titre of complement fixing antibody was rising. In a series of mucocutaneous diseases associated with mycoplasma infection, an outbreak of acute respiratory disease coupled with various skin rashes was attributed by Feizi et al (1967) to *M. pneumoniae*. A relevant finding is the presence of mycoplasma-like particles in allergic vasculitis studied by electron microscopy (Sussman et al, 1973).

Infective endocarditis

Much of this monograph discusses disease patterns that are exemplified by infective endocarditis. Osler (1885) described the disease most beautifully and now almost a century later it is explained by the interrelationship between infection, immunology and coagulation (Cole, 1975).

Either the streptococcus or a virus seem to provoke an immune reaction resulting in rheumatoid factor production and consequent immune complex disease. However, a non-infective thrombotic process, often due to endothelial injury, seems to encourage the infection. As mentioned elsewhere, the peripheral manifestations include stripping and proliferation of endothelial cells (see page 88) — the endocarditis lenta cell — and a consumption coagulopathy.

It should be possible to learn from a study of endocarditis how injury to the endothelium of the heart valves prepares the tissues for infection and how the persistence of such infection provokes a persistent immunological reaction.

Disseminated intravascular coagulation

The literature on disseminated intravascular coagulation is particularly well endowed with tales of fulminant vasculitis following infection and is discussed in Chapter 10. Table 8.1 gives a list of infections thought to be responsible for disseminated intravascular coagulation; meningococcal septicaemia is, of course, the best known. The role of infection and disseminated intravascular coagulation in the rejection of renal transplants is discussed on page 234, and in most of these patients rejection episodes occur without warning and in the absence of obvious precipitating factors.

Viruses

Sometimes rejection coincides with viral infection such as 'flu' (Simmons et al, 1970; Briggs et al, 1972; David et al, 1972). Such infection has been used to account for deaths after heart transplants with the suggestion that pure rejection processes were not responsible for the deaths. Some authors have elaborately attempted to distinguish between infection and rejection while admitting that it was impossible to tell clinically which was the true cause of the essentially vascular death. One group used inhibition of the rosette inhibition test as an indication for enhanced rejection, but they did not acknowledge that this test might be affected by severe sepsis which is known to depress bone marrow function (Cullum et al, 1972).

The distinctions between primary and secondary effects of an infection or between its triggering action and its effect on the local constitution are in fact difficult to elucidate. Disseminated intravascular coagulation is set in motion by a number of viruses — varicella, vaccinia, variola, rubella, rubiola and the arbo-viruses. Such viruses act in a number of ways — by platelet agglutination, endothelial damage, haemolysis and antigen—antibody complex formation (McKay and Margaretten, 1967).

Table 8.1. Bacterial infections contributing to intravascular coagulation.

Infection	Reference[a]
Gram-positive cocci	
Streptococcus, β haemolytic, Lancefield Group A	Antley and McMillan, 1967
	Collins and Nadel, 1965
	Dyggve, 1947
	Heal and Kent, 1953
	Hjort and Rapaport, 1964
	Little, 1959
	Rahal et al, 1968
Streptococcus, β haemolytic, Lancefield Group B	Hall, 1965 (mitral valve endocarditis)
Staphylococcal septicaemia	Powell, 1961 (49 cases)
	Rahal et al, 1968
	Rosner and Ritz, 1966
	Yoshikawa et al, 1971
Pneumococcal sepsis	Bisno and Freeman, 1970: 1 case and review of 17 cases
	Grant, 1970
	McCracken and Dickerman, 1969
	Ratnoff and Nebehay, 1962
	Rosner and Ritz, 1966
	Stossel and Levy, 1970
Streptococcus viridans	Phillips et al, 1967
Gram-positive bacilli	
Clostridium welchii	Clark and Ellison, 1959: Septic abortion
	Lutz, 1962 ,, ,,
	Phillips et al, 1967 ,, ,,
	Pritchard, 1956 ,, ,,
	Ruberberg et al, 1967 ,, ,,
Gram-negative cocci	
	Friederichsen, 1918
	Voelcker, 1894
	Waterhouse, 1911
Meningococcus	Abildgaard et al, 1967
	Daniels, 1948
	Evans et al, 1969
	Hjort and Rapaport, 1965
	Margaretten and McAdams, 1958 (52 cases)
	McGehecet et al, 1967
	Monfort and Mehrling, 1941
	Wilhelm and Cherubin, 1967
	Winkelstein et al, 1969
	Yoshikawa et al, 1971
Gram-negative bacilli	
Escherichia coli	Cavanagh and Alborrs, 1965
	Clarkson et al, 1969
	Conley et al, 1951
	Corrigan et al, 1968 (12 cases)
	Finegold et al, 1968
	Gans and Krivit, 1960
	Graeff and Beller, 1968
	Hardaway et al, 1961
	Jackson et al, 1955
	Masland and Barrows, 1962
	McBride, 1958
	McCally and Vasicka, 1962
	McKay and Shapiro, 1958

Table 8.1.—*continued*

Infection	Reference[a]
	Mookerjee et al, 1968
	Phillips et al, 1967
	Rigby and Christy, 1968
	West et al, 1966
Proteus	Bubeck, 1960
	Josey and Szeiklies, 1963
Salmonella gastroenteritis	Allen et al, 1969

[a]For references see Yoshikawa, Tanaka and Guze (1971).

The association between viruses and vasculitis is illustrated in several reports. Four cases of vasculitis due to the virus of serum hepatitis Australia antigen were described following very intensive investigation (Gocke et al, 1970; Combes et al, 1971; Trepo, Thivolet and Prince, 1972). Gocke (1975) reviewing the extrahepatic manifestations (Table 8.2) of viral hepatitis reported a personal series of 21 patients and gave references to a further 19. He also described nine patients developing a similar illness following otitis media in whom mycoplasma or some other agent was suspected. A case can be made that the papular eruption seen in children and described by Gianotti also is a vasculitis due to Australia antigen (Gianotti, 1973). A severe necrotising vasculitis of muscles and kidney which accounted for death following an influenza vaccination was reported by Wharton and Pietroni (1974). Hepatitis-B antibody has also been blamed for nine out of twelve cases of polymyalgia rheumatica (Bacon, Doherty and Zuckerman, 1975).

Table 8.2. Vasculitis from hepatitis B infection.

1. Fever, joint pains and swelling, muscle tenderness, erythema and urticaria. Often tender and each lesion lasting more than 24 hours.
2. High blood pressure, haematuria and uraemia. Peripheral neuropathy.
3. Eosinophilia.
4. Histological evidence of small vessel injury in fibrinoid, neutrophilic exudate.
5. Circulating immune complexes containing hepatitis antigen B in vessels with IgM, IgG, C_3 of fibrinogen-related antigen.

Chronic viral infections can lead to the formation of circulating immune complexes consisting of viral antigen and antibody, a fact which explains a number of animal diseases (Notkins et al, 1966), such as lactic dehydrogenase virus, lymphocytic chorio-meningitis and Moloney sarcoma in mice, Aleutian disease of mink, equine anaemia and hog cholera (Oldstone and Dixon, 1971). Characteristically such infections incite some antibody response but this is insufficient to eliminate the virus, or, in the case of chronic lymphocytic choriomeningitis, the antibodies made by the mice are ineffectual (Soothill and Steward, 1971). Other syndromes occur. Thus viruses may sometimes be responsible for lupus-like disease in certain strains of mice (see Chapter 7); and a focal proliferative glomerulonephritis with haematuria, occurring at the height of an upper respiratory tract infection, has been attributed to viral infection (Berger, 1969; Mauer et al, 1973).

Aleutian disease in mink is the best understood of those viral diseases that cause vasculitis. The mink lose weight and develop anaemia, ulceration of mucosae, generalised lymphadenopathy and hepatosplenomegaly. There is a disseminated plasmacytosis and a widespread necrotising vasculitis due to the deposition of antigen—antibody complexes (Henson et al, 1969; Porter, Larsen and Porter, 1973). The reason why viruses persist in these animals has not been explained.

Several viral diseases broadly classified as haemorrhagic fever cause severe haemorrhages in the lungs and the gastrointestinal tract. One well documented study of 169 patients dying of such diseases in Thailand (Halstead, 1970) recorded fever, shock, haemoconcentration, elevated transaminases, hypoproteinaemia, acidosis, azotaemia and abnormalities of haemostasis. Such a response depends on the development of heterologous dengue antibody passively acquired in utero or produced endogenously. It is usual, therefore, for the immune complex disease to develop during a second infection acquired shortly after the primary infection. It is probable that antibody tags on to virus to form complexes which are themselves antigenic (Halstead, 1970).

References

Allen, A. C. (1954) *The Skin. A Clinicopathological Treatise.* St. Louis: C. V. Mosby.
Andriasian, G. K. (1967) *Precongress Abstracts of the 13th International Congress of Dermatology, Berlin.* p. 72. Munich: Springer.
Ash, J. E. & Spitz, S. (1945) *Pathology of Tropical Diseases. An Atlas.* Philadelphia: W. B. Saunders.
Bacon, P. A., Doherty, S. M. & Zuckerman, A. J. (1975) Hepatitis-B antibody in polymyalgia rheumatica. *Lancet,* **ii,** 476.
Bazex, A., Salvador, R., Dupre, A. & Parant, M. (1960) On some cutaneous manifestations of a fever, demonstrated at the level of the lesions of a Prowazek—Poppof—Fraenkel nodule and rickettsiform mass. *Bulletin de la Société Française de Dermatologie et de Syphiligraphie,* **67,** 74.
Berger, J. (1969) IgA glomerular deposits in renal disease. *Transplantation Proceedings,* **1,** 939.
Bloch, B. (1921) Les trichophytides. *Annales de Dermatologie et de Syphiligraphie,* **2,** 55.
Briggs, J. D., Timbury, M. C., Paton, A. M. & Bell, P. R. F. (1972) Viral infection of renal transplantation rejection. *British Medical Journal,* **iv,** 520.
Cannell, H., Churcher, G. M. & Milton-Thompson, G. J. (1969) Stevens—Johnson syndrome associated with Mycoplasma pneumoniae infection. *British Journal of Dermatology,* **81,** 196.
Cok, P. (1975) The enigma of infective endocarditis. *Hospital,* **1,** 128.
Cole, P. (1975) The enigma of infective endocarditis. *Hospital Update,* **1,** 128.
Combes, B., Stastny, P., Shorey, J., Eigenbrodt, E., Varrera, A., Hull, A. & Carter, N. (1971) Glomerulonephritis with deposition of Australia antigen—antibody complexes in glomerular basement membrane. *Lancet,* **ii,** 234.
Cremer, G. (1953) A special granulomatous form of mycosis on the lower legs caused by Trichophyton rubrum castellani. *Dermatologica* (Basel), **107,** 28.
Cullum, P. A., Bewick, M., Shilkin, K., Tee, D. E. H., Ayliffe, P., Hutchinson, D. C. S., Laws, J. W., Mason, S. A., Reid, L., Hugh-Jones, P. & Macarthur, A. M. (1972) Distinction between infection and rejection in lung transplantation. *British Medical Journal,* **ii,** 71.
Danielsson, D., Norberg, R. & Svanbom, M. (1975) Circulating immune complexes in a patient with prolonged gonococcal septicaemia. *Acta Dermato-venereologica,* **55,** 301.
David, D. S., Millian, S. J., Whitsell, J. C., Schwartz, G. H., Riggio, R. R., Rubin, A. L. & Stenzel, K. H. (1972) Viral syndromes and renal homograft rejection. *Annals of Surgery,* **175,** 257.
Feizi, T., Maclean, H., Sommerville, R. F. & Selwyn, J. G. (1967) Studies on an epidemic of respiratory disease caused by mycoplasma pneumoniae. *British Medical Journal,* **i,** 457.
Ferguson-Smith, J. F. (1963) Erythema nodosum in association with pustular ringworm. *British Medical Journal,* **i,** 1592.
Fleming, P. C., Krieger, E., Turner, J. A. P., Watbey, E. I., Quinn, P. A. & Bannatyne, R. M. (1967) Febrile mucocutaneous syndrome with respiratory involvement associated with isolation of mycoplasma pneumoniae. *Journal of the Canadian Medical Association,* **97,** 1458.
Foy, H. M., Kenney, G. E. & Koler, J. (1966) Mycoplasma pneumoniae in Stevens—Johnson syndrome. *Lancet,* **ii,** 550.
Gianotti, F. (1973) Papular acrodermatitis of childhood; An Australia antigen disease. *Archives of Disease in Childhood,* **48,** 794.
Gocke, D. J. (1975) Extrahepatic manifestations of viral hepatitis. *American Journal of Medical Science,* **270,** 49.
Gocke, D. J., Hsu, K., Morgan, C., Bombardieri, S., Lockshin, M. & Christian, C. L. (1970) Association between polyarteritis and Australia antigen. *Lancet,* **ii,** 1149.

Gordon, A. M. & Lyell, A. (1970) Mycoplasmas and their association with skin diseases. *British Journal of Dermatology,* **82**, 414.

Halmy, K. & Pintye, I. (1968) Gomba antigennel végzett agar-gel diffusiós vizsgalatok vasculitises betegeknél. *Bórgyögyászti és venerologia szlemle,* **44**, 12.

Halstead, S. B. (1970) Observations related to the pathogenesis of dengue fever; hypotheses and discussion. *Yale Journal of Biological Medicine,* **42**, 350.

Henson, J. B., Gorham, J. R., Padgett, G. A. & Davis, W. C. (1969) Pathogenesis of the glomerular lesions in Aleutian disease of mink: immunofluorescent studies. *Archives of Pathology,* **87**, 21.

Katz, H. I., Wooten, J. W., Davis, R. G. & Griffin, J. P. (1967) Stevens—Johnson syndrome, report of a case associated with culturally proven mycoplasma pneumoniae infection. *Journal of the American Medical Association,* **99**, 504.

Lassus, A., Förström, H., Pihá, H. J. & Kiistala, U. (1969) Anticomplementary reactions and their relationships to some autoimmune phenomena in syphilis infection. *Acta Dermato-venereologica,* **49**, 519.

Ludlam, G. B., Bridges, J. B. & Benn, E. C. (1964) Association of Stevens—Johnson syndrome with antibody for mycoplasma pneumoniae. *Lancet,* **i**, 958.

Lyell, A., Gordon, A. M., Dick, H. M. & Sommerville, R. G. (1967) Mycoplasmas and erythema multiforme. *Lancet,* **ii**, 1116.

McKay, D. G. & Margaretten, W. (1967) Disseminated intravascular coagulation in virus diseases. *Archives of Internal Medicine,* **120**, 129.

Mauer, M. S., Sutherland, D. E. R., Howard, R. J., Fish, A. J., Najarian, J. S. & Michael, A. F. (1973) The glomerular mesangium. III. Acute immunomesangial injury. A new model of glomerulonephritis. *Journal of Experimental Medicine,* **137**, 553.

Medeiros, A. A., Marty, S. D., Tosh, F. E. & Chin, T. D. Y. (1966) Erythema nodosum and erythema multiforme as clinical manifestations of histoplasmosis in a community outbreak. *New England Journal of Medicine,* **274**, 415.

Mustakallio, K. K., Lassus, A. & Wager, O. (1967) Auto-immune phenomena in syphilitic infection: rheumatoid factor and cryoglobulins in different stages of syphilis. *International Archives of Allergy and Applied Immunology,* **31**, 417.

Nicolau, St G., Noaghea, G. & Bucur, G. (1967) Capilaritele necrozante si infectia rukettsiana latenta. *Dermato-venereologica,* **12**, 385.

Notkins, A. L., Mahar, S., Scheele, C. & Goffman, J. (1966) Infectious virus antibody complex in the blood of chronically infected mice. *Journal of Experimental Medicine,* **124**, 1.

Oldstone, M. B. A. & Dixon, F. J. (1971) Chronic viral infection associated with immune complex disease. In *Progress in Immunology* (Ed.) Amos, B., p. 764. London: Academic Press.

Osler, W. (1885) Goulstonian lectures on malignant endocarditis. *Lancet,* **i**, 505.

Porter, D. D., Larsen, A. E. & Porter, H. G. (1973) The pathogenesis of Aleutian disease of mink. *American Journal of Pathology,* **71**, 331.

Shapiro, L., Teisch, J. A. & Brownstein, M. H. (1973) Dermato-histopathology of chronic gonococcal sepsis. *Archives of Dermatology,* **107**, 403.

Sieber, O. F., John, T. J., Fulginiti, V. A. & Oberholt, E. (1967) Stevens—Johnson syndrome associated with mycoplasma pneumoniae infection. *Journal of the American Medical Association,* **200**, 79.

Simmons, R. L., Weil, R., Tallent, M. B., Kjellstrand, C. M. & Najarian, J. S. (1970) Do mild infections trigger the rejection of renal allografts? *Transplantation Proceedings,* **2**, 419.

Smith, C. E. (1940) The epidemiology of acute coccidioidomycosis with erythema nodosum. *American Journal of Public Health,* **60**, 600.

Smith, J. G., Harris, J. S., Conant, N. F. & Smith, D. T. (1955) An epidemic of North American blastomycosis. *Journal of the American Medical Association,* **158**, 641.

Snyder, J. C. (1965) Typhus fever rickettsiae. In *Viral and Rickettsial Infections of Man,* 4th edition (Ed.) Horsfall, F. L. & Tamm, I. Philadelphia: J. B. Lippincott.

Soothill, J. F. & Steward, M. W. (1971) The immunopathological significance of the heterogeneity of antibody affinity. *Clinical and Experimental Immunology,* **9**, 193.

Strom, J. (1965) Ectodermosis erosiva pluriorificialis, Stevens—Johnson syndrome and other febrile mucocutaneous reactions and Behçets syndrome in cold agglutination positive infections. *Lancet,* **i**, 457.

Sussman, M., Jones, J. H., Almeida, J. D. & Lachmann, P. J. (1973) Deficiency of the second component of complement associated with anaphylactoid purpura and presence of mycoplasma in the serum. *Clinical and Experimental Immunology,* **14**, 531.

Sutter, E. (1920) Zur Kenntnis der Pathogenese der Trichophytide Skarlatiniforome, Lichenoide, und Nodose Exantheme. *Archiv für Dermatologie und Syphilis,* **18**, 271.

Torres, J., Humphreys, E. & Bisno, A. L. (1973) Rocky Mountain spotted fever in the mid-South. *Archives of Internal Medicine,* **132**, 340.

Trepo, C. G., Thivolet, J. & Prince, A. M. (1972) Australia antigen and polyarteritis nodosa. *American Journal of Diseases of Children,* **123**, 390.

Warin, R. P. (1963) Erythema nodosum and pustular ringworm. *British Medical Journal,* **ii**, 57.

Wharton, C. F. P. & Pietroni, R. (1974) Polyarteritis after influenza vaccination. *British Medical Journal,* **ii**, 331.

Wiggelinkhuizen, J., Kaschulo, R. O., Uys, C. J., Kunzten, R. H. & Dale, J. (1973) Congenital syphilis and
    glomerulonephritis with evidence for immune pathogenesis. *Archives of Disease in Childhood,* **48,** 375.
Wolbach, S. B., Todd, J. L. & Palfrey, F. W. (1922) *The Etiology and Pathology of Typhus.* Cambridge:
    Harvard University Press.
Yoshikawa, T., Tanaka, K. R. & Guze, L. B. (1971) Infection and disseminated intravascular coagulation.
    Medicine (Baltimore), **50,** 237.

DRUGS

As many as one in 20 medical admissions to hospitals have been attributed to a drug reaction (Seidl et al, 1966). Clinically recognisable reactions occur more often in the skin than in other organs, and vasculitis is one of the severest forms.

Drugs and food are often blamed for rashes such as vasculitis but are less often proved to be the cause. Sometimes infection and drugs play a combined role, there being exposure to both, as is the case in drug addicts (Citron et al, 1970). The type of rash any one drug produces and the frequency of its occurrence depends rather more on the idiosyncrasies of the recipient's constitution than on the drug. Only thus can one explain the variety of rashes induced by, for example, phenylbutazone which has been blamed for urticaria (Levin, 1953), allergic vasculitis (Schuppli, 1966), temporal arteritis (Wadman and Werner, 1967), ulcerated purpura and polyarteritis nodosa (Almeyda and Baker, 1970), livedo reticularis (Castelli et al, 1965), and erythema nodosum (Glotzer, 1953). The same applies to penicillin, which has been blamed for urticaria, serum sickness, non-thrombocytopenic purpura and erythema nodosum (reviewed by Almeyda and Levantine, 1972). In this chapter, no attempt will be made to be comprehensive in this respect and only some aspects will be discussed. Very few drugs are consistently associated with a particular pattern of rash; well known examples of these exceptions are pigmented purpuric eruptions from carbromal and fixed drug eruptions from phenolphthalein.

Some drugs and foods seem to promote urticaria in the majority of patients already predisposed to it. This is particularly the case with aspirin and indomethacin, a topic which is discussed fully by Warin and Champion (1974). Such drugs sometimes also cause vasculitis (Marsh, Almeyda and Levi, 1970) in the same way as urticariogenic foods such as strawberries will (Tondra, 1969). Several mechanisms underlie this sort of vasculitis. Stefanini and Mednicoff (1954) described anti-vessel agents in the sera of patients with anaphylactoid purpura or polyarteritis nodosa induced by drugs. The Arthus phenomenon has been most commonly blamed for purpura and anaphylactoid patterns of vasculitis whereas serum sickness-like illnesses have been attributed to immune complexes; penicillin is one of the best documented examples of the latter (Criep and Cohen, 1951).

Ackroyd (1953), working with allylisopropylacetylurea (Sedormid), and Shulman (1958) and Bridges, Fichera and Baldini (1962), using quinine showed that sera of patients suffering from purpura due to these agents contain antibodies which destroy platelets in the presence of the relevant drugs. While Ackroyd favoured an antibody to platelets, Shulman thought in terms of immune complexes damaging platelets nonspecifically. A fall in the number of platelets has long been known to be an indication of sensitivity to drugs (Bettman, 1963). Indeed, Comaish (1968) attempted to use the release of serotonin from platelets in an in vitro test of drug sensitivity.

Many drugs cause changes in blood fibrinolysis in vitro (Table 8.3) and salicylates have been blamed for consumption coagulopathy (Pinedo, Van de Putte and Loeliger, 1973).

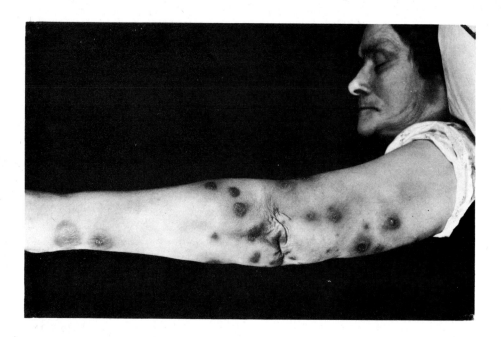

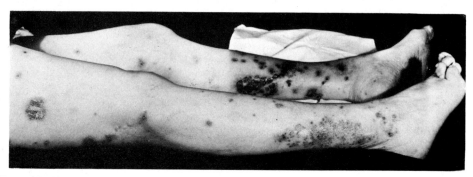

Figure 8.8. Vasculitis in a 67-year-old woman following challenge with a vaccine to fish. Initial lesions appeared at site of inoculation.

Table 8.3. Dilute blood clot lysis times in minutes with and without addition of drugs.

Drugs	Without drug × 2 specimens	With drug × 10 specimens	
		1%	5%
Acecoline	265	>1440	>1440
Aneurine hydrochloride	390	540	540
Anthisan	300	450	450
Ascorbic acid	540	540	540
Atropine sulphate	390	390	390
Brontina	360	420	420
Ca. gluconate	420	>1440	>1440
Coramine	540	600	600
Crystapen	960	960	960
Cytamen	600	660	660
Daptazole	540	780	780
Digoxin	300	480	480
Dilaudid	720	>1440	>1440
Dilavase	720	780	840
Ephynal	600	600	600
Femergin	660	660	660
Fentazin	390	1560	1560
Ferrivenin	540	>1440	>1440
Gardenal sodium	690	>1440	>1440
Inderal	660	660	660
Largactil	420	>1440	>1440
Lasix	420	420	420
Levophed	270	360	360
Librium	330	1360	1360
Lobeiline	240	280	280
Mersalyl	720	>1440	>1440
Micoren	420	550	550
Millophylline	540	1440	1440
Myocrisin	60	360	360
Phenergan	300	>1440	>1440
Piriton	540	660	660
Pyridoxine	960	240	240
Riboflavin	600	600	600
Rogitine	540	600	600
Ronicol	540	600	600
Stemetil	1440	>3600	>3600
Sympatol	330	420	420
Torecan	300	360	360
Valoid	540	>1440	>1440

The importance of drugs as a cause of vasculitis in serum sickness was extensively demonstrated by Rich (1942) using sulphonamides, and a review by Rose and Spencer (1957) convinced many people that there was a relationship between the disease and these drugs. The same applied to other drugs including chloramphenicol, penicillin, streptomycin, bismuth, gold and uracil, howbeit raising the possibility that these drugs were acting in the presence of an altered host reactivity. Drugs given for infection have the highest incidence of vasculitic side-effects and have been reviewed by Zürcher and Krebs (1973). Most reviews of vasculitis have perpetuated this concept (McCombs, Patterson and MacMahon, 1956; Winkelmann and Ditto, 1964; Copeman and Ryan, 1970), but proof of the relationship is rare.

The question of the specificity of drug reactions was raised in a description of 25 patients with necrotising vasculitis, 11 of whom were on thiazides. All the patients were elderly and had evidence of other diseases before the onset of vasculitis (Bjornberg and Gisslen, 1965). One of them had had a severe exacerbation of vasculitis induced by a test dose of hydrochlorothiazide, and another suffered the same reaction to chlorthalidone.

While steroids are frequently prescribed for vasculitis, Golding, Hamilton and Gill (1965) drew attention to a particularly high incidence of vasculitis affecting the vasa nervorum of peripheral nerves in patients on these drugs. Spagnuolo and Taranta (1961) and Ferguson and Slocumm (1961), on the other hand, considered that vasculitis became worse after discontinuing systemic steroids.

Bruinsma (1973) suggested the following criteria for assessing the probability that an adverse reaction to a drug is allergic in nature:
1. Circulating or cell-bound antibodies may be demonstrable.
2. The reaction occurs after a sensitising period of administration. Although the amount of antigen is important in causing sensitisation, minimal doses may thereafter elicit a reaction.
3. After recovery the same reaction can as a rule be precipitated by a single dose.
4. The reaction conforms to a known allergic pattern, as for instance urticaria, anaphylaxis or exanthema. The reaction is different from those which would be expected on the basis of the pharmacological action of the drug.

Many drug eruptions are clearly related in some way to the illness for which they are given and they produce no further reaction when the patient is well. Drug eruptions tend to affect ill people rather than healthy controls who can be given the drug safely in equivalent dosage. Bruinsma (1973) believed that proteins altered by age or by illness combine with the drug to produce complete allergens. The reactivity of the tissues alters will illness (see page 118), and such reactivity includes factors such as the anatomy of stasis.

The Shwartzman phenomenon is a good example of these temporary changes in local vascular behaviour which encourage even grosser responses to minor injury from drugs. This altered reactivity, unlike allergy, is limited to a period usually of about three months, after which recovery seems to be complete and the Shwartzman reaction can no longer be induced. It can be explained by stasis and by alteration in coagulation and fibrinolysis.

Proof that a particular rash is caused by a drug is, of course, difficult to obtain. Challenge with the suspected drug is a dangerous practice when vasculitis is suspected (Figure 8.9). For example, Meyler (1968) described two cases with sulphonamide reactions, illustrating that fever, leucocytosis, a purpuric rash and polyneuritis can develop within 24 hours of ingesting tablets to which the patient is known to be sensitive. Also, Wahlberg and Wikstrom (1963) gave ^{131}I to a woman suspected of iodine sensitivity and she deteriorated the same day and died a few days later from vasculitis.

In an article on so-called 'collagen diseases' as a manifestation of sensitivity to drugs, Symmers (1958) described eight cases of vasculitis. One man developed a myositis and glomerulonephritis while taking sulphadiazine, and a young woman developed a neuropathy, urticaria, fever and glomerulonephritis during a course of chlorpromazine. In both, patch tests produced erythema and induration. A positive haemorrhagic and oedematous patch test has been observed in an elderly lady who had a fulminant necrotising vasculitis from aspirin, and positive patch tests with sulphonamides have been described in two cases of thrombotic purpura due to sulphathiazole. More recently, Billings et al (1974) described three patients who developed vasculitis within a week of taking alclofenac, an analgesic with anti-inflammatory properties.

As indicated in many other sections of this book, the vascular reactions that should be regarded as vasculitis are part of a spectrum and it is particularly the case with drug eruptions that little advantage accrues from making a distinction between different morphological varieties of vasculitis. Bruinsma (1973) also emphasised that no sharp demarcation is possible, either histologically or clinically between, for instance, allergic vasculitis and polyarteritis nodosa. Bruinsma's list of drugs causing such reactions is reproduced in Table 8.4. Clinical differentiation between thrombocytopenic and non-thrombocytopenic vasculitis is not always possible. Drugs causing purpura are listed in Table 8.5.

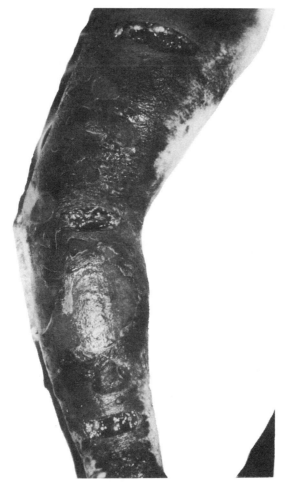

Figure 8.9. Severe gangrene due to warfarin sodium.

The term livedo reticularis or livedo racemosa is applied to an enhancement of the normal reticulate vascular markings of the skin. As mentioned in Chapters 3 and 12, such markings are dependent on the anatomy of the vasculature of the skin and on a tendency for blood flow to be slower in those parts of the epidermal blood supply which are farthest from the arterioles and veins entering and leaving the deep dermis. Anything that contributes to such stasis in the periphery will therefore produce livedo reticularis. This applies equally to the inflammatory effect of immune complexes silted out in the areas of stasis. Many drugs may contribute to this, but amantadine hydrochloride is one that has been particularly associated with livedo reticularis (Shealy, Weeth and Mercier, 1970; Vollum, Parkes and Doyle, 1971).

Table 8.4. List of drugs with main type of purpura.

	Thrombocytopenic purpura	Vascular purpura
Acetazolamide	x	o
Acetylsalicylic acid	x	x
Allopurinol	x	x
p Aminosalicylic acid	x	x
Apronal	x	x
Arsenicals	x	x
Bromisoval	o	x
Carbimazole	x	x
Carbromal	o	x
Chloramphenicol	x	x
Chlorpropamide	x	o
Chlordiazepoxide and related diazepines	x	x
Chlorothiazide and related benzothiadiazines	x	x
Chlorpromazine and related phenothiazines	x	x
Cytostatics	x	o
Digitoxin	x	o
Ethacrynic acid	x	o
Furosemide	x	x
Gold salts	x	x
Indomethacin	x	x
Iodine		x
Isoniazid	x	x
Measles vaccine	x	o
Meprobamate	x	x
Methyldopa	x	x
Nitrofurantoin	x	o
Oestrogens	x	x
Oxyphenbutazone	x	o
Phenylbutazone	x	o
Phenytoin and related compounds	x	o
Piperazine	o	x
Propranolol	x	o
Quinine	x	x
Quinidine	x	x
Reserpine	o	x
Rifamycin	x	o
Rifampicin	x	o
Smallpox vaccine	x	o
Streptomycin	x	o
Sulphonamides	x	x
Thiouracil and derivatives	x	x
Tolbutamide	x	x

x = yes; o = not recorded in the literature.

Table 8.5. List of drugs most frequently implicated in drug-induced vasculitis.

> Sulphonamides
> Guanethidine
> Phenylbutazone and oxyphenbutazone
> Allopurinol
> Thiouracil and derivatives
> Indomethacin
> Phenytoin and related compounds
> Iodides and bromides
> Chlorothiazide and related benzothiadiazines

Erythema nodosum

Bruinsma (1973) emphasised that the incidence of erythema nodosum due to drugs is extremely low and that there are no documented cases in which readministration resulted in clinically and histologically identical lesions. There is a suspicion that oral contraceptives, sulphonamides, salicylates, bromides and iodides cause erythema nodosum but as in pregnancy, in which erythema nodosum may also occur (Daw, 1971; Wetherill, 1971), tissues of the front of the leg are in some way temporarily 'prepared' or sensitised so that otherwise undetected potentially noxious agents have an effect. The discussion on page 286 is relevant in this respect — erythema nodosum possibly being a limited form of thrombophlebitis (Montgomery, 1967) induced by amounts of circulating immune complexes which normally would not elicit pathological change.

Necrosis from anticoagulants

Haemorrhagic skin infarction secondary to oral anticoagulants is another syndrome in which intravascular coagulation is the predominant feature. Everett and Overholt (1969) reviewed the literature and referred to 150 cases reported since the original description by Flood et al (1943) and the incrimination of anticoagulants by Verhagen (1954). Dihydroxycoumarin, phenprocoumarin and warfarin sodium (Figure 8.9) have all been incriminated. Ninety per cent of the cases have been women, and gangrene of the breast occurred in at least 25 cases of those reported in the literature (Kahn, Stern and Rhodes, 1971). Venous thrombosis was found in all cases.

Martin and Phillips (1970) compared the process to purpura fulminans and the Shwartzman phenomenon, as did Lieb (1964) after looking at the histology. The histology of the lesion shows perivascular accumulations of inflammatory cells involving predominantly the venules, with extensive thrombosis of draining veins but virtually no involvement of arterioles (Lipp et al, 1969).

The purpura fulminans picture developed acutely about three to ten days after therapy was instituted and bears little relationship to the effect that the anticoagulants have on the prothrombin time. There is evidence of a hypercoagulable state (Nudelman and Kempson, 1966) and the condition responds to heparin (Beller, 1961) provided the initial bleeding is stopped by vitamin K (Nalbandian et al, 1971). A direct toxic action by coumarin on endothelium has been shown (Neumayr and Schmid, 1948; McCarter, Bingham and Meyer, 1944) and electron microscopy of capillaries after warfarin therapy shows loss of cytoplasmic ground substance and changes in organelles suspiciously like degeneration (Kahn, Stern and Rhodes, 1971).

The breast seems to be particularly susceptible to venous thrombosis as in Mondor's disease, and mammary gangrene has been reported in diabetes mellitus (Switzer, 1950) and in Wegener's granulomatosis. There is another complication of coumarin therapy worthy of note — purple toes. This curious purplish erythema develops three weeks or so after starting therapy with phenindione or warfarin sodium (Feder and Auerbach, 1961).

References

Ackroyd, J. F. (1953) Allergic purpura, including purpura due to foods, drugs and infections. *American Journal of Medicine*, **14**, 605.
Almeyda, J. & Baker, H. (1970) Drug reactions xii. Cutaneous reactions to antirheumatic drugs. *British Journal of Dermatology*, **83**, 707.
Almeyda, J. & Levantine, A. (1972) Drug reactions xix. Adverse cutaneous reactions to the penicillins — ampicillin rashes. *British Journal of Dermatology*, **87**, 293.
Beller, F. K. (1961) Therapy of the so-called coumarin necrosis. *Medical Biology*, **4**, 116.
Bettman, J. W. (1963) Drug hypersensitivity purpuras. *Archives of Internal Medicine*, **112**, 840.

Billings, R. A., Burry, H. C., Emslie, F. S. & Kerr, G. D. (1974) Vasculitis with alclofenac therapy. *British Medical Journal*, **iv**, 263.

Bjornberg, A. & Gisslen, H. (1965) Thiazides: A cause of necrotising vasculitis? *Lancet*, **ii**, 982.

Bridges, J. M., Fichera, J. & Baldini, M. (1962) The effect of anti platelet antibodies on the in vitro uptake of 5-hydroxytryptamine by blood platelets. *Blood*, **20**, 760.

Bruinsma, W. (1973) *A Guide to Drug Eruptions*. Amsterdam: Excerpta Medica.

Castelli, E., Bernadi, P., Bonavita, E. & Montini, T. (1965) La livedo rassengna critica, un casodi livedo reticularis in cardiopatica: un casodi livedo racemosa da fenilbutazone. *Giornale di Clinica Medica*, **46**, 253.

Citron, B. P., Halpern, M. & McCarron, M. (1970) Necrotising angiitis associated with drug abuse. *New England Journal of Medicine*, **283**, 1003.

Comaish, S. (1968) The blood platelets in immune hypersensitivity. *Acta Dermato-venereologica*, **48**, 592.

Copeman, P. W. M. & Ryan, T. J. (1970) The problems of cutaneous angiitis with reference to histopathology and pathogenesis. *British Journal of Dermatology*, **82** (Supplement 5), 2.

Criep, L. H. & Cohen, S. G. (1951) Purpura as a minifestation of penicillin sensitivity. *Annals of Internal Medicine*, **34**, 1219.

Daw, E. (1971) Recurrent erythema nodosum of pregnancy. *British Medical Journal*, **ii**, 44.

Everett, B. D. & Overholt, E. L. (1969) Haemorrhagic skin infarction secondary to oral anticoagulants. *Archives of Dermatology*, **100**, 588.

Feder, W. & Auerbach, R. (1961) 'Purple toes' an uncommon sequelae of oral coumarin drug therapy. *Annals of Internal Medicine*, **55**, 911.

Ferguson, R. H. & Slocumm, C. H. (1961) Peripheral neuropathy in rheumatoid arthritis. *Bulletin of Rheumatic Diseases*, **11**, 251.

Flood, E. P., Redish, M. H., Bociek, S. J. & Shapiro, S. (1943) Thrombophlebitis migrans disseminata. Report of a case in which gangrene of the breast occurred. *New York State Journal of Medicine*, **43**, 1121.

Glotzer, S. (1953) Phenylbutazone therapy. *Journal of the American Medical Association*, **151**, 1023.

Golding, J. R., Hamilton, M. G. & Gill, R. S. (1965) Arteritis of rheumatoid arthritis. *British Journal of Dermatology*, **77**, 207.

Kahn, S., Stern, H. D. & Rhodes, G. A. (1971) Cutaneous and subcutaneous necrosis as a complication of coumarin congener therapy. *Plastic and Reconstructive Surgery*, **48**, 160.

Levin, S. J. (1953) Severe urticaria and angio-oedema resulting from phenylbutazone (Butazolidin). *Journal of the Michigan State Medical Society*, **52**, 1210.

Lieb, L. (1964) Uber die Kumarinnekrose und ihre Beziehung zum Shwartzmansanarelli Phanomen. *Zentralblatt für Chirurgie*, **89**, 81.

Lipp, H., Pitt, A., Masterton, J. P., Kay, H. B. & Anderson, S. T. (1969) A case of coumarin induced skin necrosis. *Medical Journal of Australia*, **2**, 351.

Marsh, F., Almeyda, J. & Levi, I. (1970) Quoted by Almeyda, J. & Baker, H. (1970) Drug reactions. XII. Cutaneous reactions to anti-rheumatic drugs. *British Journal of Dermatology*, **83**, 707.

Martin, B. F. & Phillips, J. D. (1970) Gangrene of female breast with anticoagulant therapy. *American Journal of Clinical Pathology*, **53**, 622.

McCarter, J. C., Bingham, J. B. & Meyer, O. O. (1944) Studies on haemorrhagic agent 3,3'-Methyenebis (4-hydroxy coumarin). *American Journal of Pathology*, **20**, 631.

McCombs, R. P., Patterson, J. F. & MacMahon, H. E. (1956) Syndromes associated with "allergic" vasculitis. *New England Journal of Medicine*, **255**, 251.

Meyler, L. (1968) *Drug Induced Diseases*. p. 1. Paris: Excerpta Medica Foundation.

Montgomery, H. (1967) *Dermatopathology*, Vol. 2, p. 677. New York: Hoeber Medical Division, Harper and Row.

Nalbandian, R. M., Beller, F. K., Kamp, A. K., Henry, R. L. & Wolf, P. L. (1971) Coumarin necrosis of skin healed successfully with heparin. *Obstetrics and Gynecology*, **38**, 395.

Neumayr, A. & Schmid, J. (1948) Kapillar Permeabilität und Antithrombon. *Schweizer medizinische Wochenschrift*, **78**, 616.

Nilsson, I. M. & Isaacson, S. (1972) New aspects of the pathogenesis of thrombo-embolism. *Progress in Surgery*, **11**, 46.

Nudelman, H. L. & Kempson, R. L. (1966) Necrosis of the breast. A rare complication of anticoagulant therapy. *American Journal of Surgery*, **111**, 728.

Pinedo, H. M., Van de Putte, L. B. A. & Loeliger, E. A. (1973) Salicylate induced consumption coagulopathy. *Annals of the Rheumatic Diseases*, **32**, 66.

Rich, A. R. (1942) Additional evidence of the role of hypersensitivity in the aetiology of perarteritis nodosa. Another case associated with sulphonamide reaction. *Bulletin of the Johns Hopkins Hospital*, **71**, 375.

Rose, G. A. & Spencer, H. (1957) Polyarteritis nodosa. *Quarterly Journal of Medicine*, **26**, 43.

Schuppli, R. (1966) Hautschadigungen durch Uberdosierung von Merfen. *Dermatologica*, **133**, 5.

Seidl, L. G., Thornton, G. F., Smith, J. W. & Cluff, L. E. (1966) Studies on the epidemiology of adverse drug reactions iii. Reactions in patients on a general medical service. *Bulletin of the Johns Hopkins Hospital*, **119**, 299.

Shealy, C. N., Weeth, J. B. & Mercier, D. (1970) Livedo reticularis in patients with Parkinsonism receiving amantadine. *Journal of the American Medical Association,* **212,** 1522.

Shulman, N. R. (1958) Immunoreactions involving platelets. I. Asteric and kinetic model for formation of a complex from a human antibody. Quinidine as a haptene; and platelets; and for fixation of complement by the complex. *Journal of Experimental Medicine,* **107,** 665.

Spagnuolo, M. & Taranta, A. (1961) Poststeroid panniculitis. *Annals of Internal Medicine,* **54,** 1181.

Stefanini, M. & Mednicoff, I. B. (1954) Demonstration of antivessel agents in serum of patients with anaphylactoid purpura and periarteritis nodosa. *Journal of Clinical Investigation,* **33,** 967.

Switzer, P. K. (1950) Gangrene of the breast associated with diabetes mellitus. *Journal of the State of Carolina Medical Association,* **46,** 42.

Symmers, W. St C. (1958) In *Sensitivity Reactions to Drugs.* A symposium organised for the Council for International Organisations of Medical Sciences (Ed.) Rosenheim, G. M. L. & Moulton, R. p. 209. Oxford: Blackwell.

Tondra, J. M. (1969) Gangrene of the skin due to allergic reaction. *Plastic and Reconstructive Surgery,* **43,** 392.

Verhagen, H. (1954) Local haemorrhage and necrosis of skin and underlying tissues during anticoagulant therapy with dicoumarol or dicumacyl. *Acta Medica Scandinavica,* **148,** 453.

Vollum, D. I., Parkes, J. D. & Doyle, D. (1971) Livedo reticularis during amantadine treatment. *British Medical Journal,* **ii,** 627.

Wadman, B. & Werner, I. (1967) Therapeutic hazards of phenylbutazone and oxyphenbutazone in polymyalgia rheumatica. *Lancet,* **i,** 597.

Wahlberg, J. E. & Wikstrom, K. (1963) A case of periarteritis nodosa with skin manifestations, probably provoked by iodide administration. *Acta Dermato-venereologica,* **43,** 556.

Warin, R. P. & Champion, R. H. (1974) *Urticaria.* London: W. B. Saunders.

Wetherill, J. H. (1971) Recurrent erythema nodosum of pregnancy. *British Medical Journal,* **iii,** 535.

Winkelmann, R. K. & Ditto, W. B. (1964) Cutaneous and visceral syndromes of necrotising or allergic angiitis. A study of 38 cases. *Medicine* (Baltimore), **43,** 59.

Zürcher, K. & Krebs, A. (1973) Hautnebenwirkung interner Arzneimittel. (Cutaneous side effects of systemic drugs.) ii. Teileiner Synopsis. *Dermatologica,* **147,** Supplement 1.

FOODS

A leading article in the *Lancet* (1969) drew attention to the huge quantities of chemical substances ingested by everyone in this country — an average of 3 lb per person per year (Table 8.6). The total number of known food additives exceeds 20 000. Levantine and Almeyda (1972) emphasised in a review for dermatologists that some of these are known poisons even in small amounts, and in humans the long-term effects are unknown.

The role of foods as a cause of vasculitis, as in urticaria, was emphasised in recent studies from Sweden on the yellow colouring agent tartrazine (Juhlin, Michaelsson and Zetterstrom, 1972; Michaelsson and Juhlin, 1973; Michaelsson, Pettersson and Juhlin, 1974). In 1959 Lockey recorded asthma and urticaria in a patient taking oral steroids in which the yellow aniline dye tartrazine was used as a colouring agent, and in 1971 he drew attention to reactions to hidden agents in food, beverages and drugs. By 1972, 18 such cases of asthma and urticaria had been described, and Michaelsson and Juhlin (1973) reported a further 39 patients.

Criep (1971) described a young nurse who for five years had had episodes of menorrhagia, purpura and bleeding from her ears, nose, gums and bowel. Full haematological and serological investigations revealed no defects in the clotting mechanism, in platelet behaviour or in blood fibrinolysis. Detailed listing of her food intake showed that butter and margarine could be incriminated. Careful double-blind studies eventually showed that tartrazine was responsible. Scratch patch tests produced erythema, induration, vesiculation and petechiae at 24 hours. Passive transfer tests were negative and no precipitating antibodies to tartrazine could be found in the patient's serum. Tartrazine seemed to have no effect on the patient's platelets in vitro.

Michaelsson, Pettersson and Juhlin (1974) described seven patients with non-thrombocytopenic purpura and a leucocytoclastic histology in whom dyes and sodium benzoate were probable contributors to the rash, and certainly an oral test dose coincided with recurrences. One patient also had angio-oedema, another erythema multiforme and mouth ulcers, and two others had associated thrombosis of deep or superficial veins. Fibrinolytic therapy with phenformin and ethylestrenol was helpful in several of these patients.

Table 8.6. Classification of additives in foods, as reported by the National Science Foundation (1965).

Preservatives	33
Anti-oxidants	28
Sequestrants	45
chelating agents	
metal scavengers	
emulsifiers	
stabilising agents	
Surface active agents	111
Stabilisers, thickeners	39
Bleaching and maturing agents	24
Buffers, acids, alkalis	60
Food colours	34
Non-nutritive and special	
dietary sweeteners	4
Nutritive supplement	117
Flavourings — synthetic	1610
Flavourings — natural	502
Miscellaneous	157
yeast foods	
texturisers	
firming agents	
binders	
anti-caking agents	
enzymes	
Total number of additives	2764

Michaelsson, Pettersson and Juhlin (1974) used thurfyl nicotinate (Trafuril) to test the skin of their patients since they found it a reliable method of inducing purpura in susceptible patients; in one case it invariably did so even when no food additives were being taken. The value of this test requires some comment. In normal subjects thurfyl nicotinate, sometimes used as a treatment for chilblains, produces redness and slight oedema of the skin. Some patients with urticaria show an exaggerated response, and altered reactions have been described in several populations such as psoriatics (Holti, 1964) and diabetics (Razka and Ostman, reported by Juhlin and Michaelsson, 1971). Juhlin and Michaelsson (1971) in one study found that thurfyl nicotinate produced an isomorphic response in several diseases; for instance, eczema in eczematous subjects and purpura in purpuric subjects. It is not surprising therefore that in their study of purpura induced by food additives it was a means of enhancing the response. In order to interpret these results one should also take into account studies using the same tests in urticaria.

Juhlin, Michaelsson and Zetterstrom (1972) recorded that seven of eight aspirin-sensitive patients reacted with urticaria and asthma after ingesting tartrazine and that several also reacted to benzoic acid derivatives. This phenomenon of aspirin sensitivity had received more detailed investigation in the past (Moore-Robinson and Warin, 1967;

Samter and Beers, 1967). Rarely a true allergy may be responsible and then especially to aspirin anhydride, as can be demonstrated experimentally (DeWeck, 1971). In the majority of cases, however, it is simply by temporary enhancement of an urticarial tendency by several unrelated drugs including aspirin, indomethacin, phenazone and tartrazine.

Samter and Beers (1967) considered a pharmacological explanation through kinin receptors, while Yurchak, Wicher and Arbesman (1970) discussed the equal likelihood that earlier activation of complement or a failure of enzyme inhibition is responsible. These agents induce urticaria within one to two hours, whereas purpura takes some 12 hours to appear. Susceptible subjects are more likely to show prolonged wealing from histamine or kallikrein inoculation and a prolonged reaction to thurfyl nicotinate. Reactions are maximal during active phases of chronic urticaria and may return to normal a few months after recovery.

Smith (1971) described sensitivity in asthmatic subjects to several other analgesics — acetominophen, mefenamic acid and dextropropoxyphene — but he and Michaelsson and Juhlin (1973) were unable to explain the variations in the pattern of reactivity and the frequency of negative responses. The thurfyl nicotinate reaction, like any isomorphic response or Koebner reaction, must be interpreted in the light of the reactivity of the skin at the time of active disease, perhaps with altered reactivity following infection. Just as one would not always blame chronic urticaria on the aspirin which can be shown to induce it, so one should not blame vasculitis solely on the tartrazine which can be shown to elicit it. As a routine, however, it would be sensible to advise patients with micro-vascular disease to avoid these drugs. But it would be wrong to blame vasculitis on tartrazine as it would be to blame the thurfyl nicotinate which can be used to reveal it — and should equally be avoided.

The fact that phenformin and ethylestrenol can be used to inhibit purpura induced by food additives suggests that fibrinolytic mechanisms are involved or are protective in some way. Thune et al (1976) found that thurfyl nicotinate inhibits skin fibrinolysis, and Ryan (1973) has emphasised that such inhibition is a localising factor in any vasculitis. Aspirin enhances fibrinolysis, possibly by encouraging release of an activator, and the later development of vasculitis might be due to its exhaustion. Thune et al (1976) have inhibited the Trafuril response using an inhibitor of prostaglandins, and in Ryan's view thurfyl nicotinate releases prostaglandins from the epidermis and in consequence inhibits repair mechanisms such as the release of fibrinolytic activators. There is also evidence that fibrinolytic activity generates histamine (Inderbitzin, 1961). Certainly early exhaustion of fibrinolytic activity could encourage vasculitis.

Margarine disease

One of the most extensive epidemics of vasculitis ever described took place in Holland and Germany in 1960. The disease took the form of a toxic erythema often with a purpuric element. The epidemic was blamed on an emulsifier used in margarine but exactly how it produced the disease could not be ascertained; it was clearly not a simple immunological problem (Mali and Malten, 1961).

Pseudolupus and pseudoscleroderma

Various forms of mixed connective tissue disease are described and seem to be immunological in nature. Two disorders which have been blamed on ingested or inhaled agents — venocuran and polyvinyl chloride, are discussed briefly on page 153.

References

Criep, L. H. (1971) Allergic vascular purpura. *Journal of Allergy and Clinical Immunology,* **48,** 7.

DeWeck, A. L. (1971) Immunological effects of aspirin anhydride, a contaminant of commercial acetyl-salicylic acid preparations. *International Archives of Allergy and Applied Immunology,* **41,** 393.

Holti, G. (1964) Vascular phenomena diagnostic of latent psoriasis. *British Journal of Dermatology,* **76,** 503.

Inderbitzin, T. (1961) The mechanisms involved in histamine release and histamine increase in allergic skin reactions. *International Archives of Allergy and Applied Immunology,* **18,** 85.

Juhlin, L. & Michaelsson, G. (1971) Abnormal cutaneous reactions to a nicotinic acid ester. *Acta Dermato-venereologica,* **51,** 448.

Juhlin, L., Michaelsson, G. & Zetterstrom, O. (1972) Urticaria and asthma induced by food and drug additives in patients with aspirin sensitivity. *Journal of Allergy and Clinical Immunology,* **50,** 92.

Lancet (1969) Leading article. Food additives. *Lancet,* **ii,** 369.

Levantine, A. & Almeyda, J. (1972) Cutaneous reactions to anticonvulsants. *British Journal of Dermatology,* **87,** 646.

Lockey, S. D. (1959) Allergic reactions due to F.D. & C. Yellow No. 5. Tartrazine and aniline dye used as a colouring and identifying agent in various steroids. *Annals of Allergy,* **17,** 719.

Lockey, S. D. (1971) Reactions to hidden agents in foods, beverages and drugs. *Annals of Allergy,* **29,** 481.

Mali, J. W. H. & Malten, K. E. (1961) The epidemic of polymorph toxic erythema in the Netherlands in 1960. *Acta Dermato-venereologica,* **46,** 123.

Michaelsson, G. & Juhlin, L. (1973) Urticaria induced by preservatives and dye additives in food and drugs. *British Journal of Dermatology,* **88,** 525.

Michaelsson, G., Juhlin, L. & Zetterstrom, O. (1972) Urticaria induced by food and drug additives in patients with aspirin hypersensitivity. *Journal of Allergy and Clinical Immunology,* **50,** 92.

Michaelsson, G., Pettersson, L. & Juhlin, L. (1974) Purpura caused by food and drug additives. *Archives of Dermatology,* **109,** 49.

Moore-Robinson, M. & Warin, R. P. (1967) Effect of salicylates in urticaria. *British Medical Journal,* **iv,** 262.

National Academy of Sciences and the National Science Foundation (1965) National Research Council Publication 1270, Washington.

Samter, M. & Beers, R. F. Jr (1967) Concerning the nature of intolerance to aspirin. *Journal of Allergy,* **40,** 281.

Smith, A. P. (1971) Response of aspirin allergic patients to challenge by some analgesics in common use. *British Medical Journal,* **ii,** 494.

Thune, P., Ryan, T. J., Powell, S. M. & Ellis, J. R. (1976) The cutaneous reactions to kallikrein, prostaglandin and thurfyl nicotinate in chronic urticaria and the effect of polyfloretin phosphate. *Acta Dermato-veneriologica* (Stockholm) **56,** in press.

Yurchak, A. M., Wicher, K. & Arbesman, C. E. (1970) Immunologic studies on aspirin. *Journal of Allergy,* **40,** 281.

9. The Localisation of Granulomatous Diseases and Vasculitis in the Nasal Mucosa

M. W. KANAN AND T. J. RYAN

It is not known with certainty why the nasal mucosa is often involved and severely mutilated during the course of several chronic infectious diseases, some forms of vasculitis and disorders of intravascular coagulation. In Chapter 8 the question is raised why infections, drugs and food additives localise and produce vasculitis in certain areas. It may also be asked why the response of the target organ to noxious agents is in some cases urticaria, in others vasculitis and in yet others granuloma formation. The nose is a good example of such an organ and the wide range of triggers alighting there includes infectious organisms, allergens, toxins and cryoglobulins.

In this chapter a review of the clinicopathological and experimental aspects of this problem is presented and an attempt made to show how studies of the localising features and vascular behaviour of the nasal mucosa have lent support to most of the hypotheses discussed in other chapters in this monograph.

CLINICOPATHOLOGICAL ASPECTS

Irrespective of the diversity of the causative agents, most of the mutilating granulomatous diseases encountered by dermatologists and otorhinolaryngologists tend to involve the nasal mucosa (Table 9.1).

Infectious granulomata

Lupus vulgaris

Among 1200 Danish cases of lupus vulgaris, Forchammer (1911) reported primary involvement of the face in 81 per cent, the site first affected being the nose in 51 per cent,

195

Table 9.1. Organisms causing chronic granulomatous disease of the nose: their characteristics, geographical distribution and the animals they infect.

Disease and causative organism	Geographical distribution	Susceptible animals	Portal of entry and mode of dissemination
Lupus vulgaris: *Mycobacterium tuberculosis* (2.5—3.5 × 0.3 μm) Acid-fast bacillus. Alcohol-fast. Stains with Sudan black. Gram pos.	Ubiquitous, rare in tropics.	Human strain fatal in g. pigs. Rabbits and mice affected less. *M. bovis* virulent to all. Chicken not affected by both strains.	Inhalation, ingestion and skin inoculation. Lymph and blood-borne spread.
Leprosy: *Mycobacterium leprae.* (1—8 × 0.2—0.5 μm) AFB less alcohol-fast. Not stained by Sudan black. Gram pos. Uncultivable.	Tropics, sub-tropics and endemic in Malta, Cyprus and countries on the Adriatic, Med. and Black seas.	Ear of hamster, mouse footpad and armadillo.	Undecided. Cutaneous? Dissemination by blood and nerves.
Rhinoscleroma: *Klebsiella rhinoscleromatis.* (1.6—2.4 × 0.8 μm) Gram neg.	Central Europe, Russia, China, India, Indonesia, North Africa, Central and South America.	Mice.	Unknown. ? Inhalation (upper resp. tract). Localised extension.
Venereal syphilis: *Treponema pallidum.* (6—15 × 0.09—0.18 μm) Close, rigid (8—20 coils spirochaete). Rotar and flexion movements. Uncultivable.	Ubiquitous in urban communities.	Apes, rabbits and hamsters.	Genital and extra-genital, skin and mucosa. Transplacental. Blood-borne dissem.
Non-venereal endemic syphilis (bejel): same as venereal syphilis. Uncultivable.	Arid deserts of Asia and Africa.	Apes, rabbits and hamsters.	Mouth (communal drinking, food utensils and kissing).
Yaws: ,, ,, Uncultivable.	Tropical, humid jungles of Central Africa, Asia, Australia and South and Central America.	Monkeys, rabbits and hamsters.	Abrasions or bite in skin by direct contact by vector (hippelates fly). Blood-borne dissem.
Mucocutaneous leishmaniasis: *Leishmania braziliensis.* (2—4 × 0.5—2.5 μm)	Endemic in Central and South America (damp forests).	Monkey, dog, g. pigs, bat, white rat, squirrel and hamster.	Through a bite by local sandfly (phlebotomus) in skin. Dissemination by lymph and blood.
Lutz's mycosis: *Paracoccidioides braziliensis.* (10—60 μm diameter) Spherical and budding.	Brazil, South and Central America, occasionally U.S.A., Italy, Portugal, Morocco and Bulgaria.	Inoc. into g. pigs — specific orchitis. In hamsters and mice — dissemination.	Undecided. ? Lungs, skin, GI tract & bucco-pharyngeal mucosa. Blood-borne and lymphatic dissem.
Rhinosporidiosis: *Rhinosporidium seeberi.* Dimorphic fungus. Sporangium = 2.5 mm diam. Endospores 6—7 μm diam. Uncultivable.	Endemic in India and Ceylon. Sporadic elsewhere.	Natural infection in nose of cattle and horses. Experimental inoc. failed.	Unknown. ? Direct inoc. in nose. Dissem. only 2 cases (blood-borne).

Table 9.1.—*continued*

Disease and causative organism	Geographical distribution	Susceptible animals	Portal of entry and mode of dissemination
Rhinophycomycosis: *Entomophthora coronata.* 5—25 µm diam. PAS positive. Grows better at 25°C.	Tropics and sub-tropics.	Inoculation experiments in young animals failed.	Portal of entry unknown. ? by inhalation.
Glanders: *Actinobacillus mallei.* Short coccoid, rod-shaped bacillus. Gram neg.	Eastern Europe, Asia Minor, Asia and North Africa.	Natural disease of solipeds. Horse, mule, donkey and occasionally sheep. Accidental in man by contact with animals or lab. material.	In animals through intest. wall by contaminated fodder with nasal discharge and sputum. Dissem. blood-borne.

the cheek in 28 per cent and the ears in two per cent. Between 1896 and 1906, he had also seen lesions in the nasal and oral mucosa of 72 per cent of 800 cases of this disease. Similarly in a large number of cases of mucosal lupus vulgaris seen at the London Hospital, Sequeira, Ingram and Brain (1947) found the nose to be involved in the majority. According to Degos (1953), endonasal lupus vulgaris usually is the starting point of the disease, the nose being affected in 75 per cent of cases. He also stated that when lupus involves the buccopharyngeal mucosa, the lips, the face and the eyes it usually does so as a result of direct or lymphatic spread from disease in the nasal cavity. Horwitz (1966), in his thesis on 'lupus vulgaris in Denmark, 1895—1954', re-emphasised the tendency to cephalic localisation by quoting its occurrence in 92 per cent of a series of 208 patients of both sexes. In his view, the head and neck are common sites for lupus vulgaris because the disease originates in cervical adenitis or the nasal mucosa.

Sarcoidosis

This granulomatous disease, believed to be related to tuberculosis, also seems to involve the nasal mucosa. Wayoff (1960) drew attention to the relative frequency of endonasal sarcoidosis and recommended biopsy of the nasal mucosa as a diagnostic aid.

Leprosy

The nasal mucosa is thought to be affected quite early in lepromatous leprosy. According to Prabhu (1946), the endonasal lesion may start on the turbinates or on the septum and then usually spreads to the cartilage and the small nasal bones causing considerable deformity (Figure 9.1). Involvement of other mucosae of the respiratory tract is secondary to the nose. Thus Wise (1954) found leprosy to be the commonest cause of septal perforation, and Dharmendra and Sen (1948), in a study of 4072 cases of leprosy, found that nasal scrapings were positive in 92 per cent of patients with the lepromatous form. Job, Karat and Karat (1966) studied the histopathological changes in various stages of leprous rhinitis in 33 patients and concluded that lepra bacilli seem to grow profusely and by preference in the mucosal lining of the nose.

In a recent study of endonasal lesions in 31 patients with early lepromatous leprosy from Dichpalli, India (McDougall et al, 1975), some important findings emerged. A

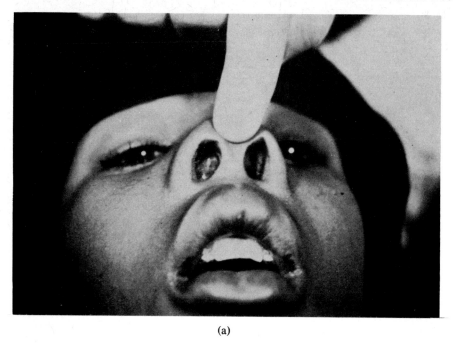

(a)

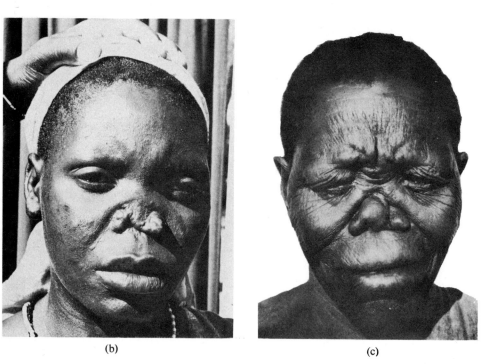

(b)   (c)

Figure 9.1. Three examples of nasal pathology: (a) septal swelling in rhinoscleroma, (b) and (c) deformity from destruction of nasal cartilage and small nasal bones in leprosy.

highly bacillated, granulomatous infiltrate occurred consistently in the lamina propria of the septum and of the inferior and middle turbinates. Uniformly stained and granular acid-fast bacilli were frequently seen in the endothelial cells, and the walls and the lumina of the venules and venular capillaries (Figure 9.2). Less frequently, such bacilli were found in the secretory cells and ducts of the mucous glands. It was evident that lepra bacilli arc discharged into the nasal cavity mainly within migrating neutrophils, monocytes and macrophages passing through 'septic' breaks in the surface epithelium.

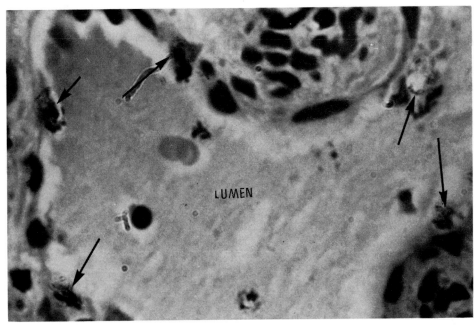

Figure 9.2. Aggregates of lepra bacilli (arrows) phagocytosed by endothelial cells and lying free in the lumen of nasal venule in the lamina propria. × 300.

To some extent bacilli are phagocytosed by epithelial cells overlying the granulomatous infiltrate (Figure 9.3) but not by the basal cells of the stratified squamous epithelium. Occasionally some acid-fast bacilli can be seen flowing out of the secretory duct onto the mucosal surface. These findings are thought to be relevant to the mode of dissemination of lepra bacilli in the environment.

Rhinoscleroma

This disease starts mainly in the submucosa of the nasal septum spreading slowly forward to cause fibrosis, stenosis, ulceration and a deformity known as 'Hebra nose'. The lesion may spread backwards to involve the nasopharynx, larynx and occasionally the bronchi (Kerdel-Vegas et al, 1963) (Figure 9.1).

Treponemal diseases

Venereal syphilis. In the late secondary stage of the disease, gummatous lesions of the nasal septum with consequent deformity used to be common, although in late congenital

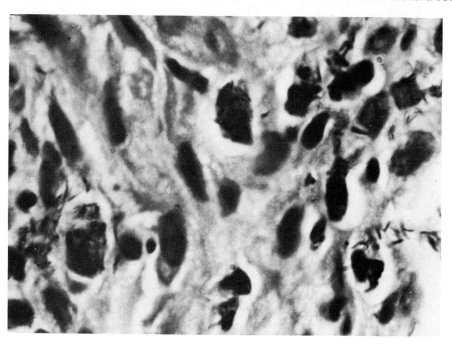

Figure 9.3. Bacillated macrophages bordering an epithelial rete of the nasal mucosa on either side. Lepra bacilli are clearly seen interiorised in the overlying epithelial prickle cells. $\times$ 320.

syphilis they were even more common (Stokes, 1943; Sullivan, 1964; Lomholt, 1968). As in lupus vulgaris, a few organisms can be demonstrated in the lesions, but unlike lupus, which destroys the cartilaginous parts of the nose, syphilis mutilates the bony septum and other nasal bones.

Yaws. In the late gummatous form of the disease described as gangosa, the alae nasi and the supporting structures of the nose, nasopharynx and palate are mutilated (Fordyce and Arnold, 1906; Mink and McLean, 1906; Guitierrez, 1925). However, treponemata are hardly ever recovered from late cutaneous or mucosal lesions of yaws (Furtado, 1973).

Bejel (non-venereal endemic syphilis). This was first described by Hudson in 1936 as a form of non-venereal mucocutaneous syphilis common among the bedouins of the Euphrates valley in Syria. In his comprehensive monograph, Hudson (1958) stated that when he first visited the market place in Deir-Ez-Zor in Syria with his team, it was common to see eroded and saddle noses and to hear cleft palate-like voices caused by perforation and erosion of the hard palate. Among 1238 bedouin patients whom he had seen with bejel, 695 had lesions identical to gangosa of yaws in the centre of their faces. The gangosa type of lesion in bejel (Figure 9.4, a and b) was also reported recently by Kanan, Abbas and Girgis (1971) among the bedouins in the outskirts of Kuwait, Arabia. In spite of positive serological tests for syphilis, no treponemes could be found histologically in Levaditi-stained serial sections from such lesions (Olsen, 1958).

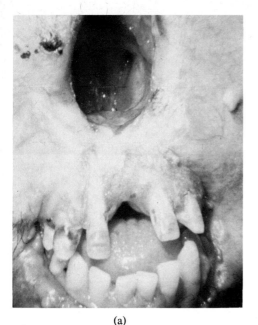 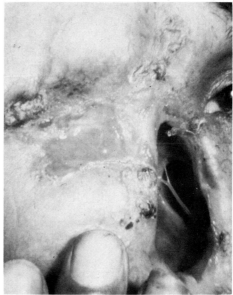

(a)   (b)

Figure 9.4. (a) Late gangosa-type lesion in bejel showing destruction of the nasal septum, turbinates and the right eye.
(b) Nasal cavity replaced by a hole in the centre of the face in bejel and loss of the upper lip and the upper two central incisor teeth. Untreated syphilis, yaws and leprosy may lead to the same deformity.

Mucocutaneous leishmaniasis

The organism *Leishmania brasiliensis* sets up inflammation initially at the site of a phlebotomus bite. After months or years, secondary lesions sometimes develop in mucous membranes especially of the nasal septum and nasopharynx (Harman, 1972). The earliest mucosal lesion starts usually as hyperaemia of the septal mucosa, and this subsequently ulcerates and leads eventually to septal perforation. The nasal bones, however, escape destruction so that when the bridge sinks the appearance of a parrot's beak or a camel's nose is produced. The ulceration may become mutilating and involve the middle of the face (Pierini, 1969).

Busquets (1948), in an investigation of numerous patients of all ages with visceral leishmaniasis, showed that 81.8 per cent had positive nasal smears, while Roccuzzo and Lomeo (1950) found a positive nasal smear in all the affected children they studied.

Fungal diseases

Rhinosporidiosis. This is a chronic granulomatous disease caused by an endo-sporulating phycomycete, *Rhinosporidium seeberi.* Of the 88 cases reviewed by Karunaratne (1936), 71 were nasal, 10 conjunctival, three involved the lacrymal sac and there were three cases affecting the ear, uvula and penis, respectively. However, in seven North American cases (Caldwell and Roberts, 1938), the lesions were in the nose in every instance, apparently on the nasal septum. Usually the nasal lesion is a pink or red polypoid mass or masses with papillary projections located most frequently on the right side near the junction of the cartilaginous and bony portions of the nasal septum, well above the floor of the nostril (Caldwell and Roberts, 1938).

Rhinophycomycosis. This is caused by another phycomycete, *Entomophthora coronata,* which involves the nasal septum and sinuses and can destroy the nose, palate and lips (Clark, 1968). It occurs in otherwise apparently healthy individuals and is found almost exclusively in tropical and subtropical regions. The mode of infection is still unknown; inhalation is a possibility which has been studied but no proof has been obtained. However, radiological examination of the chest in one case showed lesions that might have been caused by mycotic infection (Tio, Moeljono and Njo-Injo, 1966).

Paracoccidiodomycosis (Lutz's mycosis). The mucocutaneous variant of this fungal granuloma usually begins in the region of the mouth where small papules and ulcerations appear and spread, ultimately destroying the nose, lips and facies (Andrews and Domonkos, 1963).

Histoplasmosis. In this systemic mycosis, the primary lesion is usually in the lungs, but cutaneous and mucocutaneous forms do occur and endonasal localisation with perforation of the nasal septum has been reported (Miller et al, 1947).

Non-infectious granulomatous vasculitis

Wegener's granulomatosis

In 1936 Wegener described three cases of a widespread granulomatous vasculitis similar to polyarteritis nodosa in which rhinitis was the initial symptom. Walton (1958) reviewed the disease in a thesis and pointed out that, in about two-thirds of the cases, it begins in the nose, where it produces persistent purulent rhinorrhoea, nasal obstruction, antral pain and epistaxis. This leads not only to extensive mucosal ulceration and cartilaginous or osseous destruction in the nose and palate, but also to widespread pulmonary consolidation. Sooner or later, widespread hypersensitivity reactions in the form of inflammatory granulomatous and necrotising lesions occur in the small blood vessels, and progressively produce renal or respiratory failure and death. The average survival period is five months, but there have been reports of five cases which remitted and survived for up to four years.

Wegener's disease is now a well recognised form of vasculitis which tends to be diagnosed whenever lesions of the upper respiratory tract, and especially of the nasal cavity, form a prominent feature. However, it overlaps with other forms of vasculitis and other granulomatous respiratory diseases (Burton and Burton, 1972). Whatever the aetiology, the anterior nasal septum and the facial aspect of the nose are often destroyed (Figure 9.5, a and b) (see Chapter 13, p. 313).

Lethal mid-line granuloma

This is a locally destructive granulomatous process which involves the nose and paranasal sinuses. Death occurs eventually from cachexia or haemorrhage (Friedmann, 1955). A reticulum cell sarcoma may account for some cases while others may represent incomplete forms of Wegener's granulomatosis (Godman and Churg, 1954). Shillitoe et al (1974) recorded no significant immunological difference between Wegener's granulomatosis and midline granuloma (Table 9.2). The systemic nature of both these forms of granulomatosis was emphasised by Mills (1965) who recorded elevation of the ESR and hypergammaglobulinaemia.

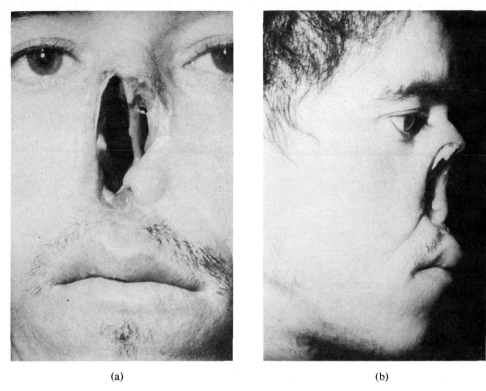

(a)   (b)

Figure 9.5. (a) Mutilating deformity of the nose in chronic nonspecific granulomatous disease usually seen in lethal midline granuloma or Wegener's granulomatosis. (b) Profile of the same deformity.

Other forms of vasculitis and autoimmune disease

Perforation of the nasal septum was reported by Leites and Benenson (1949) to have occurred in six children who were severely ill with rheumatic carditis. The perforation had been preceded by atrophic changes and haemorrhages in the septal mucosa.

In the recent literature attention has been drawn to the involvement of the endonasal tissues with frequent perforation of the nasal septum in systemic vascular diseases. Like Winkelmann and Ditto (1964), the author has seen it occur in Schönlein—Henoch purpura, and in one of his patients with a peculiar and unidentified recurrent cutaneous vasculitis, repeated nasal bleeding with eventual perforation of the septum was a prominent feature (Figure 9.6).

Strom (1965) reported that involvement of endonasal tissues occurs also in severe cases of Behçet's syndrome, while Vachtenheim and Grossmann (1969) were the first to record nasal septum perforation in systemic lupus erythematosus. More recent medical correspondence has featured another such example (Simpson, 1974) and two similar cases in young patients were reported by Snyder et al (1974); other patients were reported by Rothfield (1974) and Moasabhoy and Seeler (1974). The latter authors recorded ulceration of the nasal septum in eight out of 150 patients with SLE, but perforation in only two. Perforation of the nasal septum has been reported also in Sjögren's syndrome by Doig et al (1971).

Table 9.2. Comparison of immunological data in Wegener's granulomatosis and midline granuloma.

	Wegener's granulomatosis	Midline granuloma
Serum immunoglobulins		
IgG: Mean ($\pm$S.E.) mg per 100 ml	1216 ($\pm$146)	1165 ($\pm$217)
IgA: Mean ($\pm$S.E.) mg per 100 ml	537 ($\pm$83)	782 ($\pm$273)
IgM: Mean ($\pm$S.E.) mg per 100 ml	186 ($\pm$42)	153 ($\pm$24)
C3: Mean ($\pm$S.E.) mg per 100 ml	245 ($\pm$31)	218 ($\pm$25)
Lymphocyte transformation		
to PHA	45%[a]	31%
to PPD, SKSD, Candida, Herpes	5/26[b]	3/11
Macrophage migration inhibition		
to PPD, Candida, Herpes	3/17[c]	6/11
Delayed hypersensitivity		
to PPD, SKSD, Candida	2/21[d]	1/9
Autoantibodies		
Rheumatoid factor, thyroid, gastric, adrenal, smooth muscle, DNA, mitochondria, reticulin	4/7[e]	1/3
Immune complexes	1/7[f]	1/3

[a] Stimulation index as % of mean normal adult value.
[b] No. of antigens yielding stimulation index >2/no. of antigens used.
[c] No. of antigens inducing migration index < 80/no. of antigens used.
[d] No. of antigens causing induration >5 mm at 48 h/no. of antigens used.
[e] No. of patients with autoantibodies/no. of antigens used.
[f] No. of patients with complexes/no. of patients tested.

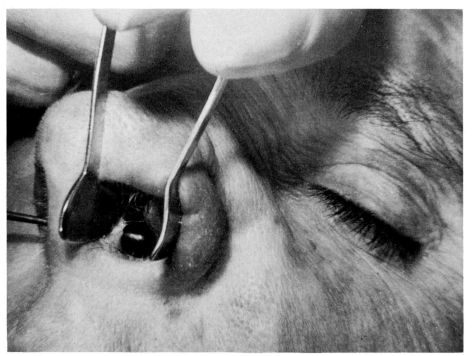

Figure 9.6. Perforation of the anterior nasal septum with a metal rod shown through the hole. From a case of vasculitis of unidentified nature.

Disorders of intravascular coagulation

In cryoglobulinaemia symptoms are usually explained in terms of cryoglobulins being precipitated intravascularly from plasma or serum when they are cooled, but the precise method of cell damage is uncertain. Nasal septum perforation has been seen recently in a patient with cryoglobulinaemia (Cream, personal communication, 1975).

In a peculiar case reported recently by Brödthagen et al (1968), a 62-year-old woman with idiopathic hypercoagulability of the blood presented with chronic progressive cutaneous lesions and painful ulcerations in the peripheral parts of her body (Figure 9.7). The ulceration of her nasal septum progressed to such an extent that its anterior 4 cm was lost. The outstanding histological findings in cutaneous biopsy specimens were the markedly dilated capillaries with intraluminal hyaline thrombi and the almost complete absence of any inflammatory reaction (Figure 9.8).

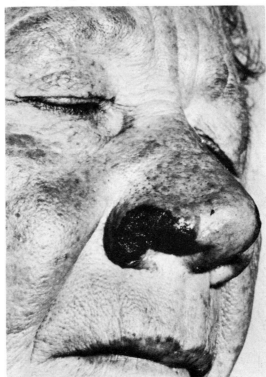

Figure 9.7. Endonasal lesion involving the septum and extending anteriorly to destroy the right ala nasi. A case of mucocutaneous intravascular coagulation.

GRANULOMATOUS DISEASES IN THE ANIMAL NOSE

Veterinarians rarely encounter in the animal such destructive nasal lesions as are seen in the human. The main granulomatous infections which cause nasal lesions in animals are glanders and rhinosporidiosis.

Glanders

This is a contagious disease of solipeds — usually horses, mules and donkeys. In the acute form there is a high fever, cough and nasal discharge with rapidly spreading

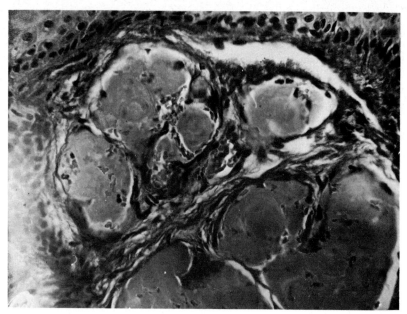

Figure 9.8. Cutaneous lesion from the case in Figure 9.7 showing a non-inflammatory histology. Dilated dermal capillaries and venules clogged with haemolysed red blood cells. White cells are absent from the microscopical scene. H.E. × 400.

ulcers on the nasal mucosa and nodules in the skin of the lower limbs or abdomen. In the chronic form, nasal lesions appear on the lower parts of the turbinates and on the cartilaginous nasal septum (Blood and Henderson, 1963). Man can occasionally contract this infection, which is usually fatal, when working with the organism in the laboratory or through close contact with affected animals (McGilvray, 1944).

Rhinosporidiosis

As in man, this can cause a chronic endonasal granulomatous lesion in the anterior third of the nasal cavity. Yeast-like bodies resembling rhinosporidium spores are usually found in an infiltrate composed largely of eosinophils. This type of rhinosporidiosis has been reported from the USA, Australia, India and South America. Clinically the disease resembles the nasal obstruction caused by the blood fluke, *Schistosoma nasalis,* and the enzootic nasal granuloma in cattle and sheep (Albiston and Gorrie, 1935; Saunders, 1948; Robinson, 1951; Choudbury, 1955; Biswal and Das, 1956; Hore, 1966).

EXPERIMENTAL ASPECTS OF NASAL LOCALISATION OF INFECTIVE AGENTS

In experimental leprosy

Rees (1966) reduced the immunological capacity of the experimental mouse by thymectomy and whole-body x-irradiation, and was then able to produce a disease pattern resembling human lepromatous leprosy. Reappraisal of this work (Rees, McDougall and Weddell, 1974) showed that, irrespective of whether the animals were inoculated in the footpad, intraperitoneally or intravenously, the nose eventually became heavily infected and bacilli were abundant in the nasal mucus.

In experimental leishmaniasis

Guinea-pig leishmaniasis, caused naturally by *Leishmania enriettii*, has been claimed by Muniz and Medina (1948) to affect the skin exclusively. Paraense (1953) inoculated the organism into the ear of 20 guinea-pigs and showed that a local leishmanial nodule developed at the site of inoculation, and after a varying period metastatic lesions developed in the feet, ears and external genitalia. He also examined sections from the snout of one animal killed 344 days after inoculation and found a thickened band of infiltrate with parasitised macrophages on one side of the septum but no involvement of the epithelium.

Previously, Paraense (1952) had demonstrated leishmanial lesions in the nasal mucosa of eight out of ten guinea-pigs inoculated intraperitoneally with *L. enriettii*. He also described necrosis of the epithelium with 'septic' catarrhal inflammation and abundant leishmanial bodies in the exudate. In some animals parasites were seen, free or within macrophages, in the lumen of capillaries and venules. Recently Kanan (1975) has produced leishmanial lesions in the nasal mucosa and external genitalia in a whole batch of seven guinea-pigs (Figure 9.9) six weeks after intravenous inoculation with *L. enriettii*. Abundant numbers of leishmanial protozoa were demonstrated in histological sections from the lamina propria of the nasoturbinals, some having been phagocytosed by the overlying epithelium (Figure 9.10, a and b).

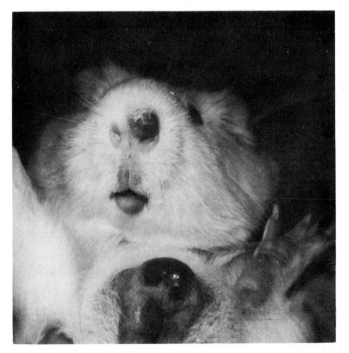

Figure 9.9. Experimental mucocutaneous nodules in the left nostril and the scrotum of a male guinea-pig inoculated intravenously with *L. enriettii* seven weeks previously.

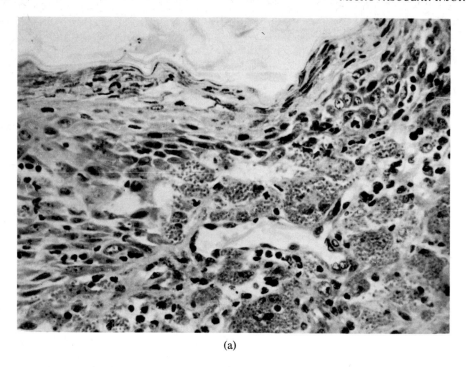

(a)

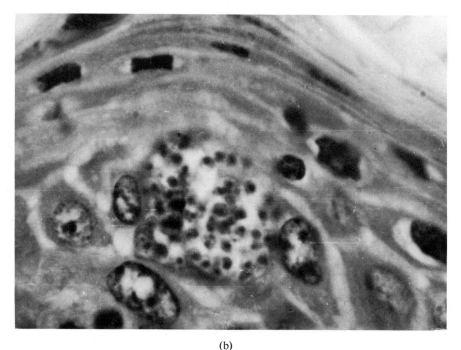

(b)

Figure 9.10. (a) Anterior mucosa of nasoturbinal with highly parasitised monocytes and histiocytes with *L. enriettii* in lamina propria. A few mononuclear cells and polymorphs are intermingled. H. & E. × 225. (b) Phagocytosis of many leishmanial protozoa by the overlying prickle cells of the anterior nasoturbinal. H. & E. × 360.

In experimental treponematosis

Experimental syphilis in the rabbit has been seen to localise at the sites of inoculation. Syphilitic lesions developing at sites remote from that of experimental inoculation were first reported by Grouven (1907, 1910). However, syphilitic involvement of the nasal mucosa in the experimental rabbit was first described by Grouven in 1908 and later by Uhlenhuth and Mulzer (1910). Reasoner (1916), who continued Nichols' investigations (1914), emphasised involvement of the nasal mucosa after intravenous inoculation of the rabbit with a neurophilic strain of *Treponema pallidum*. He also reported the presence of the treponema in the nasal discharge.

Brown and Pearce (1920) emphasised the occurrence of syphilitic lesions in the mucous membranes and mucocutaneous junctions in 20 per cent of their experimental rabbits. On the other hand, yaws was successfully produced in experimental monkeys by Ashburn and Craig (1907). Their work was continued by Schobl who successfully produced destructive lesions of the nose similar to those of gangosa in man by inoculating yaws material into the face of Philippine monkeys (Figure 9.11). He made no attempt to inoculate yaws treponemata intravenously.

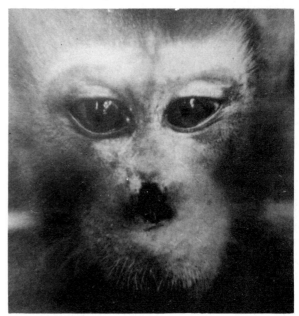

Figure 9.11. Typical gangosa-type lesion of experimental yaws in a Philippine monkey.

PATHOGENESIS

The pathogenesis of granulomatous diseases in the nasal mucosa is obviously multifactorial. Here we are concerned with those factors involved in the endonasal localisation of such diseases. The question must be asked whether they begin in the nose or whether they pick out that site during haematogenous dissemination from foci in other organs.

Mode of transport

The nasal mucosa as a portal of entry for micro-organisms has been investigated by many workers. McMahon (1933) showed that carbon particles in suspension cannot penetrate the intact ciliated or squamous epithelium of the rabbit's turbinates despite repeated and frequent instillation over a period lasting from thirty minutes to six hours. But Linton (1933) demonstrated that provided the dosage is adequate a sufficiently virulent strain of *Streptococcus haemolyticus* is able to penetrate unaided the normal mucosa of guinea-pigs and rabbits.

The work of Cannon and Walsh (1937), however, showed that, when virulent staphylococci are instilled intranasally into normal rabbits and guinea-pigs, they do not pass directly through the epithelium of the upper respiratory tract but are aspirated into the lungs where they enter the blood.

Bacteria that elicit chronic granuloma formation behave differently to those causing acute inflammation. The former are, on the whole, of low virulence, do not secrete an exotoxin and, although a few have been grown in vitro with difficulty, the majority cannot be cultured (Table 9.1). It is unlikely, therefore, that they can enter the normal nasal mucosa from without. Cochrane (1959) stated that he had never seen a primary endonasal lesion in leprosy and he emphasised that patients brought to his attention with nasal lesions were either proved to be misdiagnosed or shown to have unrevealed lesions of cutaneous leprosy elsewhere. Another strong argument against the concept proposed by Sticker (1897), that the nose is a portal of entry for lepra bacilli, stems from the frequently reported statement that the nose is not involved in tuberculoid leprosy.

Lutz's mycosis is considered by many to start most commonly in the buccopharyngeal mucosa, although the idea that the primary lesion is in the lungs has recently been gaining support (Padilha-Gonclaves, 1969). It has to be admitted that the portal of entry in rhinoscleroma and rhinosporidiosis has yet to be identified but, as the lesions are strictly confined to the nasal mucosa and the upper respiratory tract, it is tempting to assume a direct mucosal portal of entry.

Most agents producing granulomata in the nasal mucosa seem to arrive via the bloodstream. In lupus vulgaris, for example, it had been thought by Dowling and Wetherly-Mein (1954) that a considerable number of the lesions follow primary implantation in the skin of tubercle bacilli from the exterior. However, Horwitz (1959, 1966) believed that lesions develop frequently as a result of haematogenous dissemination from a primary complex in another organ. This was not without good reason for chest x-rays were taken of 201 patients who had lupus vulgaris as the only evidence of active tuberculous disease; 66 of them (33 per cent) showed pulmonary calcifications and in another 11, fibrotic lesions of tuberculous origin were seen. It was presumed that these pulmonary lesions were tuberculous because Edwards (1957) had found that histoplasmosis did not occur in Denmark. Another reason for considering primary inoculation of the skin an unlikely cause of lupus vulgaris is the rarity of the disease on the hands and forearms, especially among the farming population, many of whom must have often milked or attended tuberculous cattle (Horwitz, 1966).

In the case of leprosy, it has been shown repeatedly that, irrespective of the portal of entry, at some point in the disease acid-fast bacillaemia is a significant feature (Crow, 1912; Rivas, 1912; Honeij, 1915; Hollman, 1916; Rhodes-Jones, 1963). Recently, Drutz, Chen and Lu Wen-Hsiang (1972) have convincingly demonstrated acid-fast bacillaemia in 25 out of 32 patients with leprosy. In six of these with untreated lepromatous leprosy, acid-fast bacilli were continuously present at a concentration of 10^5/ml of blood, both extracellularly and in neutrophils, monocytes and large circulating histiocytes. They thought that the bacilli enter the bloodstream by invading skin arterioles, capillaries and venules. Furthermore, work in the experimental mouse by Rees (1966) lends support to the view that endonasal lesions in lepromatous leprosy are the outcome of haematogenous spread.

In mucocutaneous leishmaniasis, according to Pierini (1969), a high percentage of cases have nasal, pharyngeal and buccal mucous membrane lesions as a result of haematogenous spread. A similar mode of spread was postulated for Lutz's mycosis by Padilha-Gonclaves (1969). Although the causative fungus is 20 to 60 μm in diameter, Fialho (1960) reported the emergence of minute forms by rapid reproduction, and these can pass through the pulmonary filter into the general circulation. In syphilis, treponemata have been demonstrated in the blood even in the later stages of the disease, and the infectivity of the blood has been confirmed when transfused into healthy recipients (Stokes, 1943).

It is conceivable that whatever the portal of entry of the causative organism and wherever the site of the primary lesion, be it in the skin, lungs, intestine or lymph nodes, some of the viable micro-organisms are carried to the blood capillaries within wandering macrophages. When these cells rupture, the organisms pass on freely in the venules and into the general circulation. Less frequently they may enter the local lymphatics and reach the circulation via the thoracic duct, provided they escape being trapped and destroyed by the draining lymph nodes. Should the causative agent be small, it can escape by way of the pulmonary veins and the left side of the heart into the general circulation.

Large-sized micro-organisms, on the other hand, are usually unable to escape through the walls of the local venules, and were they ever to do so they would be trapped in the alveolar capillaries. It is not surprising, therefore, that haematogenous dissemination of large fungi, such as rhinosporidiosis (40 to 300 μm in diameter) has been extremely rare. Only two such cases have been reported (Rajam et al, 1955; Agrawal, Sharma and Shrivastava, 1959), small endospores (2.5 to 7 μm in diameter) being responsible. In Lutz's mycosis, with fungal bodies 20 to 60 μm in diameter, haematogenous dissemination has been reported to occur by means of rapidly reproduced minute buds (Fialho, 1960). This matter of particle size has been investigated in the experimental animal by injecting plastic beads (Bio-Rad Laboratories) of 37 to 70 μm into the tail vein of the mouse. Two to four days later embolic foreign body granulomata were found in the lungs only (Von Lichtenberg, 1962).

Mode of localisation

It is quite conceivable that circulating micro-organisms will be trapped in greater numbers by organs with blood stasis and more permeable microvessels. Majno (1965) speculated that the preference of certain disease processes for particular organs may also depend on the local vascular pattern, particularly on the distribution of the venules. This is supported by the finding that endotoxins injected intravenously tend to accumulate in the walls of venules, possibly as a result of physiological leakage followed by retention at the level of the basement membrane. Venules are more susceptible to many kinds of injury and hence are a site of predilection for haemorrhage, thrombosis and diapedesis as well as for allergic and cold injury. This topic also forms the basis of several papers on the localisation of immune complexes and other noxious agents in vasculitis of the skin (Copeman and Ryan, 1971; Ryan, 1973).

In the human nose Cauna and Hinderer (1969) and Cauna (1970) have shown that the subepithelial and periglandular capillaries of the lamina propria of the septum and turbinates possess a fenestrated endothelial lining enclosed by a porous basement membrane. The venules also have a highly porous basement membrane, but they are lined by a continuous endothelium.

On the other hand, Dawes and Prichard (1953) in an extensive study of the nasal mucosal angioarchitecture in animals, emphasised that in the side facing the inhaled airstream the veins are larger and more numerous than the arteries. Kanan, Ryan and Weddell (1975), in experiments on rats, mice, guinea-pigs and goats, showed that colloidal carbon C11/1143a, administered intravenously as a single dose of 8 to 16 g body weight, leaks into the nasal lamina propria through the superficial capillaries and venules; this occurs predominantly in the anterior dorsal part of the septum and turbinates (Figures 9.12 and 9.13). This phenomenon, in their opinion, is due in part to the overall porosity of the vessels in these areas, which is similar to that described by Cauna and Hinderer (1969) and Cauna (1970) in the human nose. They also believed that the constant bombardment of the anterior nasal mucosa by an alternately cool inspired and warm expired air creates a state of relative stasis in the superficial capillaries and venules. This in turn may well increase the permeability of the barrier between the vessels and the surrounding connective tissue.

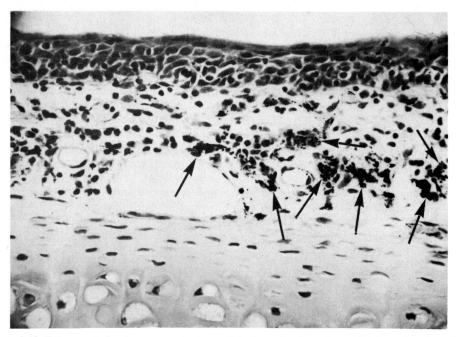

Figure 9.12. Entrapment of carbon aggregates (arrows) in the walls of venular capillaries and perivascular macrophages of the anterior nasal mucosa. H. & E. × 200.

In another experiment, Kanan (1975) quantified the tissue uptake of intravenously administered radioactive colloidal gold (^{198}Au) and found it to be significant in the anterior regions of the nasal septum and turbinates. This uptake was enhanced by exposure of the animal to a cold atmosphere at $+10°C$ to $+6°C$ for a period of 24 hours (Table 9.3). In a different controlled experiment designed to study the effect of sex hormones on this uptake, he found that in female rats ovariectomy depressed the uptake whereas oestrogen enhanced it (Table 9.4).

The role of the fibrinolytic—anti-fibrinolytic system in phagocytosis

The injection of various colloidal particles into the bloodstream soon causes the formation of platelet aggregates (Figure 10.8) (Tait and Elvidge, 1926; Salvidio and Cosby, 1960; Stehbens and Florey, 1960; Cohen, Braunwald and Gardner, 1965; French

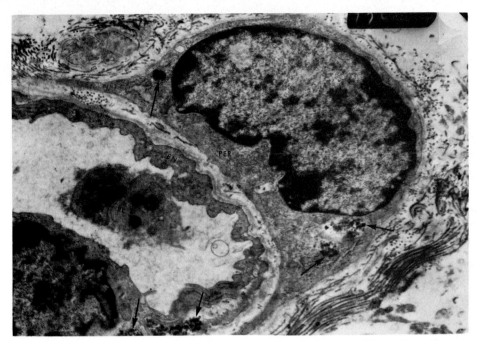

Figure 9.13. Carbon particles (arrows) which have escaped through the permeable venular wall are seen phagocytosed by the pericyte (PER). EN = endothelium; PL = platelet.

1967; Van Aken, Goote and Vreeken, 1968). Before phagocytosis of these particles by the reticuloendothelial system, the aggregates must pass through the capillary networks of other organs, especially the lung (Stehbens and Florey, 1960). The work of Van Aken and Vreeken (1969) lends support to the idea that these aggregates are dissociated in the microcirculation by activated fibrinolysis. The micro-obstruction caused by the trapped aggregates causes anoxaemia of the vessel wall (Tagnon et al, 1946; Kwaan and McFadzean, 1956) and this probably releases plasminogen activator from the endothelium to produce increased fibrinolytic activity (Astrup and Albrechtsen, 1957; Todd, 1964). This activated fibrinolysis leads to the local formation of fibrinogen degradation products (FDP) which may influence platelet aggregation (Kowalski et al, 1964; Jerushalmy and Zucker, 1965; Larrieu, Inceman and Marder, 1967).

As far as the liver and spleen are concerned, their low content of fibrinolytic activity (Astrup and Albrechtsen, 1957), together with particle accumulation attributable

Table 9.3. Distribution of intravenous ^{198}Au in the rat (24 hours).[a]

Tissue 100 mg	Room temperature (23°C) 6 male Wistar rats Mean value counts/min	Cold room (5—7°C) 10 male Wistar rats Mean value counts/min
Nose tip	2	1.8
Anterior septum	150	359
Posterior septum	26	83
Inferior turbinate	136	268
Lip	1.6	3.6
Liver	33 125	32 994

[a]Radioactive gold localised in the nose is compared to that in other tissues, in rats kept in a cold room at 23°C. Higher levels were recorded in the anterior septum of the nose in animals exposed to the cold.

Table 9.4. Influence of female sex hormone on distribution of intravenous ^{198}Au in the ovariectomised rat (24 hours).[a]

Tissue 100 mg	4 ovariectomised rats kept at 23°C mean value	6 ovariectomised rats + oestrogen kept at 23°C mean value	4 ovariectomised rats + progesterone kept at 23°C mean value
Nose tip	7	9	2
Anterior septum	106	406	114
Posterior septum	26	107	33
Inferior turbinate	63	242	84
Lip	3.5	20	3.5
Liver	22 415	37 555	25 767

[a]Preliminary observations showed that following intravenous inoculation of carbon, larger amounts of carbon were deposited in the nose of pregnant animals. This table summarises the results of a quantitative estimation of the localisation of radioactive gold. The largest counts were found in the anterior septum of the animals with the highest levels of oestrogen.

mainly to the phagocytic capacity and specific structure of the RES, may well go a long way towards explaining the specific accumulation of such particles in their cells. On the other hand, the high fibrinolytic activity in non-RES sites, especially in the lung, probably leads to enhanced disaggregation of thrombocyte-particle aggregates under physiological conditions.

The catchment area in the nasal mucosa seems to behave differently to other non-RES sites in this respect, and the reason lies partly in the peculiar micro-anatomy of stasis and partly in diminished fibrinolytic activity due to constant exposure of the area to the cold inspired airstream. Jensen et al (1953) demonstrated raised blood antifibrinolytic activity in rats and human subjects exposed to cold. This may be relevant not only to the accumulation in special sites of particulate matter administered intravenously to the experimental animal, but also to the entrapment of infective and other biological particles which provoke granulomatous diseases and various forms of vasculitis in the endonasal tissues.

Kahn's flare-up reaction

Kahn, working in retirement in Michigan, became particularly interested in the nose during his continuing studies on syphilis. In a paper on Wegener's granulomatosis, he proposed that, should the agents to which the nose is constantly exposed by inhalation happen to be deposited there from the bloodstream, then a local flare-up reaction might occur and even lead to destruction of the organ.

His hypothesis is similar to that of Polak, Frey and Turk (1970), who induced flare-up reactions at the site of previous allergic contact dermatitis by parenteral administration of the sensitiser. They concluded that cells at the site of the reaction produce antibody which reacts with circulating antigen. Kahn (1936) showed that an important defensive reaction in immunity is the localising response manifested by tissues not only against infecting micro-organisms but equally against antigens and allergens. The studies carried out in his laboratory indicated that at least three factors are necessary to elicit specific local flare-up reactions to microbial or protein antigens:
1. A given degree of immunity.
2. An inflammatory focus, visible or invisible, associated with antigen or antibody localised in a tissue.

3. The presence of a given concentration of the same antigen in the bloodstream.

Williams (1949), supported by Kahn (1954), believed that the mucous membranes of the nose and pharynx are bombarded constantly by infective agents, dust and other airborne particles and become immunologically hyper-reactive. This concept of a hyper-reactive state in the normal nasal mucosa gains support from the finding of IgG, IgA, IgM and IgD-positive cells in the lamina propria (Brandtzaeg, Fjellanger and Gjeruldsen, 1967; Lai A Fat, Cormane and Van Furth, 1974).

Local tissue temperature and granuloma formation

Apart from the problem of initial localisation, the reason why blood-borne infective agents survive and proliferate at sites of stasis has yet to be decided. Purtilo et al (1974) showed that transformation of lymphocytes in vitro was depressed both at 33°C and at 28°C, and, as this happened to human and to armadillo lymphocytes, they concluded that cool temperatures probably depress cell-mediated immunity in vivo.

Infective agents producing granulomas seem to survive, multiply and flourish in tissues where the temperature is lower than the normal body temperature. Indeed, it has been thought that lepra bacilli grow abundantly in the cooler sites of the body (Binford, 1956; Brand, 1959) and by preference in the mucosal lining of the nose (Job, Karat and Karat, 1966), where the temperature at the surface is reckoned to vary between 30.4 and 32°C (Eggston and Wolff, 1947). It has been shown that lepra bacilli multiply most rapidly in mouse footpads kept at an air temperature of 20°C, but under these conditions, the temperature of the footpad tissue averages 27 to 30°C (Shepard, 1965). Even so, Samuel et al (1973) showed that lepra bacilli multiply equally well at 33°C and at 37°C in human macrophages cultured in vitro.

The role that cooling plays in localising lupus vulgaris, leprosy and sarcoidosis to the nose was emphasised by Haxthausen (1930). In Lutz's mycosis, MacKinnon (as quoted by Padilha-Gonclaves, 1969), inoculated guinea-pigs intracardially but obtained disseminated lesions only when the animals were kept at an ambient temperature lower than 37°C.

In their experimental work on treponematosis, Turner and Hollander (1957) showed that 19 rabbits, kept in a cool environment (18 to 21°C), produced a maximum number of lesions within 20 days of inoculation, whereas 18 similarly inoculated rabbits, which were kept in a warm environment (29 to 31°C), developed lesions poorly or hardly at all. Turner and Hollander also obtained similar results in the hamster; the incubation period tended to be longer in the animals housed in the warm room, and a larger proportion of those kept in a warm environment showed no evidence of infection. Infected lymph nodes from animals kept under cool conditions were consistently larger and contained more treponemes than those from hamsters living in the warm room. In guinea-pig leishmaniasis, the lesions are restricted to the cool, unhairy areas of the body.

Whether the cooler temperature in the nasal mucosa encourages the growth of granuloma-producing micro-organisms directly or whether it depresses the killing capacity of the local macrophages remains a controversial issue. In this connection it is relevant to compare the behaviour of the professional macrophages in the RES with that of the potential phagocytes in the non-RES sites, especially in the nasal mucosa. Although the latter, which include the endothelial cells, pericytes and fibroblasts, have been shown to ingest these micro-organisms, they usually fail to kill them owing to lack of lysosomal organelles. Hence obligatory intracellular parasites seem to use such cells as hideaways where they can survive and flourish.

Organ oxygen tension

Chandler et al (1964) studied the effect of hyperbaric oxygen on the development of tuberculosis in different organs of the rabbit. They found that disease occurred much less frequently or severely in the lungs of the treated animals than in those of untreated controls, while in the spleen and the liver the disease was more extensive in the treated group. The increased severity of the disease in the spleen and the liver in the treated animals suggested to them that perhaps the usual resistance of these organs to tuberculosis is due in part to too low an oxygen tension for optimum growth of tubercle bacilli. Their work supports the in vitro finding of Novy and Soule (1925), that an oxygen concentration above 30 per cent impedes the growth of tubercle bacilli. Thus it would seem that the Po_2 in an organ may be a decisive factor in its resistance to a particular micro-organism.

In a recent investigation in goats, Kanan and Silver (1975) used microprobes to measure tissue oxygen tension and found an area of relative hypoxia in the mucosa of the anterior nasal septum and of the maxillo-and nasoturbinals, a few microns deep to the surface epithelium. It is too early to evaluate the significance of this finding as a factor in the survival and pathogenicity of micro-organisms which frequently localise in this area, but it adds further support to the concept that chronic stasis is a hallmark of this part of the nose. If this finding can be extrapolated to other animals including man, it may also explain the peculiar biological behaviour of the nasal mucosa towards blood-borne particulate matter (Kanan and Ryan, 1975).

THE NOSE AS AN EXPERIMENTAL MODEL

In this chapter the nasal mucosa has been shown to be a useful experimental model for the study of the pathogenesis and mode of localisation of granulomatous disease, vasculitis and other intravascular disorders. However, it is probable that other sites may develop similar behaviour and thus become affected by a persistent and recurrent vasculitis. Thus, when this occurs in the skin, as in nodular vasculitis of the lower leg, anatomical changes and the effect of stasis, cooling and factors such as endocrine status all become important contributors to the local constitution.

A constant theme in this monograph is the concept that vasculitis occurs when triggers settle at prepared sites. At all times the nose may be more nearly 'prepared' than many other tissues.

References

Agrawal, S., Sharma, K. D. & Shrivastava, J. B. (1959) Generalized rhinosporidiosis with visceral involvement. *Archives of Dermatology,* **80,** 22.
Albiston, H. E. & Gorrie, C. J. R. (1935) A preliminary note on bovine nasal granuloma in Victoria. *Australian Veterinary Journal,* **11,** 72.
Andrews, G. C. & Domonkos, A. N. (1963) In *Diseases of the Skin.* p. 277. Philadelphia, London: W. B. Saunders.
Ashburn, P. M. & Craig, C. F. (1907) Observation upon Treponema pertenuis Castellani of yaws and the experimental production of the disease in monkeys. *Philippine Journal of Science,* **441,** 465.
Astrup, T. & Albrechtsen, O. K. (1957) Estimation of the plasminogen activator and the trypsin inhibitor in animal and human tissues. *Scandinavian Journal of Clinical and Laboratory Investigation,* **9,** 233.
Binford, C. H. (1956) Comprehensive programme for inoculation of human leprosy into laboratory animals. *U.S. Public Service Report,* no. 71. p. 995.
Biswal, G. & Das, L. N. (1956) Observations on the treatment of nasal schistosomiasis in cattle and buffaloes in Orissa. *Indian Veterinary Journal,* **33,** 204.

Blood, D. C. & Henderson, J. A. (1963) In *Veterinary Medicine,* 2nd edition. London: Bailliere, Tindall & Cox.

Brand, P. W. (1959) Temperature variation and leprosy deformity. *International Journal of Leprosy,* **27,** 1.

Brandtzaeg, P., Fjellanger, I. & Gjeruldsen, S. T. (1967) Localisation of immunoglobulins in human nasal mucosa. *Immunochemistry,* **4,** 57.

Brödthagen, H., Larsen, V., Brockner, J. & Amris, C. J. (1968) Cutaneous manifestations in capillary dilatation and endovascular fibrin deposits. *Acta Dermato-venereologica,* **48,** 277.

Brown, W. H. & Pearce, L. (1920) Experimental syphilis in the rabbit. V. Syphilitic affections of the mucous membranes and the mucocutaneous borders. *Journal of Experimental Medicine,* **32,** 497.

Burton, J. L. & Burton, P. A. (1972) Pulmonary eosinophilia associated with vasculitis and extravascular granulomata. *British Journal of Dermatology,* **87,** 412.

Busquets, A. P. (1948) The methods of culture in the diagnosis of Mediterranean visceral leishmaniasis. *Medicina Clinica* (Barcelona), **11,** 110.

Caldwell, G. T. & Roberts, J. D. (1938) Rhinosporidiosis in the United States. *Journal of the American Medical Association,* **110,** 1641.

Cannon, P. R. & Walsh, T. E. (1937) Studies on the fate of living bacteria introduced into the upper respiratory tract of normal and intranasally vaccinated rabbits. *Journal of Immunology,* **32,** 49.

Cauna, N. (1970) Electron microscopy of the nasal vascular bed and its nerve supply. *Annals of Otology, Rhinology and Laryngology,* **3,** 443.

Cauna, N. & Hinderer, K. H. (1969) Fine structure of blood vessels of the human nasal respiratory mucosa. *Annals of Otology, Rhinology and Laryngology,* **78,** 865.

Chandler, P. J., Allison, M. J., Margolis, G. & Gerszten, E. (1965) The effects of intermittent hyperbaric oxygen therapy on the development of tuberculosis in the rabbit. *American Review of Respiratory Diseases,* **91,** 855.

Choudbury, B. (1955) Nasal granuloma in the state of West Bengal — studies on sixty-eight cases. *Indian Veterinary Journal,* **31,** 403.

Clark, B. M. (1968) The epidemiology of phycomycosis. In *Ciba Foundation Symposium on Systemic Mycosis* (Ed.) Wolstenholme, G. E. W. & Porter, R. p. 179. London: J. and A. Churchill.

Cochrane, R. G. (1959) In *Leprosy in Theory and Practice,* p. 171. Bristol: John Wright.

Cohen, P., Braunwald, J. & Gardner, F. H. (1965) Destruction of canine and rabbit platelets following intravenous administration of carbon particles or endotoxin. *Journal of Laboratory and Clinical Medicine,* **66,** 263.

Copeman, P. W. M. & Ryan, T. J. (1970) The problem of cutaneous angiitis with reference to histopathology and pathogenesis. *British Journal of Dermatology,* **82** (Supplement 5), 2.

Copeman, P. W. M. & Ryan, T. J. (1971) Cutaneous angiitis patterns of rashes explained by 1) flow properties of blood 2) anatomical disposition of vessels. *British Journal of Dermatology,* **85,** 205.

Crow, G. B. (1912) Acid-fast bacilli in the circulating blood of lepers. *United States Naval Medical Bulletin,* **6,** 25.

Dawes, J. D. K. & Prichard, M. M. L. (1953) Studies of the vascular arrangements of the nose. *Journal of Anatomy,* **87,** 311.

Degos, R. (1953) Lupus tuberculeux. In *Dermatologie. Collection Médico-chirurgicale à revision Annuelle.* Paris: Editions Médicales Flammarion.

Dharmendra, O. & Sen, N. R. (1948) Frequency of the presence of leprosy bacilli in nasal smears of leprosy patients. *Leprosy in India,* **20,** 180.

Doig, J. A., Whaley, K., Dick, W. C., Nuki, G., Williamson, J. & Buchanan, W. W. (1971) Otolaryngological aspects of Sjögren's syndrome. *British Medical Journal,* **iv,** 460.

Dowling, G. B. & Wetherley-Mein, G. (1954) In *Modern Trends in Dermatology* (Ed.) MacKenna, R. M. B. London: Butterworth.

Drutz, D. J., Chen, T. S. N. & Wen-Hsiang, L. (1972) The continuous bacteremia of lepromatous leprosy. *New England Journal of Medicine,* **287,** 159.

Edwards, Ph. Q. (1957) Histoplasmin testing in different geographic areas. *Lancet,* **ii,** 707.

Eggston, A. A. & Wolff, D. (1947) In *Histopathology of Ear, Nose and Throat.* Baltimore: Williams & Wilkins.

Fialho, A. (1960) In *Ergebnisse der allgemeinen Pathologie und pathologischen Anatomie* (Ed.) Gohrs, P., Giese, W. & Meessen, H. Berlin: Springer-Verlag.

Forchammer, H. (1911) "Bekampfung der Tuberculose". Proceedings of the Sittings of the Lupus Congress of the German Central Committee, Berlin, April 21. *British Journal of Dermatology,* **23,** 338 (abstract).

Fordyce, J. A. & Arnold, W. F. (1906) A case of undetermined tropical ulceration involving the nose, pharynx and larynx with histological findings and some general considerations regarding clinically similar cases in Oceania and elsewhere. *Journal of Cutaneous Diseases including Syphilis,* **24,** 1.

French, J. E. (1967) Blood platelets: Morphological studies on their properties and life cycle. *British Journal of Haematology,* **13,** 595.

Friedman, L. (1955) The pathology of malignant granuloma in the nose. *Journal of Laryngology and Otology,* **69,** 331.

Furtado, T. (1973) Some problems of late yaws. *International Journal of Dermatology*, **12**, 123.
Godman, G. & Churg, J. (1954) Wegener's granulomatosis: pathology and review of the literature. *Archives of Pathology*, **58**, 533.
Grouven, C. (1907) Ueber positive syphilisimpfung am Kaninchenauge. *Medizinische Klinik* (Berlin), **3**, 774.
Grouven, C. (1908) Ueber Klinish erkenn bare Allgemeinsyphilis beim Kaninchen. *Dermatologische Zeitschrift*, **15**, 209.
Grouven, C. (1910) Experimentelles zur Kaninchen-syphilis. *Dermatologische Zeitschrift*, **17**, 161.
Guitierrez, P. D. (1925) Late or tertiary manifestations of yaws. *Archives of Dermatology and Syphilology*, **12**, 465.
Harman, R. R. M. (1972) In *Textbook of Dermatology* (Ed.) Rook, A., Wilkinson, D. S. & Ebling, F. J. G. Oxford: Blackwell.
Haxthausen, H. (1930) In *Cold in Relation to Skin Diseases*. Copenhagen: Levin and Munksgaard.
Hollman, H. T. (1916) B. leprae in the circulating blood of lepers. *Public Health Bulletin*, **75**, 15.
Honeij, J. A. (1915) Leprosy — the presence of acid-fast bacilli in the circulating blood and excretions. *Journal of Infectious Diseases*, **17**, 376.
Hore, D. E. (1966) Nasal granuloma in Victorian dairy cattle. *Australian Veterinary Journal*, **42**, 273.
Horwitz, O. (1959) Localisation and pathogenesis of lupus vulgaris. *Acta Tuberculosa Scandinavica*, Supplement **47**, 175.
Horwitz, O. (1966) In *Applied Epidemiology. I. Epidemiology and Natural History of Lupus Vulgaris in Denmark, 1895-1954*. Copenhagen: The Danish Tuberculosis Index.
Hudson, E. H. (1936) Bejel: non-venereal syphilis. *Archives of Dermatology and Syphilology*, **33**, 994.
Hudson, E. H. (1958) In *Non-Venereal Syphilis. A Sociological and Medical Study of Bejel*. Edinburgh, London: E. & S. Livingstone.
Jensen, H., Chamovitz, D. L., Volkringer, E., Gray, E., James, B. A., Gosney, J. E. & Kocholaty, W. (1953) Antifibrinolytic activity in plasma after exposure to cold and after chymotrypsin administration. *Blood*, **8**, 324.
Jerushalmy, Z. & Zucker, M. B. (1965) Some effects of fibrinogen degradation (FDP) on blood platelets. *Thrombosis et Diathesis Haemorrhagica*, **15**, 413.
Job, C. K., Karat, A. B. A. & Karat, S. (1966) The histopathological appearance of leprous rhinitis and pathogenesis of septal perforation in leprosy. *Journal of Laryngology and Otology*, **80**, 718.
Kahn, R. L. (1936) In *Tissue Immunity*. Springfield: Charles C. Thomas.
Kahn, R. L. (1954) Tissue immunity — Its possible relationship to midline facial granulomatous ulceration. *University of Michigan Medical Bulletin*, **20**, 208.
Kanan, M. W. (1975) Mucocutaneous leishmaniasis in guinea-pigs inoculated intravenously with Leishmania enriettii. *British Journal of Dermatology*, **92**, 663.
Kanan, M. W. & Ryan, T. J. (1975) Endonasal localisation of blood borne viable and non-viable particulate matter. *British Journal of Dermatology*, **92**, 475.
Kanan, M. W. & Silver, I. A. (1975) Oxygen tension and surface temperature of the endonasal tissues in the goat. *Journal of Laryngology and Otology*, in press.
Kanan, M. W., Abbas, M. & Girgis, H. Y. (1971) Late mutilating bejel in the nomadic Bedouins of Kuwait. *Dermatologica*, **143**, 277.
Kanan, M. W., Ryan, T. J. & Weddell, A. G. M. (1975) The behaviour of the nasal mucosa and other tissues toward blood borne colloidal carbon in experimental animals. *Pathologia Europaea*, **10**, 263.
Karunaratne, W. A. E. (1936) The pathology of rhinosporidiosis. *Journal of Pathology and Bacteriology*, **42**, 193.
Kerdel-Vegas, F., Convit, J., Gordon, B. & Goihman, M. (1963) In *Rhinoscleroma*. Springfield, Illinois: Charles C. Thomas.
Kowalski, E., Kopec, M., Wegrzynowicz, Z., Hurwic, M. & Budzynski, A. Z. (1964) Influence of fibrinogen degradation products (FDP) on platelet aggregation, adhesiveness and viscous metamorphosis. *Thrombosis et Diathesis Haemorrhagica*, **10**, 406.
Kwaan, H. C. & McFadzean, A. J. S. (1956) On plasma fibrinolytic activity induced by ischaemia. *Clinical Science*, **15**, 245.
Lai A. Fat, R. F. M., Cormane, R. H. & Van Furth, R. (1974) An immunohistopathological study on the synthesis of immunoglobulins in normal and pathological skin and in adjacent mucous membranes. *British Journal of Dermatology*, **90**, 123.
Larrieu, M. J., Inceman, S. & Marder, V. (1967) Action of fibrinogen degradation products on platelet function. *Nouvelle Revue Francaise d'Hématologie*, **7**, 691.
Leites, B. G. & Benenson, Z. S. (1949) Perforation of the nasal septum in severe forms of rheumatism in children (7 case reports). *Pediatria*, **3**, 60.
Linton, C. S. (1933) Resistance of the upper respiratory mucosa to infection. *Annals of Otology*, **42**, 64.
Lomholt, G. (1968) In *Textbook of Dermatology* (Ed.) Rook, A., Wilkinson, D. S. & Ebling, F. J. G. p. 682. Oxford, Edinburgh: Blackwell.
Majno, G. (1965) Ultrastructure of the vascular membrane. In *Handbook of Physiology* (Ed.) Hamilton, W. F. & Dow, P. Sec. 2, **3**, 2375. Washington D.C.: American Physiological Society.

McDougall, A. C., Rees, R. J. W., Weddell, A. G. M. & Kanan, M. W. (1975) The histopathology of lepromatous leprosy in the nose. *Journal of Pathology*, **115**, 215.

McGilvray, C. D. (1944) The transmission of glanders from horse to man. *Journal of the American Veterinary Association*, **104**, 255.

McMahon, B. J. (1933) The spread and phagocytosis of particulate matter in nasal mucous membrane of the rabbit. *Annals of Otology*, **42**, 660.

Miller, H. E., Keddie, F., Johnstone, H. G. & Bustick, W. L. (1947) Histoplasmosis: cutaneous and muco-membranous lesions, mycologic and pathologic observations. *Archives of Dermatology and Syphilology*, **56**, 715.

Mills, C. P. (1965) Wegener's granulomatosis. *British Journal of Dermatology*, **77**, 203.

Mink, O. J. & McLean, N. T. (1906) Gangosa. *Journal of the American Medical Association*, **47**, 1166.

Moasabhoy, H. & Seeler, R. A. (1974) Nasal-septum perforation in systemic lupus erythematosus. *New England Journal of Medicine*, **291**, 51.

Muniz, J. & Medina, H. (1948) Leishmaniose tegumentar do cobaio (leishmania enriettii). *'O Hospital'* (Rio de Janeiro), **33**, 7.

Nichols, H. J. (1914) Observations on a strain of spirochaeta pallida, isolated from the nervous system. *Journal of Experimental Medicine*, **19**, 362.

Novy, F. G. & Soule, M. H. (1925) Microtic respiration. II. Respiration of the tubercle bacillus. *Journal of Infectious Diseases*, **36**, 168.

Olsen, R. E. (1958) In *Non-Venereal Syphilis. A Sociological and Medical Study of Bejel* (Ed.) Hudson, E. H. Chapter 17. Edinburgh, London: E. & S. Livingstone.

Padilha-Gonclaves, A. (1969) In *Essays on Tropical Dermatology* (Ed.) Simons, R. D. G. Ph. & Marshall, J. Vol. 1. p. 261. Amsterdam: Excerpta Medica Foundation.

Paraense, W. L. (1952) Infection of the nasal mucosa in guinea-pig leishmaniasis. *Annals da Academia Brasiléira de Ciéncias*, **24**, 307.

Paraense, W. L. (1953) The spread of Leishmania enriettii through the body of the guinea-pig. *Transactions of the Royal Society of Tropical Medicine and Hygiene*, **47**, 556.

Pierini, L. E. (1969) In *Essays on Tropical Dermatology* (Ed.) Simons, R. D. G. Ph. & Marshall, J. Vol. 1. p. 175.

Polak, L., Frey, J. R. & Turk, J. L. (1970) Studies on the effect of systemic administration of sensitisers to guinea-pigs with contact sensitivity to inorganic metal compounds. V. Studies on the mechanism of the "flare-up" reaction. *Clinical and Experimental Immunology*, **7**, 739.

Prabhu, M. N. (1946) Leprosy of the upper respiratory passages. *Leprosy in India*, **18**, 10.

Purtilo, D. T., Walsh, G. P., Storrs, E. E. & Banks, I. S. (1974) Impact of cool temperatures on transformation of human and armadillo lymphocytes (Dasypus novemcinctus, Linn.) as related to leprosy. *Nature*, **248**, 450.

Rajam, R. V., Viswanathan, G. S., Rao, A. R., Rangiah, P. N. & Anguli, V. C. (1955) Rhinosporidiosis — a study with report of a fatal case of systemic dissemination. *Indian Journal of Surgery*, **17**, 269.

Reasoner, M. A. (1916) Some phases of experimental syphilis with special reference to the question of strains. *Journal of the American Medical Association*, **67**, 1799.

Rees, R. J. W. (1966) Enhanced susceptibility of thymectomized and irradiated mice to infection with Mycobacterium leprae. *Nature* (London), **211**, 657.

Rees, R. J. W., McDougall, A. C. & Weddell, A. G. M. (1974) The nose in mice with experimental human leprosy. *Leprosy Review*, **45**, 112.

Rhodes-Jones, R. (1963) An investigation into bacillaemia in leprosy. *Leprosy Review*, **34**, 26.

Rivas, D. (1912) Bacteremic nature of leprosy. *Journal of the American Medical Association*, **59**, 298.

Robinson, V. B. (1951) Nasal granuloma — A report of two cases in cattle. *American Journal of Veterinary Research*, **12**, 85.

Roccuzzo, M. & Lomeo, G. (1950) The presence of leishman bodies in the mucosa and nasal mucosa of children suffering from internal leishmaniasis. *Bollettino de Societa Italiana di Biologia Sperimentale*, **26**, 353.

Rothfield, N. F. (1974) Nasal-septum perforation in systemic lupus erythematosus. *New England Journal of Medicine*, **291**, 51.

Ryan, T. J. (1973) In *The Physiology and Physiopathology of the Skin* (Ed.) Jarrett, A. Vol. 1. London, New York: Academic Press.

Salvidio, E. & Crosby, W. H. (1960) Thrombocytopenia after intravenous injection of India ink. *Journal of Laboratory and Clinical Medicine*, **56**, 711.

Samuel, D. R., Godal, T., Myrang, B. & Song, Y. K. (1973) Behaviour of mycobacterium leprae in human macrophages in vitro. *Infection and Immunology*, **8**, 446.

Saunders, L. Z. (1948) Systemic fungus infections in animals: a review. *Cornell Veterinarian*, **38**, 213.

Schöbel, O. (1928) Experimental yaws in Philippine monkeys and a critical consideration of our knowledge concerning framboesia tropica in the light of recent experimental evidence. *Philippine Journal of Science*, **35**, 209.

Sequeira, J. H., Ingram, J. T. & Brain, R. T. (1947) In *Diseases of the Skin*. London: J. & A. Churchill Ltd.

Shepard, C. C. (1965) Temperature optimum for Mycobacterium leprae in mice. *Journal of Bacteriology,* **96,** 1271.

Shillitoe, E. J., Lehner, T., Lessof, M. & Harrison, D. F. N. (1974) Wegener's granulomatosis. *Lancet,* **i,** 805.

Simpson, J. B. (1974) Nasal septum perforation in systemic lupus erythematosus. *New England Journal of Medicine,* **290,** 859.

Snyder, G. G. III, McCarthy, K. E. & Toomey, J. M. (1974) Nasal septal perforation in systemic lupus erythematosus. *Archives of Otolaryngology,* **99,** 456.

Stehbens, W. E. & Florey, H. W. (1960) The behaviour of intravenously injected particles in chambers in rabbits' ears. *Quarterly Journal of Experimental Physiology,* **45,** 252.

Sticker, G. (1897) Mittheilungen über lepra nach erfahrungen in Indian und Aegypten. *Munchener Medizinische Wochenschrift,* **44,** 39.

Stokes, J. H. (1943) In *Modern Clinical Syphilology.* Philadelphia, London: W. B. Saunders.

Strom, J. (1965) Ectodermosis erosiva pluriorificialis, Stevens—Johnson's syndrome and other febrile mucocutaneous reactions and Behçet's syndrome in cold agglutination-positive infections. *Lancet,* **i,** 457.

Sullivan, W. A. (1964) Syphilitic gumma misdiagnosed midline granuloma. *Archives of Internal Medicine,* **114,** 336.

Tagnon, H. J., Levenson, S. M., Davidson, C. S. & Taylor, F. H. L. (1946) The occurrence of fibrinolysis in shock, with observations on the prothrombin time and the plasma fibrinogen during haemorrhagic shock. *American Journal of the Medical Sciences,* **211,** 88.

Tait, J. & Elvidge, A. R. (1926) Effect upon platelets and on blood coagulation of injecting foreign particles into the bloodstream. *Journal of Physiology,* **62,** 129.

Tio, T. H., Moeljono, D. & Njo-Injo, T. E. (1966) Subcutaneous phycomycosis. *Archives of Dermatology,* **93,** 550.

Todd, A. S. (1964) Localisation of fibrinolytic activity in tissues. *British Medical Bulletin,* **20,** 210.

Turner, T. B. & Hollander, D. H. (1957) *The Biology of the Treponematoses.* WHO Monograph Series No. 35. Geneva: World Health Organization.

Uhlenhuth, P. & Mulzer, P. (1910) Allgemein-syphilis bei Kaninchen und Affen nach intravenoser Impfung. *Arbeiterversicherung Klinik Gesundhtsamte* (Berlin), **34,** 222.

Vachtenheim, J. & Grossmann, J. (1969) Perforation of the nasal septum in systemic lupus erythematosus. *British Medical Journal,* **ii,** 5649.

Van Aken, W. G. & Vreeken, J. (1969) Accumulation of macromolecular particles in the reticuloendothelial system (RES) mediated by platelet aggregation and disaggregation. *Thrombosis et Diathesis Haemorrhagica,* **22,** 496.

Van Aken, W. G., Goote, Th. M. & Vreeken, J. (1968) Platelet aggregation. An intermediary mechanism in carbon clearance. *Scandinavian Journal of Haematology,* **5,** 333.

Von Lichtenberg, F. (1962) Host response to eggs of S. mansoni. I. Granuloma formation in the unsensitized laboratory mouse. *American Journal of Pathology,* **41,** 711.

Walton, E. W. (1958) Giant cell granuloma of the respiratory tract (Wegener's granulomatosis). *British Medical Journal,* **ii,** 265.

Wayoff, M. (1960) Endonasal localisation of Besnier—Boeck—Schaumann disease. *Revue de Médecine* (Nancy), **85,** 745.

Wegener, F. (1936) Uber ganeralasierte, septische Gefasserkrankungen. *Verhandlungen der Deutschen Gesellschaft für Pathologie,* **29,** 202.

Williams, H. L. (1949) Lethal granulomatous ulceration involving the midline facial tissues. *Annals of Otology, Rhinology and Laryngology,* **58,** 1013.

Winkelmann, R. K. & Ditto, W. B. (1964) Cutaneous and visceral syndromes of necrotising or allergic angiitis. A study of 38 cases. *Medicine* (Baltimore), **43,** 59.

Wise, H. S. (1954) Genesis of nasal perforation in lepromatous leprosy; its prevention and care. *Archives of Otology,* **59,** 306.

10. Coagulation and Fibrinolysis

In an article entitled 'Vessel wall and thrombogenesis — Endotoxin', McKay (1973) wrote of a reaction that "is a definitive disease process which is the result of two minor episodes of acute inflammation of the circulating blood. The identifying feature of this reaction is thrombosis of the microcirculation . . ." He suggested that antigen—antibody complexes, endotoxin and particulate matter all acted similarly in this reaction and that the eventual thrombosis was the result of interplay between clotting and fibrinolytic mechanisms, leucocytes, complement, platelets, adrenal glucocorticoids, adrenal catecholamines and alpha adrenergic mechanisms (Figure 10.1). A primary event is fibrin deposition but this is initially balanced by fibrinolysis and by the removal of many of the components of the coagulation cascade by the reticuloendothelial system (known also as the mononuclear phagocytic system). Should a further insult to the vessel occur, the fibrinolytic enzymes may still be depleted and the reticuloendothelial system overloaded. Heavy deposits of fibrin entwined with platelets and leucocytes complete the block of the vessel which is, at the same time, partly in spasm as a result of alpha adrenergic and corticosteroid activity.

Vasculitis comprises all of the above, and the fact that McKay was describing the Shwartzman phenomenon should not prejudice this view. It is sometimes said that the Shwartzman phenomenon is not seen in man and that Shwartzman's original experiments have not been conducted in man. Nevertheless, the mechanisms underlying Shwartzman's experiments are now well understood (see page 252), and certainly each can be demonstrated in man. Furthermore all of them have been demonstrated in vasculitis.

References

McKay. D. G. (1973) Vessel wall and thrombogenesis — endotoxin. *Thrombosis et Diathesis Haemorrhagica,* **29**, 11.

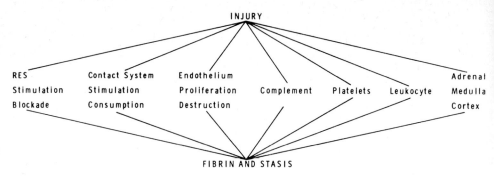

Figure 10.1. Diagram showing the interplay of various factors which, following injury, result in coagulation.

FIBRIN: ITS DEMONSTRATION IN VASCULITIS

Fibrin is a common component of vasculitis (Figures 10.2 and 10.3), and is a major constituent of fibrinoid. It stains red with eosin, reddish brown with the coupled tetrazonium reaction after heating and benzylation, and blue with Mallory's phospho-tungstic acid—haematoxylin. These are features, but not proof, of fibrin (Pearse, 1960). Gitlin et al (1957) studying such diseases as polyarteritis nodosa, lupus erythematosus and rheumatic nodules, concluded that fibrin, shown up by a fluorescent antibody method, was present in significant amounts in the injured vessel wall. Ruiter (1962), studying cutaneous vasculitis using several different stains, was led to believe that fibrinoid represents the minimum lesion and that collagen fibres are split up and coated with fibrin in this disease. He described a solid form of fibrin similar to that seen in thrombi, and an amorphous form which more readily coats the collagen fibres. One of the main difficulties is that conventional stains for fibrin fail to show up quite large fragments produced by lysis which may have pathological significance. There are, for instance, permeability and chemotactic factors extractable from lymph nodes, liver (Willoughby and Spector, 1964a, b) and skin (Inderbitzin, 1964; Inderbitzin, Keel and Blumenthal, 1966) which cause massive deposits of a material resembling fibrin yet have no affinity for fibrin stains.

Conversion of fibrinogen into soluble fibrin by thrombin is not the only mechanism by which a clot can be formed. Some forms of partially degraded fibrinogen, altered by both fibrinolysis and coagulation, can be shown by electron microscopy to be similar to fibrin (Horn, Hawiger and Collins, 1969). Electron microscopy of vasculitis (Ruiter and Molenaar, 1970) and of malignant hypertension (Ashton, 1972) has revealed fibrin in the lumen, between endothelial cells as well as in the vessel wall and surrounding tissues.

Important contributions to the acceptance of the role of fibrin in vasculitis have come from experiments by Vassalli, Simon and Rouiller (1963) in which the use of immuno-fluorescent stains confirmed that fibrinogen and fibrin, or its degradation products, were early features of vasculitis and contributed to renal damage. Later, McKay, Gitlin and Graig (1959) and McKay, Margaretten and Csavossy (1966), made use of both fluorescein-labelled antibodies to fibrinogen and electron microscopy, and found evidence that the occlusive deposits in the Shwartzman phenomenon are due to fibrin. Subsequently Scott (1968), using trypan blue and electron microscopy to study the generalised Shwartzman reaction suggested that fibrinoid is composed of modified fibrin impregnating collagen, and a derivative of fibrinogen and fibrin, which need not have the characteristic transverse banding that is sometimes used as the sole criterion for fibrin. This amorphous material is commonly observed in vasculitis and in conditions like thrombotic thrombocytopenic purpura (Feldman et al, 1966).

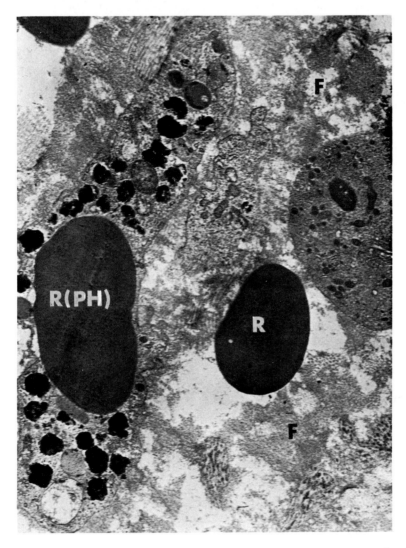

Figure 10.2. Necrotising angiitis of the skin. Fibrin (F) is a prominent feature. Red cells are both free-lying (R) and phagocytosed R (PH). $\times$ 12 000.

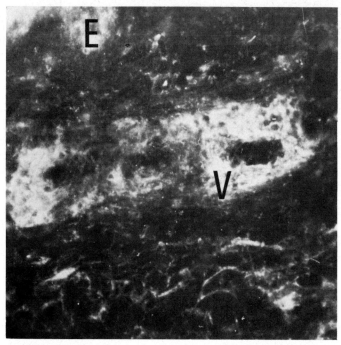

Figure 10.3. Vasculitis of the skin in which immunofluorescence for fibrin shows heavy staining in a small venule (V) lying close to the epidermis (E).

References

Ashton, N. (1972) The eye in malignant hypertension. *Transactions of the American Academy of Ophthalmology and Otolaryngology,* **76,** 17.

Feldman, J. D., Mardiney, M. R., Unanue, E. R. & Cutting, H. (1966) The vascular pathology of thrombotic thrombocytopenic purpura. *Laboratory Investigation,* **15,** 927.

Gitlin, D., Craig, J. M. & Janeway, C. A. (1957) Studies on the nature of fibrinoid in the collagen diseases. *American Journal of Pathology,* **33,** 55.

Horn, R. G., Hawiger, J. & Collins, R. D. (1969) Electron microscopy of fibrin-like precipitate formed during the paracoagulation reaction between soluble fibrin monomer complexes and protamine sulphate. *British Journal of Haematology,* **17,** 463.

Inderbitzin, T. (1964) Studies on the permeability increasing factors (PIF). *International Archives of Allergy and Applied Immunology,* **24,** 332.

Inderbitzin, T., Keel, A. & Blumental, G. (1966) The identity of the permeability factors from lymph node cells (LNPF) with the permeability increasing factors (PIF). *International Archives of Allergy and Applied Immunology,* **29,** 417.

McKay, D. G., Gitlin, D. & Graig, J. M. (1959) Immune-chemical demonstration of fibrin in the generalised Shwartzman reaction. *Archives of Pathology,* **67,** 270.

McKay, D. G., Margaretten, W. & Csavossy, I. (1966) An electron-microscope study of the effect of bacterial endotoxin on the blood vascular system. *Laboratory Investigation,* **16,** 511.

Pearse, A. G. E. (1960) *Histochemistry.* London: J. & A. Churchill Ltd.

Ruiter, M. (1962) Vascular fibrinoid in cutaneous "allergic" arteriolitis. *British Journal of Dermatology,* **38,** 85.

Ruiter, M. & Molenaar, J. (1970) Ultrastructural changes in arteriolitis. *British Journal of Dermatology,* **83,** 14.

Scott, G. B. D. (1968) Trypan blue and the generalised Shwartzman reaction. The nature and formation of fibrinoid material in the pulmonary arteries. *British Journal of Experimental Pathology,* **49, 251.**

Vassalli, P., Simon, G. & Rouiller, C. (1963) Electron microscopic study of glomerular lesion resulting from intravascular fibrin formation. *American Journal of Pathology,* **43,** 579.

Willoughby, D. A. & Spector, W. G. (1964a) The lymph node permeability factor: A possible mediator of the delayed hypersensitivity reaction. *Annals of the New York Academy of Sciences,* **116,** 874.

Willoughby, D. A. & Spector, W. G. (1964b) The production of eosinophilic deposits resembling fibrinoid by injection of lymph node extracts. *Journal of Pathology and Bacteriology,* **88,** 557.

FIBRIN: ITS CONSEQUENCES

The presence of fibrinoid means that both clotting and fibrinolysis are active within and without the vessel. It represents a dynamic and continuous process, not an irreversible one, for although it is a considerable stimulus to new collagen deposition (Triantaphyllopoulos and Triantaphyllopoulos, 1969; Niewiarowski, 1973) and may progress to scarring, it may be cleared within a few weeks in malignant hypertension (Pickering, 1971).

Emphasis on the role of fibrin in coagulation and haemostasis may have diverted attention from its effect on tissue growth and repair. However, as long ago as 1908 Nolf postulated that its presence between cells affects their nutrition. Fibrinogen diffuses freely through the tissues and there is no shortage of clotting agents for its conversion into fibrin. More recently Astrup (1966) and many other workers have described it as a scaffold upon which much cellular activity can take place, while others have regarded it as a lattice-work through which cells can climb and have emphasised this aspect in neoplasia (O'Meara and Thornes, 1961), in wound healing (Figure 10.4) and in

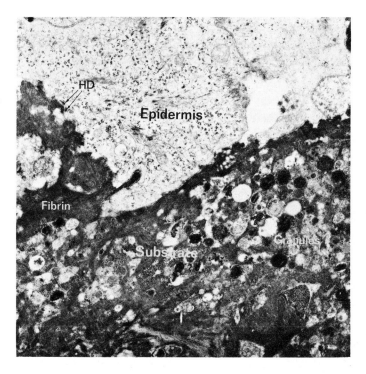

Figure 10.4. Fibrin is a scaffold for epithelial growth. A small wound of the skin of the human forearm is illustrated in which there is migration of the epidermis over a substrate of fibrin. Most of the dark fibrillar material is fibrin. Hemidesmosomes (HD) are visible. Clearance of the fibrin is dependent on macrophages at sites such as epidermal wounds where fibrinolysis is inhibited.

experimental epidermal growth (Nishioka and Ryan, 1971). The phagocytosis and lysis of fibrin by neoplastic cells (Back et al, 1966), the effect of fibrinolysis on the spread of cancer (Clifton, 1966), and the influence of coagulation processes on cancer in general (O'Meara and Thornes, 1961) have all been the subject of study and speculation.

Perhaps more relevant to the subject of vasculitis have been studies by rheumatologists on the inflammatory role of fibrin. Glynn (1963), Riddle, Bluhm and Barnhart (1965), Bluhm, Riddle and Barnhart (1966) and Barnhart et al (1968), for example, were impressed by the ill effects of fibrin in inflamed joints, while the attraction of white cells to fibrin was studied by Curran and Clark (1964), Hurley (1964) and, amongst others, Nishioka and Ryan (1971) who used millipore filters in the hamster cheek pouch chamber. Barnhart (1965) considered that fibrin was often both attractive to and of necessity cleared by neutrophils. Several authors have considered that fibrin is an enhancer of phagocytosis by coating otherwise indigestible material (Knisely, Bloch and Warner, 1948; Bloch and Coyas, 1964; Curran and Clark, 1964; Vassalli and McCluskey, 1964). In inflammatory events fibrin is found where the type of injury and the cellular necrosis are more intense (Wilhelm, 1971); it is not induced by a specific type of injury. Its effect is to prolong the inflammatory response (Ryan, Nishioka and Dawber, 1971) and, by virtue of vessel block, to prevent replenishment of local demands for nutriment as well as for inhibitors and activators of biochemical processes and blood-borne cells.

Fibrin degradation products and incompletely polymerised fibrinogen may not only account for incomplete amorphous materials in fibrinoid but also be of greater significance because they are chemotactic (Barnhart, 1968) and promote permeability (Copley et al, 1966). Furthermore, fibrin degradation products potentiate the action of several mediators of inflammation, at least in vitro (Malofiejew, 1972). Ryan, Nishioka and Dawber (1971) have therefore suggested that fibrin is an intrinsic part of delayed or prolonged inflammation, and thereby, at least from observations on the skin, makes a significant contribution to diseases of that tissue.

Currently there is much interest in the demonstration of fibrin in a number of diseases of the skin: dermatitis herpetiformis (Jakubowicz, Dabrowski and Maciejewski, 1971), psoriasis, lichen planus (Salo et al, 1972) and lupus erythematosus (Salo, Tallberg and Mustakallio, 1972). The question is asked whether it is a cause or effect. The same question is also asked about its role in other disease processes such as glomerulonephritis (see Chapter 7). The answer must be that fibrin can contribute to pathology for all the reasons stated above and that it matters little at what stage it appears in the pathogenic sequence. If it is present it will act as a pathogen even if at the same time it is encouraging or initiating the processes of repair or contributing to haemostasis.

While polymerisation of fibrinogen to fibrin is taking place, the polymer is adhesive and attractive to a variety of cells including fibroblasts and platelets (Niewiarowski, 1973), but once transformation to fibrin is complete these cells are no longer affected. Polymer when mixed with platelets is contractile, and its contraction is thought to allow orientation of the fibres and may be important in wound healing. Fully formed fibrin is cross-linked in the presence of fibrin stabilising factor. Contractility is inhibited by prostaglandin E_1, and once stabilised, fibrin is less resistant to proteolytic enzymes and is less contractile. It is of interest that the collagen contained in highly purified insoluble bovine tendon enhances fibrinolysis (Engel and Alexander, 1973) and may prevent excessive fibrin deposition and hence excessive fibroblast activity.

Anticoagulants inhibit classic skin hypersensitivity to tuberculin (Nelson, 1965) and allergic contact dermatitis (Cohen et al, 1967). Their action in the latter may depend in part on the substantial amounts of fibrin-like material that accumulate in the dermis in allergic contact dermatitis (Colvin et al, 1973); they are found, in fact, in a predominantly intervascular distribution, seemingly sparing the vessels themselves (Colvin et al, 1973). Both lymphocytes (Maillard, Pick and Turk, 1972) and macrophages (Unkeless, Gordon and Reich, 1974) release an activator of plasminogen when they are antigenically stimulated, demonstrating the interrelation of cell-mediated immunity and coagulation factors.

References

Astrup, T. (1966) Tissue activators of plasminogen. *Federation Proceedings,* **25,** 42.

Back, N., Shields, R. R., De Witt, G., Branshaw, R. H. & Ambrus, C. M. (1966) Uptake of fibrinogen and fibrinolytic enzymes by neoplastic tissue. *Journal of the National Cancer Institute,* **36,** 171.

Barnhart, M. I. (1965) Importance of neutrophilic leukocytes in the resolution of fibrin. *Federation Proceedings,* **24,** 846.

Barnhart, M. I. (1968) Role of blood coagulation in acute inflammation. *Biochemical Pharmacology,* Supplement **229.**

Barnhart, M. I., Riddle, J. M., Bluhm, G. B. & Quintana, C. (1968) Fibrin promotion and lysis in arthritic joints. *Annals of the Rheumatic Diseases,* **26,** 206.

Beevers, D. G. (1972) Cutaneous lesions in multiple myeloma. *British Medical Journal,* **iv,** 275.

Bloch, E. H. & Coyas, S. I. (1964) The transit of large molecules and particulate matter across individual endothelial cells analysed in living animals with television microphotometry. *Angiology,* **15,** 353.

Bluhm, G. B., Riddle, J. M. & Barnhart, M. I. (1966) Significance of fibrin and other particles in rheumatoid joint inflammation. *Henry Ford Hospital Medical Bulletin,* **14,** 119.

Carrington, C. B. & Liebow, A. A. (1968) Limited forms of angiitis and granulomatosis of Wegener's type. *American Journal of Medicine,* **41,** 497.

Clifton, E. E. (1966) Effect of fibrinolysis on spread of cancer. *Federation Proceedings,* **25,** 89.

Cochrane, C. G., Weigle, W. O. & Dixon, F. J. (1959) The role of polymorphonuclèar leukocytes in the induction and cessation of the Arthus vasculitis. *Journal of Experimental Medicine,* **110,** 480.

Cohen, S., Benacerraf, B., McCluskey, R. T. & Ovary, Z. (1967) Effect of anticoagulants on delayed hypersensitivity reactions. *Journal of Immunology,* **98,** 351.

Colvin, R. B., Johnson, R. A., Mihm, M. C. Jr & Dvorak, H. F. (1973) Role of the clotting system in cell mediated hypersensitivity. 1) Fibrin deposition in delayed skin reactions in man. *Journal of Experimental Medicine,* **138,** 686.

Copley, A. L., Hanig, J. P., Luchini, B. W. & Allen, R. L. Jr (1966) Capillary permeability enhancing action of fibrinopeptides isolated during fibrin monomer formation. *Federation Proceedings,* **25,** 446.

Curran, R. S. & Clark, A. E. (1964) Phagocytosis and fibrinogenesis in peritoneal implants in the rat. *Journal of Pathology and Bacteriology,* **88,** 489.

Engel, A. M. & Alexander, B. (1973) Effects of collagen on fibrinolysis. *Thrombosis et Diathesis Haemorrhagica,* Supplement **56,** 63.

Glynn, L. E. (1963) Symposium on inflammation and role of fibrin in the rheumatic diseases. *Bulletin of Rheumatic Diseases,* **14,** 323.

Hurley, J. V. (1964) Substances promoting leukocyte emigration. *Annals of the New York Academy of Sciences,* **116,** 918.

Jakubowicz, K., Dabrowski, J. & Maciejewski, W. (1971) Deposition of fibrin like material in early lesions of dermatitis herpetiformis. *Annals of Clinical Research,* **3,** 34.

Knisely, M. H., Bloch, E. H. & Warner, L. (1948) Selective phagocytosis. *Gelskab Biologiske Skrifter,* **4,** 1.

Kulaga, V. V., Talovskaya, Zh. S. & Suponitsky, V. Ya. (1971) The study of morphology of mast cells in allergic vasculitis of the skin. *Vestnik Dermatologii i Venerologii,* **45,** 26.

Maillard, J. L., Pick, E. & Turk, J. L. (1972) Interaction between "sensitised" lymphocytes and antigen in vitro. V. Vascular permeability induced by skin reactive factor. *International Archives of Allergy,* **42,** 50.

Malofiejew, M. (1972) The biological and pharmacological properties of some fibrinogen degradation products. *Scandinavian Journal of Haematology,* Supplement **13,** 303.

Nelson, D. S. (1965) The effects of anticoagulants and other drugs on cellular and cutaneous reactions of antigen in guinea pigs with delayed type hypersensitivity. *Immunology,* **9,** 219.

Niewiarowski, S. (1973) Interaction of fibrin with various cells. *Thrombosis et Diathesis Haemorrhagica,* **56,** 51.

Nishioka, K. & Ryan, T. J. (1971) Inhibitors and proactivators of fibrinolysis in human epidermis. *British Journal of Dermatology,* **85,** 561.

Nolf, P. (1908) Contribution à l'étude de la coagulation du sang, la fibrinolyse. *Archives Internationales de Physiologie et de Biochemie,* **6,** 306.

O'Meara, R. A. Q. & Thornes, R. D. (1961) Some properties of the cancer coagulative factor. *Irish Journal of Medical Science,* **423,** 106.

Pickering, G. W. (1971) Reversibility of malignant hypertension. *Lancet,* **i,** 413.

Riddle, J. M., Bluhm, G. B. & Barnhart, M. I. (1965) Inter-relationship between fibrin, neutrophils and rheumatoid synovitis. *Journal of the Reticulo-Endothelial Society,* **2,** 420.

Ryan, T. J., Nishioka, K. & Dawber, R. P. R. (1971) Epithelial—endothelial interactions in the control of inflammation through fibrinolysis. *British Journal of Dermatology,* **84,** 501.

Salo, O. P., Tallberg, Th. & Mustakallio, K. K. (1972) Demonstration of fibrin in skin diseases. I. Lichen ruber planus and lupus erythematosus. *Acta Dermato-venereologica,* **52,** 291.

Salo, O. P., Kousa, M., Mustakallio, K. K. & Lassus, A. (1972) Demonstration of fibrin in skin diseases. II. Psoriasis. *Acta Dermato-venereologica,* **52,** 295.

Triantaphyllopoulos, D. C. & Triantaphyllopoulos, E. (1969) Fibrin deposition and growth of connective tissue. *Thrombosis et Diathesis Haemorrhagica,* **21,** 144.
Unkeless, J. C., Gordon, S. & Reich, E. (1974) Secretion of plasminogen activator by stimulated macrophages. *Journal of Experimental Medicine,* **139,** 834.
Vassalli, P. & McCluskey, R. T. (1964) Pathogenic role of fibrin deposition in immunologically induced glomerulonephritis. *Annals of the New York Academy of Sciences,* **116,** 1052.
Wilhelm, D. L. (1971) Increased vascular permeability in acute inflammation. *Revue Canadienne de Biologie,* **30,** 153.

Intravascular coagulation and thrombosis in various diseases

The resolution of the current argument about the role of intravascular coagulation in various diseases already depends on points of view: whether one believes that fibrin is itself evidence of pathological coagulation, whether platelet involvement is more important, or whether any particular significance should be placed on the distribution of fibrin either intravascularly or in the tissues.

Kincaird-Smith (1970) has been a main proponent of the role of intravascular coagulation in the pathogenesis of renal failure by causing progressive vascular or glomerular occlusion, and Urizar and Herdman (1970) have highlighted the problem particularly with regard to anaphylactoid purpura. In a study of 3000 renal biopsies over a ten-year period, occlusion of glomerular capillaries, arterioles and interlobular arteries emerged as the most prominent lesion and the usual cause of deterioration of renal function. It was demonstrated as an initial lesion in many conditions including glomerulonephritis, malignant hypertension, thrombotic microangiopathy, allograft rejection, scleroderma and lupus nephritis (Kincaird-Smith, 1970).

A number of points relevant to the interpretation of vasculitis in the skin arise from these renal studies. Thus, a feature of capillaries in acute coagulation is a rather prominent and swollen endothelial cell projecting into the lumen and often becoming exfoliated (Vassalli, Simon and Rouiller, 1963; Kincaird-Smith, 1970). It is similar to the endocarditis lenta cell, and Ruiter and Mandema's (1965) description of severe vascular proliferation in sub-acute bacterial endocarditis is relevant in this report (see also Chapter 8). Reduplication of endothelial cells is frequent in this disease, the capillaries being lined with several layers of them and alternating with layers of fibrinoid basement membrane-like material.

This picture is also seen in renal allografts and in kidneys in which thromboplastin has been inoculated intravascularly. Such observations have led to the successful treatment of renal allograft rejection, malignant hypertension, glomerulonephritis and thrombotic thrombocytopenic purpura by using both inhibitors of platelet aggregation and anti-coagulants (Kincaird-Smith, Laver and Fairley, 1970). Similar observations have been made on lung transplants and Table 3.1 illustrates the proposed sequence of events. Raised levels of fibrin degradation products in the serum of patients with rheumatoid arthritis and systemic lupus erythematosus occur most significantly in those who have the most obvious vascular injury in the kidneys (Kanyerezi, Lwanga and Bloch, 1971).

Frank disseminated intravascular coagulation during rapid renal homograft rejection was recorded by Starzl et al (1970). Similarly, Papilian, Ciobanu and Stroescu (1967) described intravascular deposition of fibrin in three cases of systemic lupus erythematosus, and in these patients thrombosis in the general circulation consumed clotting factors to such an extent that haemorrhage resulted. These authors suggested that this was an acute example of a process which occurs in a low-grade way in most patients with systemic lupus erythematosus.

Regan, Lackner and Karpatkin (1974) observed that 12 out of 21 patients with lupus erythematosus had a platelet defect such that in vitro aggregation induced by connective tissue was prevented. Three of these patients had a circulating anticoagulant and elevated fibrin degradation products. In such patients aspirin therapy is contraindicated.

Cummings and Taleisnik (1971), reviewing 12 cases of peripheral gangrene in rheumatoid arthritis, found that thrombosis was extensive and that the histological picture ranged from adventitial infiltration by neutrophils in the acute case to mononuclear cells in an older lesion. Castleman (1963) also found in rheumatoid arthritis widespread intravascular thrombosis due this time to thrombotic thrombocytopenic purpura. Earlier workers, reviewing pathological material from rheumatic fever (Van Glahn and Pappenheimer, 1926), found fibrin deposition in peripheral vessels in 21 per cent of cases, while Sokoloff (1963) found frank thrombosis to be common in both rheumatic fever and rheumatoid arthritis. Similar occlusion by fibrin in children with lupus erythematosus, anaphylactoid purpura, dermatomyositis and scleroderma was discussed by Kornreich (1967).

There have also been discussions about the overlap of thrombophlebitis with nodular vasculitis (Wilkinson, 1954), and clear descriptions of a thrombosing angiitis in diseases such as Wegener's granulomatosis (Kraus et al, 1965). Other reports provide good evidence of disseminated intravascular coagulation in cases labelled as acute allergic vasculitis (Johnson and Merskey, 1966) or anaphylactoid purpura (Garofalo, Minerva and Baltieri, 1972). Perks, Green and Gleeson (1974) described a patient who had purpura hyperglobulinaemia of Waldenström's related to an IgA paraprotein and suffered four episodes of embolism and marked superficial thrombophlebitis of the legs.

Taylor and Jacoby (1949) and Melczer and Venkei (1947) both found disturbance of in vitro coagulation in cases of polyarteritis nodosa and were at pains to show similarities between that disease and purpura fulminans.

Hardaway, McKay and Williams (1954) described a syndrome consisting of hypotensive shock, acute renal failure and a bleeding tendency occurring after incompatible blood transfusion or in the presence of severe sepsis. Reviewing the subject many years later, Hardaway (1971) defined disseminated intravascular coagulation (DIC) as "acute, transient coagulation occurring in the flowing blood throughout the vascular tree and which may obstruct the microcirculation. It may or may not result in accumulation of fibrin but does involve the transformation of fibrinogen into fibrin. It includes the agglutination of platelets and red cells and the sticking of leucocytes".

This excessive coagulation consumes all clotting factors, activates fibrinolysis and ultimately may lead to bleeding. In fact one often diagnoses the syndrome because of uncontrolled bleeding from many sites. At a local level coagulation may also be associated with bleeding; for instance, the splinter haemorrhage of the nail-fold as often as not begins as a local intracapillary thrombosis (see Chapter 3, Figure 3.3).

Disseminated intravascular coagulation has been discussed mainly by non-dermatologists, hence for some time the skin has received little attention. Haim et al (1970) described four cases of DIC in which cutaneous symptoms were the presenting signs, and more recently Colman's group (Robboy et al, 1973) has suggested that a skin biopsy may be the most reliable investigation since fibrin in the skin capillaries can so easily be demonstrated in this disorder. Colman and Rodriguez-Erdmann (1970) believed that DIC is a pathophysiological state seen in a variety of diseases, and McKay (1965) defined it as an intermediary mechanism of disease that contributes to systemic lupus erythematosus, glomerulonephritis, polyarteritis nodosa, rheumatoid arthritis, rheumatic fever, dermatomyositis and scleroderma.

Two types of disseminated intravascular coagulation have been observed. The first consists of a low grade, chronic progressive process which is incomplete and is associated with thrombocytopenia, cryofibrinogenaemia, granular deposits of fibrin macromolecules on the basement membrane of the renal glomeruli, and Raynaud's phenomenon. The second type may be superimposed on the first and consists of a sudden, acute, disseminated thrombosis in arterioles, capillaries and venules. It is also associated with shock, a haemorrhagic tendency, decrease in circulating components of the haemostatic mechanism, and focal necrosis in a variety of organs including the lungs, heart, kidney, adrenals, pancreas and other viscera.

References

Castleman, B. (1963) Case 58 of the Case Reports of the Massachusetts General Hospital. *New England Journal of Medicine*, **269**, 577.
Colman, R. W. & Rodriguez-Erdmann, F. (1970) Terminology of intravascular coagulation. *New England Journal of Medicine*, **282**, 99.
Cummings, J. K. & Taleisnik, J. (1971) Peripheral gangrene as a complication of rheumatoid arthritis. *Journal of Bone and Joint Surgery*, **53A**, 1001.
Garofalo, E., Minerva, A. & Baltieri, G. (1972) Porpora anafilattoide a coccarda di seidmayer. *Minerva Pediatrica*, **24**, 817.
Haim, S., Tatarski, I., Zeltzer, M. & Amikam, S. (1970) Disseminated intravascular coagulation presenting with cutaneous symptoms. *Dermatologica*, **141**, 239.
Hardaway, R. M. (1971) Disseminated intravascular coagulation. *Thrombosis et Diathesis Haemorrhagica*, **46**, 209.
Hardaway, R. M., McKay, D. G. & Williams, J. H. (1954) Lower nephron nephrosis (ischemuric nephrosis). *American Journal of Surgery*, **87**, 41.
Johnson, A. J. & Merskey, C. (1966) Diagnosis of diffuse intravascular clotting. Its relation to secondary fibrinolysis and treatment with heparin. *Thrombosis et Diathesis Haemorrhagica*, Supplement **20**, 161.
Kanyerezi, B. R., Lwanga, S. K. & Bloch, K. J. (1971) Fibrinogen degradation products in serum and urine of patients with systemic lupus erythematosus. *Arthritis and Rheumatism*, **14**, 267.
Kincaird-Smith, P. (1970) The pathogenesis of the vascular and glomerular lesions of rejection in renal allografts and their modification by antithrombotic and anticoagulant drugs. *Australian Annals of Medicine*, **3**, 207.
Kincaird-Smith, P., Laver, M. C. & Fairley, K. F. (1970) Dipyridamole and anticoagulants and renal disease due to glomerular and vascular lesions. A new approach to therapy. *Medical Journal of Australia*, **3**, 145.
Kornreich, H. (1967) Systemic rheumatic disorders of childhood. *Bulletin of Rheumatic Diseases*, **441**, 445.
Kraus, Z., Vortel, V., Fingerland, A., Salavec, M. & Krch, V. (1965) Unusual cutaneous manifestations in Wegener's granulomatosis. *Acta Dermato-venereologica*, **45**, 288.
McKay, D. G. (1965) *Disseminated Intravascular Coagulation. An Intermediary of Disease*. New York: Hoebner Medical Division, Harper and Row.
Melczer, N. & Venkei, T. (1947) Uber die Hautformen der Periarteriitis Nodosa. *Dermatologica*, **94**, 214.
Pandolfi, M., Robertson, B., Isacson, S. & Nilsson, I. M. (1968) Fibrinolytic activity of human veins in arms and legs. *Thrombosis et Diathesis Haemorrhagica*, **20**, 247.
Papilian, M., Ciobanu, V. & Stroescu, O. (1967) Sindromul de coagulopatie prin consom in cursul bolii lupicé. *Medicina Internazionale*, **19**, 827.
Perks, W. H., Green, F. & Gleeson, M. H. (1974) A case of purpura hyperglobulinaemia of Waldenström studied by skin immunofluorescence. *British Journal of Dermatology*, **91**, 563.
Regan, M. G., Lackner, H. & Karpatkin, S. (1974) Platelet function and coagulation profile in lupus erythematosus. Studies in 50 patients. *Annals of Internal Medicine*, **81**, 462.
Robboy, S. J., Mihm, M. C., Colman, R. W. & Minna, J. D. (1973) The skin in disseminated intravascular coagulation. Prospective analysis of 36 cases. *British Journal of Dermatology*, **88**, 221.
Ruiter, M. & Mandema, E. (1965) Hochgradige mit ungewohnlichen Hautmanifestationen einhergehende Gefassendothelwucherung bei subakuter bakterieller endokarditis. *Hautartz*, **16**, 205.
Sokoloff, L. (1963) Pathophysiology of peripheral blood vessels in collagen diseases. In *Peripheral Blood Vessels* (Ed.) Orbison, J. L. & Smith, D. E. p. 297. Baltimore: Williams and Wilkins.
Starzl, T. E., Boehmig, H. J., Amemiya, H., Wilson, C. B., Dixon, F. J., Giles, G. R. Simpson, K. M. & Halgrimson, C. G. (1970) Clotting changes, including disseminated intravascular coagulation, during rapid renal homograft rejection. *New England Journal of Medicine*, **283**, 383.
Taylor, A. W. & Jacoby, N. M. (1949) Acute polyarteritis nodosa in childhood. *Lancet*, **ii**, 792.
Urizar, R. E. & Herdman, R. C. (1970) Anaphylactoid purpura. III. Early morphologic glomerular changes. *American Journal of Clinical Pathology*, **53**, 258.
Van Glahn, W. C. & Pappenheimer, A. M. (1926) Specific lesions of peripheral blood vessels in rheumatism. *American Journal of Pathology*, **2**, 235.

Vassalli, P., Simon, G. & Rouiller, C. (1963) Electron microscopic study of glomerular lesion resulting from intravascular fibrin formation. *American Journal of Pathology,* **43,** 579.

Warren, B. A. & de Bono, A. H. B. (1969) The ultrastructure of early rejection phenomena in lung homografts in dogs. *British Journal of Experimental Pathology,* **50,** 593.

Wilkinson, D. S. (1954) The vascular basis of some nodular eruptions of the legs. *British Journal of Dermatology,* **66,** 201.

THE CAUSES OF INTRAVASCULAR COAGULATION

If one considers the three types of injury responsible for activating coagulation (Colman, Robboy and Minna, 1972) then one must agree that they are all present in vasculitis as well as in disseminated intravascular coagulation: (1) injury to endothelial cells, (2) tissue injury, and (3) red cell and platelet injury.

The considerable knowledge that we now have about the triggers and the predisposing factors in disseminated intravascular coagulation (DIC) can be applied equally well to the problem of local fibrin deposition leading to consumption of clotting factors and activation of fibrinolysis locally. The picture of fibrin deposition with extravasation and exudation of fluid elements of the blood is one aspect of vasculitis which clearly overlaps with DIC on the one hand and with a more inflammatory leucocytoclastic picture on the other. Colman stated that a somewhat artificial line is drawn between Schönlein—Henoch purpura and purpura fulminans (Colman and Kish, 1969), a point exemplified by Kisker, Glueck and Kauder's (1968) description of a case of anaphylactoid purpura progressing to gangrene which did well on heparin.

The triggers of DIC are similar to those encountered in vasculitis and are listed in Table 10.1. In a series of articles Copeman and Ryan (1970) suggested that a mechanistic classification of vasculitis is preferable to a morphological one and they proposed a classification based on fibrin deposition (Table 6.1).

In vitro studies by Robbins and Stetson (1959) showed that coagulation could be accelerated by immune complexes. They titrated antigenic bovine gamma globulin and bovine serum albumin against rabbit antisera. Supernatant fluids taken from the region of antigen excess produced marked acceleration of clotting when added to normal rabbit blood in silicone. When the ratio of antigen to antibody was one to one or when antibody was in excess the complexes were without activity. Soluble complexes showed some activity; whole blood rather than cell-free plasma was necessary to produce this effect. Simpson, Robertson and Stalker (1973) have studied the consumption of coagulation factors in whole blood in rabbits after injecting antigen and found evidence of DIC.

With respect to coagulation one need not draw too sharp a distinction between the various types of immunological reaction. Anaphylaxis, the Arthus reaction and delayed hypersensitivity all encourage clotting and platelet aggregation. In rabbits the drop in the platelet count that occurs in anaphylaxis can be prevented by heparin (Johansson, 1961) and not surprisingly anaphylaxis is accompanied by a prolonged coagulation time and by consumption of prothrombin proconvertin antihaemophilic globulin, and Factor V. Consumption of fibrinogen occurs late in the reaction perhaps because the release of heparin by mast cells prevents disseminated clotting but cannot prevent immediate platelet reactions to antigen. The fibrin clot forms once heparin has disappeared from the bloodstream (Johansson, 1961).

In many 'allergic' subjects and in atopy a fall in the number of circulating platelets is a common finding when the subjects are provoked by foods or inhalants to which they are

Table 10.1. Triggers of disseminated intravascular coagulation as listed by Colman et al (1972) from experience at the Massachusetts General Hospital, July 1967 to January 1970.

Disease state	Primary disease or event	Precipitating or complicating factor
Tissue injury		
Obstetrical		
pregnancy	1	1
Surgical		
extensive surgery	1	1
arterial or venous surgery	0	5
dilation and curettage of uterus	0	1
Neoplastic		
carcinoma		
adenocarcinoma prostate	5	0
bronchogenic carcinoma	1	0
leukaemia		
acute promyelocytic	3	0
acute myeloblastic	2	0
acute myelomonocytic	2	0
acute lymphoblastic	1	0
associated with chemotherapy	0	10
Endothelial injury		
Gram-negative septicaemia (endotoxaemia)		
Neisseria meningitidis	6	0
N. gonorrhoeae	1	0
Klebsiella sp.	1	2
Serratia sp.	1	0
Proteus mirabilis	0	1
Pseudomonas aeruginosa	1	1
Escherichia coli	1	0
Salmonella sp.	1	0
Gram-positive septicaemia		
Pneumococcus pneumoniae	1	0
Staphylococcus aureus	2	1
S. albus	1	0
Streptococcus sp.	2	0
Viraemia		
myocarditis and pneumonitis	1	0
meningitis	1	0
Prolonged hypotension	3	17
Platelet or red cell injury		
Immunologic		
purpura fulminans	1	2
Haemolysis		
haemolytic anaemia, Coombs' positive	0	1
micro-angiopathic haemolytic anaemia,		
Aspergillus fumigatus septicaemia	2	0
possible haemolysis	0	5
Reticuloendothelial system injury		
Liver injury		
acute fulminant hepatitis	1	0
cirrhosis	0	5
other	1	2
Post-splenectomy	0	3
Totals	44	58

The numbers in the table represent the number of patients presenting with a trigger.

sensitive. This is the basis of the thrombocyte test in which a 20 per cent fall is regarded as positive (Rajka, 1961). It may explain such tales as that of the patient of Tondra (1969) who developed urticaria followed by purpura gangrenosum after eating strawberries. Storck (1951) studied patients with Schönlein—Henoch purpura in whom he considered bacterial infection was a significant feature. Challenge of his patients with bacterial products caused a drop in the platelet count and a rise in heparin levels in the blood. Ruiter (1956) described a case in which a 30 per cent drop in the platelet count occurred within 30 minutes of a test dose of butobarbitone. Of course, these patients had vasculitis — a prolonged reaction — although the platelet phenomenon was brief, lasting a mere one and one-half hours.

Histological examination of renal cortical necrosis following inoculation of immune complexes has confirmed that widespread clotting occurs and that it can be prevented by heparin (Lee, 1963). Moreover, if animals are made anaphylactic by giving antigen to which they are sensitised, lung capillaries fill with thrombus.

McKinnon et al (1957) demonstrated incorporation of immune complexes into thrombus, and Lüscher (1970) suggested that their damaging effect is exerted through platelet aggregation. Quick, Ota and Baronofsky (1964) had, in fact, previously demonstrated clumping of circulating platelets and ultimately a fall in the platelet count in a study of anaphylaxis. Similar conclusions were drawn from an investigation into the effects of endotoxin on blood coagulation (McKay, Shapiro and Shanberge, 1958).

From the clinical point of view there is, on the one hand, the large amount of data suggesting that various forms of vasculitis can be due to immune complexes (see Chapter 7), and on the other hand, a usually quite separate set of data suggesting that clotting has occurred in such diseases. Handel et al (1975) found evidence of partially aggregated fibrin in the blood of four out of fourteen cases of necrotising vasculitis. There are, however, increasing numbers of reports of complement consumption in DIC (see Chapter 6).

References

Colman, R. W. & Kish, L. S. (1969) Fulminant purpura and severe coagulation disturbance. *New England Journal of Medicine*, **281**, 153.

Colman, R. W., Robboy, S. J. & Minna, J. D. (1972) Disseminated intravascular coagulation (D.I.C.). An approach. *American Journal of Medicine*, **52**, 679.

Copeman, P. W. M. & Ryan, T. J. (1970) The problems of cutaneous angiitis with reference to histopathology and pathogenesis. *British Journal of Dermatology*, **82** (Supplement 5), 2.

Handel, D. W., Roenigk, H. H., Shainoff, J. & Deodhar, S. (1975) Necrotising vasculitis. *Archives of Dermatology*, **111**, 847.

Irwin, J. W., Weille, S., York, I. M. & Rappaport, M. A. (1959) The pulmonary microcirculation of living rabbits during passive anaphylaxis. In *Microcirculation* (Ed.) Reynolds, S. R. M. & Zweifach, B. W. p. 92. Urbana: University Press.

Johansson, S. A. (1961) On the protective effect of heparin in cases of anaphylactic shock. *Acta Dermato-venereologica*, **41**, 500.

Juhlin, L., Michaelsson, G. & Zetterstrom, O. (1972) Urticaria and asthma induced by food and drug additives in patients with aspirin sensitivity. *Journal of Allergy and Clinical Immunology*, **50**, 92.

Kisker, C. T., Glueck, H. & Kauder, E. (1968) Anaphylactoid purpura progressing to gangrene and its treatment with heparin. *Journal of Pediatrics*, **73**, 748.

Lee, L. (1963) Antibody reactions in pathogenesis of bilateral renal cortical necrosis. *Journal of Experimental Medicine*, **117**, 365.

Lüscher, E. F. (1970) Immune complexes and platelet aggregation. *Series Haematologica*, **3**, 121.

McKay, D. G., Shapiro, S. S. & Shanberge, J. N. (1958) Alterations in blood coagulation system induced by bacterial endotoxin II in vivo. *Journal of Experimental Medicine*, **107**, 369.

McKinnon, G. E., Andrews, E. C. Jr, Heptinstall, R. H. & Germuth, F. G. Jr (1957) An immunologic study on occurrence of intravascular antigen antibody precipitation and its role in anaphylaxis in the rabbit. *Bulletin of the Johns Hopkins Hospital*, **101**, 258.

Quick, A. J., Ota, R. K. & Baronofsky, I. D. (1964) Thrombopenia of anaphylactic and peptone shock. *American Journal of Physiology*, **145**, 273.

Rajka, G. (1961) Prurigo Besnier (atopic dermatitis) with special reference to the role of allergic factors. *Acta Dermato-venereologica*, **41**, 1.

Robbins, J. E. & Stetson, C. A. (1959) An effect of antibody—antigen interaction on blood coagulation. *Journal of Experimental Medicine*, **109**, 1.

Ruiter, M. (1956) Purpura rheumatica, allergic cutaneous arteriolitis, a type of. *British Journal of Dermatology*, **68**, 16.

Simpson, J. G., Robertson, A. J. & Stalker, A. L. (1973) The effect of immune complexes on coagulation and fibrinolysis. *7th European Conference on Microcirculation, Part II, Clinical Aspects of Microcirculation* (Ed.) Ditzel, J. & Lewis, D. H. p. 260. Basel: S. Karger.

Storck, H. (1951) Uber hämorrhagische phänomene in der Dermatologie. *Dermatologica*, **102**, 197.

Storck, H., Hoigne, R. & Koller, F. (1955) Thrombocytes in allergic reactions. *International Archives of Allergy*, **6**, 372.

Tondra, J. M. (1969) Gangrene of the skin due to allergic reaction. *Plastic and Reconstructive Surgery*, **43**, 392.

INFECTIVE AGENTS AS TRIGGERS

Many viruses, rickettsiae or bacteria promote coagulation by endothelial damage (Colman, Robboy and Minna, 1972) (see Chapter 8).

In viraemia (McKay and Margaretten, 1967), heat stroke (Bachman, 1967; Sohal et al, 1968), meningococcaemia (Mason et al, 1970) and gram-positive endotoxaemia (Thomas, Denney and Floyd, 1953), the endothelium may be disrupted and Hageman factor activated. In gram-negative septicaemia with endotoxaemia, necrotic endothelial cells may even detach and circulate (Gaynor, Bouvier and Spaet, 1970; Bouvier, 1973) (Figure 10.5).

> The commonest and most significant sign of complicated vasculitis is bleeding from the skin, mucous membranes, genito-urinary tract, lung or gastro-intestinal tract. As often as not, this is due to hypercoagulation.

Figure 10.5. A reminder that hypercoagulation is responsible for the bleeding that so often complicates vasculitis.

Bacteria are in some cases specific activators of clotting but another phenomenon important in disseminated intravascular coagulation is activation of the Hageman factor XII by surfaces. Intravascular catheters, extracorporeal circulation or dialysis are important in this respect (Hardaway, 1971). Particulate matter such as kaolin, red cell membranes, large molecular weight dextrans, cold-precipitable proteins, bacteria, and amniotic or placental membrane all may act as surface activators.

Bacterial endotoxin in the circulating blood results in 'blockade' of the reticulo-endothelial system (Beeson, 1947). In this context, 'blockade' signifies a reduced phagocytic capacity to remove particulate matter, colloidal substances and certain endogenous materials from the circulating blood.

Bacterial toxins

Loeb (1903) wrote of the influence of certain bacteria on the coagulation of the blood. All of the following are relevant to this topic. Filtrates of pathogenic coagulase-positive staphylococci cause platelet aggregation, platelet thrombosis and fibrin clots. Staphylo-coagulase reacts with prothrombin, even in the absence of calcium and Factors V and VII to produce a form of thrombin which is not inhibited by heparin or by the antithrombin of the serum (Biggs and MacFarlane, 1962). Several gram-negative organisms produce endotoxins that cause platelet aggregation and coagulation — shown conclusively to be the case in studies of the Shwartzman phenomenon using such organisms. Observations in vivo of swelling of endothelial cells, increased leucocyte stickiness, and the formation of fibrin and platelet thrombi in response to endotoxin are also convincing (Branemark and Urbaschek, 1967).

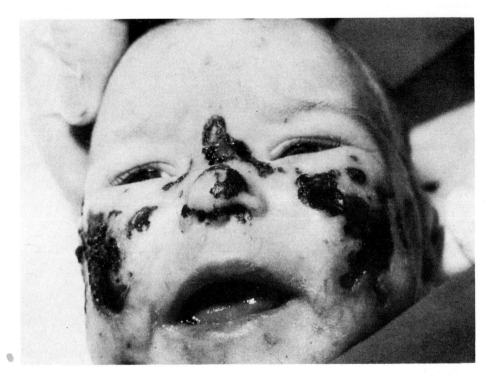

Figure 10.6. Skin necrosis in a baby admitted with meningococcal septicaemia and cold exposure.

There are numerous reports of severe purpura with gangrene following bacterial infection. Corrigan, Ray and May (1968) have reviewed the changes in blood coagulation associated with septicaemia and examples include: staphylococcal infection (Hofstad, 1959; Frederiks and Huffstadt, 1970); *Streptococcus* — scarlet fever (Dick, Miller and Edmondson, 1934); *Meningococcus* (Leoni, 1969; Gerard et al, 1973 gave 15 references to DIC with meningococcal septicaemia and discussed 19 of their own patients) (Figure 10.6); *Pseudomonas* (Forener et al, 1958); *Citrobacter* (Grant, Horowitz and Lorian, 1969); *Candida albicans* (Phillipidis et al, 1971; Prochazka et al, 1971); *Aspergillus* (Daughten and Pearson, 1968); trypanosomiasis (Barrett-Connor, Ugoretz and Braude, 1973) (with this organism parenteral feeding is often a factor); malaria (Dennis et al, 1967; Borochovitz, Crossley and Metz, 1970) (blood fibrinolytic activity is consistently low in malaria, probably because of vascular injury (Petchclai, Pratumvinit and Benjaponges, 1975)).

Important evidence of coagulation occurring in every case of meningococcal septicaemia comes from a new method of detecting circulating fibrin (Kisker and Rush, 1973) (see page 344). Using an isotope label, these authors demonstrated circulating fibrin in six patients and showed that platelet aggregation and consumption of clotting factors may not correlate too well with fibrin formation. They suggested that the production of such factors may equal their consumption. Such observations parallel the discussion on the role of immune complexes in DIC because one of the main stumbling blocks to accepting intravascular coagulation as an important feature of the various autoimmune diseases is the failure to demonstrate thrombocytopenia, the consumption of prothrombin and the presence of several fibrin degradation products in all or in some series (Corrigan, 1970).

Corrigan, Ray and May (1968) found that patients with allergic diseases often had elevated rather than reduced levels of clotting factors and platelets in their blood. But this too may be transient or occur in the recovery phase of undoubted DIC.

There are a number of diseases in which DIC has been postulated and for which heparin therapy is advocated and yet evidence of consumption of clotting factors and fibrinogen may not be found, examples being the haemolytic uraemic syndrome (Gilchrist et al, 1965; Katz, Lurie and Kaplan, 1969) and thrombotic thrombocytopenic purpura (Lerner, Rapaport and Meltzer, 1967; Kwaan et al, 1968). Similarly a mild chronic form of DIC is recognised in which circulating levels of fibrin degradation products are not raised and blood samples may not show much change in clotting factors (Kwaan, 1972).

References

Bachman, F. (1967) Evidence for hypercoagulability in heat stroke. *Journal of Clinical Investigation,* **46,** 1033.
Barrett-Connor, E., Ugoretz, R. J. & Braude, A. L. (1973) Disseminated intravascular coagulation in trypano-somiasis. *Annals of Internal Medicine,* **131,** 574.
Beeson, P. B. (1947) Effect of reticuloendothelial blockade on immunity to the Shwartzman phenomenon. *Proceedings of the Society for Experimental Biology and Medicine,* **64,** 146.
Biggs, R. & MacFarlane, R. G. (1962) *Human Blood Coagulation and its Disorders,* 3rd edition. Oxford: Blackwell.
Borochovitz, D., Crossley, A. L. & Metz, J. (1970) Disseminated intravascular coagulation with fatal haemorrhage in cerebral malaria. *British Medical Journal,* ii, 710.
Bouvier, C. A. (1973) Endothelium and the G.S.R. *Bibliographie Anatomique,* **12,** 92.
Branemark, P. I. & Urbaschek, B. (1967) Endotoxins in tissue injury. Vital microscopic studies on the effect of endotoxin from E. coli on the microcirculation. *Angiology,* **18,** 667.
Colman, R. W., Robboy, S. J. & Minna, J. D. (1972) Disseminated intravascular coagulation (D.I.C.). An approach. *American Journal of Medicine,* **52,** 679.
Corrigan, J. J. (1970) Studies on the coagulation fibrinolytic systems in 'autoimmune' disease. *American Journal of Diseases of Children,* **120,** 324.
Corrigan, J. J. Jr, Ray, W. L. & May, N. (1968) Changes in blood coagulation system associated with septicaemia. *New England Journal of Medicine,* **279,** 851.
Daughten, R. M. & Pearson, H. (1968) Disseminated intravascular coagulation associated with aspergillus endocarditis. *Journal of Pediatrics,* **73,** 576.
Dennis, L. H., Eichelberger, J. W., Inman, M. N. & Conrad, M. E. (1967) Depletion of coagulation factors in drug resistant Plasmodium falciparum malaria. *Blood,* **29,** 713.
Dick, G. F., Miller, E. M. & Edmondson, H. (1934) Severe purpura with gangrene of lower extremity following scarlet fever, recovery after amputation. *American Journal of Diseases of Children,* **47,** 374.
Forener, C. E., Frei, E., Edgcomb, J. H. & Utz, J. P. (1958) Pseudomonas septicaemia, observations on 23 cases. *American Journal of Medicine,* **25,** 877.
Frederiks, E. & Huffstadt, A. J. C. (1970) Purpura fulminans. *British Journal of Plastic Surgery,* **23,** 90.
Gaynor, E., Bouvier, C. C. & Spaet, T. H. (1970) Vascular lesions: possible pathogenetic basis of the generalised Schwartzman reaction. *Science,* **170,** 989.
Gerard, P., Morian, M., Bachy, A., Malvaux, P. & De Meyer, R. (1973) Meningococcal purpura. Report of 19 patients treated with heparin. *Journal of Pediatrics,* **82,** 780.
Gilchrist, G. S., Ekert, H., Lieberman, E., Fine, R. N. & Grushkin, C. (1965) Heparin therapy in the hemolytic—uremic syndrome. *New England Journal of Medicine,* **273,** 754.

Grant, M. D., Horowitz, H. I. & Lorian, V. (1969) Gangrenous ulcer and septicaemia due to citrobacter. *New England Journal of Medicine,* **280,** 1286.

Hardaway, R. M. (1971) Disseminated intravascular coagulation. *Thrombosis et Diathesis Haemorrhagica,* **46,** 209.

Hofstad, T. (1959) Pyoderma gangrenosum. *Acta Dermato-venereologica,* **39,** 481.

Katz, J., Lurie, A. & Kaplan, B. (1969) Haemolytic—uraemic syndrome and heparin therapy. *Lancet,* **ii,** 700.

Kisker, C. T. & Rush, R. (1973) Circulating fibrin and meningococcaemia. *Journal of Pediatrics,* **82,** 787.

Kwaan, H. C. (1972) Disseminated intravascular coagulation. *Medical Clinics of North America,* **56,** 177.

Kwaan, H. C., Gallo, G., Potter, E., Cutting, H. & Stanzler, R. (1968) The nature of the vascular lesion in thrombotic thrombocytopenic purpura. *Annals of Internal Medicine,* **68,** 1169.

Leoni, A. (1969) A case of disseminated skin gangrene in the course of infantile meningococcal sepsis. *Giornale Italiano di Dermatologia,* **44,** 347.

Lerner, R. G., Rapaport, S. I. & Meltzer, J. (1967) Thrombotic thrombocytopenic purpura, serial clotting studies, relation to the generalised Shwartzman reaction and remission after adrenal steroid and dextran therapy. *Annals of Internal Medicine,* **68,** 1180.

Loeb, L. (1903) The influence of certain bacteria on the coagulation of the blood. *Journal of Medical Research,* **10,** 407.

Mason, J. W., Kleeberg, U., Dolan, P. & Colman, R. W. (1970) Human plasma kallikrein and Hageman factor in endotoxin shock. *Annals of Internal Medicine,* **73,** 545.

McKay, D. G. & Margaretten, W. (1967) Disseminated intravascular coagulation in virus diseases. *Archives of Internal Medicine* (Chicago), **120,** 129.

Petchclai, B., Pratumvinit, U. & Berjaponges, W. (1975) Decreased fibrinolytic activity and malaria. *Lancet,* **i,** 1143.

Phillipidis, P., Naman, J. L., Maarten, S. S. & Valdes-Dapena, M. A. (1971) Disseminated intravascular coagulation in Candida albicans septicemia. *Journal of Pediatrics,* **78,** 683.

Prochazka, J. V., Lucas, R. N., Beauchamp, C. J. & Strauss, R. G. (1971) Systemic candidiasis with disseminated intravascular coagulation. *American Journal of Diseases of Children,* **122,** 255.

Sohal, R. S., Sun, S. C., Colcolough, H. L. & Burch, G. E. (1968) Heatstroke. An electron microscopic study of endothelial cell damage and disseminated intravascular coagulation. *Archives of Internal Medicine,* **122,** 43.

Thomas, L., Denney, F. W. & Floyd, J. (1953) Studies on the generalised Shwartzman reaction. III. Lesions of myocardium and coronary artery accompanying the reaction in rabbits prepared by infection with group A staphylococci. *Journal of Experimental Medicine,* **92,** 751.

Other factors: part constitutional, part trigger

Malignant tumours

A recent symposium from the Mayo Clinic included several papers on the abnormal coagulation seen in patients with malignant disease (Bowie and Owen, 1974). Cancer cells stimulate coagulation and this is the basis of thrombophlebitis migrans in malignant disease (Sproul, 1938; Cruickshank, 1956; Lieberman et al, 1960). Blood-borne neoplastic cells may be responsible (Williams, 1954) as may a coagulation factor associated with carcinomatous tissue (O'Meara and Thornes, 1961; Wood, 1964; Warren, 1968). There is a high incidence of DIC in leukaemia which may be due to release of thromboplastin especially during treatment with drugs that destroy leukaemic cells (Thomas, Hasselback and Perry, 1960; Leavey, Kahn and Brodsky, 1970). Copeman (1970) has emphasised that malignancy often underlies vasculitis, and there are many mechanisms whereby malignant tissue can encourage inflammation of the vessel wall (see also Figure 6.7).

References

Bowie, E. J. N. & Owen, C. A. (1974) Symposium on the intravascular coagulation—fibrinolysis (ICF) syndrome. *Proceedings of the Mayo Clinic,* **9,** 635.

Carrier, E. B. (1922) Studies on the physiology of capillaries. *American Journal of Physiology,* **61,** 528.

Copeman, P. W. M. (1970) Investigations into the pathogenesis of acute cutaneous angiitis. *British Journal of Dermatology,* **82** (Supplement 5), 51.

Cruickshank, A. H. (1956) Venous thrombosis in internal organs associated with thrombosis of leg veins. *Journal of Pathology and Bacteriology,* **71,** 383.

Leavey, R. A., Kahn, S. B. & Brodsky, I. (1970) Disseminated intravascular coagulation, a complication of chemotherapy in acute myelomonocytic leukaemia. *Cancer,* **26,** 142.

Lieberman, J. S., Borrero, J., Urdanetta, E. & Wright, I. S. (1960) Thromboembolism associated with neoplasm. Review of seventy-seven cases. *Circulation,* **22,** 780.

O'Meara, R. A. Q. & Thornes, R. D. (1961) Some properties of the cancer coagulative factor. *Irish Journal of Medical Science,* **423,** 106.

Sproul, E. E. (1938) Carcinoma and venous thrombosis; frequency of association of carcinoma in body or tail of pancreas with multiple venous thrombosis. *American Journal of Cancer,* **34,** 566.

Thomas, J. W., Hasselback, R. C. & Perry, W. H. (1960) A study of the hemorrhagic diathesis in leukaemia and allied diseases. *Canadian Medical Association Journal,* **83,** 639.

Warren, B. A. (1968) Observations on tumour embolism in small veins. *Biorheology,* **5,** 89.

Williams, A. A. (1954) Malignant disease associated with vascular phenomena. *British Medical Journal,* **ii,** 82.

Wood, S. Jr (1964) Experimental studies of the intravascular dissemination of ascitic V₂ carcinoma cells in the rabbit with special reference to fibrinogen and fibrinolytic agents. *Bulletin der Schweizerischen Akademie der Medizinische Wissenschaften,* **20,** 92.

Pregnancy

This is another factor influencing DIC. Supporting evidence includes: the ease with which the Shwartzman phenomenon can be induced in pregnant animals; the presence of fibrin in the pre-eclamptic kidney (Morris et al, 1964); the increase of cryofibrinogen in pregnancy (McKay and Corey, 1964); and the disturbance of clotting and fibrinolysis in pregnancy toxaemia (Wardle and Menon, 1969; Bonnar, McNicol and Douglas, 1971) (see also Chapters 6 and 9).

References

Bonnar, J. (1973) Blood coagulation and fibrinolysis in human pregnancy. *Bibliographie Anatomique,* **12,** 58.

Bonnar, J., McNicol, G. P. & Douglas, A. S. (1971) Coagulation and fibrinolytic systems in pre-eclampsia and eclampsia. *British Medical Journal,* **ii,** 12.

McKay, D. G. & Corey, A. E. (1964) Cryofibrinogenemia in toxemia of pregnancy. *Obstetrics and Gynecology,* **23,** 508.

Morris, R. H., Vassalli, P., Beller, F. K. & McCluskey, R. T. (1964) Immunofluorescent studies of renal biopsies in the diagnosis of toxemia of pregnancy. *Obstetrics and Gynecology,* **24,** 32.

Wardle, E. N. & Menon, I. S. (1969) Slow state of intravascular coagulation and reduced fibrinolysis in toxaemia. *British Medical Journal,* **ii,** 625.

Liver disease

Liver disease may contribute to DIC by releasing fibrinogen (Tytgat, 1970) and various other agents such as inhibitors of fibrinolysis or anti-heparin factors. In one series of 45 cases, 24 per cent had either mild cirrhosis or previous hepatitis or had undergone splenectomy (Colman, Robboy and Minna, 1972).

A damaged liver may fail to clear Factors X and XII from the circulation (Deykin, 1965; Deykin et al, 1968), and in patients with massive liver necrosis absence of fibrinolysis has been reported (Meili, Frick and Straub, 1969). Figure 10.7 shows widespread fibrin deposition and recanalisation of thrombi in skin vessels of an Indian woman who died of profuse rectal haemorrhage after her acutely necrotic liver had released an excess of anti-heparin factors. She had had a two-year illness, the main features of which had been a necrotising vasculitis of the skin. Meili, Frick and Straub (1969) had the opportunity to examine clotting factors in eight patients during massive hepatic necrosis due to *Amanita phalloides* poisoning. Circulating amounts of all clotting factors of hepatic origin fell early and simultaneously, and there was complete absence of fibrinolysis. However, no fibrin was demonstrable in the tissues.

Flute (1971) went as far as to suggest that all patients in hepatic coma should be assumed to have intravascular coagulation.

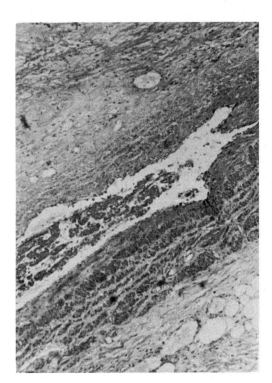

Figure 10.7. Recanalised vessel and fibrin in the deep dermis of a patient who had repeated episodes of DIC.

References

Colman, R. W., Robboy, S. J. & Minna, J. D. (1972) Disseminated intravascular coagulation (D.I.C.). An approach. *American Journal of Medicine,* **52,** 679.
Deykin, D. (1965) The hepatic clearance of the thrombosis inducing capacity of serum. *Journal of Clinical Investigation,* **44,** 1040.
Deykin, D., Cochios, F., DeCamp, G. & Lopez, A. (1968) Hepatic removal of activated factor by the perfused rabbit liver. *American Journal of Physiology,* **214,** 414.
Flute, P. T. (1971) Haemostasis in fulminant hepatic failure. *British Medical Journal,* **i,** 215.
Meili, E. O., Frick, P. G. & Straub, P. W. (1969) Coagulation changes during massive hepatic necrosis due to Amanita phalloides poisoning. *Helvetica Medica Acta,* **35,** 304.
Tytgat, G. (1970) Accelerated fibrinogen consumption in cirrhosis of the liver. *Clinical Research,* **18,** 419.

Paralysis of the reticuloendothelial system

Blocking or paralysis of the reticuloendothelial system is one of the most important contributory factors not only to well documented DIC but also to vasculitis (see page 125). Fibrin, once formed, is removed either by fibrinolysis or by the reticuloendothelial system. Fibrinolysis is easily exhausted or inhibited and also requires a healthy endothelium to activate it; consequently the reticuloendothelial system is most important in prolonged inflammatory disease, in which it is the only means of removing fibrin. Walsh and Barnhart (1969) have been the main proponents of this theme and have demonstrated failure in the clearance of coagulation and fibrinolytic products after injection of reticuloendothelial system blocking agents (see also Lee, Prose and Cohen, 1966; Bleyl, Kuhn and Graeff, 1969; Kwaan, 1972). Likewise, Wiedmeier et al (1969) demonstrated in the blood a marked fall in the number of platelets and in the level of fibrinogen with marked hypercoagulability after intravascular infusion of colloidal thorium dioxide and silicon dioxide. In a masterly review, Saba (1970) emphasised that the predominant role of cells lining the vascular tree is phagocytic and that serum factors are necessary for this activity. The paralysis of this system is therefore influenced particularly by the availability of such factors and hence by blood flow.

Some of the severest examples of DIC occur in diabetes mellitus (Kwaan, Colwell and Suwanwela, 1972; Cooper et al, 1973; Timperley, Preston and Ward, 1974; Nicholson and Tomkin, 1974). Switzer (1950) described gangrene of the breast, probably with a similar pathogenesis, in a diabetic. There are many reasons for the diabetic's susceptibility, including abnormalities of vascular endothelium, platelet adhesiveness and fibrinogen levels, but reduced reticuloendothelial phagocytosis (Bagdade, Root and Bulger, 1974) and acidosis may be among the most significant.

Hardaway (1971) maintained that acidosis is the most important factor relating stasis, ischaemia and coagulation. A fall in pH to 6.8, for instance, greatly accelerates clotting and inhibits heparin, but in shock, noradrenaline contributes further to this state of affairs (Hardaway et al, 1962). Hardaway, McKay and Holowell (1961) suggested that vasoconstriction, stasis, acidosis and coagulation create a vicious circle, all encouraging each other.

Ketosis is the main factor impairing the migration of neutrophils through abraded diabetic skin (Perillie, Nolan and Finch, 1962) and suppressing phagocytic activity (Bybee and Rogers, 1964), but hyperosmolarity reduces leucocyte stickiness and emigration (Ainsworth and Allison, 1970). Detailed studies by Mowat and Baum (1971) failed to explain why neutrophils show impaired chemotaxis in diabetes mellitus.

Antoniades et al (1973) injected human Factor XII-like material into rats in a study of the effects of feeding, fasting and diabetes mellitus. Diabetic and obese rats showed enhanced susceptibility to intravascular coagulation which was quickly improved by insulin. The levels of saturated long-chain fatty acids in the blood were considered to be the determining factor.

References

Ainsworth, S. K. & Allison, F. Jr (1970) Studies on the pathogenesis of acute inflammation. IX. The influence of hyperosmolarity secondary to hyperglycaemia upon the acute inflammatory response induced by thermal injury to ear chambers of rabbits. *Journal of Clinical Investigation,* **49,** 433.
Antoniades, H. N., Iatridis, P. G., Westmoreland, N., Simon, J. D., Hayes, K. C. & Surgenor, D. M. (1973) Effects of nutritional, endocrine and metabolic state on the development of intravascular coagulation induced by human serum preparations with procoagulant activity. *Thrombosis et Diathesis Haemorrhagica,* **29,** 33.

Bagdade, J. D., Root, R. K. & Bulger, R. J. (1974) Impaired leucocyte function in patients with poorly controlled diabetes. *Diabetes,* **23,** 9.

Bleyl, U., Kuhn, W. & Graeff, H. (1969) Retikuloendotheliale clearance intravasaler fibrinmonomere in der milz. *Thrombosis et Diathesis Haemorrhagica,* **22,** 87.

Bybee, J. D. & Rogers, D. E. (1964) The phagocytic activity of polymorphonuclear leucocytes obtained from patients with diabetes mellitus. *Journal of Laboratory and Clinical Medicine,* **64,** 1.

Cooper, M. R., Turner, R. A., Hutaff, L. & Prichard, R. (1973) Diabetic ketosis complicated by disseminated intravascular coagulation. *Southern Medical Journal,* **66,** 653.

Hardaway, R. M. (1971) Disseminated intravascular coagulation. *Thrombosis et Diathesis Haemorrhagica,* **46,** 209.

Hardaway, R. M., McKay, D. G. & Holowell, O. W. (1961) Vascular spasm and disseminated intravascular coagulation; influence of the phenomena one on the other. *Archives of Surgery,* **83,** 173.

Hardaway, R. M., Neimes, R. E., Burns, J. W., Mock, H. P. & Trenchak, P. T. (1962) Role of nor-epinephrine in irreversible shock. *Annals of Surgery,* **156,** 57.

Kwaan, H. C. (1972) Disseminated intravascular coagulation. *Medical Clinics of North America,* **56,** 177.

Kwaan, H C., Colwell, J. A. & Suwanwela, N. (1972) Disseminated intravascular coagulation in diabetes mellitus, with reference to the role of increased platelet aggregation. *Diabetes,* **21,** 108.

Lee, L., Prose, P. M. & Cohen, M. H. (1966) The role of the reticuloendothelial system in diffuse low grade intravascular coagulation. *Thrombosis et Diathesis Haemorrhagica,* **20,** 87.

Mowat, A. G. & Baum, J. (1971) Chemotaxis of polymorphonuclear leukocytes from patients with diabetes mellitus. *New England Journal of Medicine,* **284,** 621.

Nicholson, G. & Tomkin, G. H. (1974) Successful treatment of disseminated intravascular coagulopathy complicating diabetic coma. *British Medical Journal,* **iv,** 450.

Perillie, P. E., Nolan, J. P. & Finch, S. C. (1962) Studies of the resistance to infection in diabetes mellitus. Local exudative cellular response. *Journal of Laboratory and Clinical Investigation,* **59,** 1008.

Saba, T. M. (1970) Physiology and physiopathology of the reticuloendothelial system. *Archives of Internal Medicine,* **126,** 1031.

Switzer, P. K. (1950) Gangrene of the breast associated with diabetes mellitus. *Journal of the South Carolina Medical Association,* **46,** 48.

Timperley, W. R., Preston, F. E. & Ward, J. D. (1974) Cerebral intravascular coagulation in diabetic ketoacidosis. *Lancet,* **i,** 952.

Walsh, R. T. & Barnhart, M. I. (1969) Clearance of coagulation and fibrinolysis products by the reticulo-endothelial system. *Thrombosis et Diathesis Haemorrhagica,* Supplement **36,** 83.

Wiedmeier, V. T., Johnson, S. A., Siegesmund, K. & Smith, J. J. (1969) Systemic effects of R.E.S. blocking agents in the dog. *Journal of the Reticulo-Endothelial Society,* **6,** 202.

The role of stasis

In a study of microvascular behaviour and platelet aggregation in transparent chambers implanted in man, Branemark et al (1972) observed that platelet aggregates occurred in acidotic diabetics in response to minor injury and stasis. They noted that the aggregation was usually reversible, and that stasis by itself could occur for several hours without subsequent pathology.

In cutaneous vasculitis, fibrinoid is frequently found at sites of stasis induced by belts, braces or scratches (Ruiter, 1962; Copeman and Ryan, 1971) (see Figure 12.15).

Stasis is a major cause of thrombosis. The triad of Virchow — stasis, endothelial injury and changes in the blood — explains not only deep vein thrombosis but also microvascular thrombosis. As mentioned above stasis by itself is not always a cause of thrombosis, but it can certainly contribute to ischaemia and must interfere with the local demands for certain enzymes normally carried by the bloodstream — plasminogen for instance. Blood flow determines in part not only platelet—endothelial interaction (Mustard, Jorgansen and Packham, 1972) but also, as mentioned above, the provision of serum factors on which reticuloendothelial function depends. It is not surprising, therefore, that abnormal vascular channels in a disease such as Kaposi's sarcoma may be associated with DIC (Carey, Colman and Mihm, 1971).

The role of stasis has been discussed in leg ulcers associated with sickle cell anaemia. The latter trait is present in 10.8 per cent of the population of Kingston, Jamaica and in 25 per cent of the leg ulcer population there (Sergeant and Gueri, 1970). (Leg ulcers, on the other hand, are present in 6.8 per cent of patients with congenital spherocytosis (Gendel, 1948)). The histology is usually one of thrombosis with fibrinoid necrosis and is sometimes leucocytoclastic (Berge, Brehmer-Andersson and Rorsman, 1970). Often, an initial mild inflammation leads to anoxia and consequently to sickling. The vicious circle of Hardaway (see page 299) is thus enhanced in the haemoglobino-pathies. As streptokinase—streptodornase cures the ulcers, fibrin deposition probably plays a pathogenic role (Cooper and Wacker, 1954). Fibrinolysis is impaired in sickle cell disease in which fibrinogen levels are raised, and although anoxia partly explains this, Green, Kwaan and Ruiz (1970) blamed intercurrent infection and suggested that fibrinolysis is inhibited. In addition, platelet counts are raised and may have a significant role to play.

The thrombotic and haemorrhagic complications of polycythaemia vera are common in those patients who have elevated platelet counts, even when the haematocrit is maintained within the normal range by therapy (Dawson and Ogston, 1970). Indeed thrombophlebitis was the presenting symptom in association with an elevated platelet count and a normal haematocrit in six of 16 patients in one series (Edwards and Cooley, 1970).

Injured red cells contribute to DIC in malaria (Dennis et al, 1967), microangiopathic haemolytic anaemia (Brain, 1970), mismatched plasma (Lopas, Birndorf and Robboy, 1971) or blood (Krevans et al, 1957), or experimental intravascular haemolysis (Birndorf, Lopas and Robboy, 1971). Peruvian surgeons reduce the incidence of DIC in open heart surgery by bleeding those patients who have high haematocrits due to altitude (Hardaway, 1966).

References

Berge, G., Brehmer-Andersson, E. & Rorsman, H. (1970) Thalassaemia minor and painful ulcers of lower extremities. *Acta Dermato-venereologica,* **50,** 125.
Birndorf, N., Lopas, H. & Robboy, S. J. (1971) Intravascular coagulation and renal failure; production in the monkey with autologous red cell stroma. *Laboratory Investigation,* **25,** 314.
Brain, M. C. (1970) Microangiopathic haemolytic anaemia. *Annual Review of Medicine,* **21,** 133.
Branemark, P. I., Breine, U., Langer, L. & Skalak, R. (1972) Microvascular behaviour of platelets in man. *Thrombosis et Diathesis Haemorrhagica,* **51,** 182.
Carey, R. W., Colman, R. W. & Mihm, M. C. (1971) Kaposi sarcoma, pulmonary nodules, septicaemia and disseminated intravascular coagulation. *New England Journal of Medicine,* **285,** 279.
Cooper, C. D. & Wacker, W. E. C. (1954) Successful therapy with streptokinase—streptodornase of ankle ulcers associated with Mediterranean anaemia. *Blood,* **9,** 241.
Copeman, P. W. M. & Ryan, T. J. (1971) Cutaneous angiitis patterns of rashes explained by 1) flow properties of blood; 2) anatomical disposition of vessels. *British Journal of Dermatology,* **85,** 205.
Dawson, A. A. & Ogston, D. (1970) The influence of the platelet count on the incidence of thrombotic and haemorrhagic complications in polycythaemia vera. *Postgraduate Medical Journal,* **46,** 76.
Dennis, L. H., Eichelberger, J. W., Inman, M. N. & Conrad, M. E. (1967) Depletion of coagulation factors in drug resistant plasmodium falciparum malaria. *Blood,* **29,** 713.
Edwards, E. A. & Cooley, M. H. (1970) Peripheral vascular symptoms as the initial manifestation of poly-cythaemia vera. *Journal of the American Medical Association,* **214,** 1463.
Gendel, B. R. (1948) Chronic leg ulcer in disease of the blood. *Blood,* **3,** 1283.
Green, D., Kwaan, H. C. & Ruiz, G. (1970) Impaired fibrinolysis in sickle cell disease. *Thrombosis et Diathesis Haemorrhagica,* **24,** 10.
Hardaway, R. M. (1966) *Syndromes of Disseminated Intravascular Coagulation with Special Reference to Shock and Haemorrhage.* Springfield, Illinois: Charles C. Thomas.
Krevans, J. R., Jackson, D. P., Conley, C. L. & Hartman, R. C. (1957) The nature of the hemorrhagic defect accompanying hemolytic transfusion reactions in man. *Blood,* **12,** 834.

Lopas, H., Birndorf, N. I. & Robboy, S. J. (1971) Experimental transfusion reactions and disseminated intravascular coagulation produced by incompatible plasma in monkeys. *Transfusion*, **11**, 196.

Mustard, J. F., Jorgensen, L. & Packham, M. A. (1972) Blood flow and platelet interaction with surfaces. *Thrombosis et Diathesis Haemorrhagica*, **51**, 151.

Ruiter, M. (1962) Vascular fibrinoid in cutaneous "allergic" arteriolitis. *Journal of Investigative Dermatology*, **38**, 85.

Sergeant, G. & Gueri, M. (1970) Sickle cell trait and leg ulceration. *British Medical Journal*, **i**, 820.

Platelets

Relevant to the view of platelet involvement in DIC is a contemporary discussion about thrombotic thrombocytopenic purpura. Several authors have expressed the belief that platelet aggregation will trigger intravascular thrombosis (Evenses and Jeremic, 1970; Umlas and Kaiser, 1970). Fiddes and Penny (1970) also held this view and believed that DIC occurs in thrombotic thrombocytopenic purpura, for they observed a transient increase in circulating fibrin degradation product and an excellent response to heparin. Neame (1973), however, suggested that disseminated intravascular platelet aggregation should be distinguished from DIC because the two processes do not always overlap.

Of special relevance to polyarteritis nodosa is the regular occurrence of aneurysmally dilated arterioles in thrombotic thrombocytopenic purpura (Umlas and Kaiser, 1970) (see Chapter 13). Such aneurysms in any of these diseases can best be explained by ischaemic necrosis of the smooth muscle in the vessel wall, usually as a consequence of distal obstruction. Particulate matter, as occurs in antigen—antibody reactions or rapid renal allograft rejection (Starzl et al, 1970), may activate the Hageman factor but, as is illustrated in Figure 10.8, experiments on the nose discussed in Chapter 9 have shown

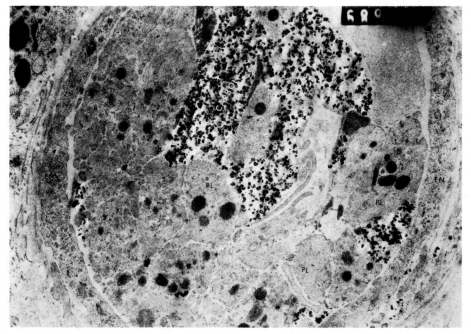

Figure 10.8. Aggregated platelets (PL) with carbon in a venule in the nose of a rat a few minutes after intravenous inoculation of carbon into the tail. EN = endothelium.

that it encourages platelets to aggregate. In an interesting patient with hyperacute allograft rejection and with activation of Hageman factor, kallikrein and fibrinolysis, heparin blocked intravascular coagulation and fibrin deposition. As soon as the heparin was stopped, DIC was unmasked (Colman, Robboy and Minna, 1972). Fortunately, in most patients with allograft rejection intravascular coagulation and fibrinolysis are localised to the allograft (Colman et al, 1969).

One has to be careful when using the term 'disseminated' intravascular coagulation that one means fibrin clot as opposed to platelet thrombi. Neame (1973), in a serial haemostatic and electron-microscopic study of thrombotic thrombocytopenic purpura, found normal fibrinogen levels and mild fibrinolysis. At many sites disseminated platelet aggregation was not accompanied by fibrin deposition. This distinction was stressed also by Lerner, Rapaport, and Meltzer (1967), Frick (1969), and Harker and Slichter (1972). Nevertheless, some overlap has been admitted by Neame (1973). One probable secondary phenomenon is the depression of plasminogen activator production by the walls of vessels involved by extensive microthrombi, as is seen in thrombotic thrombocytopenic purpura (Kwaan et al, 1968).

Damage to endothelium, particularly of venules, is an important factor in initiating coagulation. The accumulation of fibrin and platelets at sites of injury is well documented and may be observed directly in vivo in preparations such as the hamster cheek pouch (Berman, 1964) or in man (Branemark et al, 1972) and also in rabbit's ear windows — Cliff (1966) used immune complexes to study leucocyte stickiness. It is useful to point out that ischaemia and reperfusion can damage endothelial cells, as described in Chapter 5 (Cherry, Ryan and Ellis, 1974).

Harker and Slichter (1972) made a valuable contribution to the solution to this problem in a study of both platelet and fibrinogen consumption in a number of diseases. Normal haemostasis, as in surgical injury or thrombosis in veins, consumes both platelets and fibrinogen. DIC in widespread neoplasia, obstetric complications or bacteraemia also consumes both, but as these authors pointed out, compensatory increase in production may make detection difficult. Consumption of fibrinogen but not of platelets occurs when fibrinolysis is enhanced by urokinase infusions or snake bites. Perhaps most relevant to vasculitis, because it occurred in four such patients in their series, was the observation that platelet consumption without consumption of fibrinogen occurred from immune injury. This effect was also produced by prosthetic surfaces in surgery. Reversal is achieved by dipyridamole inhibition of platelet function or by adrenocortical steroids but not by anticoagulants. These authors also distinguished between platelet involvement alone in arterial disease and combined fibrin and platelet deposition in venous thrombosis.

References

Berman, H. J. (1964) Platelet agglutinability as a factor in hemostasis. *Bibliotheca Anatomica*, **4**, 736.
Branemark, P. I., Breine, U., Langer, L. & Skalak, R. (1972) Microvascular behaviour of platelets in man. *Thrombosis et Diathesis Haemorrhagica*, **51**, 182.
Cherry, G., Ryan, T. J. & Ellis, J. P. (1974) Decreased fibrinolysis in reperfused ischaemic tissue. *Thrombosis et Diathesis Haemorrhagica*, **32**, 659.
Cliff, W. J. (1966) The acute inflammatory reaction in the rabbit ear chamber with particular reference to the phenomena of leukocyte migration. *Journal of Experimental Medicine*, **124**, 543.
Colman, R. W., Robboy, S. J. & Minna, J. D. (1972) Disseminated intravascular coagulation (D.I.C.). An approach. *American Journal of Medicine*, **52**, 679.
Colman, R. W., Braun, W. E., Busch, G. I., Dammin, G. J. & Merrill, J. P. (1969) Coagulation studies in hyperacute and other forms of renal allograft rejection. *New England Journal of Medicine*, **281**, 685.
Colman, R. W., Girey, G., Galvanek, E. G. & Busch, G. (1972) Human renal allografts: the protective effects of heparin, kallikrein activation and fibrinolysis during hyperacute rejection. In *Coagulation Problems in Transplanted Organs* (Ed.) Von Kaulla, K. N. p. 87. Springfield, Illinois: Charles C. Thomas.

Evenses, J. A. & Jeremic, M. (1970) Platelets and the triggering mechanism of intravascular coagulation. *British Journal of Haematology,* **19,** 33.

Fiddes, P. J. & Penny, R. (1970) Fibrin degradation products in thrombotic thrombocytopenic purpura. *Australian Annals of Medicine,* **4,** 350.

Frick, P. G. (1969) Primary thrombocythaemia. Clinical, haematological and chromosomal studies of thirteen patients. *Helvetica Medica Acta,* **35,** 20.

Harker, L. A. & Slichter, S. J. (1972) Platelet and fibrinogen consumption in man. *New England Journal of Medicine,* **287,** 999.

Kwaan, H. C., Gallo, G., Potter, E., Cutting, H. & Stanzler, R. (1968) The nature of the vascular lesion in thrombotic thrombocytopenic purpura. *Annals of Internal Medicine,* **68,** 1169.

Lerner, R. G., Rapaport, S. I. & Meltzer, J. (1967) Thrombotic thrombocytopenic purpura, serial clotting studies, relation to the generalised Shwartzman reaction and remission after adrenal steroid and dextran therapy. *Annals of Internal Medicine,* **68,** 1180.

Neame, P. B. (1973) Disseminated intravascular platelet aggregation and thrombotic thrombocytopenic purpura. *Lancet,* **ii,** 1320.

Starzl, T. E., Boehmig, H. J., Amemiya, H., Wilson, C. B., Dixon, F. J., Giles, G. R., Simpson, K. M. & Halgrimson, C. G. (1970) Clotting changes, including disseminated intravascular coagulation during rapid renal homograft rejection. *New England Journal of Medicine,* **283,** 383.

Umlas, J. & Kaiser, J. (1970) Thombolytic thrombocytopenic purpura (T.T.P.) a disease or syndrome? *American Journal of Medicine,* **49,** 723.

FIBRINOLYSIS

Some investigators (Copley et al, 1959; Illig, 1961; Muller, 1969; Todd, 1971; Todd, 1973) have held a concept of an oscillating balance between fibrin deposition and fibrinolysis such that blood vessels tend to be lined with fibrin, which is, however, continuously being removed. Indeed, the endothelial cell does secrete an activator of fibrinolysis (Todd, 1959; Pandolfi, 1970), so that plasminogen carried in the blood-stream with fibrinogen is activated to form its plasmin. Moreover the lysed component of fibrin contributes to the slippery surface of the blood vessel and thereby promotes flow. However, this concept of continuing haemostasis and continuous intravascular clotting is not accepted by all authors (Hjort, 1966). Experimental injury of the vessel wall encourages fibrin deposition and this is enhanced not only by infusions of thrombin but equally by infusions of inhibitors of fibrinolysis. In experiments on dog mesentery, fibrin deposition was depressed by depleting coagulation factors or by the topical application of urokinase (Guest, Bond and Crawford, 1973).

Locally in the tissues, there are also varying degrees of activation and inhibition both of clotting and of fibrinolysis. The results of various studies in the author's laboratory have emphasised the role of inhibitors of fibrinolysis released by damaged epidermis. The epidermis contains a soluble and probably freely diffusible agent that inhibits fibrinolysis in vitro (Table 10.2) (Nishioka and Ryan, 1971). In vivo damage to the epidermis by stripping with cellotape (Turner, Kurban and Ryan, 1969), or by short wave ultraviolet irradiation (Grice, Ryan and Magnus, 1970) is associated with decreased fibrinolysis in the upper dermis.

Any consideration of small vessel pathology must take into account the complex interaction between the vessel and the tissue it supplies (Ryan, 1973). In this respect epithelial and endothelial control of fibrin deposition and fibrinolysis may be important. There can be no doubt that fibrinolytic agents and their inhibitors diffuse widely around the vessels of the upper dermis and the amount of fibrin lying there must depend on the contribution of such agents by all the cells in the neighbourhood.

Table 10.2. Semiquantitative inhibitory activity of subcellular fraction.

Fraction	Inhibitory activity
Heavy mitochondria	×2
Light mitochondria	×1
Microsome	×2
Soluble	>×128

Fractions obtained by homogenisation and centrifugation of epidermis were used to inhibit urokinase on a fibrin plate. Strong inhibition was obtained in the soluble fraction.

The possible role of long-chain fatty acids in coagulation has been mentioned above. Ogston, Ogston and Ratnof (1969) have shown that their presence in sebum is responsible for surface activation of clotting, and Dawber, Nishioka and Ryan (1971) discussed their role as activators of fibrinolysis (Figure 10.9).

In vasculitis fibrin is deposited and fibrinolysis is impaired. This can be seen in Table 10.3 which lists fibrin deposition and vascular fibrinolytic activity as estimated in selected inflammatory skin disorders in a study of the roles of the coagulation and the fibrinolytic systems in inflammation. Immunofluorescence with anti-fibrin and anti-fibrinogen conjugates and Todd's technique of fibrinolysis autography were performed on frozen biopsies. Fibrin deposits and fibrinolytic activity were graded 0 to 4+. The results shown in this table demonstrate that fibrin deposition and loss of fibrinolytic activity are common to the inflammatory processes in a number of diseases of the skin. Turner, Kurban and Ryan first reported this at a combined meeting of the British Microcirculation Society and the Dowling Club (Dermatology) in 1970 and their

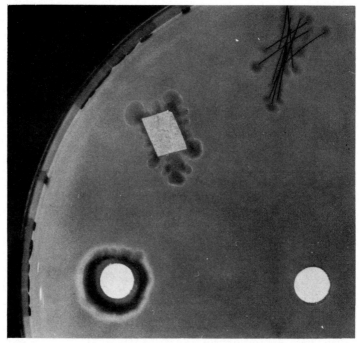

Figure 10.9. Fibrin plate lysed by sebum and its ingredients. Top: cut scalp hairs. Centre: paper after application to forehead. Lower left: paper impregnated with fatty acid fraction of sebum. Lower right: control paper.

Table 10.3. Fibrin deposition and vascular fibrinolytic activity in inflammatory dermatoses (for explanation see text).

Diagnosis	No.	Fibrin			Fibrinolytic activity		
		0	1—2+	3—4+	0	1—2+	3—4+
Normal	15	15	0	0	0	0	15
Vasculitis	35	1	7	27	21	1	3
Lupus erythematosus	12	0	3	9	8	4	0
Lichen planus	4	0	0	4	3	1	0
Bullous pemphigoid	8	0	0	8	6	2	0
Dermatitis herpetiformis	5	0	2	3	3	2	0
Erythema multiforme	6	1	3	2	3	3	0

published results (Ryan, Nishioka and Dawber, 1971) and those more detailed and controlled studies of Cunliffe et al (1971) together with independent studies by Isacson et al (1970) and Parish (1972) confirm this observation (reviewed by Cunliffe, 1976).

Pandolfi, Isacson and Nilsson (1969) observed low fibrinolytic activity in the walls of veins in patients with thrombosis. Furthermore, the vessels of persons predisposed to vasculitis have decreased amounts of activator even in areas unaffected by pathology. Thrombotic complications in patients with ulcerative colitis are more frequent in those with decreased fibrinolytic activity (Swan, Williams and Cooke, 1970). Nilsson et al (1961) reported a 28-year-old man with widespread thrombosis of most veins in whom an inhibitor of fibrinolysis was present in excess, and Brodthagen et al (1968) described a patient with widespread vasculitis who had a similar inhibitor (Figure 10.10). The

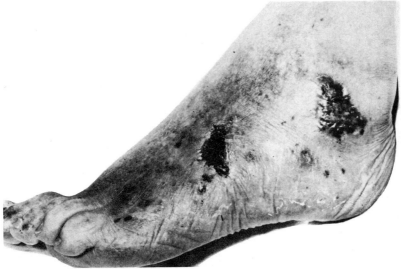

Figure 10.10. Necrosis of skin in a patient with DIC ascribed to an inhibitor of fibrinolysis. The exposed areas such as the ear and nose were particularly affected. See also Figures 4.29a, 9.7, 14.5a, 15.2, and 15.16.

therapeutic use of inhibitors of fibrinolysis such as ε-aminocaproic acid (EACA) also may occasionally produce a widespread thrombotic state (Naeye, 1962; Charytan and Purtilo, 1969; Rowell, 1974) or a disastrous local thrombosis (Colman, Robboy and Minna, 1972). Moreover, DIC occurs more readily in animals treated with EACA than in man (Margaretten et al, 1964) and small injuries in the femoral veins of rats develop fibrin only if inhibitors of fibrinolysis are administered (Ashford and Frieman, 1968).

The endothelial cell synthesises both plasminogen activator and Factor VIII (Bloom, Giddings and Wilks, 1973; Jaffe, Hoyee and Nachman, 1973; Hoyer, De Los Santos and Hoyer, 1973). Injury to endothelium releases these agents into the circulation. It has been suggested by Ekberg and Nilsson (1975), Ekberg, Nilsson and Linell (1975) and by Todd (personal communication, 1975) that the levels of these agents in the blood may be of prognostic value. They indicate not only the intensity of the injury but the degree of exhaustion of the endothelial cell. Serial daily estimations of blood levels of such agents indicate exhaustion prior to attacks of disease, as for instance in Behçet's disease (Suguira and Saito, 1974).

In sickle cell disease vasculitis may also be partly dependent on impairment of fibrinolysis (Green, Kwaan and Ruiz, 1970) and the same has been said of vasculitis of the lepromatous form of leprosy (Myers, 1969; Ryan, Nishioka and Dawber, 1971). Six of the biopsies from erythema nodosum leprosum reported by Wemambu et al (1969) were also examined for fibrinolytic activity; five failed to show any but they had heavy deposits of IgG and complement; one case showed only slight depression and no deposits of complement or IgG.

In Behçet's disease venous thrombosis has been reported secondary to impaired fibrinolysis, and stimulants of fibrinolysis are advocated as therapy. As indicated in Chapter 13, there is a case for widening the spectrum of Behçet's syndrome to include a disease in which venous thrombosis is the only significant finding. In such patients, fibrinolysis is impaired (Brakman, Mohler and Astrup, 1966). This is in contrast to the findings in the bleeding disease hereditary haemorrhagic telangiectasia, in which fibrinolysis is locally increased and in which inhibitors of fibrinolysis are therapeutically helpful (Kwaan and Silverman, 1973) (Figure 10.11).

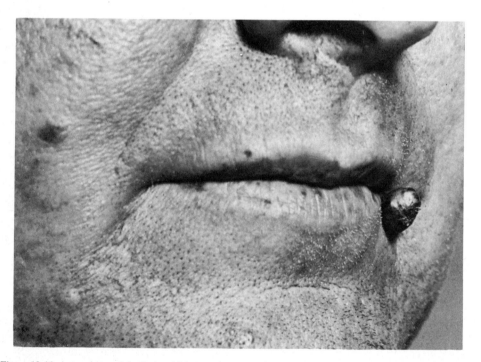

Figure 10.11. An angioma of the lip in which greatly increased fibrinolytic activity could be demonstrated. The patient had hereditary haemorrhagic telangiectasia.

The debate about the role of fibrinolysis in diseases such as the respiratory distress syndrome is of interest. Some authors have expressed their belief that impaired fibrinolysis is responsible for this disease, while others have disagreed with this view. Margolis, Orzalesi and Schwartz (1973) could find conclusive evidence of coagulation in only two out of 11 cases and even in these two, fibrin degradation products were present in normal amounts. Ekelund et al (1973) found normal or increased fibrinolysis in the lungs of babies in whom there clearly was fibrin deposition. Thus, skin is not the only organ to provoke a debate about the exact relationship between fibrin deposition and fibrinolysis.

The phenomenon of bleeding in coagulation disorders is particularly difficult to assess. Systemic or local consumption of coagulation factors may result in bleeding; but excessive fibrinolysis may do the same, in which case fibrin would not be much in evidence. Thus, Ruiter (1964) observed that where local haemorrhage predominates, fibrinoid was less distinct and often absent, and Haustein (1969) described a case of 'vasculitis allergica Ruiter' in which purpura seemed to be caused by increased fibrinolytic activity in the blood and could be controlled by an antifibrinolytic agent. Excessive fibrinolysis occurs in a number of conditions (Table 10.4).

Table 10.4. Conditions associated with excessive fibrinolysis.

1. Malignancy such as carcinoma of the prostate
   (Tagnon et al, 1953; Brown, Campbell and Thompson, 1962)
   Carcinoma of the pancreas
   (Ratnoff, 1952)
   Giant cell carcinoma of the lung, or Hodgkin's disease (Davidson et al, 1969)
2. Polycythaemia, leukaemia
   (Mikata et al, 1959; Brown, Campbell and Thompson, 1962)
3. Cirrhosis of the liver
   (Grossi, Moreno and Rousselot, 1961; Fletcher et al, 1964)
4. Shock (Weiner, Reid and Roby, 1950; Reid, Weiner and Roby, 1953;
   Hodgkinson and Luzadre, 1954)
5. Mental and physical stress
   (Sherry et al, 1959; Sawyer et al, 1960; Schneck and Van Kaulla, 1961).
6. Acute urticaria (Braun, Nitzschner and Peschel, 1970; Ryan, Nishioka and Dawber, 1971)
7. Haemorrhagic vasculitis (Haustein, 1969)

In Chapters 3 and 4 is discussed a spectrum of pathology in which urticaria, vasculitis and coagulation are seen to overlap. Two important factors influencing this spectrum are blood flow and fibrinolysis. In urticaria, fibrinolysis is thought to be increased, although for various reasons this is difficult to prove (Braun, Nitzschner and Peschel, 1970; Ryan, Nishioka and Dawber, 1971). In vasculitis, however, injury to the endothelial cell and its subsequent necrosis lead to impaired fibrinolysis. Because coagulation impairs fibrinolysis, while blood stasis modifies the pathology and in particular reduces the immigration of white cells to the site, it can be seen that in any one patient the vasculitis may at various times be more urticarial, more fibrinolytic and more haemorrhagic, or alternatively be more thrombotic, less fibrinolytic and less cellular.

The mast cell is an important determinant of the site involved and of the position of the pathology within the spectrum, since histamine and heparin promote diffusion of fibrinolytic activators and blood contents through the tissues. In this way a more urticarial and less thrombotic reaction is encouraged, and tissues such as the upper dermis that are rich in coagulation activators and fibrinolytic inhibitors are flooded with agents that prevent fibrin deposition.

McKay (1973) suggested that impaired fibrinolysis, reticuloendothelial paralysis and arterial vasoconstriction due to catecholamines are the three most important changes in the tissues that 'prepare' the microvasculature so that minor injury, by causing thrombosis, results in severe pathology. One need look no further than this for an explanation of most cases of vasculitis and for an explanation of diseases associated with vasculitis, particularly those described in Chapter 13. The concept of generalised and localised forms of coagulation parallels that of the Shwartzman phenomenon, and McKay's observations on this reaction are particularly relevant.

References

Ashford, T. P. & Frieman, D. G. (1968) Platelet aggregation at sites of minimal endothelial injury. *American Journal of Pathology,* **53,** 599.

Bloom, A. L., Giddings, J. C. & Wilks, C. J. (1973) Factor 8 on the vascular intima; possible importance in haemostasis and thrombosis. *Nature, New Biology,* **241,** 217.

Brakman, P., Mohler, E. & Astrup, T. (1966) A group of patients with impaired plasma fibrinolytic system and selective inhibition of tissue activator induced fibrinolysis. *Scandinavian Journal of Haematology,* **3,** 389.

Braun, H., Nitzschner, H. & Peschel, H. (1970) Fibrinolyse untersuchungen bei chronisch rezidivierender urtikaria mit niedrigem fibrinogen spiegel. *Zeitschrift für Haut und Geschlectskrankheiten underen Grenzgebiete,* **45,** 761.

Brodthagen, H., Larsen, V., Brockner, J. & Amris, C. J. (1968) Cutaneous manifestations in capillary dilatation and endovascular fibrin deposits. *Acta Dermato-venereologica,* **48,** 277.

Brown, R. C., Campbell, D. C. & Thompson, J. H. (1962) Increased fibrinolysin with malignant disease. *Archives of Internal Medicine,* **109,** 201.

Charytan, C. & Purtilo, D. (1969) Glomerular capillary thrombosis and acute renal failure after epsilon aminocaproic acid therapy. *New England Journal of Medicine,* **280,** 1102.

Colman, R. W., Robboy, S. J. & Minna, J. D. (1972) Disseminated intravascular coagulation (D.I.C.). An approach. *American Journal of Medicine,* **52,** 679.

Copley, A. L., Steichele, D., Spradau, M. & Thorley, R. S. (1959) Anti-coagulant action of fibrin surfaces on mammalian blood. *Nature,* **183,** 683.

Cunliffe, W. J. (1976) Fibrinolysis and cutaneous vasculitis. *Clinical and Experimental Dermatology,* **1,** 1.

Cunliffe, W. J., Dodman, B., Holmes, R. L. & Forster, R. A. (1971) Local fibrinolytic activity in patients with cutaneous vasculitis. *British Journal of Dermatology,* **84,** 420.

Davidson, J. F., McNicol, G. P., Frank, G. L., Anderson, T. J. & Douglas, A. (1969) Plasminogen activator-producing tumour. *British Medical Journal,* **i,** 88.

Dawber, R. P. R., Nishioka, K. & Ryan, T. J. (1971) Fibrinolytic activity of skin surface lipids. *Lancet,* **i,** 193.

Ekberg, M. & Nilsson, I. M. (1975) Factor VIII and glomerulonephritis. *Lancet,* **i,** 1111.

Ekberg, M. R., Nilsson, I. M. & Linell, F. (1975) Significance of increased factor VIII in early glomerulo-nephritis. *Annals of Internal Medicine,* **83,** 337.

Ekelund, H., Pandolfi, M., Ostberg, G. & Bjernstad, A. (1973) Fibrinolytic activity in the lung tissue from neonates with hyaline membrane disease. *Acta Paediatrica Scandinavica,* **62,** 149.

Fletcher, A. P., Bierderman, O., Moore, D., Alkjaersig, N. & Sherry, S. (1964) Abnormal plasminogen—plasmin system activity (fibrinolysis) in patients with hepatic cirrhosis; its cause and consequences. *Journal of Clinical Investigation,* **43,** 681.

Green, D., Kwaan, H. C. & Ruiz, G. (1970) Impaired fibrinolysis in sickle cell disease. *Thrombosis et Diathesis Haemorrhagica,* **24,** 10.

Grice, K., Ryan, T. J. & Magnus, I. A. (1970) Fibrinolytic activity in lesions produced by monochromatic ultraviolet irradiation in various photodermatoses. *British Journal of Dermatology,* **83,** 637.

Grossi, D. E., Moreno, A. H. & Rousselot, L. M. (1961) Studies on spontaneous fibrinolytic activity in patients with cirrhosis of the liver and its inhibition by epsilon aminocaproic acid. *Annals of Surgery,* **153,** 383.

Guest, M. M., Bond, T. P. & Crawford, M. A. (1973) A possible role of leucocytes in hemostasis. *Bibliographia Anatomique,* **12,** 131.

Haustein, U. F. (1969) Purpura hyperfibrinolytica als pathogenetisches prinzipeines haemorrhagieschen mikrobides miescher. *Dermatologische Monatsschrift,* **155,** 771.

Hjort, P. F. (1966) Continuous hemostasis and continuous intravascular clotting. Fact or myth. *Thrombosis et Diathesis Haemorrhagica,* **20,** 15.

Hodgkinson, C. F. & Luzadre, J. H. (1954) Etiology and management of hypofibrinogenemia of pregnancy. *Journal of the American Medical Association*, **154**, 557.

Hoyer, L. W., De Los Santos, R. P. & Hoyer, J. R. (1973) Antihemophilic factor antigen. Localization in endothelial cells by immunofluorescent microscopy. *Journal of Clinical Investigation*, **52**, 2737.

Illig, L. (1961) *Die Terminale Strombahn*. Berlin: Springer Verlag.

Isacson, S., Linell, F., Moller, H. & Nilsson, I. M. (1970) Coagulation and fibrinolysis in chronic panniculitis. *Acta Dermato-venereologica*, **50**, 213.

Jaffe, E. A., Hoyee, L. W. & Nachman, R. L. (1973) Synthesis of antihaemophilic factor antigen by cultured human endothelial cells. *Journal of Clinical Investigation*, **52**, 2757.

Kwaan, H. C. & Silverman, S. (1973) Fibrinolytic activity in lesions of hereditary haemorrhagic telangiectasia. *Archives of Dermatology*, **107**, 571.

Margaretten, W., Csavossy, I. & McKay, D. G. (1967) An electron microscopic study of thrombosis induced disseminated intravascular coagulation. *Blood*, **29**, 169.

Margaretten, W., Zunker, H. O. & McKay, D. G. (1964) Production of the generalised Shwartzman reaction in pregnant rats by intravenous infusion of thrombin. *Laboratory Investigation*, **13**, 552.

Margolis, C. Z., Orzalesi, M. M. & Schwartz, A. D. (1973) Disseminated intravascular coagulation in the respiratory distress syndrome. *American Journal of Diseases of Children*, **125**, 344.

McKay, D. G. (1973) Vessel wall and thrombogenesis endotoxin. *Thrombosis et Diathesis Haemorrhagica*, **29**, 11.

Mikata, I., Hasegawa, M., Igarashi, T., Shirakura, N. & Hoshida, M. (1959) Plasmin in haemorrhagic blood diseases. *Keio Journal of Medicine*, **8**, 279.

Myers, W. M. (1969) Impairment of plasma fibrinolytic activity in leprosy patients. *International Journal of Leprosy*, **37**, 343.

Naeye, R. L. (1962) Thrombotic state after haemorrhagic diathesis: possible complications of therapy with epsilon amino caproic acid. *Blood*, **19**, 697.

Nilsson, I. M., Krook, H., Sternby, N. H., Soederberg, E. & Doederstrom, N. (1961) Severe thrombotic disease in a young man with bone marrow and skeletal changes with a high content of an inhibitor of the fibrinolytic system. *Acta Medica Scandinavica*, **169**, 323.

Nishioka, K. & Ryan, T. J. (1971) Inhibitors and proactivators of fibrinolysis in human epidermis. *British Journal of Dermatology*, **85**, 561.

Ogston, D., Ogston, C. M. & Ratnoff, O. D. (1969) Studies on clot promoting activity of skin. *Journal of Laboratory and Clinical Medicine*, **73**, 70.

Pandolfi, M. (1970) Persistence of fibrinolytic activity in fragments of human veins cultured in vitro. *Thrombosis et Diathesis Haemorrhagica*, **24**, 43.

Pandolfi, M., Isacson, S. & Nilsson, I. M. (1969) Low fibrinolytic activity in the walls of veins in patients with thrombosis. *Acta Medica Scandinavica*, **186**, 1.

Parish, W. E. (1972) Cutaneous vasculitis: antigen—antibody complexes and prolonged fibrinolysis. *Proceedings of the Royal Society of Medicine*, **65**, 276.

Ratnoff, O. D. (1952) Studies on a proteolytic enzyme in human plasma. VII. A fatal haemorrhagic state associated with excessive plasma proteolytic activity in a patient undergoing surgery for carcinoma of the head of the pancreas. *Journal of Clinical Investigation*, **31**, 521.

Reid, D. C., Weiner, A. E. & Roby, C. C. (1953) Intravascular clotting and afibrinogenaemia. Presumptive lethal factors in syndrome of amniotic fluid embolism. *American Journal of Obstetrics and Gynecology*, **66**, 564.

Ruiter, M. (1964) Arteriolitis (vasculitis) 'allergic' cutis (superficialis). A new dermatological concept. *Dermatologica*, **129**, 217.

Ryan, T. J. (1973) In *Physiology and Pathophysiology of the Skin* (Ed.) Jarrett, A. London: Academic Press.

Ryan, T. J., Nishioka, K. & Dawber, R. P. R. (1971) Epithelial—endothelial interactions in the control of inflammation through fibrinolysis. *British Journal of Dermatology*, **84**, 501.

Sawyer, W. D., Fletcher, A. P., Alkjaersig, N. & Sherry, S. (1960) Studies on the thrombolytic activity of human plasma. *Journal of Clinical Investigation*, **39**, 426.

Schneck, S. A. & Van Kaulla, K. N. (1961) Fibrinolysis and the nervous system. *Neurology*, **11**, 959.

Sherry, S., Lindemeyer, R. I., Fletcher, A. P. & Alkjaersig, N. (1959) Studies on enhanced fibrinolytic activity in man. *Journal of Clinical Investigation*, **88**, 810.

Sugiura, S. & Saito, K. (1974) Fibrinolytic activity in Behçet's disease. *Japanese Journal of Ophthalmology*, **18**, 275.

Swan, C. H., Williams, J. A. & Cooke, W. T. (1970) Fibrinolysis in colonic diseases. *Gut*, **11**, 588.

Tagnon, H. J., Whitmore, W. F. Jr, Schulman, P. & Kravitz, S. C. (1953) Significance of fibrinolysis occurring in patients with metastatic cancer of the prostate. *Cancer*, **6**, 63.

Todd, A. S. (1959) The histological localisation of fibrinolysin activator. *Journal of Pathology and Bacteriology*, **78**, 281.

Todd, A. S. (1971) Endothelial fibrinolysis and blood flow. *Lancet*, **i**, 1179.

Todd, A. S. (1973) Endothelium and fibrinolysis. *Bibliographia Anatomique*, **12**, 98.

Turner, R. H. (1969) The fibrinolytic system in human skin. *Biorheology*, **6**, 258.

Turner, R. H., Kurban, A. D. & Ryan, T. J. (1969) Fibrinolytic activity in human skin following epidermal injury. *Journal of Investigative Dermatology,* **53,** 458.

Weiner, A. E., Reid, D. C. & Roby, C. C. (1950) Coagulation defects associated with premature separation of normally implanted placenta. *American Journal of Obstetrics and Gynecology,* **60,** 379.

Wemambu, S. N. C., Turk, J. L., Waters, M. F. R. & Rees, R. J. W. (1969) Erythema nodosum leprosum: a clinical manifestation of the Arthus phenomenon. *Lancet,* **ii,** 933.

THE SHWARTZMAN REACTION (McKAY, 1965, 1973)

The local Shwartzman reaction

Shwartzman (1931) produced his reaction in the skin by an intracutaneous injection of bacterial endotoxin, followed 24 hours later by an intravenous injection of the same bacterial endotoxin. The reaction is morphologically similar to the Arthus reaction with haemorrhagic necrosis at the prepared skin site. The first injection of endotoxin into the skin produces a mild local inflammation with dilatation of capillaries and venules and the accumulation of polymorphonuclear leucocytes in and around the vessels. In control animals, this reaction subsides during the next three days. When an intravenous injection of the same bacterial product is given, however, an enhanced inflammatory reaction develops at the site of the first injection. The initial change is the appearance of slight swelling and purpura which enlarges and coalesces to produce a black haemorrhagic necrotic lesion reaching its largest size three to six hours after the intravenous injection. In the local reaction the intradermal injection is referred to as 'preparatory', and the intravenous injection as 'provocative'.

The preparatory injection leads to diapedesis of polymorphonuclear leucocytes resulting in a large perivascular accumulation of these cells (Stetson, 1952). Within one hour after the provocative injection is given, many of the vessels in the prepared skin site show occlusion of their lumens by masses of leucocytes and platelets, a relatively nonspecific inflammatory process. As is so often the case in vasculitis, capillaries and venules show this occlusive cellular mass, while arteries and arterioles are generally not involved. Necrosis of the occluded vessels follows within one or two hours, probably from ischaemia and from the release of lysosomes from the neutrophils. The final stage includes the deposition of fibrin in the vessel lumen and the extravasation of red blood cells from the damaged vessels — these account for the haemorrhagic character of the lesion. The importance of intravascular coagulation in this reaction is demonstrated by the fact that it can be prevented by heparinising the animal just prior to the provocative injection (Cluff and Berthrong, 1953) or by the use of warfarin (Muller-Berghaus and Schneberger, 1971). Identical pathology can be induced by a combination of thrombin infusion at the same time as inhibition of fibrinolysis by ε-amino-caproic acid (Margaretten, Csavossy and McKay, 1967).

To a limited extent, antigen—antibody complexes can substitute for bacterial endotoxin in producing the local Shwartzman reaction. In hypersensitive rabbits, intravenous injection of the antigen, after local preparation of the skin with endotoxin, produces the reaction (Stetson, 1951; Schlang, 1952). Antigen—antibody complexes can also be used as substitutes for bacterial endotoxin for the provocative intravenous injection in producing the local Shwartzman reaction (Shwartzman, 1931, 1937). It is of interest to note that antigen—antibody complexes will not substitute for the preparing injection at the skin site. In these experiments the antigen—antibody complex is able to exert its effect only through its ability to induce disseminated intravascular coagulation.

The generalised Shwartzman reaction

McKay (1973) wrote: "Perhaps the best illustration of the ability of the antigen—antibody complex to induce disseminated intravascular clotting comes from those special instances where it induces the generalised Shwartzman reaction. As with the local, the generalised reaction is ordinarily produced by two properly spaced injections of bacterial endotoxin, with the one difference being that both injections are given intravenously. Following the first injection fibrin thrombi appear in the capillary vessels of the lungs, liver and spleen. After the second injection an increased number of thrombi appear in these organs and in addition in the renal glomerular capillaries (McKay and Shapiro, 1958). If the animal survives it often exhibits bilateral renal cortical necrosis. 'Blockade' of the reticuloendothelial system (RES) is induced by the first injection, and 'blockade' of the RES by such diverse substances as cortisone acetate, thorium dioxide suspension (Thorotrast), and trypan blue will take the place of the first injection. In these latter experiments only the provocative injection is required to produce the renal lesion. The physiological state of pregnancy is also preparatory and by some means other than reticuloendothelial blockade (McKay, 1963). In essence this reaction is composed of two episodes of disseminated intravascular coagulation. In this case 'blockade' signifies a reduced phagocytic capacity to remove particulate matter, colloidal substances and certain endogenous materials from the circulating blood. Among the endogenous materials removed by the RES, particularly the Kupffer cells of the liver, are certain of the active coagulation factors including tissue thromboplastin and active Factors IX and XI."

The major consequence of the blockade of the mononuclear phagocytic system is the alteration it produces when the second injection of endotoxin is given. The reduced phagocytic capacity allows an increased amount of the active coagulation factors to circulate for a longer period of time and, in effect, increases the amount of clotting induced by the second dose of endotoxin.

The first evidence that antigen—antibody complexes could substitute for bacterial endotoxin in this reaction came from the studies of McCluskey et al (1960). Intravenous administration of soluble antigen—antibody complexes into mice resulted in a transient glomerulonephritis. Because of its known anti-inflammatory effect, cortisone acetate was given in high doses in order to modify the severity of the glomerulonephritis. The cortisone acetate diminished the severity of the nephritis, but in addition, in four or five mice that received cortisone and complexes and were sacrificed one day later, there was a striking accumulation of amorphous eosinophilic material filling many glomerular capillary loops. This material stained with Weigert's fibrin stain and stained blue with Mallory's phosphotungstic acid haematoxylin (PTAH). Smaller amounts of the material were found in two of the mice from the same group killed four days after treatment, and similar material was occasionally found in small amounts in animals given complexes alone and sacrificed shortly after the last injection. The history of the glomerular deposits, the known clot-promoting effect of soluble antigen—antibody complexes, and the known ability of cortisone to 'prepare' for the generalised Shwartzman reaction leave little doubt that this phenomenon was present in these animals.

This has been further explored in the rabbit by Lee (1963). The intravenous injection of antigen into specifically immunised rabbits or the infusion of soluble antigen—antibody complexes produced the generalised Shwartzman reaction only when the rabbits' reticuloendothelial systems were 'blockaded'. The prior administration of heparin prevented the appearance of the glomerular thrombi. Cryofibrinogen appeared in the plasma after the administration of antigen—antibody complex.

In summary, antigen—antibody complexes shorten the coagulation time of blood and plasma in vitro, and induce the thrombi characteristic of the Arthus, the local, and the generalised Shwartzman reactions. Thus, under these conditions in experimental animals they are capable of inducing disseminated intravascular coagulation as well as local thrombosis, and, in their basic effects on the haemostatic mechanism, antigen—antibody complexes (in excess of antigen) bear a close resemblance to bacterial endotoxin. Local factors such as impaired fibrinogen or stasis which increase the tendency for fibrin to be formed or to persist, account for many aspects of this phenomenon. Essentially, the generalised Shwartzman reaction is a result of two minor episodes of acute inflammation in the microcirculation resulting in thrombosis. Vasculitis has most of the features ascribed to this reaction (Copeman, 1970).

The prepared state of the vasculature in the Shwartzman phenomenon is the same as that observed in the 'anatomy of stasis' described by Cherry and by Kanan in Chapters 5 and 9 on skin flaps and the nose. It is a state of partial reticuloendothelial blockade, impaired fibrinolysis and increased sensitivity of contractile protein to catecholamines.

If one regards most vasculitis as venulitis (Copeman, 1975) and the Shwartzman phenomenon as a mechanism underlying it, then like Copeman, one soon achieves a simplified view of the numerous morphological diseases described in the literature. Venulitis is one disease; it is a consequence of the anatomy of stasis and hence it is a product of those factors which contribute to the preparation for and provocation of venular injury. In considering chronic intravascular coagulation syndromes one may not be able to make a distinction between a generalised or localised process especially if the picture is incomplete and falls short of gross fibrin deposition. It is likely that such chronicity occurs almost as a regular feature in certain sites such as the nose or the coiled papillary vessels of the lower leg in atrophie blanche. These are preparatory in the same sense as pregnancy is preparatory.

References

Chapman, L. F., Goodell, H. & Wolffe, H. G. (1959) Changes in tissue vulnerability induced during hypnotic suggestions. *Journal of Psychosomatic Research,* **4,** 99.
Cluff, L. E. & Berthrong, M. (1953) Inhibition of local Shwartzman reaction by heparin. *Bulletin of the Johns Hopkins Hospital,* **92,** 353.
Copeman, P. W. M. (1970) Investigations into the pathogenesis of acute leukaemia antigen. *British Journal of Dermatology,* **82** (Supplement 5), 2.
Copeman, P. W. M. (1975) Cutaneous angiitis. *Journal of the Royal College of Physicians,* **9,** 103.
Lee, L. (1963) Antigen antibody reactions in pathogenesis of bacterial renal cortical necrosis. *Journal of Experimental Medicine,* **117,** 365.
Margaretten, W., Csavossy, I. & McKay, D. G. (1967) An electron microscope study of thrombosis induced disseminated intravascular coagulation. *Blood,* **29,** 169.
McCluskey, R. T., Benacerr, A. F. B., Potter, J. L. & Miller, F. (1960) Pathologic effects of intravenously administered soluble antigen-antibody complexes. I. Passive serum sickness in mice. *Journal of Experimental Medicine,* **111,** 181.
McKay, D. G. (1963) A partial synthesis of generalized Shwartzman reaction. *Federation Proceedings,* **22,** 1373.
McKay, D. G. (1965) *Disseminated Intravascular Coagulation. An Intermediary of Disease.* New York: Hoebner Medical Division, Harper and Row.
McKay, D. G. (1973) Vessel wall and thrombogenesis endotoxin. *Thrombosis et Diathesis Haemorrhagica,* **29,** 11.
McKay, D. G. & Shapiro, S. S. (1958) Alterations in blood coagulation system induced by bacterial endotoxin. II. In vivo (generalized Shwartzman reaction). *Journal of Experimental Medicine,* **107,** 353.
Muller-Berghaus, G. & Schneberger, R. (1971) Hageman factor activation in the generalised Shwartzman reaction induced by endotoxin. *British Journal of Haematology,* **21,** 513.
Schlang, H. A. (1952) Shwartzman phenomenon. II. Suppressive action of nitrogen mustard on antigen-antibody provocation. *Proceedings of the Society for Experimental Biology and Medicine,* **79,** 639.
Shwartzman, G. (1931) Phenomenon of local skin reactivity to serum precipitates. *Proceedings of the Society for Experimental Biology and Medicine,* **29,** 193.

Shwartzman, G. (1937) Phenomenon of local skin reactivity to bacterial filtrates: its relation to anaphyla-
toxins, Forssman antibodies and serum toxicity. *Journal of Infectious Diseases,* **61,** 293.
Stetson, C. A. Jr (1951) Studies on mechanism of Shwartzman phenomenon: similarities between reactions to
endotoxins and certain reactions of bacterial allergy. *Journal of Experimental Medicine,* **94,** 521.
Stetson, C. A. Jr (1952) Pathogenesis of Shwartzman and Arthus phenomena and their relation to human
'rheumatic fever'. In *Rheumatic Fever. A Symposium.* Minneapolis: University of Minnesota Press.

11. Psychosomatic Vasculitis

The role of the psyche in inflammation is not easy to measure, but clearly in some patients it is important. A patient reported by Ryan (1964) as having non-thrombocytopenic purpura with a leucocytoclastic histology is illustrated in Figures 11.1, 3.5 and 12.16. For some 15 years this woman was affected by a most disabling purpura with a pronounced urticarial element. It was always difficult to assess the relative effects of cold or shyness in this patient. Within a few minutes of exposure to the public's gaze, or while watching her accident-prone son disappear with wild acceleration in his new Jaguar car, weals would appear over most of her uncovered skin and, within half an hour, most of them would develop a purpuric centre. This patient produced a marked reaction when inoculated intradermally with her own platelets. The rapidity of onset of her rash brings to mind a patient who also showed sensitivity to cold and was described as purpura urticans by Forman (1953). This type of reaction, which at times is so obviously provoked by anxiety, is not far removed from that seen in psychogenic purpura or in the stigmatists. One such woman has recently caused much interest in Lisbon where, during the course of a Friday afternoon, she became pale and sweaty and at 5 p.m. exhibited spontaneous bleeding from the dorsa of her feet, even when wearing stockings, and a lesion on her forehead which clearly started as a spontaneous weal.

There are many variations on this theme and the stigmatists are merely examples of a pattern of reaction that can be induced by hypnosis or may occur in the hysteric with Charcot's oedême bleu; it also includes the psychogenic purpuras and autoerythrocyte sensitisation (known also as the painful bruising syndrome).

The best kept records of a stigmatist were those on Therése Neumann of Konnersreuth, Germany, who was the subject of a review by Klauder (1938) in which he separated the fraudulent artefact from the genuine eruption. Therése Neumann clearly was an hysteric and, as is the case in so many persons in this group, she had menstrual disturbances and spontaneous bleeding which in her case was from the stomach, eyes, skin and ears. She showed great concern about the suffering of others, a feature which is a characteristic not only of the saints but also of patients with the painful bruising syndrome. Klauder reported: "Soon after the appearance of stigmas she began having trances and ecstasies and at that time bloody tears first appeared; later new stigmas appeared over the heart and on the feet. On Nov. 6 1926, during ecstasy, bleeding appeared on the palms and the soles. In the beginning there was a constant but slow oozing of blood from the stigmas; later only some of them bled, and only on Friday, during the Passion of Holy Week was there bleeding from all stigmas.

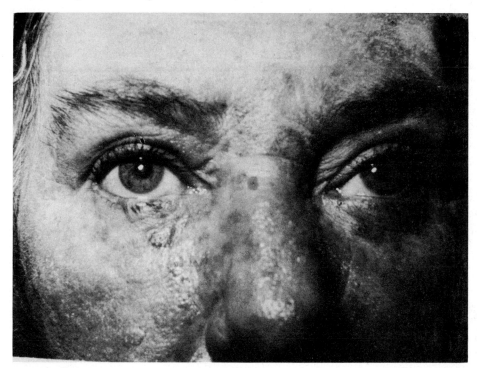

Figure 11.1. Purpura urticans provoked by anxiety. This patient is also illustrated in Figures 3.5 and 12.16.

As recorded by Ewald the stigmas were not penetrating wounds, although there was a subjective sensation of penetration. On the dorsa of the hands and the feet they were the size of a 10 pfennig piece and were slightly raised and presented a dark crust, despite the absence of bleeding for three months prior to the time of the examination. The crusts did not become detached and fall off. Their surfaces were dry and glazed. When blood oozed through the crust the appearance was that of a fresh clot of blood; at other times the colour was dark. Signs of inflammation were absent. The skin at the periphery of the crusts was thin and drawn in . . . Seidle, who witnessed bleeding of the stigmas, described the appearance of an oedematous elevation above the level of the skin, as though it had been separated from the upper epithelial layers of the skin. Through a magnifying glass serum was seen to appear in a manner comparable to the formation of a drop of perspiration. It became bloody and rolled away. When examined microscopically it was seen actually to be blood."

Dr Seidle also observed that during ecstasy Thérése Neumann's tears became bloody and that she also vomited blood. When Klauder examined her stigmas some nine years later, the one on the dorsum of her right hand was a flat dry dark clot. It was slightly elevated, was almost perfectly square with a mean diameter of about 1.5 cm, and had a dry and shiny surface which apparently had not been adherent to the fishnet glove that had just been removed. The skin around the clot was normal in colour, looked wrinkled and was firmly adherent to the clot. There was no evidence of inflammation, ulceration or destruction of tissue.

The frequency with which observers have watched spontaneous bleeding develop in the stigmatists makes external trauma unlikely. In patients with psychogenic purpura or painful bruising there is even less reason to postulate artefacts. Squareness and linearity is a feature of many other spontaneous lesions during their healing phase and is particularly common in infarcted lesions following vasculitis. It is not necessarily an indication of external injury as in dermatitis artefacta. Psychogenic purpura need not be confined to the upper dermis, for the author observed one boy who had a blue swollen foot and an intense desire to have it amputated; on biopsy extensive zosteriform vesiculation and haemorrhage were seen to extend through the full thickness of the skin (Figure 11.2).

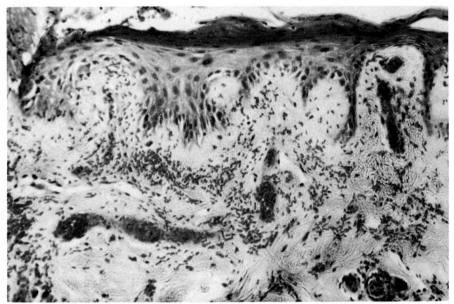

Figure 11.2. Haemorrhagic vasculitis in the skin of a blue and swollen foot (Charcot's oedême bleu) in a boy desiring amputation because of pain. Several explorations of his foot revealed no explanation of the pain.

Agle and Ratnoff (1962) made a psychiatric study of autoerythrocytic sensitisation which they entitled 'purpura as a psychosomatic entity'. Previously Gardner and Diamond (1955) had described a sensitivity to red cells and to erythrocyte stroma and had reported in such patients crops of ecchymoses, gastrointestinal bleeding, haematuria, abdominal pain and neurological abnormalities. Agle and Ratnoff described nine such patients all of whom also had menorrhagia, tingling and numbness of their extremities and face, as well as painful spontaneous bleeding (Table 11.1). Later they reported 27 'angry' women with psychogenic purpura, nine of whom did not react to intracutaneous testing (Ratnoff and Agle, 1968). They re-emphasised the severe anxiety experienced by these patients, the provocation by emotional stress and the fact that psychological factors may influence the site of the skin lesion and the positivity of skin tests. Further data on these patients are listed in Tables 11.2 to 11.10. Schindler (1929) also recorded 16 patients in whom hysteria and bleeding were related but the bleeding was incidental in most.

Table 11.1. Symptoms in nine cases of autoerythrocyte sensitisation.

Ecchymoses	9
Menorrhagia	9
Gastrointestinal bleeding	5
Epistaxis	3
Haematuria	3
Bleeding after surgical procedures	3
Tingling and numbness of extremities or face	8
Abdominal pain	6

Table 11.2. Haemorrhagic manifestations in autoerythrocyte sensitisation.

	Time of onset				
	Before purpura		After purpura		
	Skin test		Skin test		Total
	Pos.	Neg.	Pos.	Neg.	
Number of patients	18	9	18	9	27
Symptom					
Meno-metrorrhagia	8	4	4	5	21
Gastrointestinal bleeding[a]	4	1	10	2	17
Epistaxis	5	3	7	1	16
Haematuria	4	0	5	4	13
'Always bruised easily'	5	0	—	—	5
Haemoptysis[a]	0	0	3	1	4
Bleeding after minor surgery	1	1	1	1	4
Gingival bleeding	0	2	0	1	3

[a]Nearly always minor in character.

Table 11.3. 'Neurologic' manifestations in autoerythrocyte sensitisation.

	Time of onset				
	Before purpura		After purpura		
	Skin test		Skin test		Total
	Pos.	Neg.	Pos.	Neg.	
Number of patients	18	9	18	9	27
Symptom					
Severe headaches	7	2	9	5	23
Transient paraesthesias	3	1	11	5	20
Transient paresis	0	1	8	3	12
Cutaneous hypoaesthesia or anaesthesia	1	0	7	1	9
Seizures	0	0	3	2	5
Ataxic gait	0	0	5[a]	0	5
Episodic aphonia	2	2	0	0	4
Other speech defects	0	2	1[a]	1	4
Tremor	0	0	2[a]	0	2

[a]In one of these patients, the symptoms may have been related to cerebellar disease.

Table 11.4. Syncopal episodes in autoerythrocyte sensitisation.

	Time of onset				
	Before purpura		After purpura		
	Skin test		Skin test		Total
	Pos.	Neg.	Pos.	Neg.	
Number of patients	18	9	18	9	27
Symptom					
Repeated syncope	2	3	11	3	19
Transient faintness	3	1	3	1	8
Transient vertigo	1	0	4	1	6

Table 11.5. 'Ocular' manifestations in autoerythrocyte sensitisation.

	Time of onset				
	Before purpura		After purpura		
	Skin test		Skin test		Total
	Pos.	Neg.	Pos.	Neg.	
Number of patients	18	9	18	9	27
Symptom					
Diplopia[a]	0	0	7	4	11
Blurred vision[b]	0	0	3	3	6
Constricted visual fields	0	1	2	1	4
Episodic puffy eyes	0	0	3	1	4
Transient blindness	0	1	1	0	2
Scotomata with headaches	0	0	0	2	2
Orbital pain with headaches	0	0	1	0	1

[a]Monocular in six.
[b]Usually transient.

Table 11.6. Chest, abdominal and urinary tract complaints in autoerythrocyte sensitisation.

	Time of onset				
	Before purpura		After purpura		
	Skin test		Skin test		Total
	Pos.	Neg.	Pos.	Neg.	
Number of patients	18	9	18	9	27
Symptom					
Abdominal pain or distress	6	3	5	4	18
Bouts of nausea and vomiting	3	1	10	4	18
Diarrhoeal episodes	3	5	4	3	15
Severe constipation	3	1	2	0	6
Chest pain or distress[a]	6	4	7	2	19
Dyspnoea[a]	3	1	8	4[b]	16
Palpitations[a]	1	1	1	0	3
Dysuria and frequency	6	4	5	2	17
Urinary tract infection[c]	3	1	0	1	5

[a]Episodic.
[b]In one patient, dyspnoea was associated with pulmonary tuberculosis.
[c]Probably underestimated.

Table 11.7. Muscle and joint symptoms in autoerythrocyte sensitisation.

	Before purpura Skin test		After purpura Skin test		Total
	Pos.	Neg.	Pos.	Neg.	
Number of patients	18	9	18	9	27
Symptom					
Joint pains	4	2	10	6	22
Backache	1	1	6	4	12
Joint swelling	1	1	5	4	11
Aches in extremities	1	0	4	3	8
'Rheumatic fever'[a]	5	2	0	0	7
Muscle cramps	1	0	3	3	7
'Neuritis' or 'neuralgia'	0	1	3	0	4
Neck stiff or painful with headaches	1	0	1	1	3

[a]In only one did this diagnosis seem appropriate.

Table 11.8. Cutaneous manifestations in autoerythrocyte sensitisation.

	Skin test[a]		Total
	Pos.	Neg.	
Number of patients	18	9	27
Symptom			
Drug rashes	7	5	12
Urticaria not related to drugs	8	4	12
Erythematous blotches	2	1	3
Cutaneous ulcers[b]	2	0	2
Burning or itching skin	2	0	2
Atopic dermatitis	1	1	2

[a]Data on time of onset were incomplete.
[b]Perhaps factitious in one.

Agle and Ratnoff (1962) rightly discussed the stigmatists, but they also mentioned various case reports of bleeding into the skin which were unrelated to religious experience and were mainly associated with extreme anxiety, sometimes induced during hypnosis. Hersle and Mobacken (1969) drew attention to the many other clinical features present in 32 cases of autoerythrocyte sensitisation. More recently Klein, Gonen and Smith (1975) included accident proneness as a feature of psychogenic purpura and at the same time discussed the rarity of the syndrome in males.

It is the author's experience, too, that spontaneous bruising or purpura may or may not be the main feature of a syndrome which occurs in women of an anxious disposition (Figure 11.3). Two of his patients were distressed by their blue and painful extremities. A story of ill-treatment during childhood, nose bleeds, heavy menstruation, abortions, postpartum haemorrhage, frigidity or votes of chastity has occurred in nearly every case.

The features which occur are listed in Table 11.1; sometimes they are associated, but in other patients they occur separately. Sensitivity to agents inoculated into the skin is usual (Figure 11.4). In some cases this agent is red cell stroma (Gardner and Diamond,

Table 11.9. Miscellaneous symptoms in autoerythrocyte sensitisation[a]

	Time of onset				
	Before purpura		After purpura		
	Skin test		Skin test		Total
	Pos.	Neg.	Pos.	Neg.	
Number of patients	18	9	18	9	27
Symptom					
Weight fluctuation[b]	—	—	13	6	19
Nervousness	1	0	6	5	12
Asthenia	3	1	6	1	11
Insomnia	0	0	8	1	9
Fatigue	1	0	4	3	8
Raynaud's phenomenon	6	1	0	0	7
Anorexia	1	1	4	1	7
Hyperventilation	2	0	4	0	6
Dependent oedema	1	0	4	0	5
Dysphagia	3	0	2	0	5
Anterior neck pain[c]	2	1	0	2	5
Systemic drug reactions	3	1	0	0	4
Fever	1	0	3[d]	0	4
Tinnitus	0	0	1	1	2

[a]The symptoms were usually episodic.
[b]Usually weight loss; data on the time of onset of the weight loss were inadequate.
[c]Described as a 'lump in the throat' by one patient.
[d]An additional patient had factitious fever.

Table 11.10. Operative procedures in patients with autoerythrocyte sensitisation.

| | Skin test | | Total |
	Pos.	Neg.	
Number of patients	18	9	27
Appendectomy	8	5	13
Hysterectomy	8	4	12
Other gynaecological operations[a]	6	4	10
Dilatation and curettage[a]	3	6	9
Almost all teeth pulled	5	2	7
Exploratory laparotomy	3	3	6
Repeated cystoscopies	4	2	6
Minor breast operations[a]	4	1	5
Cholecystectomy	2	3	5
Laminectomy	0	2	2
Bilateral mastectomy	1	0	1
Other major operations[a]	4	4	8

[a]Number of patients; the procedures were often multiple.

1955), in others it is haemoglobin (Kremer et al, 1967), an agent extracted from red cell stroma, or phosphatidyl serine (Hersle and Mobacken, 1969). The histology is that of vasculitis (Nelson, 1971) or a leucocytoclastic angiitis (Hersle and Mobacken, 1969). There is some clinical and histological resemblance to delayed pressure urticaria (Ryan, Shim-Young and Turk, 1968) as was seen in two females in one of the authors' series. Deficiency of platelet factor III can occur and was reported by Di Grande (1971) and Young (1972).

Table 11.11. Emotional characteristics of patients with autoerythrocyte sensitisation.

	Skin test		Total
	Pos.	Neg.	
Number of patients	18	9	27
Depression	13	7	20
Suicidal attempt	3	2	5
Overt sexual problems	12	6	18
Hostility	12	3	15
Masochism or martyrism	11	4	15
Anxiety	9	5	14
'Hysteria'	10	4	14
Emotional lability	7	4	11
Divorced[a]	6	3	9
Obsessive-compulsive behaviour	6	2	8
Temper tantrums	5	3	8
'Tom boy' as child	7	1	8
Litigiousness	8	0	8
Addiction	5	2	7
Hallucinations	4	3	7
Dissociative episodes	4	2	6

[a]Of 23 married, 5 remarried.

Figure 11.3. Painful bruise developing spontaneously in a nurse.

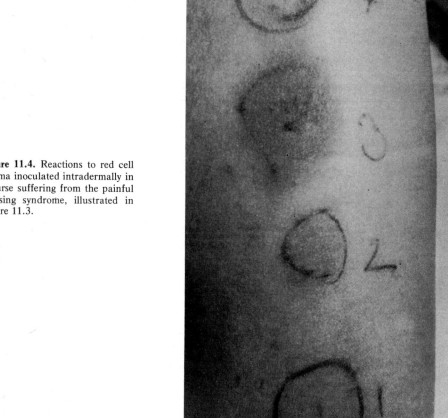

Figure 11.4. Reactions to red cell stroma inoculated intradermally in a nurse suffering from the painful bruising syndrome, illustrated in Figure 11.3.

Agle, Ratnoff and Wasman (1969) discussed autoerythrocytic sensitisation, pointing out the role suggestion plays in eliciting a positive response to red cell stroma and presumably to DNA, platelets or phosphatidyl serine. It has been noted, too, by several investigators that positive skin tests are obtained only intermittently. Bleeding into the skin can be induced by hypnosis, and Stefanini and Baumgart (1972) have shown how frequently it is not possible to induce a purpuric lesion unless the patient anticipates the result.

Gardner and Diamond (1955), Hersle and Mobacken (1969), and the author have been interested in the disassociation of pain and bruising. Some patients complain of severe, painful bruising, whereas others not only develop bruising which is either painful or painless but also experience severe pains elsewhere at the same time. In fact quite severe bruising can be painless and non-tender if sufficient pain is experienced elsewhere.

The overlap with the stigmatists is further illustrated by the frequency of hysterical convulsions, hallucinations and syncope in patients with painful bruising or psychogenic purpura (Agle and Ratnoff, 1962). Enjoyment of the hardship is a characteristic which, as these authors emphasised, is a masochistic tendency associated with an attitude of 'grin and bear it'.

It is impossible to estimate to what degree anxiety and stress are responsible for any one rash. On the whole the transient immediate forms of inflammation are those most easily attributable to the emotions. Blushing, pallor and cholinergic urticaria are clearly dependent on the psyche, and there have been many reports of emotionally induced urticaria (Warin and Champion, 1974). In the severer forms of vasculitis emotional factors play a less significant role, the triggers by comparison being the more virulent agents such as immune complexes and bacterial elements. The psyche may modify or enhance, prepare or provoke, but it is doubtful whether it is ever the sole cause of severe vasculitis.

THE NERVOUS SYSTEM IN THE INFLAMMATORY REACTION

The following paragraphs summarise an important review by Chapman and Goodell (1964) of the participation of the nervous system in the inflammatory reaction. Their observations were largely based on the researches of Harold G. Wolff at the New York Hospital, Cornell University Medical College.

The nervous system may react strongly to a threatening situation, but equally strong reactions may occur to very mild stimuli in anxious individuals. The reactions, such as flight, are protective, but much that is the result of fright may be damaging. Responses may be inappropriate and prolonged. For instance, ever since Pavlov experimented on his dogs, it has been recognised that gastrin secretions may be inappropriately enhanced or prolonged and ultimately damage the stomach. Stomach, colon, nose or lungs may react in this way to anxiety, developing gastric ulceration, colitis, vasomotor rhinitis or asthma respectively. Similarly, essential hypertension, coronary thrombosis or migraine have a well documented psychosomatic component. When discussing the role of past experience in developing an emotional response, Wolff (1970) stated: "It is possible to call an individual a coward in a precisely modulated tone so that the decibels may be accurately measured and hence the energy transmitted through the ear drum and the middle ear to the organ of Corti is as nicely quantified as any stimulus in biological research. Such pains at quantification, however, would not reward the investigator with a uniformity of response from person to person and even from time to time in the same person. Energy fed via receptors into the nervous system actuates an integrative process which ultimately interprets the event in the light of individual proclivities and past experience as threatening, neutral or pleasurable and to what degree. Thus the stimulus gains its force from its meaning. It would appear therefore that the search for a standard stimulus is a 'will-o-the-wisp'. The important concern is more the relevance than the quantity of a stimulus situation".

None of this, however, explains psychogenic purpura. Different groups of persons working in the psychosomatic field speak in their own jargon, and the concepts of the psychiatrist or theologian are not easy for the physiologist to re-interpret. The fact that these patients do show anxiety, masochism and disturbance of sexual drive does not explain the peripheral purpuric lesion.

Early work on peripheral innervation and the acute inflammatory response included studies on anaesthetisation of mucous membranes and stimulation or section of nerves to the rabbit ear. Cutting the sympathetic vasoconstrictor nerve speeded up the blood flow through the ear when rubbed and placed in a hot bath, whereas sectioning the vasodilator nerves resulted in vasoconstriction and stasis or gangrene of the ear when warmed in the same way (Samuel, cited by Adami, 1909). The streptococcus similarly produced a more rapid but transient injury in a vasodilated ear, but necrosis in a vasoconstricted ear (Roger, cited by Adami, 1909).

Early observations included decreased redness both of the conjunctiva in response to mustard oil (Bruce, 1910) and of the cocainised frog tongue to iodine (Krogh, 1929). But more important were the observations of Lewis et al (1927) on the axon reflex — redness of the skin in response to local injury which they showed was entirely dependent on functioning afferent nerves. Such a finding could easily be related to the vasodilatation that occurs when a peripheral sensory nerve is stimulated antidromically. This was demonstrated by Goltz (1874) using the sciatic nerve and by Stricker (1876) stimulating dorsal roots. Bayliss (1902, 1923) was able to exclude the activity of sympathetic nerves in the response and used limb volume increase as a valid measure of a purely afferent nerve stimulus.

Much of the subsequent interest concerned the nature of the chemical mediators, released from the afferent nerve endings, which take a few seconds following antidromic stimulus to mediate the vasodilatation (Bayliss, 1923; Langley, 1923, a and b). Histamine could explain this reaction, but its mere presence does not rule out a precursor any more than does inhibition of the antidromic effects by antihistamines. There is more histamine in the skin after an antidromic stimulus and in inflammation in general, but Chapman and Wolff, in their review, supported Dale's concept that acetylcholine is a more likely candidate as a mediator of antidromic vasodilatation.

Major difficulties are the speed with which acetylcholine is inactivated, and the failure of atropine or eserine to influence significantly the antidromic effects. Kibjakow (1931) observed that the vasodilator substance released into the blood in areas of antidromic vasodilatation was, in fact, fairly stable. Wybauw (1936, 1938) isolated an acetylcholine-like substance from the blood but this could have been released from sympathetic cholinergic fibres. As a result of studies on salivation and on thermoregulatory sweating, the kinin—kallikrein system was favoured as a mediator of vasodilatation (Unger and Parrot, 1938; Hilton and Lewis, 1955a, b, 1958; Fox and Hilton, 1958). It was therefore concluded that acetylcholine released from postganglionic nerves in turn released proteolytic enzymes.

At the time of Chapman and Wolff's review, ATP release from dorsal root nerve endings was the newest candidate for antidromic vasodilatation. It had been demonstrated in nerve endings by Holton and Holton (1952) and was shown to be released on antidromic stimulation (Holton, 1959).

It is suggested below that, so far as psychogenic purpura is concerned, the fibrinolytic system must also be considered as a mediator. In this respect it could be activated by any one of the postulated mediators — histamine, acetylcholine, kinins or ATP.

The first question that must be answered is whether a thought, anxiety or fear can cause vasculitis. If they can, the question inevitably arises whether such an influence is carried by known nerve pathways acting on the vasculature. In pathology such as the stigma, or the weal induced by hypnosis, one must explain the ability to determine the site of the lesion. In this respect, humoral factors such as adrenal hormones or the neuroendocrine system in the hypothalamus are unlikely mediators. They explain fright and flight, flushing, pallor and faintness, and are important in systemic diseases such as essential hypertension or coronary thrombosis, but they cannot satisfactorily explain local phenomena in the skin. The alteration in blood flow that occurs in a subject's limb when he is doing mental arithmetic may be more relevant (Abramson and Ferris, 1940; Burch, 1948; Allwood et al, 1959), but this is not very specific. Luria and Vinogradova (1959) suggested that any new stimulus, visual, tactile or auditory, causes vasoconstriction of the fingers and vasodilatation of the face.

Like Chapman and Wolff, the author prefers to blame antidromic afferent sensory nerve impulses for the more bizarre inflammatory disease in psychosomatic medicine. There is important clinical evidence to support this in disease of dorsal root nerve endings (Figure 11.5). Osler and McCrae (1920) writing about 'neurotic purpura' stated:

"One variety is met with in cases of organic disease. It is so called myelopathic purpura, which is seen occasionally in tabes dorsalis, particularly following attacks of lightening pains, and as a rule, involving the area of skin in which pains have been most intense. Cases have been met with in acute transverse myelitis and occasionally in severe neuralgia".

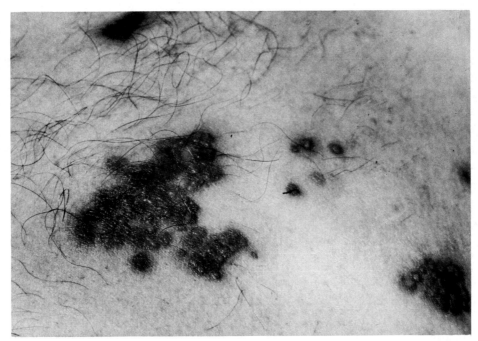

Figure 11.5. Vesiculation and haemorrhage into the skin in herpes zoster.

There can be little doubt that axon reflex vasodilatation can influence inflammatory events. The role of the central nervous system in modifying the axon reflex was illustrated by Reed, Pidgeon and Becker (1961) who showed that 54 out of 68 subjects with spinal cord injury had decreased axon reflex vasodilatation in response to stroking below the level of the lesion. In 24 of these 68 subjects there was a decreased flare response to histamine inoculation. Swanson, Buchan and Alvord (1963) demonstrated a decreased flare response in patients with absence of pain fibres in the spinal cord. Relevant studies were those of Andersen, Eccles and Sears (1962, 1964) in which depolarisation of the spinal cord followed stimulation of the cerebral cortex. However, the most detailed analysis of the effect of the central nervous system on the inflammatory response was carried out by Chapman, Goodell and Wolff (1959a, b) and Chapman and Goodell (1964). They showed that the axon reflex flare lowers the pain threshold and enhances inflammation, and in skin perfusion studies they isolated higher levels of kinins and proteases from the flare zone. Similar experiments on dermographism have been carried out by Winkelmann, Wilhelm and Horner (1965) and by Greaves and Sondergaard (1970) who have obtained histamines, kinins and prostaglandins in the perfusates.

In order to study more central effects, Bilisoly, Goodell and Wolff (1954) showed that a lowered pain threshold, an increase in tissue vulnerability and an augmented axon reflex vasodilatation occurred in the arms when the legs were heated. Cold exposure and the consequent reflex vasoconstriction diminished inflammation. The pathways involved in such experiments reach at least the level of the thermoregulatory centres of the mid-brain. Evidence that still higher cerebral centres can influence the inflammatory response was obtained by the use of hypnosis (Chapman, Goodell and Wolff, 1959a, b). Thus hypnotised subjects were told that one arm was sensitive, vulnerable and painful and that the other was normal or anaesthetic. Of 12 subjects with one arm 'sensitive' and the other 'normal' nine showed raised skin temperature and increased kinins in perfusates only in the 'sensitive' arm. Of 27 subjects in whom 'sensitive' and 'anaesthetic' arms were compared, 20 were more reactive in their 'sensitive' arm, inflammation being suppressed in the other. Suggestion under hypnosis that a cold metal rod on the skin would burn resulted in an acute inflammatory response at the point of contact with the rod.

As mentioned above, there is a literature on wealing and purpura in response to suggestion under hypnosis (Barber, 1963; Paul, 1963). One of the main features of such a response is that it has, to some extent, to be learned. The subjects have to be susceptible to auto-suggestion, and the responding organ must have some experience of the inflammation. Normal skin is less likely to respond to suggestion than is habitually diseased skin. Dennis and Phillipus (1965) showed that atopic subjects can alter the blood flow in their skin very readily, even without hypnosis. Most such studies have shown that it is the vascular component of inflammation that is most responsive. Black (1963) could diminish redness and oedema in the Prausnitz—Kustner and Mantoux reactions, but not the cellular infiltrate. Ikemi and Nagagawa (1962) could similarly alter the highly oedematous and acutely vasodilated response to poison ivy. Five subjects tested under hypnosis developed a cutaneous reaction from the application of water and four out of five had no response to the ivy although they were known to be very sensitive. To explain such behaviour, one has to suppose that nerve endings may release an excess of agents capable of inducing severe inflammation and that the normal tissues are habitually bathed to some degree in these agents; but suppression of their release greatly diminishes the response to injury by other agents.

Brunner (1948), Chapman, Goodell and Wolff (1959a, b), and Cormia (1952) believed that acetylcholine or some similar agent could be incriminated in this manner. Present in normal skin but increased in amount to atopic skin and in lichen simplex (Scott, 1962), an agent such as acetylcholine might well enhance the action of mediators of inflammation. It is rapidly destroyed by cholinesterases, and suppression of its release from the increased number of dorsal root nerve endings present in a lesion such as lichen simplex could depress the reactivity of such skin. Beahrs, Harris and Hilgard (1970) believed that only abnormal skin is likely to show a response to suggestion. In the case of the stigmatists and in psychogenic purpura a history of injury is usual and the skin has subsequently learned to be abnormal. Holti (1955) made several observations on this learning capacity of the skin. It is largely a vascular phenomenon such that increased blood flow can be demonstrated for many months at sites of previous relatively mild injury in the past — by histamine inoculation, ultraviolet radiation or the Mantoux reaction, for example. Moody (1948) concluded that the production of swelling, bruising and bleeding during abreaction were all, so far as circumstantial evidence goes to show, somatic repetitions of previous experience. It may not be so easy to produce a lesion which the subject never had before. Whatever its identity, the mediator of the reaction induced by hypnosis is one that increases permeability besides causing vasodilatation. Such effects can be demonstrated by inducing blistering by cantharidin; Kepecs, Robin and Brunner (1951) showed that the exudation produced in this way was little affected by the pulse rate or the blood pressure but that, in highly suggestible subjects prone to emotional outbursts of weeping, it was greatly increased during an excited phase. Di Palma, Reynolds and Foster (1942) and Milberg (1947) also studied the erythema response to pressure on the skin and found it to be clearly related to such stimuli as mental arithmetic or other threatening situations.

The less clearly defined relationship between local blood flow, skin permeability and electrical conductivity is also altered in a similar fashion by hypnosis, by anxiety and by acupuncture (Cade and Woolley Hart, 1971; Woolley Hart, 1972; Bergsmann and Woolley Hart, 1973).

References

Abramson, D. I. & Ferris, F. B. (1940) Response of blood vessels in the resting hand and forearm to various stimuli. *American Heart Journal*, **19**, 541.

Adami, J. G. (1909) *An Introduction to the Study of Pathology*. London: Macmillan.

Agle, D. P. & Ratnoff, O. D. (1962) Purpura as a psychosomatic entity; a psychiatric study of autoerythrocyte sensitisation. *Archives of Internal Medicine*, **109**, 685.

Agle, D. P., Ratnoff, P. D. & Wasman, M. (1969) Studies in autoerythrocyte sensitisation. The induction of purpura lesions by hypnotic suggestion. *Psychosomatic Medicine*, **29**, 491.

Allwood, M., Barcroft, H., Hayes, J. P. L. A. & Hirsjarui, E. A. (1959) The effect of mental arithmetic on the blood flow through normal sympathectomised and hyperidrotic hands. *Journal of Physiology*, **148**, 108.

Andersen, P., Eccles, J. C. & Sears, T. A. (1962) Presynaptic inhibitory action of cerebral cortex on the spinal cord. *Nature*, **194**, 740.

Andersen, P., Eccles, J. C. & Sears, T. A. (1964) Cortically evoked depolarization of primary afferent fibers in the spinal cord. *Journal of Neurophysiology*, **27**, 63.

Barber, T. X. (1963) The effects of hypnosis on pain. A critical review of experimental and clinical findings. *Psychosomatic Medicine*, **25**, 303.

Bayliss, W. M. (1902) Further researches on antidromic nerve impulses. *Journal of Physiology*, **28**, 276.

Bayliss, W. M. (1908) The excitation of vasodilator nerve fibers in depressor reflexes. *Journal of Physiology*, **37**, 264.

Bayliss, W. M. (1923) *The Vasomotor System*. London: Longmans, Green.

Beahrs, J. O., Harris, D. R. & Hilgard, E. R. (1970) Failure to alter skin inflammation by hypnotic suggestion in five subjects with normal skin reactivity. *Psychosomatic Medicine*, **32**, 627.

Bergsmann, O. & Woolley Hart, A. (1973) Differences in electrical skin conductivity between acupuncture points and adjacent skin areas. *Journal of Acupuncture*, **1**, 27.

Bilisoly, F. N., Goodell, H. & Wolff, H. G. (1954) Vasodilatation, lowered pain threshold, and increased tissue vulnerability. *Archives of Internal Medicine*, **94**, 759.

Black, S. (1963) Inhibition of immediate type hypersensitivity response by direct suggestion under hypnosis. *British Medical Journal*, **i**, 925.

Black, S., Humphrey, J. H. & Niven, J. S. F. (1963) Inhibition of Mantoux reaction by direct suggestion under hypnosis. *British Medical Journal*, **i**, 1619.

Bruce, A. N. (1910) Uber die Beziehung der sensiblen Neruenendigungen zum Entzundungsvorgang. *Archiv für experimentelle Pathologie und Pharmakologie*, **63**, 424.

Brunner, M. (1948) Biological basis of psychosomatic disease of the skin. *Archiv für Dermatologie und Syphilis*, **57**, 374.

Burch, G. (1948) The cardiovascular system and the effector in psychosomatic phenomena. *Journal of the American Medical Association*, **136**, 1011.

Cade, C. M. & Woolley Hart, A. (1971) The measurement of hypnosis and autohypnosis by determination of electrical skin resistance. *Journal of the Society for Psychical Research*, **46**, 81.

Chapman, L. F. & Goodell, H. (1964) The participation of the nervous system in the inflammatory reaction. *Annals of the New York Academy of Sciences*, **116**, 990.

Chapman, L. F., Goodell, H. & Wolff, H. G. (1959a) Changes in tissue vulnerability induced during hypnotic suggestion. *Journal of Psychosomatic Research*, **4**, 99.

Chapman, L. F., Goodell, H. & Wolff, H. G. (1959b) Augmentation of the inflammatory response by the CNS. *Archives of Neurology*, **1**, 557.

Cormia, F. E. (1952) Experimental histamine pruritus. I. Influence of physical and psychological factors on threshold reactivity. *Journal of Investigative Dermatology*, **19**, 21.

Dennis, M. & Phillipus, M. J. (1965) Hypnotic and non-hypnotic suggestion and skin response in atopic patients. *American Journal of Clinical Hypnosis*, **7**, 342.

Di Grande, Elaine (1971) Psychogenic purpura. *Archives of Dermatology*, **104**, 444.

Di Palma, J. R., Reynolds, S. R. M. & Foster, F. I. (1942) Quantitative measurement of reactive hyperaemia in human skin. *American Heart Journal*, **23**, 377.

Forman, L. (1953) Purpura urticans with regional distribution (early manifestation of vascular sensitisation) and polyarthritis. *Proceedings of the Royal Society of Medicine*, **46**, 547.

Fox, R. H. & Hilton, S. M. (1958) Bradykinin formation in human skin as a factor in heat vasodilation. *Journal of Physiology*, **142**, 219.

Gardner, F. H. & Diamond, L. K. (1955) Autoerythrocyte sensitisation: a form of purpura producing painful bruising following autosensitisation to red blood cells in certain women. *Blood*, **10**, 675.

Goltz, F. (1874) Uber gefasserweiternde nerven. *Pflugers Archiv für die gesamte Physiologie des Menschen und der Tiere*, **9**, 185.

Greaves, M. W. & Sondergaard, J. (1970) Urticaria pigmentosa and factitious urticaria. Direct evidence for release of histamine and other smooth muscle contracting agents in dermographic skin. *Archives of Dermatology*, **101**, 418.

Hersle, K. & Mobacken, H. (1969) Autoerythrocyte sensitisation syndrome (painful bruising syndrome). Report of two cases and review of the literature. *British Journal of Dermatology*, **81**, 574.

Hilton, S. M. & Lewis, G. P. (1955a) The cause of the vasodilatation accompanying activity in the submandibular salivary gland. *Journal of Physiology*, **128**, 235.

Hilton, S. M. & Lewis, G. P. (1955b) The mechanism of functional hyperaemia in the submandibular salivary gland. *Journal of Physiology*, **129**, 235.

Hilton, S. M. & Lewis, G. P. (1958) Vasodilatation in the tongue and its relationship to plasma kinin formation. *Journal of Physiology*, **144**, 532.

Holti, G. (1955) Measurements of vascular responses in skin at various time intervals after damage with histamine and ultraviolet radiation. *Clinical Science*, **14**, 143.

Holton, F. A. & Holton, P. (1952) The possibility that ATP is a transmitter at sensory nerve endings. *Journal of Physiology*, **119**, 50.

Holton, P. (1959) The liberation of adenosine triphosphate on antidromic stimulation of sensory nerves. *Journal of Physiology*, **145**, 494.

Ikemi, Y. & Nagagawa, S. (1962) A psychosomatic study of contact dermatitis. *Kyushi Journal of Medical Science*, **13**, 335.

Kepecs, J. G., Robin, M. & Brunner, M. J. (1951) Relationship between certain emotional states and exudation into skin. *Psychosomatic Medicine*, **13**, 10.

Kibjakow, A. W. (1931) Zur frage des vasodilatations mechanismus bei der reizng antidromer. Nerven I über die gefasserweiternden eigenschaften des blutes beim reiz der hinteren sensiblen wurzeln. *Pflugers Archiv für die gesamte Physiologie des Menschen und der Tiere*, **228**, 30.

Klauder, J. V. (1938) Stigmatization. *Archives of Dermatology and Syphilology*, **37**, 650.

Klein, R. F., Gonen, J. Y. & Smith, C. M. (1975) Psychogenic purpura in a man. *Psychosomatic Medicine*, **37**, 41.

Kremer, W. B., Mengel, C. E., Nowlin, J. J. & Nagaya, H. (1967) Recurrent ecchymoses and cutaneous hyper-reactivity to haemoglobin. A form of autoerythrocyte sensitisation. *Blood*, **30**, 62.

Krogh, A. (1929) *The Anatomy and Physiology of Capillaries*. New Haven, Connecticut: Yale University Press.

Langley, J. N. (1923a) Antidromic action. *Journal of Physiology*, **57**, 428.

Langley, J. N. (1923b) The vascular dilatation caused by the sympathetic and the course of vasomotor nerves. *Journal of Physiology*, **58**, 70.

Langley, J. N. (1923c) Antidromic action. III. Stimulation of the peripheral nerves of the cat's hind foot. *Journal of Physiology*, **58**, 49.

Lewis, T., Harris, K. E. & Grant, R. T. (1927) Influence of the cutaneous nerves on various reactions of the cutaneous vessels. *Heart*, **14**, 1.

Luria, A. R. & Vinogradova, I. (1959) An objective investigation of the dynamics of the semantic system. *British Journal of Psychology*, **50**, 89.

Milberg, I. L. (1947) The reactive hyperaemic response of the uninvolved skin of patients with psoriasis. *Journal of Investigative Dermatology*, **9**, 31.

Moody, R. L. (1948) Bodily changes during abreaction. *Lancet*, **i**, 964.

Nelson, C. T. (1971) Autoerythrocyte sensitisation syndrome. *Archives of Dermatology*, **103**, 549.

Osler, W. & McCrae, T. (1920) *The Principles and Practice of Medicine*. New York, London: D. Appleton and Company. p. 743.

Paul, G. L. (1963) The production of blisters by hypnotic suggestion: another look. *Psychosomatic Medicine*, **25**, 233.

Ratnoff, O. D. & Agle, D. P. (1968) Psychogenic purpura: a re-evaluation of the syndrome of autoerythrocyte sensitization. *Medicine*, **47**, 475.

Reed, W. B., Pidgeon, J. & Becker, S. W. (1961) Studies on the triple response of Lewis in patients with spinal cord injury. *Journal of Investigative Dermatology*, **37**, 135.

Schindler, R. (1929) *Nervensystem und Spontane Blutungen mit Besonderer Berucksichtigung der Hysterischen Diathesen*. Berlin: S. Karger.

Scott, A. (1962) Acetylcholine in normal and diseased skin. *British Journal of Dermatology*, **74**, 317.

Stefanini, M. & Baumgart, E. T. (1972) Purpura factitia: an analysis of criteria for its differentiation from auto-erythrocyte sensitisation purpura. *Archives of Dermatology*, **106**, 238.

Stricker, S. (1876) Untersuchung uber die Geffasserwurzeln des Ischiadicus. *Sitzungsberichte, Kaiserl Akademie der Wissenschaften Wien*, **3**, 173.

Swanson, A. G., Buchan, G. C. & Alvord, E. D. (1963) Absence of Lissauer's tract and small dorsal root axons in familial, congenital universal insensitivity to pain. *Transactions of the American Neurological Association*, **88**, 99.

Unger, G. & Parrot, L. L. (1938) Sur la nature de la substance liberée au cours de la vasodilatation dite antidiomique. *Compte Rendu des Séances de la Société de Biologie*, **128**, 753.

Warin, R. P. & Champion, R. H. (1974) *Urticaria*. London: W. B. Saunders.

Winkelmann, R. K., Wilhelm, C. M. & Horner, F. A. (1965) Experimental studies on dermographism. *Archives of Dermatology*, **92**, 436.

Wolff, S. (1970) Emotions and the autonomic nervous system. *Archives of Internal Medicine*, **126**, 1024.

Woolley Hart, A. (1972) The role of the circulation in measurements of skin conductivity. *British Journal of Dermatology*, **87**, 213.

Wybauw, L. (1936) Transmission humorale de la vasodilatation provoquée par l'excitation du bout périphérique des racines postérieures lombaires chez le chat. *Compte Rendu des séances de la Société de Biologie*, **123**, 524.

Wybauw, L. (1938) Contribution a l'étude du role vasomoteur et trophique des nerfs sensitifs: les vaso-dilatateurs 'antidromiques' et le méchanismé de leur actions. *Archives Internationales de Physiologie*, **46**, 293.

Young, A. W. (1972) Painful purpura. *Archives of Dermatology*, **105**, 450.

COAGULATION AND FIBRINOLYSIS

The type of lesion that dominates the literature on the psyche and the skin may be acute, painful, and oedematous, or bleeding. Exudative lesions are the primary concern of this book. Like Osler's discussion of the visceral lesions of purpura (Osler, 1914), in exudative lesions, the blood elements, either the red blood corpuscles alone, the serum alone or both combined, pass out of the vessels. For an explanation one must therefore look at the vessel wall and its nerve endings which regulate permeability and hold the key to the bleeding.

Bleeding is difficult to explain. Correll (1968) electrically stimulated the brains of cats and also transected the brain at various levels. As cerebral stimulation shortened the clotting time, even in heparin-treated animals, he postulated the production of an anti-heparin factor. Previously Schneider and Zangari (1951) had demonstrated a 25 per cent reduction in the clotting time after a painful stimulus. Moreover, agitation, anxiety, tension, fear and anger are all known to shorten the clotting time, whereas a slowing down of mental processes, depression and dejection prolong it. As early as 1914 Cannon and Mendenhall (1914) in the fourth of a series of articles on factors influencing coagulation demonstrated a 'hastening of coagulation in pain and emotional excitement' which Hardaway (1971) blamed on splanchnic stimulation and release of factors from the liver.

Some of the world's experts on clotting and fibrinolysis have failed to find any evidence of a disturbance of coagulation in psychogenic purpura (Agle and Ratnoff, 1962; Rizza and Sharp in the author's series of unpublished data). However, blood from a cubital vein is not representative of the local lesion, and clotting studies are certainly not the same as fibrinolytic studies in the local lesion (see Chapter 10). Nevertheless, in a report by Reed and Firkin (1957), excess fibrinolysis was blamed for autoerythrocytic sensitisation, and Rowell (1974) reported two patients in whom painful bleeding was associated with excess fibrinolysis and who responded to antifibrinolytic therapy.

Schneider and Zangari (1951) pointed out that when clotting time increased in their anxious subjects fibrinolytic activity also tended to increase. Macfarlane and Biggs (1946) had previously noted increased fibrinolytic activity in the anxious, and Chapman,

Goodell and Wolff (1959) subsequently suggested that neurogenic influences release metabolites that convert plasminogen already present in extracellular fluid to the active proteolytic enzyme plasmin. The enhancement of blood and tissue fibrinolysis by acetylcholine, histamine and kinins was demonstrated in the dog by Holemans (1965) (Figure 11.6). Shwartzman (1965) observed a greater degree of haemorrhage and a prolongation of bleeding time at sites injected with histamine or 48/80 than at control sites. Other descriptions of plasminogen activator release by acetylcholine may be found in reports by Kwaan, Lo and McFadzean (1957, 1958), Soulier and Koupernik (1948), and Sherry et al (1959).

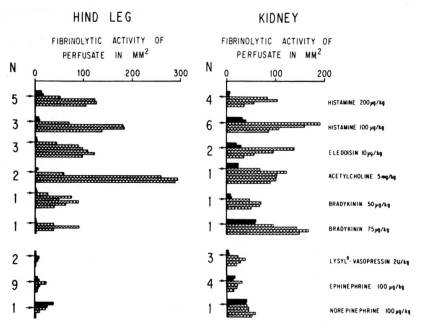

Figure 11.6. Fibrinolytic activity measured in perfusates from hind leg and kidney of the dog after infusion of various mediators of inflammation. Clearly the mediators of immediate inflammatory responses also release activators of fibrinolysis.

Ryan, Nishioka and Dawber (1971) were impressed by a tendency for increased local fibrinolysis to be present in acute exudative inflammatory responses, and they found that acetylcholine, histamine and kinins caused increased local fibrinolysis in sections of human skin. In some conditions, such as delayed pressure urticaria, it was misleading to find depressed fibrinolytic activity in the whole blood, for at the local site fibrinolysis was sometimes normal or even increased.

The clearest evidence of the effect of a stimulus from the central nervous system on local fibrinolysis came from Sherry et al (1959) and Schneck and von Kaulla (1961). Sherry et al (1959) studied the effect of electric shock while Schneck and von Kaulla (1961) used pitressin injection and pneumoencephalography as the central insult; in both studies increased fibrinolysis was demonstrated in forearms in which the circulation was totally occluded. Arterial occlusion by itself had a less pronounced effect.

In all experiments on stress and fibrinolysis one must not only distinguish between the early tendency to increased fibrinolysis and a later tendency for it to decrease (Innes and Sevitt, 1964; Chakrabarti, Hocking and Fearnley, 1969) but also recognise the difference between decreased activity in whole blood (Levi, 1972) and increased local extravascular activity. In this respect the role of the psyche has an early local effect quite different from that on the whole organism spread over many days. The postulated excessive stimulation of fibrinolysis is something that has to be learned and occurs in skin previously subjected to a similar experience.

It should be borne in mind, however, that others have placed more emphasis on the aggregation of platelets, which is enhanced when the subject is stressed mentally or physically (Harrison, Emmons and Mitchell, 1967; Cash, 1972).

Jacques (1964) observed that haemorrhage during anticoagulant treatment could be induced in experimental animals by exposing them to stress and he suggested that this was because of endocrine and neural influences on the vascular bed, in addition to the humoral and coagulation factors. Lucas and Jacques (1965) produced a similar haemorrhagic state by emotional stress mediated by LSD and these authors referred to bleeding episodes induced in haemophilia by anxiety and suppressed by hypnosis (Lucas et al, 1962).

In Chapter 3 it is suggested that urticaria, vasculitis and intravascular coagulation are part of a spectrum. It is probable that the psyche can induce the more urticarial bleeding lesion at a local level, but, if the stimulus is prolonged, a shift towards the DIC end of the spectrum is likely to occur as fibrinolysis becomes exhausted and whole blood begins to show a decreased clotting time. This is not necessarily the case, for nervousness in the cow caused by tightly securing it to a fence has been shown to cause its blood to clot sooner, but subsequently the clotting process seemed to proceed more slowly (Scott Blair, 1960).

Psychogenic purpura in its extreme form is represented by the stigmatists. It is said to be non-inflammatory, and to be either non-healing or to heal with an atrophic paper-like scar. The exacerbations are acute, painful, abrupt and somewhat urticarial responses.

Elsewhere, Ryan, Nishioka and Dawber (1971) have emphasised that inflammation in which fibrinolysis is excessive differs from that in which fibrinolysis is inhibited and fibrin is deposited. Cellular infiltrates and bluish scars tend to follow fibrin deposition, but in conditions such as porphyria cutanea tarda (Grice, Ryan and Magnus, 1970), and probably also the stigma, in which fibrinolysis is not inhibited, a rather haemorrhagic blister forms which is singularly free of leucocytes and may heal with an atrophic scar. On the other hand, Sharp (personal communication, 1974) suggested that painful purpura, with its relatively brisk neutrophil response, congestion of venules and oedema, behaves more like a venous infarct and, for that reason, the painful bruising is persistent and healing poor. The psyche and trauma, in his view, act on a local constitutional abnormality in the dermis.

Any discussion of the psychosomatic control of bleeding must also take note of the relative lack of bleeding seen when the skin is injured by daggers and nails during some eastern religious ceremonies. The 'tools' used are often so sharp, pointed and tapered that vascular injury is minimal (Figure 11.7). Nevertheless, in some ceremonies there is such violent associated movement that the amount of bleeding is still surprisingly small.

While increased bleeding into the skin as in stigmatisation and the painful bruising syndrome is associated with pain, suppressed bleeding, as in religious ceremonies or in an hypnotic trance is by contrast relatively painless. This is circumstantial evidence that the afferent nervous system, pain and the control of bleeding share common pathways. In experiments on the inflammatory response it is always the exudative element that is most easily suppressed. It is this facet of the response that can be most easily correlated with excessive local fibrinolysis enhanced possibly by mediators released from dorsal root nerve endings.

Finally, it should be emphasised that pathology that seems to be the consequence of an emotion or a thought rarely occurs solely as a psychogenic response. More usually the pathology is the result of many factors such as injury from infection or an allergen; in effect it is the response that is influenced by the psyche (Holmes, Goodell and Wolff, 1950; Prigal, 1960; Lask, 1966). As is so often mentioned in this monograph, there is a difference between provocation and preparation. A tissue that has been prepared by previous inflammation may be more easily provoked by a thought. As indicated by Kanan in Chapter 9, the nose may be such a prepared tissue and, of course, vasomotor rhinitis is one of the commonest symptoms in the anxious.

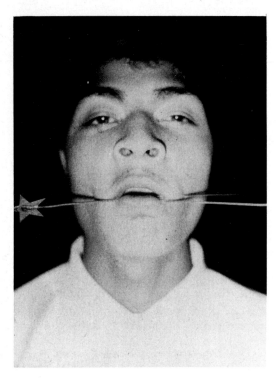

Figure 11.7. Seemingly painless and bloodless injury to the skin during a Malay ceremony in honour of the Dowling Club's visit to Cape Town.

References

Agle, D. P. & Ratnoff, O. D. (1962) Purpura as a psychosomatic entity: a psychiatric study of autoerythrocyte sensitisation. *Archives of Internal Medicine,* **109,** 685.

Cannon, W. B. & Mendenhall, W. L. (1914) Factors affecting the coagulation time of blood. IV. The hastening of coagulation in pain and emotional excitement. *American Journal of Physiology,* **34,** 251.

Cash, J. D. (1972) Platelets fibrinolysis and stress. *Thrombosis et Diathesis Haemorrhagica,* Supplement **15,** 93.

Chakrabarti, R., Hocking, E. D. & Fearnley, G. R. (1969) Reaction pattern to three stresses — electropexy, surgery and myocardial infarction — of fibrinolysis and plasma fibrinogen. *Journal of Clinical Pathology,* **22,** 659.

Chapman, L. F., Goodell, H. & Wolff, H. G. (1959) Augmentation of the inflammatory response by the C.N.S. *Archives of Neurology,* **1,** 557.

Correll, J. W. (1968) Central neural structures and pathway: important for control of blood clotting. Evidence of antiheparin factor. *Bibliographia Anatomique,* **10,** 433.

Grice, K., Ryan, T. J. & Magnus, I. A. (1970) Fibrinolytic activity in lesions produced by monochromatic ultraviolet irradiation in various photodermatoses. *British Journal of Dermatology,* **83,** 637.

Hardaway, R. M. (1971) Disseminated intravascular coagulation. *Thrombosis et Diathesis Haemorrhagica,* **46,** 209.

Harrison, M. J. G., Emmons, P. R. & Mitchell, J. R. A. (1967) The variability of human platelet aggregation. *Journal of Atherosclerosis Research,* **7,** 197.

Holemans, R. (1965) Enhancement of fibrinolysis in the dog by injections of vasoactive drugs. *American Journal of Physiology,* **208,** 511.

Holmes, T. H., Goodell, H., Wolf, S. & Wolff, H. G. (1950) *The Nose: An Experimental Study of Reactions within the Nose in Human Subjects.* Springfield, Illinois: Charles C. Thomas.

Innes, D. & Sevitt, S. (1964) Coagulation and fibrinolysis in injured patients. *Journal of Clinical Pathology,* **17,** 1.

Jacques, L. B. (1964) Stress and multiple-factor etiology of bleeding. *Annals of the New York Academy of Sciences,* **115,** 78.

Kwaan, H. C., Lo, R. & McFadzean, A. J. S. (1957) On the production of plasma fibrinolytic activity within veins. *Clinical Science,* **16,** 241.

Kwaan, H. C., Lo, R. & McFadzean, A. J. S. (1958) On the lysis of thrombi experimentally produced within veins. *British Journal of Haematology,* **4,** 51.

Lask, A. (1966) *Asthma, Attitude and Medicine.* Philadelphia: Lippincott.

Lee, L., Prose, P. M. & Cohen, M. H. (1966) The role of the reticuloendothelial system in diffuse low grade intravascular coagulation. *Thrombosis et Diathesis Haemorrhagica,* Supplement **20,** 87.

Levi, L. (1972) Definition and evaluation of stress. *Thrombosis et Diathesis Haemorrhagica,* Supplement **51,** 7.

Lucas, O. N. & Jacques, L. B. (1965) Spontaneous hemorrhage precipitated by an emotional stress drug in anticoagulant treated rats. *Thrombosis et Diathesis Haemorrhagica,* **13,** 235.

Lucas, O. N., Carroll, R. T., Finkelmann, A. & Tocantins, L. M. (1962) Tooth extractions in hemophilia. Control of bleeding without use of blood, plasma or plasma fractions. *Thrombosis et Diathesis Haemorrhagica,* **8,** 209.

Macfarlane, R. G. & Biggs, R. (1946) Observations on fibrinolysis spontaneous activity associated with surgical operations, trauma, etc. *Lancet,* **ii,** 862.

Osler, W. (1914) The visceral lesions of purpura and allied conditions. *British Medical Journal,* **i,** 517.

Prigal, S. J. (1960) The interrelationship of allergy, infection and the psyche. A unified field theory for the allergist. In *Fundamentals of Modern Allergy.* New York: McGraw Hill.

Reed, C. S. G. & Firkin, B. G. (1957) Autoerythrocyte sensitisation with a circulating fibrinolytic factor. *Australian Annals of Medicine,* **6,** 58.

Rowell, N. R. (1974) A painful bleeding syndrome associated with increased fibrinolytic activity. *British Journal of Dermatology,* **91,** 591.

Ryan, T. J., Nishioka, K. & Dawber, R. P. R. (1971) Epithelial—endothelial interactions in the control of inflammation through fibrinolysis. *British Journal of Dermatology,* **84,** 501.

Schneck, S. A. & von Kaulla, K. N. (1961) Fibrinolysis and the nervous system. *Neurology,* **11,** 959.

Schneider, R. A. & Zangari, V. M. (1951) Variations in clotting, relative viscosity and other physical properties of blood accompanying physical and emotional stress in the normotensive and hypertensive subject. *Psychosomatics,* **13,** 289.

Scott Blair, G. W. (1960) *Rheology of Blood Coagulation in Flow Properties of Blood.* p. 172. Oxford: Pergamon.

Sherry, S., Lindemeyer, R. I., Fletcher, A. P. & Alkjaersig, N. (1959) Studies on enhanced fibrinolytic activity in man. *Journal of Clinical Investigation,* **88,** 810.

Shwartzman, R. M. (1965) The reaction of canine skin to histamine and 48/80. *Journal of Investigative Dermatology,* **44,** 39.

Soulier, J. P. & Koupernik, C. (1948) Constance de la fibrinolyse au course du choc acetyl-cholinique. *Sang,* **19,** 362.

12. Constitution: Venous Stasis and Cold

Venous stasis 'prepares' the tissues, making them more vulnerable to noxious agents. In many forms of cutaneous vasculitis in man, notably the necrotising or polymorphonuclear variety, it is in the venous compartment of the skin that the pathological inflammatory processes are seen (Copeman and Ryan, 1970, 1971). This is true also for experimental cutaneous angiitis in the rabbit (Copeman, 1970) (Table 12.1). The present monograph is thus essentially a discourse on venulitis as defined by Copeman (1975).

Table 12.1. Venular features of cutaneous vasculitis in man and rabbit.

Man	Rabbit
Dependency (haemodynamic back pressure)	Arthus-type reaction (immune complex)
Cold (blood viscosity)	Local Shwartzman phenomenon
External pressure ('natural' + experimental)	Localisation of lesions (immune complexes) by
Vasoactive substances (experimental)	negative pressure, suction, vasoactive substances

The commonest sites for angiitis are areas of stasis. Thus the legs are more commonly affected than other parts of the body. In the upright position, blood flow tends to be slowed in the venous compartment of dependent areas, and in the long-term this posture produces an anatomical system of capillaries and venules that shows evidence of stasis even when the body is horizontal (Ryan, 1969). Moreover, children and adults spend as much as ten hours per day sitting (Wright, 1973) and this posture also slows the circulation in the legs (Boyd et al, 1952). The overall effect is for venous hypertension in the leg to cause a gradual dilatation of the smaller veins and venules, and to discourage the normal emptying of the capillaries while encouraging congestion of the papillae.

Papillary vessels in the legs are normally elongated and coiled and have a wider lumen than those in the skin elsewhere (Figure 12.1). The histopathology of any skin vessels,

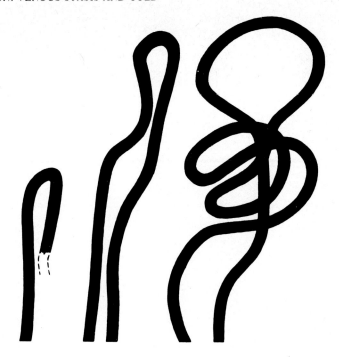

Figure 12.1. Papillary vessels in the upper dermis. On the left is a normal vessel; the two on the right are commonly observed varieties in the lower leg.

but especially those in the legs, reflects their special vulnerability to environmental influences (Chapter 4). Using capillary microscopy, one can observe blood flow in the skin of the leg and see that stasis is a very marked feature. Particularly in widened horizontal venules of the subpapillary plexus (Figure 12.2), flow may be virtually nil for several minutes on end, even in normal skin (Ryan, 1973).

The capillaries and venules of the skin have numerous anastomoses (Ryan, 1973) (Figure 12.3) and thus, when there is stasis in one area of the system, blood under a certain head of pressure is diverted through alternative channels (Figure 12.4). This diversion may be merely within a capillary loop, or the loop may be bypassed altogether. Much of the pathology which occurs in the skin depends on this pattern of short-circuit routes or systems in parallel. A mild degree of congestion in the venous arm of the papillary vessel is a normal feature of skin and was noted by Carrier (1922) and some degree of stasis in a capillary venule is both physiologically normal and necessary for its survival (Ashton, 1960). It is only during recent years that venules have received the attention and credit that they deserve. Physiologists such as Haddy (1960) observed that when the veins in the dog hind limb are constricted by a histamine perfusion there is an associated increase in permeability of the capillaries; Rowley's (1968) findings were similar. This stimulated interest in the effect of mediators of inflammation, which seem to be most active in the venules. It took a surprisingly long time from Arnold (1875) to modern authors such as Majno, Palade and Schoefl (1961) for the site of maximum permeability of the vascular system to be recognised as venular.

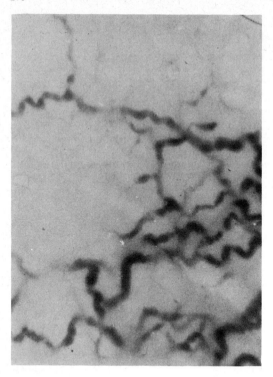

Figure 12.2. Dilated horizontal sub-papillary venous plexus as seen through a capillary microscope. Vessels are near to the surface because the upper dermis is atrophic and without papillary vessels. As a consequence the transparency of the skin is such that blood flow is easily observed in such vessels.

Leakiness, stickiness to leucocytes, variation in lumen diameter and new vessel growth are all most pronounced in the venous compartment of the microvascular system. Moreover, manipulation of venous outflow compared to arterial inflow has a disproportionately greater effect on transcapillary exchange.

The features of this special vulnerability of the venous system have been summarised by Hauck (1976) as follows:

1. As the vessels dilate the blood flow through them inevitably slows; under such circumstances red cells clump together and it becomes more difficult for blood to pass through channels.
2. Normal plasma concentration of fibrinogen influencing the post-capillary tendency to red cell aggregation.
3. Normally plasma leaks from blood as it flows through the far end of the capillaries and the small vessels of the venous tree. As this portion is lost the blood becomes concentrated, contains relatively more fibrinogen and develops an unstable flow — in fact it can become very sluggish or stop — even in normal conditions. Thus these small vessels beyond capillaries do not make a very good job of letting the blood through or keeping it in good shape. Moreover they do not control a proper distribution of fluid between and within the vessels.

When several factors work together to encourage intravascular clotting, endothelial injury or a considerable rise in blood viscosity, the blood flow in the superficial microvascular system of the skin often ceases long enough to cause ischaemic necrosis of the epidermis. This is seen in a number of skin diseases, including chilblains and other forms of perniosis, collagen diseases such as scleroderma, rheumatoid arthritis, lupus erythematosus and dermatomyositis, and those disorders classified as vasculitis.

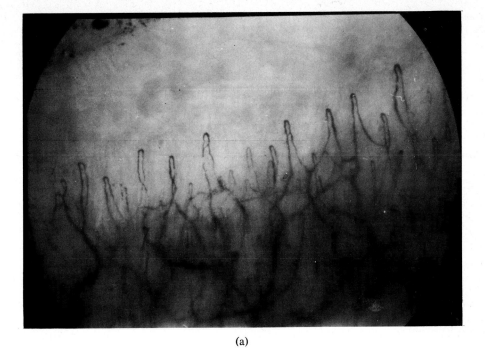

(a)

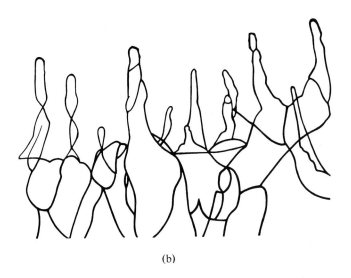

(b)

Figure 12.3. Nail-fold capillaries (a) with drawing (b) to illustrate numerous cross communications. There are anastomotic channels even in the papillary vessels.

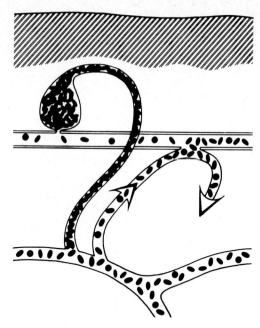

Figure 12.4. Illustration of congestion in superficial vessels resulting in diversion of blood through deeper channels.

References

Arnold, J. (1875) Über das Verhalten der Wandungen der Blütgefasse bei der Emigration weisser Blutkorper. *Virchows Archiv für Pathologische Anatomie und Physiologie und für klinische Medizin,* **62,** 487.

Ashton, N. (1960) Corneal vascularisation. In *The Transparency of the Cornea* (Ed.) Duke-Elder, S. & Perkins, E. S. p. 131. Oxford: Blackwell.

Boyd, A. M., Catchpole, B. N., Jepson, R. P. & Rose, S. S. (1952) Some observations on venous pressure estimations in lower limb. *Journal of Bone and Joint Surgery,* **34B,** 599.

Carrier, E. B. (1922) Studies on the physiology of capillaries. *American Journal of Physiology,* **61,** 528.

Copeman, P. W. M. (1970) Investigations into the pathogenesis of acute cutaneous angiitis. *British Journal of Dermatology,* **82** (Supplement 5), 51.

Copeman, P. W. M. (1975) Cutaneous angiitis. *Journal of the Royal College of Physicians of London,* **9,** 103.

Copeman, P. W. M. & Ryan, T. J. (1970) The problems of cutaneous angiitis with reference to histopathology and pathogenesis. *British Journal of Dermatology,* **82** (Supplement 5), 2.

Copeman, P. W. M. & Ryan, T. J. (1971) Cutaneous angiitis patterns of rashes explained by 1) flow properties of blood 2) anatomical disposition of vessels. *British Journal of Dermatology,* **85,** 205.

Haddy, F. J. (1960) Effect of histamine on small and large vessel pressure in the dog foreleg. *American Journal of Physiology,* **198,** 161.

Hauck, G. (1976) Low flow state predisposition of the venous microcirculation. In *Proceedings of the World Congress for Microcirculation, Toronto, 1975* (Ed.) Grayson, J. & Zingg, W. London: Plenum.

Majno, G., Palade, G. E. & Schoefl, G. I. (1961) Studies on inflammation. II. The site of action of histamine and serotonin along the vascular tree: a topographic study. *Journal of Biophysical and Biochemical Cytology,* **11,** 607.

Rowley, D. A. (1968) Venous constriction as the cause of increased vascular permeability produced by 5-hydroxytryptamine, histamine, bradykinin and 48/80 in the rat. *British Journal of Experimental Pathology,* **45,** 156.

Ryan, T. J. (1969) The epidermis and its blood supply in venous disorders of the leg. *Transactions of the St John's Hospital Dermatological Society,* **55,** 51.

Ryan, T. J. (1973) In *Physiology and Pathophysiology of the Skin* (Ed.) Jarrett, A. Vol. 2. London: Academic Press.

Wright, I. S. (1973) *Abstract of the 4th International Congress of Thrombosis and Haemostasis, Vienna.* p. 273.

BLOOD VISCOSITY

High blood viscosity is sometimes a systemic problem, as in myelomatosis or polycythaemia, but it is more usually a local phenomenon affecting the venous compartment of the circulation. Hyperviscosity in itself is not usually the whole explanation of disease. It is a direct result of decreased blood flow, and thus becomes important when there is a fall in cardiac output or there is peripheral stasis as in shock.

Local disease of the microvasculature leading to distorted vessels may combine with hyperviscosity to produce severe stasis, ischaemia and acidosis. Certain sites seem more susceptible to these changes than others, the retina being one and the nose another. Thus a change in vision, retinal micro-aneurysms, haemorrhages and exudates, as well as papilloedema, are frequently seen in Waldenström's macroglobulinaemia, while epistaxis from the nasal septum presumably is encouraged by the stasis so typical of that site (see Chapter 9) perhaps because, like the skin, it reacts to cooling.

Skin signs of hyperviscosity occur either peripherally as part of the response to cooling, as in Raynaud's phenomenon, or at sites of pathology such as scars, skin biopsies, perniosis, or atrophie blanche. A full review of the hyperviscosity syndrome can be found in Bloch and Maki (1973).

Slow flow and increased vascular permeability along the course of the vascular tree both promote haemoconcentration. Increases in the concentration of cells, protein and fibrinogen in the blood all add to the viscosity at such sites (Ryan and Copeman, 1969). It is usual for aggregates of blood cells to form where there is stasis and to disturb flow further, particularly at points of narrowing in the vascular tree. Aggregated red cells usually separate very readily, but interaction with platelet aggregates and fibrin may prevent this.

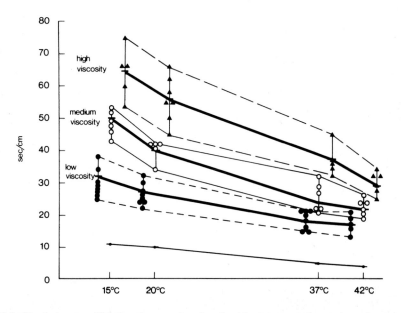

Figure 12.5. Blood viscosity. The time in seconds taken for blood to move 1 cm along 4 metres 0.5 mm diameter polythene tubing at different temperatures. At such a low rate of flow, blood with the highest viscosity is disproportionately affected by cooling to 15°C.

The problems of viscosity and flow are the subjects of several textbooks (Whitmore, 1968; Dintenfass, 1971) and need not be discussed fully in this monograph. Aspects of this phenomenon that contribute to stasis act predominantly in the venular bed (Table 12.2). Such an effect is maximal in the venules at low rates of shear. When static columns of blood in superficial vessels are exposed to cold the cooled blood thickens. In perniosis, for example, there always is gross stasis in the capillaries and venules but cooling accentuates it; stasis equally contributes to the cooling.

Table 12.2. Factors which cause an increase in blood viscosity.

Surface cooling
Low blood pressure and low blood flow velocity
Wide lumen of blood vessel
Increased permeability and hence increased haematocrit
Hyperconcentration of serum protein and fibrinogen
Rouleaux formation
Gravitational stasis

Figure 12.5 illustrates the effect of cooling on blood flow in vitro; the blood is passed through 4 metres of 0.5 mm bore polythene tubing (Figure 12.6).

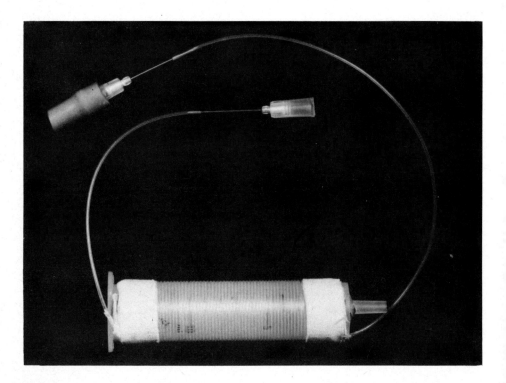

Figure 12.6. Coil of 4 metres of polythene tubing used to produce the graph for Figure 12.5.

References

Bloch, K. J. & Maki, G. (1973) Hyperviscosity syndromes associated with immunoglobulin abnormalities. *Seminars in Hematology.* **10,** 113.
Dintenfass, L. (1971) *Viscosity Factors in Blood Flow Ischaemia and Thrombosis.* London: Butterworths.
Ryan, T. J. (1973) In *Physiology and Pathophysiology of the Skin* (Ed.) Jarrett, A. Vol. 2. London: Academic Press.
Ryan, T. J. & Copeman, P. W. M. (1969) Micro-vascular pattern and blood stasis in skin disease. *British Journal of Dermatology,* **81,** 663.
Whitmore, R. L. (1968) *Rheology of the Circulation.* Oxford: Pergamon Press.

THE ANATOMY OF STASIS

Two main features characterise the anatomical pattern of the vascular tree at sites of stasis: one is dilatation and elongation of existing channels, the other is an increase in alternative or shunting vessels (Figure 12.3).

The elongated coiled papillary vessels described above and illustrated on page 32 are one of the main features of atrophie blanche (Figure 12.7) and are seen to underlie all forms of pigmented purpuric dermatoses (Davis and Lawler, 1958), including the common stasis purpura. They are somewhat susceptible to trauma, even to minor knocks which cause bleeding and thrombosis.

In some legs, the horizontal subpapillary plexus is dilated and the papillary vasculature reduced. In its grossest form this is seen as arborising telangiectasia in which leashes of fine vessels lying parallel to the surface of the skin result in purple plaques that

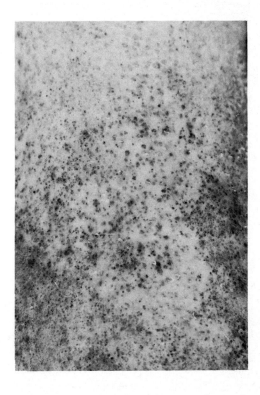

Figure 12.7. Atrophie blanche affecting shin. Each punctate lesion represents a greatly coiled capillary and the white areas are completely avascular.

present a major cosmetic problem (Figure 12.8). This pattern is associated with atrophy of the upper dermis and a decrease in the amount of supporting connective tissue; it is always more obvious in the legs but occurs also at sites of stasis induced by exposure to cold (Figure 12.9). Red cheeks show similar features, with rather degenerate connective tissue, fewer than normal papillary vessels and grossly dilated residual horizontal vessels. The stasis of acrocyanosis is also associated with a slight reduction in the number of papillary vessels, but the remaining capillaries may be dilated, particularly at their peaks where they lie nearest to the cooled surface of the skin. The predominant blueness of such tissues is due to the extreme stasis of the blood lying in columns in the dilated and easily visible horizontal venous plexus (Figure 12.10).

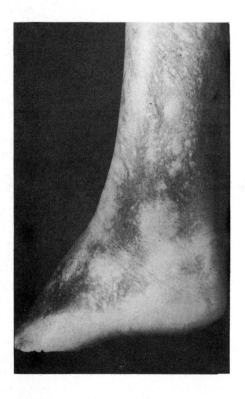

Figure 12.8. Arborising telangiectasia is a consequence of upper dermal atrophy, as well as loss of papillary vessels, but at the same time preservation and dilatation of the horizontal subpapillary venous plexus occur.

Whenever there is stasis in the papillary vessels, with or without stasis in the horizontal plexus, blood tends to be diverted through deeper alternative channels. Even in normal tissues there are ample anastomoses to take on such a shunting role; they merely have to dilate to become significant. Persistent stasis and ischaemia invariably encourage an increase in the number of actively shunting vessels. Some of these may be newly formed vessels, but much depends on whether the affected area also has some stimulus to angiogenesis. The stasis seen in carcinomatous tissue is usually associated with very considerable new vessel formation stimulated probably by metabolic demands and by the irritation of various byproducts. The same may be true of the skin flaps described in Chapter 5. Any endothelial injury in association with coagulation seems to result in endothelial proliferation provided that complete infarction does not occur.

In allograft rejection, venous block is more usual and damaging than is arterial occlusion and the distribution of autoallergic lesions depends on the distribution of veins in the affected organs (Waksman, 1960). Species variation in the morphology of lesions

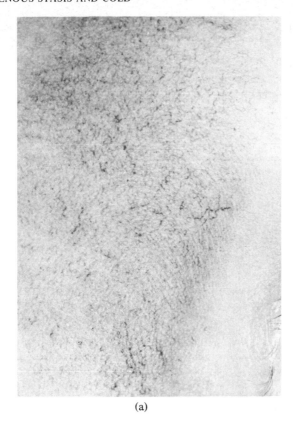

(a)

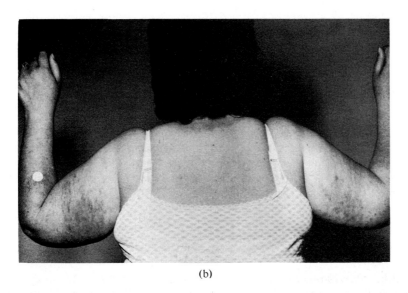

(b)

Figure 12.9. Scanty dilated venules (a) in the skin of the upper arm. (b) These are a feature of perniosis and are often seen over thick pads of fat.

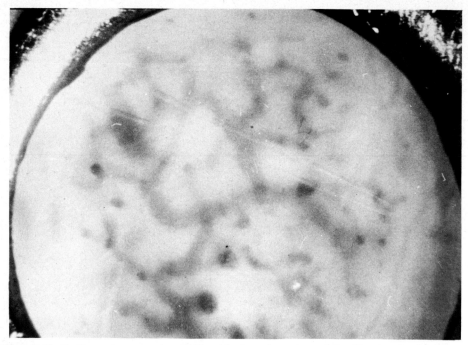

Figure 12.10. Capillary-microscope view of dilated horizontal venules and the dilated peaks of one or two papillary vessels in an area of acrocyanosis. The diameter of the ring is 2 mm.

due to tuberculin inoculation can be explained by differences in venous pattern. Delayed hypersensitivity reactions, as a class, can be expressed only where veins and venules are numerous.

Contact dermatitis is initially a venular phenomenon (Wilms-Kretschmer, Flax and Cotran, 1967). The main reason why venules are so important in inflammation is the tendency for the noxious agents provoking inflammation (in other words the triggers), to lodge at sites where there is both stasis and an increase in permeability (see Chapter 6).

One important contribution made by veins, as distinct from arteries, is the greater degree to which fibrinolysis is activated by their endothelium (Todd, 1959; Chakrabarti, Birks and Fearnley, 1963). Cuffing a limb with a sphygmomanometer temporarily increases fibrinolysis in it (Clarke, Orandi and Clifton, 1960), but it may be reduced in areas of prolonged stasis. Thus fibrinolytic activity is lower in the legs than in the arms (Pandolfi et al, 1968). Nevertheless, transient venous occlusion or prolonged elevation restores the activity in the legs to levels found in the arms. Less activator than normal is found in the endothelium of veins predisposed to thrombosis (Nilsson and Isaacson, 1972) or to vasculitis (Cunliffe et al, 1971).

In a scanning electron-microscopic study of varicose veins Mahrle and Orfanos (1972) saw endothelial exfoliation, and they related it to disturbed blood flow and to greater injury from adhesion to fibrin and platelets.

Endothelium in the skin flaps described in Chapter 5 was capable of producing activator even after six hours of stasis, and in those experiments endothelial shedding caused by the forces of reperfusion accounted for subsequent loss of fibrinolytic activity.

Some investigators have suggested that venous insufficiency is the major factor causing tissue necrosis in pedicle flaps used in plastic surgery (Braithwaite, 1950; de Haan and Stark, 1961; Fujino, 1967); others (Hynes, 1950) have blamed arterial insufficiency. But probably the truth is that both are important and each is responsible for a different pattern of tissue behaviour before the final common factor, ischaemia, is induced (Myers and Cherry, 1968) (see Chapter 5).

Oedema can be a significant feature of stasis. Thus Smith et al (1974) measured the hand volume of patients who had an arteriovenous fistula for renal dialysis. Oedema of the fistulous hand was a common finding and it was probably due to high venous pressure, exacerbated by immobility during dialysis. The oedema also accumulates in transplanted skin flaps in humans and has been thought to be a major factor in pedicle necrosis. Although it is common clinical practice to position patients in such a way that the effects of gravitation are circumvented, little experimental work has been done to justify it. In the skin flap studies by Cherry on the relationship between oedema formation and gravity it was shown that when an increased water content was the predominant factor in a dependent pedicle, the tissue survival was little affected; that is, gravity interferes with blood flow but not with ultimate survival. The histological changes in these dependent skin pedicles are discussed in Chapter 4. In other experiments, some degree of tissue swelling occurred, but this was associated with increased shunting, which did cause a survival problem.

Oedema as such, unlike arteriovenous shunting, does not contribute to venous hypertension: on the other hand, it may contribute to the organisation of the supporting tissues, and the consequent fibrosis may suppress or obliterate the vasculature.

References

Braithwaite, F. (1950) Preliminary observations on vascular channels in tube pedicles. *British Journal of Plastic Surgery*, **3**, 40.

Chakrabarti, R., Birks, P. M. & Fearnley, G. R. (1963) Origin of blood fibrinolytic activity from veins and its bearing on the fate of venous thrombosis. *Lancet*, **i**, 1288.

Clarke, R. L., Orandi, A. & Clifton, E. E. (1960) Induction of fibrinolysis by venous obstruction. *Angiology*, **11**, 367.

Cunliffe, W. J., Dodman, B., Holmes, R. L. & Forster, R. A. (1971) Local fibrinolytic activity in patients with cutaneous vasculitis. *British Journal of Dermatology*, **84**, 420.

Davis, M. J. & Lawler, J. C. (1958) Capillary alterations in pigmented purpuric disease of the skin. *Archives of Dermatology*, **78**, 723.

de Haan, C. R. & Stark, R. B. (1961) Changes in efferent circulation of tubed pedicles and in the trans-plantability of large composite grafts produced by histamine iontophoresis. *Plastic and Reconstructive Surgery*, **28**, 577.

Florey, Lord (1970) *General Pathology*, 4th edition, p. 1203. London: Lloyd Luke Medical Books.

Fujino, T. (1967) Contribution of the axial and perforator vasculature to circulation in flaps. *Plastic and Reconstructive Surgery*, **39**, 125.

Hynes, W. (1950) The blood vessels in skin tubes and flaps. *British Journal of Plastic Surgery*, **3**, 165.

Mahrle, G. & Orfanos, C. E. (1972) Endothel-veranderungen bei Varicosis (stereo-electron-mikroskopische Betunde). *Archiv für Dermatologisch Forschung*, **242**, 216.

Myers, M. B. & Cherry, G. (1968) Causes of necrosis in pedicle flaps. *Plastic and Reconstructive Surgery*, **42**, 43.

Nilsson, I. M. & Isaacson, S. (1972) New aspects of the pathogenesis of thrombo-embolism. *Progress in Surgery*, **11**, 46.

Pandolfi, M., Robertson, B., Isacson, S. & Nilsson, I. M. (1968) Fibrinolytic activity of human veins in arms and legs. *Thrombosis et Diathesis Haemorrhagica*, **20**, 247.

Smith, M., Vessey, M. P., Bounds, W. & Warren, J. (1974) Swelling of arm in patients with arteriovenous fistula. *British Medical Journal*, **iii**, 106.

Todd, A. S. (1959) The histological localisation of fibrinolysin activator. *Journal of Pathology and Bacteriology*, **78**, 281.

Waksman, B. H. (1960) The pattern of rejection in rat skin homografts and its relation to the vascular network. *Laboratory Investigation*, **12**, 46.

Wilms-Kretschmer, K., Flax, M. H. & Cotran, R. S. (1967) Fine structure of vascular response in haptene-specific delayed hypersensitivity and contact dermatitis. *Laboratory Investigation*, **17**, 334.

OPENING UP OF ARTERIOVENOUS CHANNELS

Arteriography in patients with varicose veins reveals rapid emptying of arteries, early filling of veins and incomplete filling, with delayed emptying of capillaries (Haimovici, Steinman and Caplan, 1966); any stasis seen is primarily in the capillaries. This and the fact that subjects with venous stasis can taste radiopaque material used in femoral arteriograms within 30 seconds, compared to 60 to 90 seconds in normal subjects (Piulachs and Vidal-Barraquer, 1953) suggest that arteriovenous shunting is taking place. These same authors highlighted the shunting effect of multiple small arteriovenous communications by demonstrating the high oxygen saturation of venous blood in subjects with varicose veins. The vessels responsible for shunting are probably present in normal skin as small vessels with a diameter of 30 to 60 μm and become dilated and used to significant degree only when venous pressure is raised. Trauma to the skin by causing capillary stasis is responsible for diversion of blood through such communications.

Profound hormonal changes in pregnancy have a particularly important influence on arteriovenous communications, and Menendez (1967) blamed high levels of progesterone for the opening of such shunts.

In the venous stasis syndrome, the more serious the pathology, the more obvious is the shunting. Wellbourn found shunts, visible on arteriography, in 23 out of 51 patients with leg ulcers, and most of the 51 patients with leg ulcers studied by Myers and Cherry (1971) had evidence of functioning shunts. It is not unusual for the skin at sites of venous stasis to be warm and, at the same time, to show almost total capillary stasis when viewed by capillary microscopy. Haeger and Bergman (1963) considered such warm spots to be due to arteriovenous shunts, and even varicose veins were attributed to high venous pressure from such shunts. The odd discolouration and paraesthesiae in the skin of the leg on standing have been blamed on the opening up of such shunts (Malan, 1958; Khobreh and Roy, 1966; Amir Jahed, 1968; Ryan and Wilkinson, 1974). However, red warm spots on a background of acrocyanosis can occur even in children with no evidence of varicose veins.

The development of shunts in areas of extreme stasis is well known in neoplasia (Urbach, 1961). It is also a feature of the vascular changes seen in psoriasis. A fall in blood pressure also may lead to shunting because capillaries are preferentially clogged up by aggregated blood. Lambert (1957), for instance, noted short-circuiting in muscle only when the blood pressure fell below 60 mm Hg.

Vogler and Gollman (1955) also suspected that capillary obstruction accounts for shunting of blood into superficial veins and suggested that this could lead to accelerated blood flow through the arterial and venous system with consequent hypertension. There is, in effect, a significant correlation between severe arterial disease and high plasma viscosity and high fibrinogen levels (Dormandy, Hoare and Postlethwaite, 1974).

NEW VESSEL FORMATION

In intravascular coagulation, it is usual for endothelial proliferation to occur as well as clotting, leucocyte stickiness and platelet aggregation; moreover, in some cases of repeated episodes of intravascular coagulation, the skin can produce an extraordinary degree of new vessel formation, much of which is composed of shunting vessels (see Figure 4.29).

Endothelial proliferation is an histological feature of vasculitis and, in some of the more unusual forms of angiolymphoid hyperplasia, it is the predominant finding (see Chapter 4). Such proliferation is almost invariably initiated in the venules, and usually shunts are a feature (see also Chapter 5, page 93).

Figure 12.11 illustrates the close relationship of endothelial proliferation to fibrin formation and how stasis and cold contribute to this. It also correlates the persistence of the fibrin with the presence of alternative channels. Injury to epidermis provides directive forces, and further influences are provided by the reticuloendothelial system, fibrinolysis and vasoconstriction.

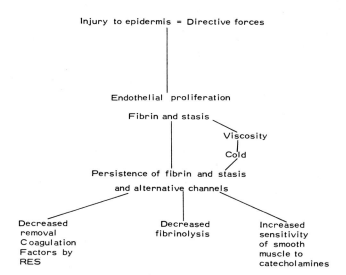

Figure 12.11. Diagram of interrelationship of new vessel formation with epidermal injury, alternative channels, cold exposure.

In the leg, gravity contributes yet another set of factors responsible for the generation of hypertrophy and alternative channels (Figure 12.12). However, modifying factors such as hypertension, anaemia or immune complex disease are also involved.

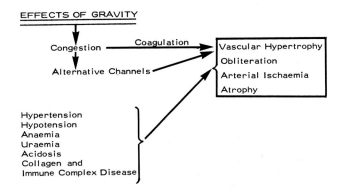

Figure 12.12. Diagram of various influences responsible for the changes in the vasculature of the legs due to gravitational stasis.

Scars are commonly affected by vasculitis and are the sole site of persistent chronic vasculitis in some patients. The selection of scar tissue has been described in Wegener's granulomatosis (Kraus et al, 1965). Atrophie blanche is an interesting example of such a locus minoris resistentiae associated with several varieties of vasculitis (see Chapter 13); the nose (see Chapter 9) is a similar site.

References

Amir-Jahed, A. K. (1968) Angiodyskinesia. *Surgery, Gynecology and Obstetrics,* **127,** 609.
Dormandy, J. A., Hoare, E. & Postlethwaite, J. (1974) Importance of blood viscosity in rheological claudication. *Proceedings of the Royal Society of Medicine,* **67,** 446.
Haeger, K. H. M. & Bergman, L. (1963) Skin temperature of normal and varicose legs and some reflections on the etiology of varicose veins. *Angiology,* **14,** 473.
Haimovici, H., Steinman, C. & Caplan, L. H. (1966) Role of arteriovenous anastomoses in vascular diseases of the lower extremity. *Annals of Surgery,* **164,** 990.
Khobreh, M. T. & Roy, P. (1966) Functional circulatory disorders of the lower extremities due to regional hemokinetic imbalance: a new clinical and angiographic concept. *Surgery,* **61,** 880.
Kraus, Z., Vortel, V., Fingerland, A., Salavec, M. & Krch, V. (1965) Unusual cutaneous manifestations in Wegener's granulomatosis. *Acta Dermato-venereologica,* **45,** 288.
Kulka, J. P. (1966) Vascular derangement in rheumatoid arthritis. In *Modern Trends in Rheumatology* (Ed.) Hill, A. G. S. London: Butterworths.
Lambert, J. (1957) Aspects et problèmes de la physiologie des anastomoses arterioveneuses. *Angeiologie et Annales de la Société Française d'Angeiologie et d'Histopathologie,* **9,** 11.
Malan, E. (1958) Vascular syndromes from dilatation of arteriovenous communications of the sole of the foot. *Archives of Surgery,* **77,** 783.
Menendez, C. V. (1967) The post phlebitic syndrome and varicose veins. *Journal of the Louisiana Medical Society,* **119,** 177.
Myers, M. B. & Cherry, G. (1971) Pathophysiology and treatment of stasis ulcers of the leg. *American Surgeon,* **37,** 167.
Piulachs, P. & Vidal-Barraquer, F. (1953) Pathogenic study of varicose veins. *Angiology,* **4,** 59.
Ryan, T. J. & Wilkinson, D. S. (1974) Angiodyskinesia and osteochondritis dissecans. *Proceedings of the Royal Society of Medicine,* **67,** 1242.
Urbach, F. (1961) The blood supply of tumours. In *Advances in Biology of the Skin* (Ed.) Montagna, W. & Ellis, R. A. Vol. 2, p. 123. Oxford: Pergamon.
Vogler, E. & Gollman, G. (1955) The significance of the terminal circulation in the development of vascular disease and disturbances of blood flow: vasographic studies. *Angiology,* **6,** 540.

THE EFFECT OF COLD ON SKIN CIRCULATION

In certain areas of skin, especially over fat pads, the skin can be cooled on a chilly day by the application of a glass vessel containing water at 20°C and such cooling persists for as long as one hour (Foged, 1929, 1930). Haxthausen (1930) emphasised that the arms and legs of women were subject to repetitive cooling effects. The skin is often red, cyanosed and traversed by numerous small dilated venules, and it is cool. The lower leg and outer aspect of the upper arm (Table 12.3) are most affected by these changes, and the vascular changes are particularly marked around the hair follicle (Figure 12.13). Haxthausen (1930) and several groups of workers cited by him have emphasised that the capillary changes of perniosis are associated with vasoconstriction of arteries and veins.

Table 12.3. Skin temperature of the upper arm.

	Anterior surface	Exterior surface	Posterior surface	Internal surface
Men	31.7°C	31.3°C	30.8°C	31.9°C
Women	31.4°C	30.0°C	29.9°C	31.5°C

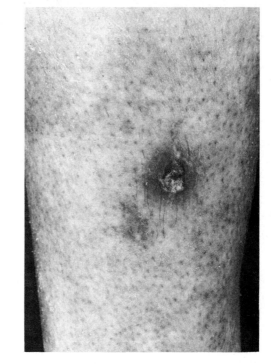

Figure 12.13. Prominent dilated vessels around hair follicles are a feature of perniosis. An area so affected has ulcerated in this patient.

Chilblains (Figure 12.14) have the histology of vasculitis, the principal feature being dilated congested vessels, endothelial proliferation, and infiltration by white cells. However, Kyrle (1915) observed similar changes even in the skin surrounding chilblains. The subcutaneous tissues tend to be thickened, and the superficial capillaries are widely dilated, aneurysmal and inclined to angiokeratomous changes. Dittrich (1929) found that cold affects the veins more than the arteries, and that they tend to be thickened. The blood in these dilated superficial vessels is almost stationary.

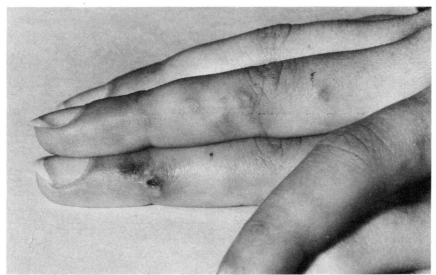

Figure 12.14. Chilblains are a form of vasculitis. In this case micropapular infarcts are a principal feature.

Perniosis is a general term useful in describing changes that have a common aetiology and pathogenesis (Table 12.4). The tendency is for arteries and veins to contract and for capillaries to dilate, and this results in the blood being trapped in the capillary bed, through which it flows sluggishly. Haxthausen (1930) suggested that in this situation there is a lowering of nutrition in the skin and a greater opportunity for microembolism. He listed the localisation of tuberculosis, leprosy and syphilis at such sites.

Table 12.4. List of conditions associated with perniosis.

Chilblains, frostbite and trench foot
Erythrocyanosis of the legs of young girls
Acrocyanosis
Cinnabar red spots
Livedo reticularis
Cutis marmorata
Erythema induratum
Angiokeratoma
Keratosis pilaris
Rosacea
Cold urticaria
Winter prurigo
Acrodermatitis pustulosa hiemalis
Ichthyosis
Lupus erythematosus
Chronic infections, tuberculosis, leprosy, syphilis, trichophytosis

As illustrated by Copeman and Ryan (1971) some rashes have a pattern determined by stasis induced by cold while others, especially experimental ones, have patterns determined by extreme pressure (Figure 12.15), suction (Figure 7.2, page 141), or the inoculation of agents that cause vasoconstriction and promote stasis. In the marbled reticulate patterns of blueness and redness seen in human skin (Figure 12.16), particularly in children when exposed to cold, it is physiological stasis that accounts for the blueness. This pattern is, in part, anatomical. In areas of skin furthest away from arterioles and draining veins, the blood tends to flow more slowly and to spend more of its transit time near the surface where it is cooled. Vasoconstriction or other causes of narrowing of the central artery will result in greater stasis at the periphery of the area of skin it supplies. Increased blood viscosity will have the same effect, and Copeman and Ryan (1971) proposed that exaggerated skin reticulation is caused as commonly by blood defects as by arterial narrowing.

Livedo reticularis is not a disease; it is a sign and symptom of a disturbed blood flow, and in the livid areas the resulting stasis is responsible for a wide range of pathology and for the localisation of haematogenous triggers of vasculitis which occurs at such sites. Renaut (1883) observed that the paler areas were supplied by deeply situated arteries and that they filled earlier than the surrounding bluish network. The bluish areas show the features of perniosis — dilated capillaries and subpapillary venous plexus and a sluggish circulation. At room temperature, 22 to 24°C, the pale and blue areas differ little in surface temperature but, when the skin is cooled, blue areas are cooler and take longer to warm up when exposed to a warm environment. By contrast, burns to the skin are always worse in the blue areas because the excess heat is less well dissipated than in the pale area with the better blood supply.

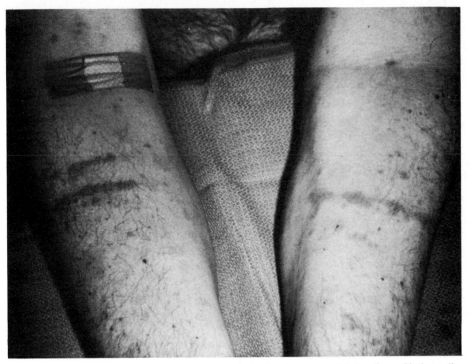

Figure 12.15. In a patient with cryoglobulinaemia constricting bands are enough to localise and induce a linear pattern of vasculitis.

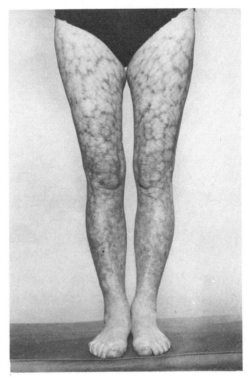

Figure 12.16. Reticulate patterns corresponding to areas of stasis in the skin. This patient is also illustrated in Figures 11.1 and 3.5.

NODULAR LESIONS ASSOCIATED WITH COLD EXPOSURE

Wilkinson (1954) described three groups of such patients:
1. Young obese women, otherwise healthy.
2. Young or middle-aged women, immobilised by rheumatoid arthritis or poliomyelitis.
3. Menopausal women with Raynaud's phenomenon and acrocyanosis.

Jepson (1951) described a group of middle-aged females with rheumatoid disease who also had cold hands and who developed painless nodules of the lower legs after exposure to cold; these initially were bright pink and later were purplish in colour and were annular or serpiginous in shape. There could also be cayenne pepper spots, seen microscopically to be dilated capillary tufts; in addition follicular perniosis and hypertrichosis were present.

Tuberculosis, syphilis and a wide variety of other diseases may be localised at sites of livedo reticularis, Raynaud's phenomenon (Figure 12.17) or perniosis, and they sometimes encourage nodular lesions in some patients. Immune complexes and hypertension are other associated complicating factors.

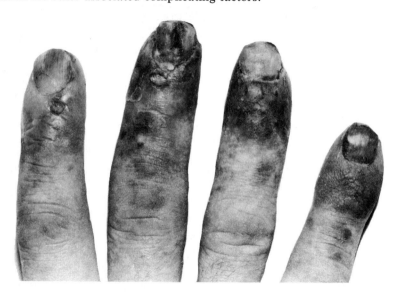

Figure 12.17. Localisation of cryoglobulins in acral areas is particularly a feature of patients with a history of peripheral vasoconstriction in response to cold.

Winter exacerbation of vasculitis is frequently mentioned in the literature, but like Osler (1914), the author blames the Victorian architecture in North Oxford for this when it happens to his patients. The contribution of cold to vasculitis is difficult to assess accurately. Winkelmann and Ditto (1964) could do no more than record that it was especially emphasised by a number of patients in their series. Haxthausen (1930) wrote a comprehensive and largely descriptive monograph on the subject. In the study reported in Chapter 9, some aspects such as the localisation of radioactive gold in the nose, can clearly be quantified. Investigators of cryoglobulinaemia have frequently recorded its obvious association, and the miniskirt has been blamed for vasculitis of the thighs of young girls (Figure 12.18) (Copeman and Ryan, 1971), and by Hamblin (1972) in a case

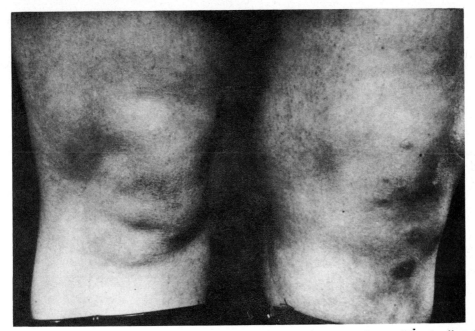

Figure 12.18. Mini-skirts and knee boots failed to protect the knees and consequently vasculitis only affected that site in this young girl. Increased girth above the knees contributed to insulation of the skin from the warm central core.

of infectious mononucleosis. Schönlein—Henoch purpura also occurs more commonly in the cold (see case report and review by Rogers et al, 1971) and charts can be drawn up like the one showing the effect of weather on painful crises in sickle-cell anaemia (Amjad, Bannerman and Judisch, 1974) (Figure 12.19). Furthermore, there is an urticarial form of leucocytoclastic angiitis known as cold vasculitis; Macmillan (1969) and Tindall, Beeker and Rosse (1969) described a familial form of this.

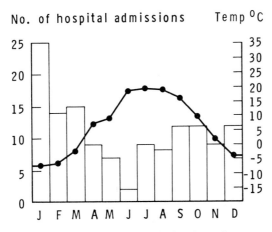

Figure 12.19. Sickle cell crises occurred more commonly during the cooler seasons of the year in one study.

References

Amjad, H., Bannerman, R. M. & Judisch, J. M. (1974) Sickling pain and season. *British Medical Journal,* **ii,** 54.

Copeman, P. W. M. & Ryan, T. J. (1971) Cutaneous angiitis patterns of rashes explained by 1) flow properties of blood 2) anatomical disposition of vessels. *British Journal of Dermatology,* **85,** 205.

Dittrich, O. (1929) Uber Froschaden. *Archiv für Dermatologie und Syphilis,* **157,** 1.

Foged, J. (1929) *Klinische Undersøgelser over Hudens Temperatur.* Quoted by Haxthausen, H. (1930).

Foged, J. (1930) Normal circulation of blood through skin (on basis of skin temperature). *Acta Rheumatologica,* **2,** 5.

Hamblin, T. J. (1972) Mononucleosis and the mini skirt, an incompatible combination. *British Medical Journal,* **iv,** 708.

Haxthausen, H. (1930) *Cold in Relation to Skin Diseases.* Copenhagen: Levin and Munksgaard.

Jepson, R. P. (1951) Raynauds' phenomenon — a review of the clinical problem. *Annals of the Royal College of Surgeons of England,* **9,** 35.

Kraus, Z., Vortel, V., Fingerland, A., Salvacec, M. & Krch, V. (1965) Unusual cutaneous manifestations in Wegener's granulomatosis. *Acta Dermato-venereologica,* **45,** 288.

Kyrle, J. (1915) *Die Schädigungen der Haut durch Beruf und gewerbliche Arbeit.* Quoted by Haxthausen, H. (1930).

Macmillan, A. L. (1969) Cold vasculitis. *Proceedings of the Royal Society of Medicine,* **60,** 12.

Osler, W. (1914) The visceral lesions of purpura and allied conditions. *British Medical Journal,* **i,** 517.

Renaut, J. (1883) *Dictionn. Encyclopaedie des Sciences Medicales,* **28,** 158. Quoted by Haxthausen, H. (1930).

Rogers, W., Bunn, S. M., Kurtzman, N. A. & White, M. G. (1971) Schönlein—Henoch syndrome associated with exposure to cold. *Archives of Internal Medicine,* **128,** 782.

Tindall, J. P., Beeker, S. K. & Rosse, W. F. (1969) Familial cold urticaria. *Archives of Internal Medicine,* **124,** 129.

Wilkinson, D. S. (1954) The vascular basis of some nodular eruptions of the legs. *British Journal of Dermatology,* **66,** 201.

Winkelmann, R. K. & Ditto, W. B. (1964) Cutaneous and visceral syndromes of necrotising or "allergic" angiitis. A study of 38 cases. *Medicine* (Baltimore), **43,** 59.

13. Complicated and Limited Forms of Vasculitis

A number of diseases that fall within the spectrum of urticaria, vasculitis, coagulation and thrombosis deserve separate analysis because as often as not they have a fairly distinct morphological or histopathological identity. Diseases such as polyarteritis nodosa or Wegener's granulomatosis were initially described as systemic diseases, but later authors classified them as *limited forms*. On the other hand, some diseases such as Behçet's syndrome were initially described as limited conditions but are now known to have more widespread manifestations. When patients with rheumatoid arthritis develop vasculitis it is described as a *complicated* form of the disease (Hart, 1966). Limitations include involvement of only one type of vessel, as in polyarteritis nodosa, or of a group of organs such as the mouth, eyes and genitalia in Behçet's disease or the respiratory tract in Wegener's granulomatosis. The pathogenesis of such diseases is not at all clear but an attempt will be made to show that they are related to vasculitis in general and that management of patients with these disorders can be rationalised.

Diseases are also limited when they are focal — a concept which is commonly applied to renal disease but could be applied equally well to skin disease. Thus atrophie blanche is a focal form of sclerosis. In the following sections various limitations and complications will be described and particular emphasis will be placed on constitutional defects which underlie certain syndromes or diseases already referred to in previous chapters.

Prognosis of these disorders is usually good if they are focal or limited, but it is bad when they are complicated or diffuse. They are all consequences of microvascular injury, and should share with all kinds of vasculitis the same programme of investigation and treatment that will be described in Chapters 14 and 15.

ARTERITIS

By arteritis is implied inflammation of the arterial wall in response to injury. Although inflammation is said to be aimed at removal of the noxious agents and the byproducts of injury so that repair can proceed, the vessel is often destroyed in the process. The clinical picture is therefore dependent on the consequent thrombosis or rupture of the artery.

The skin is so well supplied by capillaries and venules that arteries in comparison seem relatively sparse. They are found in the deeper dermis and the subcutaneous tissues and are small vessels with a thick muscular coat and internal elastic lamina. Arterioles characteristically have less elastic or muscle than arteries (see Chapter 4); they may be found in the mid-dermis where they supply the adnexa such as the sweat glands, but they are always outnumbered by capillaries and venules.

Arteriolisation is a term applied to capillaries, venules and veins which have developed thickening of their muscular coat, increased elastic tissue and fibrosis as a response to increased blood flow or to inflammation. It is important to be aware that vessels of the skin normally show a mild degree of arteriolisation and that this feature is seen especially in the skin of the lower leg in adults (see Chapter 4). For this reason the term arteritis of the skin should be used only when serial sections of deep dermal and subcutaneous vessels show clear evidence of arterial involvement. This diagnosis will be of the greatest significance only if the skin biopsy is taken from tissues not subjected to prolonged gravitational stasis.

Some of the most convincing descriptions of arteritis include details of the microscopic appearance of pinhead to millet seed-sized nodules, sometimes forming chains or strings, as of pearls, running along small arteries on the surface of viscera or muscles (see Figure 1.4, page 8) (Kussmaul and Maier, 1866; Arkin, 1930). However, such features are not so readily seen in the skin. Aneurysms are nevertheless the usual cause of focal nodularity of arteries and are found in polyarteritis nodosa, thrombotic thrombocytopenic purpura, temporal arteritis and a focal arteritis of young men with erythema nodosum described by Hines, Kelly and Barker (1960).

References

Arkin, A. (1930) A clinical and pathological study of peri-arteritis nodosa. A report of five cases. One histologically healed. *American Journal of Pathology,* **6,** 401.
Hart, F. D. (1966) Complicated rheumatoid disease. *British Medical Journal,* **ii,** 131.
Hines, E. A. J., Kelly, P. J. & Barker, N. W. (1960) Idiopathic disseminated focal arteritis: occurrence of false aneurysms in large and medium-sized arteries. *Journal of the American Medical Association,* **174,** 848.
Kussmaul, A. & Maier, R. (1866) Ueber eine bisher nicht beschriebene eigenthümliche Arterien erkrankung (Periarteritis nodosa), die mit Morbus Brightii und Rapid fortschreitender allegemeiner Muskellähmung einhergeht. *Deutsches Archiv für klinische Medizin,* **1,** 484.

POLYARTERITIS NODOSA: DIFFERENTIAL DIAGNOSIS

Whatever may have been the nature of the disease described by Kussmaul and Maier (1866), later descriptions of polyarteritis nodosa included malignant hypertension and systematised small vessel disorders — capillaritis and venulitis — such as the generalised Arthus reaction and Shwartzman phenomenon. A critical review by Pearl Zeek (1952) is referred to in Chapter 1 and it provides some justification for believing that many cases of polyarteritis nodosa described up to that time would be given some other diagnosis today. Even today, polyarteritis nodosa is probably over-diagnosed, and its prognosis and treatment remain somewhat unclear.

The diseases described in the rest of this chapter should be first excluded since they have a clearer pathogenesis and their treatment can be rationalised.

A recent case record of the Massachusetts General Hospital (Sculley and McNeely, 1974) concerned a patient with cryoglobulinaemia, strongly positive rheumatoid factor, disseminated intravascular coagulation and hypertension. With all these her disease hardly merited a diagnosis of polyarteritis nodosa.

References

Kussmaul, A. & Maier, R. (1866) Ueber eine bisher nicht beschriebene eigenthümliche Arterian erkrankung (Periarteritis nodosa) die mit Morbus Brightii und Rapid fortschreitender allgemeiner Muskellähmung einhergeht. *Deutsches Archiv für klinische Medizin,* **1,** 484.
Scully, R. F. & McNeely, B. U. (1974) Case Records of the Massachusett's General Hospital. *New England Journal of Medicine,* **291,** 1073.
Zeek, P. M. (1952) Periarteritis nodosa. A critical review. *American Journal of Clinical Pathology,* **22,** 777.

MALIGNANT HYPERTENSION

In the presence of high blood pressure and also in old age and in diabetes mellitus, lipohyaline material is deposited subendothelially in arterioles and arteries. This occurs also in malignant hypertension in which fibrinoid necrosis is an additional feature. The pathogenesis starts with ischaemic necrosis of the muscle coat, caused perhaps by prolonged vasoconstriction (Figure 13.1). The vessel then dilates focally, and its partial rupture allows plasma to seep into the wall where fibrin is then deposited (reviewed by Ashton, 1972). Many organs are affected by numerous aneurysms which can rupture, thrombose and discharge emboli and therefore produce the varied clinical picture.

Zeek (1952) emphasised that macroscopic lesions of nodular arteritis could be produced experimentally by procedures causing hypertension in the absence of immune-type hypersensitivity. She referred to kidney clamping (Goldblatt, 1950) and experiments

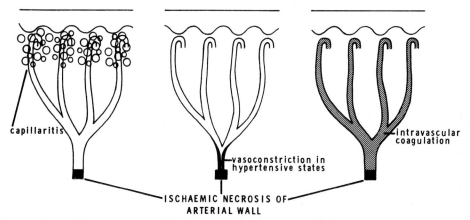

Figure 13.1. Mechanisms contributing to ischaemic necrosis of the arterial wall: no flow due to distal obstruction in capillaritis (left), vasoconstriction as in hypertension (centre) and obstruction due to intravascular coagulation (right).

administering desoxycorticosterone acetate to parabiotic rats (Hall and Hall, 1951).

In patients with hypertension, a common site for limited forms of polyarteritis is the skin where infarction results. Thus a punched-out ulcer on the upper part of the shin below the knee was described in hypertensive patients by Martorell (1945) and by Hines and Farber (1946). Commonly initiated by trauma, this begins as a small reddish spot which soon becomes cyanotic. The primary defect is capillary stasis at a site of chronic purpura with pigmentation. In the presence of hypertension, the artery supplying such a site is shut down altogether if blood flow through the capillaries it supplies is grossly impaired. Histologically, the lesion shows hyalin degeneration of the media, a greatly hypertrophied vessel wall and usually much intimal proliferation. Colomb and Vittori (1974) named such disease 'necrotic angiodermatitis' and detected atherosclerosis extending into small arteries of the skin.

Farber et al (1974) studied skin biopsies in 70 patients with essential hypertension and noted many of the features of arteritis such as endothelial proliferation and thrombotic occlusion.

One of the most significant observations favouring hypertension in the aetiology of polyarteritis nodosa is the relative absence of lesions in the lung, an organ not exposed to high arterial pressures. But such lesions are seen in pulmonary hypertension. This is usually the result of mitral valve disease or micro-embolisation which obstructs pulmonary blood flow, leading to increasing right ventricular hypertrophy as well as the rising pulmonary arterial pressure.

References

Ashton, N. (1972) The eye in malignant hypertension. *Transactions of the American Academy of Ophthalmology,* **76,** 17.

Colomb, D. & Vittori, F. (1974) Necrotic arteriosclerotic angiodermatitis of the lower limbs. Anatomicroclinical study of 34 cases. *Annales de Dermatologie et de Syphiligraphie,* **101,** 15.

Farber, E. M., Hines, E. A. Jr, Montgomery, H. & Craig, W. McK. (1947) Arterioles of skin in essential hypertension. *Journal of Investigative Dermatology,* **9,** 215.

Goldblatt, H. (1950) *Factors Regulating Blood Pressure IV.* New York: Josiah Macy Jr Foundation. p.11.

Hall, C. E. & Hall, O. (1951) Hypertensive disease produced by desoxycorticosterone acetate in parabiotic rats. *Archives of Pathology,* **51,** 249.

Hines, E. A. Jr & Farber, E. M. (1946) Ulcer of the leg due to arteriosclerosis and ischemia occurring in the presence of hypertensive disease (hypertensive-ischemic ulcers): preliminary report. *Proceedings of the Staff Meeting of the Mayo Clinic,* **21,** 337.

Martorell, F. (1945) Las ulceras supramaleolares por arteriditis de los grandes hipertenos. *Acta Institute Policlinico* (Barcelona), **1,** 6.

Zeek, P. M. (1952) Periarteritis nodosa. A critical review. *American Journal of Clinical Pathology,* **22,** 777.

INTRAVASCULAR COAGULATION

Disseminated intravascular coagulation (DIC) as a cause of arterial disease is discussed in Chapter 10, and has been mentioned in case reports of polyarteritis nodosa by Melczer and Venkei (1947), Symmers and Gillett (1951), Starobinski-Sirman (1963), and McKay (1965). Arterial aneurysmal dilatations and thrombosis with or without haemorrhage are associated phenomena. Ischaemic necrosis of the muscle wall may occur whenever there is a temporary cessation of blood flow; coagulation or spasm may cause this. Kazmeir et al (1969) reported two cases which illustrate this.

CASE 1. A 71-year-old woman presented with anorexia, recurrent fever and paraesthesiae of her hands and feet and foot drop. There was a past history of rheumatoid arthritis, hypertension and mild diabetes mellitus. She developed muscle pains and thrombophlebitis, and a biopsy taken from her leg showed arterial vessels infiltrated with polymorphonuclear leucocytes, focal obstruction of their lumina and necrosis of their walls. At the same time she had purpura of her chest wall. Coagulation studies revealed thrombocytopenia, decreased amounts of fibrinogen and decreased Factor V in her blood and a prolonged prothrombin time.

CASE 2. A 42-year-old woman presented with thrombophlebitis of her left femoral vein and painful sub-cutaneous haemorrhages in her right shoulder, abdomen, breasts and buttocks. Haematological studies showed reduced numbers of platelets and amounts of fibrinogen, Factor V and Factor VII and a prolonged prothrombin time. She responded well to heparin, but when this was discontinued her popliteal artery thrombosed and she developed widespread skin necrosis. At autopsy there were widespread infarcts caused by fibrin in the arteries, arterioles and veins. In addition there was endothelial proliferation in the small subcutaneous vessels and inflammation of the popliteal veins.

Thrombosis of veins is often recorded in polyarteritis nodosa, renal vein thrombosis being the best recognised (Miller, Hoyt and Pollock, 1954; Beard and Taylor, 1959; Mandelbaum et al, 1965). Beard and Taylor (1959) described two cases, one associated with Schönlein—Henoch purpura. Their case of polyarteritis nodosa was a girl aged 16 who had received sulphonamides for a sore throat. She developed thrombosis of her right saphenous vein and a haemorrhagic indurated rash on her elbows and knees. After an illness which involved her kidneys, colon and brain, an autopsy showed multiple venous thromboses and haemorrhages of the mucosae and the subcutaneous tissues as well as bilateral renal vein thrombosis.

Thrombosis of the vena cava has been reported from time to time, even in otherwise limited forms of cutaneous polyarteritis nodosa (Borrie, 1972), and it has been reported often in Behçet's disease (see below). The early reviews of pathological material in rheumatic fever by von Glahn and Pappenheimer (1926) mentioned prominent fibrin deposition in peripheral vessels in 21 per cent of cases. Sokoloff, Wilens and Bunim (1951) also found thrombosis to be a common feature in rheumatic diseases.

The eosinophilia so characteristic of polyarteritis nodosa is also a feature of DIC (Riddle and Barnhart, 1969).

References

Beard, M. E. J. & Taylor, D. J. E. (1959) Renal vein thrombosis in cases of polyarteritis nodosa and of Henoch—Schönlein syndrome. *Journal of Clinical Pathology,* **22,** 359.

Borrie, P. (1972) Cutaneous polyarteritis nodosa. *British Journal of Dermatology,* **87,** 87.

Kazmeir, F. J., Didisheim, P., Fairbanks, V. F., Ludwig, J., Payne, W. S. & Bowie, E. J. W. (1969) Intra-vascular coagulation and arterial disease. *Thrombosis et Diathesis Haemorrhagica,* Supplement **36,** 295.

Mandelbaum, J., Aftalion, B., Brody, C. P. & Hoffman, J. (1965) Polyarteritis with renal vein thrombosis. *New York State Journal of Medicine,* **65,** 1790.

McKay, D. G. (1965) *Disseminated Intravascular Coagulation. An Intermediary of Disease.* New York: Hoebner Medical Division, Harper and Row.

Melczer, N. & Venkei, T. (1947) Uber die Hautformen der Periarteriitis nodosa. *Dermatologica,* **94,** 214.

Miller, G., Hoyt, J. C. & Pollock, B. E. (1954) Bilateral renal vein thrombosis and nephrotic syndrome associated with lesions of polyarteritis nodosa. *American Journal of Medicine,* **17,** 856.

Riddle, J. M. & Barnhart, M. I. (1969) Eosinophil mobilisation during disseminated intravascular coagulation. *Thrombosis et Diathesis Haemorrhagica* Supplement **36,** 99.

Sokoloff, L., Wilens, S. L. & Bunim, J. J. (1951) Arteritis of striated muscle in rheumatoid arthritis. *American Journal of Pathology,* **27,** 157.

Starobinski-Sirman, J. H. (1963) Periarteritis nodosa and macroglobulinaemia. *Schweizerische medizinische Wochenschrift,* **93,** 669.

Symmers, W. S. C. & Gillett, R. (1951) Polyarteritis nodosa associated with malignant hypertension, disseminated platelet thrombosis "wire-loop" glomeruli, pulmonary silicotuberculosis and sarcoidosis-like lymphadenopathy. *Archives of Pathology,* **52,** 489.

Von Glahn, W. C. & Pappenheimer, A. M. (1926) Specific lesions of peripheral blood vessels in rheumatism. *American Journal of Pathology,* **2,** 235.

PLATELET DISORDERS

There is a group of diseases in which the arterial tree is predominantly affected and platelet consumption is a major feature. One of these diseases, described by Moschcowitz (1925), is characterised by a haemolytic anaemia, thrombocytopenia, renal disease, transient neurological symptoms and fever. It later became known as thrombotic thrombocytopenic purpura and was well reviewed by Amorosi and Ultmann (1966). The skin is often but not invariably affected by purpura and other eruptions caused by blood vessel occlusion. Thrombotic thrombocytopenic purpura has also been described in rheumatoid arthritis (Castleman, 1963) and in dermatomyositis (Boylan and Sokoloff, 1960).

Another disease described as a cause of acute renal insufficiency in infants and children was named by Gasser et al (1955) as the haemolytic-uraemic syndrome. The skin is more often spared in this condition, although the thrombocytopenia and anaemia may be severe. A familial form with a raised serum IgA level and an eosinophilia has been described by Gutenberger et al (1970) and in this variety renal failure is usual.

The severe anaemia in these diseases is accompanied by changes in red cell morphology (see page 346), consisting of fragmentation, burr cells and helmet cells, Such red cell changes have been described in the vasculitis of polyarteritis nodosa, Wegener's granulomatosis (Brain, 1970) and erythema multiforme (Lohrmann and Kubanek, 1973). A leucocytosis sometimes of leukaemoid dimensions is not unusual. Disseminated arteriolar and capillary platelet thrombosis is the main pathological feature, coupled with extensive fibrin deposition on, between and deep to endothelial cells; there is a reactive proliferation of these cells. The blood and renal picture is similar to that seen in pre-eclampsia (Zeek and Assali, 1951; Macwhinney et al, 1962). There also are IgA deposits, but these are unlikely to be due to an immunological reaction because no other immunoglobulins and complement are demonstrable (Feldman et al, 1966). Aneurysmal dilatation of arterioles is a common finding particularly in the kidney.

Orbison (1951, 1952) and Berberich et al (1974) considered that the major defect in this group of diseases is platelet consumption in excess of fibrinogen consumption. Amorisi and Ultmann (1966) included systemic lupus erythematosus and polyarteritis nodosa in the differential diagnosis, but Umlas and Kaiser (1970) regarded thrombotic thrombocytopenic purpura as a syndrome rather than a disease entity. They described several features in common with scleroderma and with necrotising vasculitis, but they could suggest no clinical sign specific to thrombotic thrombocytopenic purpura. Lindevalle (1961) claimed that the platelet masses found in arterioles and capillaries are seldom seen in the lungs. This observation is relevant both to polyarteritis nodosa which also spares the lungs, and to arterial disease in general in which platelets seem to play a more significant role than does coagulation.

Klein et al (1973) included a case of anaphylactoid purpura in their series of patients with microangiopathic haemolytic anaemia. Drummund (1967) described a patient with polyarteritis nodosa, a platelet count of 700 000/mm[3] and a neutrophil leucocytosis, in whom lung abscesses were a confusing complication. In another study, Salyer, Salyer and Heptinstall (1973) examined 29 autopsies of scleroderma and found non-occlusive intravascular fibrin deposits in the renal capillaries and arteries in all of seven patients who had microangiopathic haemolytic anaemia. Six of these patients had developed hypertension and the authors pointed out that intravascular coagulation and a rise in blood pressure are a particularly harmful combination.

References

Amorosi, E. L. & Ultmann, J. E. (1966) Thrombotic thrombocytopenic purpura: report of 16 cases and review of the literature. *Medicine,* **45,** 139.

Berberich, F. R., Cuene, S. A., Chard, R. L. & Hartmann, J. R. (1974) Thrombotic thrombocytopenic purpura: three cases with platelets and fibrinogen survival studies. *Journal of Pediatrics,* **84,** 503.

Boylan, R. C. & Sokoloff, L. (1960) Vascular lesions in dermatomyositis. *Arthritis and Rheumatism,* **3,** 379.

Brain, M. C. (1970) Microangiopathic haemolytic anaemia. *Annual Review of Medicine,* **21,** 133.

Castleman, B. (1963) Case 58. Case reports of the Massachusetts General Hospital. *New England Journal of Medicine,* **269,** 577.

Drummund, H. M. (1967) Polyarteritis nodosa. *Proceedings of the Royal Society of Medicine,* **60,** 493.

Feldman, J. D., Mardiney, M. R., Unanue, E. R. & Cutting, H. (1966) The vascular pathology of thrombotic thrombocytopenic purpura. *Laboratory Investigation,* **15,** 927.

Gasser, V. C., Gautier, E., Steck, A., Siebenmann, R. E. & Oechslin, R. (1955) Hamolytisch-uramische Syndrome. *Medizinische Wochenschrift,* **85,** 905.

Gutenberger, J., Trygstad, C. W., Stiehm, E. R., Goitz, J. M., Thatcher, L. G. & Bloodworth, J. M. B. (1970) Familial thrombocytopenia, elevated serum IgA levels and renal disease. *American Journal of Medicine,* **49,** 729.

Klein, P. J., Schaefer, H. E., Feaux de Lacroix, W. & Fischer, F. (1973) Morphological findings in micro-angiopathic haemolytic anaemia. *Haemostasis,* **1,** 304.

Lindevalle, G. (1961) Purpura thrombocytopenia thrombotica. *Acta Dermato-venereologica,* **41,** 418.

Lohrmann, H.-P. & Kubanek, B. (1973) Erythema multiforme and microangiopathic haemolysis. *Lancet,* **ii,** 261.

Macwhinney, J. B., Packer, J. T., Miller, G. & Greendyke, R. M. (1962) Thrombotic thrombocytopenic purpura in childhood. *Blood,* **19,** 181.

Moschcowitz, E. (1925) An acute febrile pleiochromic anemia, with hyaline thrombosis of the terminal arterioles and capillaries: an undescribed disease. *Archives of Internal Medicine,* **36,** 89.

Orbison, J. L. (1951) Morphology of the vascular lesions in thrombotic thrombocytopenic purpura with demonstration of aneurysms. *American Journal of Pathology,* **27,** 687.

Orbison, J. L. (1952) Morphology of thrombotic thrombocytopenic purpura with demonstrations of aneurysms. *American Journal of Pathology,* **28,** 129.

Salyer, W. R., Salyer, D. C. & Heptinstall, R. H. (1973) Scleroderma and microangiopathic hemolytic anemia. *Annals of Internal Medicine,* **78,** 895.

Umlas, J. & Kaiser, J. (1970) Thrombolytic thrombocytopenic purpura (T.T.P.) a disease or syndrome? *American Journal of Medicine,* **49,** 723.

Zeek, P. M. & Assali, N. S. (1951) Vascular changes in the decidua associated with eclampsia and toxaemia of pregnancy. *American Journal of Clinical Pathology,* **20,** 1099.

CAPILLARITIS AND VENULITIS

When capillaries and venules are occluded by haemoconcentrated blood, leucocytes, fibrin and platelets, as is a feature of many inflammatory processes, it is not unusual for flow in the supplying artery to stop and for ischaemic necrosis of the arterial wall to follow. Hence, much that is labelled capillaritis or venulitis in the spectrum of vasculitis may be followed by arterial necrosis (Figure 13.2). The various triggers of vasculitis, mentioned in other chapters in this monograph, may be associated with arteritis in this way.

Arthus (1903) described the histopathological picture of hypersensitivity to non-toxic agents, and it is similar to that seen in the spectrum of urticaria and vasculitis. Gruber (1925) suggested that polyarteritis nodosa reflects a systemic alteration in reactivity to a variety of agents acting on the vessel wall, and from about that time, the role of a similar altered reactivity in the then common rheumatic fever came under discussion.

Meanwhile a considerable amount of experimental work was carried out. Klinge (1930), for example, injected rabbits repeatedly with horse serum and thereby produced

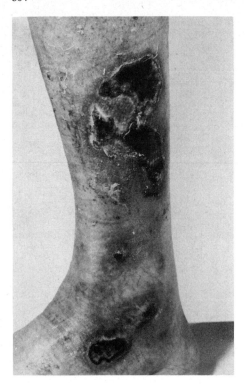

Figure 13.2. Postulated arterial infarcts which were in all probability initiated as a venulitis.

lesions that resembled polyarteritis nodosa; similar experiments were carried out by Klinge and Vaubel (1931). Metz (1921) and Vaubel (1932) produced similar lesions in the small vessels of many organs of rats by inoculating nonspecific protein. Masugi and Isibasi (1936) produced glomerulonephritis in several animal species and polyarteritis nodosa-like lesions using horse serum and egg white as antigen. The similarity between these lesions and those in serum sickness was emphasised by Clark and Kaplan (1937). Acceptance of the hypersensitivity concept followed reports by Rich (1942) on the vascular lesions in experimental sulphonamide sensitivity (Rich and Gregory, 1943); in these experiments 'abundant' small vessel lesions were produced in rabbits by intravenous injection of horse serum.

The interpretation of such experiments and their comparison with human disease have given rise to debate. Some recognise small vessel disease due to hypersensitivity but point out that such experiments do not usually produce lesions in vessels with the same calibre as those involved in human arteritis (Zeek, Smith and Weeter, 1948), nor are aneurysms formed. The widespread introduction of sulphonamides in the early 1940s was followed by many descriptions of rashes thought to be due to this drug. Vascular lesions were described (Black-Schaffer, 1945; French, 1946; Lichtenstein and Fox, 1946), and it was usually assumed that allergy to the drug was responsible.

In more recent years some of the most difficult papers to interpret have been those in which the results of immunofluorescence studies are reported. Scott and Rowell (1965) described only arteries in their much quoted study of the skin, whereas Copeman and Ryan (1970), in similar studies, believed that only veins were involved. In a paper entitled 'immune complex arteritis', Porter, Larsen and Porter (1973) reported their studies of Aleutian mink disease in which no involvement of veins had been found; they described as 'arteries' vessels with little and sometimes no internal elastic lamina and no aneurysms, and in spite of severe 'arterial' necrosis, they saw no tissue infarction. In these circumstances one wonders whether they were observing a truly arterial disease.

Although immune complexes are sometimes blamed for causing the arterial disease polyarteritis nodosa, they are initially more obviously precipitated in capillaries and venules. Biopsy material showing arteritis has often been taken late in the pathogenesis, at a time when blood flow from the arteries into the capillaries and venules was being prevented by the more distal pathology of the Arthus or Shwartzman phenomenon.

When cryoglobulin can be detected in significant amounts in rheumatoid arthritis, or when a diagnosis of lupus erythematosus can be established, there seems little justification for renaming the disease merely because small arteries are involved.

References

Arthus, M. (1903) Injections répétées de sérum de cheval chez le lapin. *Compte rendu des Séances de la Société de Biologie,* **55,** 817.
Black-Schaffer, B. (1945) Pathology of anaphylaxis due to sulfonamide drugs. *Archives of Pathology,* **39,** 301.
Clark, E. & Kaplan, B. (1937) Endocardial arterial and other mesenchymal alterations associated with serum disease in man. *Archives of Pathology,* **24,** 458.
Copeman, P. W. M. & Ryan, T. J. (1970) The problems of cutaneous angiitis with reference to histopathology and pathogenesis. *British Journal of Dermatology,* **82** (Supplement 5), 2.
French, A. J. (1946) Hypersensitivity in the pathogenesis of the histopathologic changes associated with sulfonamide chemotherapy. *American Journal of Pathology,* **22,** 679.
Gruber, G. B. (1925) Zur frage der periarteritis nodosa mit besonderer Berucksichtigung der Gallenblasen und nieren Beteiligung. *Virchows Archiv für pathologische Anatomie,* **258,** 441.
Klinge, F. (1930) Die Eisweiss überempfind Lichkeit (Gewebsanaphylaxie) der Gelenke, experimentelle pathologisch-anatomische studie zur pathogenese des Gelenksrheumatismus. *Beiträge zur pathologischen Anatomie und zur allgemeinen Pathologie,* **83,** 185.
Klinge, F. & Vaubel, E. (1931) Das Gewebsbild des fleberhaften Rheumatismus. *Virchows Archiv für pathologische Anatomie,* **281,** 701.
Lichtenstein, L. & Fox, L. J. (1946) Necrotising arterial lesions resembling those of periarteritis nodosa and focal visceral necrosis following administration of sulfathiazole. *American Journal of Pathology,* **22,** 665.
Masugi, M. & Isibasi, T. (1936) Über allergische vorgange bei allgemein infektion vom standpunkt der experimentellen forschung. *Beiträge zur pathologischen Anatomie und zur allgemeinen Pathologie,* **96,** 391.
Metz, W. (1921) Die geweblichen reaktion serscheinungen an der Gefasswand bei — ergeichen Zustanden und deren Beziehungen zur Periarteriitis nodosa. *Beiträge zur pathologischen Anatomie und zur allgemeinen Pathologie,* **69,** 85.
Porter, D. D., Larsen, A. E. & Porter, H. G. (1973) The pathogenesis of Aleutian disease of mink: III immune complex arteritis. *American Journal of Pathology,* **71,** 331.
Rich, A. R. (1942) Additional evidence of the role of hypersensitivity in the aetiology of periarteritis nodosa. Another case associated with sulphonamide reaction. *Bulletin of the Johns Hopkins Hospital,* **71,** 375.
Rich, A. R. & Gregory, J. E. (1943) The experimental demonstration that periarteritis nodosa is a manifestation of hypersensitivity. *Bulletin of the Johns Hopkins Hospital,* **72,** 65.
Scott, D. G. & Rowell, N. R. (1965) Preliminary investigation of arteric lesions using fluorescent antibody techniques. *British Journal of Dermatology,* **77,** 211.
Vaubel, E. (1932) Die Eiweiss uberempfind Lichkeit (Gewebshypergie) des Binde (11 Teile). *Beiträge zur pathologischen Anatomie und zur allgemeinen Pathologie,* **89,** 374.
Zeek, P. M., Smith, C. G. & Weeter, J. C. (1948) Studies on periarteritis nodosa. The differentiation between the vascular lesions of periarteritis nodosa and hypersensitivity. *American Journal of Pathology,* **24,** 889.

SEROPOSITIVE RHEUMATOID ARTHRITIS

Seropositive rheumatoid arthritis is a frequent cause of 'arteritis' (Figure 13.3), and there is a wide variety of skin and systemic manifestations attributed to the 'malignant'

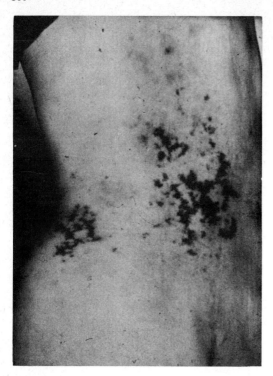

Figure 13.3. Woman aged 56 with rheumatoid arthritis and haemorrhagic infarcts on the trunk (case reported by Lindsay et al, 1973). She died from similar infarction of the caecal wall. Submucosal arteries showed evidence of repeated occlusion by thrombus and recanalisation.

or *complicated* variety (Hart, 1966). As one might expect, complicated forms have a worse prognosis, are more likely to be associated with higher titres of rheumatoid factor and are more liberally treated with dangerous drugs (Bywaters and Scott, 1963; Golding, Hamilton and Gill, 1965; Hart, 1966; Gordon, Stein and Broder, 1973). Even quite large arteries may be involved (Lindsay et al, 1973). The crops of digital vasculitic lesions around nail folds and the small painful haemorrhagic maculopapular lesions seen in rheumatoid arthritis are indistinguishable from those seen in other forms of vasculitis (Figure 13.4).

Webb and Payne (1970) quoted Scott et al (1961) in a discussion of the consequences of intestinal vascular aneurysms in this disease and described three main groups of rheumatoid vasculitis.

1. Bland proliferative endarteritis of digital vessels with little or no inflammatory reaction causes the not uncommon small nail-fold and finger-pulp infarcts, less frequently a digital mononeuritis, and occasionally digital gangrene (Bywaters, 1957). Although digital arterial narrowing and occlusion is demonstrable angiographically in these patients, it may also occur in the absence of any such clinical involvement. There is a strong though not invariable relationship to erosive rheumatoid arthritis with nodules and positive rheumatoid factor tests (Laws, Lillie and Scott, 1963).

2. Sub-acute inflammatory arteritis of small vessels causes more serious complications, the most frequent being a peripheral sensory or motor neuropathy, with lesions sometimes involving skin, skeletal muscle, heart and other organs. However, similar lesions may be found by careful pathological examination of biopsy and autopsy material in a proportion of rheumatoid arthritis cases without clinical evidence of these complications (Sokoloff, Wilens and Bunim, 1951; Cruickshank, 1954).

3. Sometimes necrotising arteritis, indistinguishable from polyarteritis nodosa, has complicated the course of rheumatoid arthritis. A severe combined sensori-motor

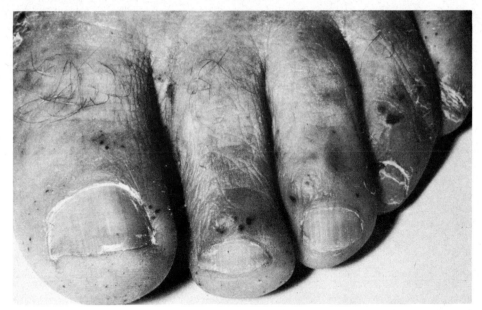

Figure 13.4. Nail-fold infarcts commonly seen in all types of vasculitis but particularly given prominence by rheumatologists.

polyneuropathy affecting both upper and lower limbs is frequently present in these cases, along with other widespread multi-system complications; this form has a high mortality (Pallis and Scott, 1965).

In the series of necrotising vasculitis reported by Winkelmann and Ditto (1964), half the patients had a positive rheumatoid factor test, and joint changes were common whether or not this factor was present. Dryness of the eyes and mouth occurred in four patients, and urethritis and conjunctivitis were also recorded. Such a relationship of vasculitis to Sjögren's syndrome was first emphasised by Waldenström. The wide spectrum of clinical features and serological abnormalities was emphasised by Hughes and Whaley (1972) who included the development of lymphoma. On the other hand, polyarteritis with bilateral enlargement of the parotid glands has been described (Schiess and Modglin, 1967).

In the group of so-called collagen diseases, vascular disease may predominate; this is the case in systemic lupus erythematosus. The high incidence of autoantibodies and immune complexes in these diseases contributes to the vascular injury. Lupus erythematosus is an accepted cause of polyarteritis nodosa-like lesions, and D'Angelo et al (1969) described acute arteritis in several organs in five patients with scleroderma; these were non-inflammatory acellular arteriolar lesions consisting of concentrically orientated fibrin and thickened intima and media. Temporal arteritis also causes infarction of the skin (Kinmont and McCallum, 1964, 1965; Bour et al, 1969; Hitch, 1970).

References

Bour, H., Renoux, M. & Grand, B. (1969) Maladie de Horton avec atteinte oculaire bilatérale nécrose cutanée et nécrose linguale. *Presse Médicale,* **77,** 233.
Bywaters, E. G. L. (1957) Peripheral vascular obstruction in rheumatoid arthritis and its relationship to other vascular lesions. *Annals of the Rheumatic Diseases,* **16,** 84.

Bywaters, E. G. L. & Scott, J. T. (1963) The natural history of vascular lesions in rheumatoid arthritis. *Journal of Chronic Diseases,* **16,** 905.

Cruickshank, B. (1954) The arteritis of rheumatoid arthritis. *Annals of the Rheumatic Diseases,* **13,** 136.

D'Angelo, W. A., Fries, J. F., Masi, A. T. & Shulman, L. E. (1969) Pathologic observations in symptomatic sclerosis (scleroderma). A study of 58 autopsy cases and 58 matched controls. *American Journal of Medicine,* **46,** 428.

Golding, J. A., Hamilton, M. G. & Gill, R. S. (1965) Arteritis of rheumatoid arthritis. *British Journal of Dermatology,* **77,** 207.

Gordon, D. A., Stein, J. L. & Broder, I. (1973) The extra-articular features of rheumatoid arthritis. *American Journal of Medicine,* **54,** 445.

Hart, F. D. (1966) Complicated rheumatoid disease. *British Medical Journal,* **ii,** 131.

Hitch, J. M. (1970) Dermatologic manifestations of giant cell (temporal cranial) arteritis. *Archives of Dermatology,* **101,** 409.

Hughes, G. R. V. & Whaley, K. (1972) Sjögren's syndrome. *British Medical Journal,* **iv,** 533.

Kinmont, P. D. C. & McCallum, D. I. (1964) Skin manifestations of giant cell arteritis. *British Journal of Dermatology,* **76,** 299.

Kinmont, P. D. C. & McCallum, D. I. (1965) The aetiology, pathology and course of giant cell arteritis. *British Journal of Dermatology,* **77,** 193.

Laws, J. W., Lillie, J. G. & Scott, J. T. (1963) Arteriographic appearances in rheumatoid arthritis and other disorders. *British Journal of Radiology,* **36,** 477.

Lindsay, M. K., Tavadia, H. B., Whyte, A. S., Lee, P. & Webb, J. (1973) Acute abdomen in rheumatoid arthritis due to necrotising arteritis. *British Medical Journal,* **i,** 592.

Pallis, C. A. & Scott, J. T. (1965) Peripheral neuropathy in rheumatoid arthritis. *British Medical Journal,* **i,** 1141.

Schiess, A. V. & Modglin, F. R. (1967) Polyarteritis nodosa involving the parathyroid gland. Report of a case. *Oral Surgery,* **24,** 617.

Scott, J. T., Hourihane, D. O., Doyle, F. H., Steiner, R. E., Laws, J. W., Dixon, A. St. J. & Bywaters, E. G. L. (1961) Digital arteritis in rheumatoid disease. *Annals of the Rheumatic Diseases,* **20,** 224.

Sokoloff, L., Wilens, S. L. & Bunim, J. J. (1951) Arteritis of striated muscle in rheumatoid arthritis. *American Journal of Pathology,* **27,** 157.

Webb, J. & Payne, W. H. (1970) Abdominal apoplexy in rheumatoid arthritis. *Australian Annals of Medicine,* **2,** 168.

Winkelmann, R. K. & Ditto, W. B. (1964) Cutaneous and visceral syndromes of necrotising or "allergic" angiitis. A study of 38 cases. *Medicine* (Baltimore), **43,** 59.

LIMITED FORMS OF POLYARTERITIS NODOSA

Cutaneous polyarteritis nodosa is a limited form of arteritis, and although such limited forms of the disease have an anatomical restriction, they commonly affect organs other than the skin. Plaut (1951), for example, claimed that the appendix commonly shows a focal arteritis, and he also found arteritis in asymptomatic disease in nephrectomy stumps, a prolapsed uterus and an occluded fallopian tube.

In cutaneous polyarteritis nodosa, the association of recurrent crops of tender nodules with livedo reticularis affecting the legs, feet and ankles is believed to represent a benign form of the disease (Orkin, 1970; Borrie, 1972) (Figure 13.5). This pattern of patchy mottling of the skin and subcutaneous nodularity has little in common with classical polyarteritis nodosa for it is not infarctive, it has a good prognosis, and internal organs are usually not affected, the legs alone being involved. The common involvement of the muscles or sensory nerves of the lower legs is not a reason for suspecting systemic disease, since such nerves are subject to the same stresses from gravitational stasis and cooling as is the rest of the cutaneous system in the periphery. In all forms of vasculitis of the lower legs superficial nerves may be involved at the height of the rash; it is only when nerves are picked out relentlessly one by one and independently of exacerbations of the rash that the prognosis is likely to be much worse (Dyk, 1973).

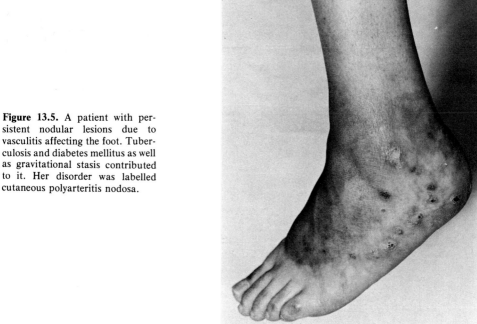

Figure 13.5. A patient with persistent nodular lesions due to vasculitis affecting the foot. Tuberculosis and diabetes mellitus as well as gravitational stasis contributed to it. Her disorder was labelled cutaneous polyarteritis nodosa.

Ketron and Bernstein (1939) reviewed 200 cases of polyarteritis nodosa recorded in the literature and reported a 25 per cent incidence of skin involvement. Others, such as Borrie (1972), have called this figure meaningless and have emphasised that skin involvement is rare in the classic disorder.

Kussmaul and Maier's (1866) first case developed some subcutaneous nodules of the trunk which were palpable rather than visible; these appeared late in the disease from which the patient eventually died. On the other hand, Lindberg (1931, 1932) described two patients with subcutaneous nodules whom he observed for four to nine years respectively, thus emphasising a cutaneous form with a good prognosis.

In recent years, Borrie (1972) has championed the term cutaneous polyarteritis nodosa for a specific clinical and histological picture composed of subcutaneous nodules due to an arteritis in the subcutis, usually accompanied by livedo reticularis in the affected area, and most commonly affecting the lower legs. A somewhat similar picture was termed livedo reticularis with nodules by Bradford, Cook and Vawter (1962). Borrie reviewed 102 cases at St Bartholomew's Hospital in which the diagnosis of polyarteritis nodosa had been made and found 18 patients with skin lesions. Histology of the skin of these patients showed eczema in one, leucocytoclastic angiitis in four, while 12 formed a remarkably cohesive clinical and histological picture, the only tissues to be affected being the skin, muscles and peripheral nerves. The histological picture showed fibrinoid necrosis of a vessel lying in the superficial subcutis, frequently an infiltrate of neutrophils, and sometimes leucocytoclasis; infarction was absent. Borrie believed that this pattern should be recognised because of its benign prognosis, but it can be argued that nodular vasculitis is a sufficient term in which to lump these patterns. Subdivisions, if any, should be based on pathogenic factors not on morphology.

A true necrotising arteritis is presumably not a transient lesion, yet many of the lesions referred to as such in the literature appear in crops and regress in a few days, while others resemble erythema nodosum; this has been reviewed by Lyell and Church (1954).

Many of the cases in the literature referred to as polyarteritis nodosa showed histological features that can be explained by gravitational stasis and/or capillaritis with venulitis, or both. Primary arterial disease is very rare, whereas crural arterial necrosis *secondary* to distal small vessel obstruction is common and, as in Borrie's (1972) case 3, may be a consequence of preceding allergic vasculitis. The interpretation of necrotising vasculitis at the junction of the dermis and subcutis in sections reproduced in the literature is difficult. Many authors have reproduced histology in which vessels are destroyed beyond recognition (Borrie, 1972).

Melczer and Venkei (1947) in a discussion of cutaneous polyarteritis produced several excellent clinical and histopathological illustrations of disseminated intravascular coagulation. Diaz-Perez and Winkelmann (1974), wishing to perpetuate the term cutaneous polyarteritis nodosa, overemphasised its morphology, and yet various clues to the mechanisms responsible for the disease in their patients were underemphasised. One patient had a prolonged prothrombin time, a high platelet count and fibrin degradation products well above normal levels (94 μg/ml), and another patient also had a high platelet count and high levels of fibrin degradation products (48 μg/ml). Fibrin was demonstrated in the tissues of two other patients and eosinophils were a feature of the lesions in eight.

References

Borrie, P. (1972) Cutaneous polyarteritis nodosa. *British Journal of Dermatology,* **87,** 87.

Bradford, W. D., Cook, C. D. & Vawter, G. F. (1962) Livedo reticularis: a form of allergic vasculitis. Report of three cases. *Journal of Pediatrics,* **60,** 266.

Diaz-Perez, J. L. & Winkelmann, R. K. (1974) Cutaneous periarteritis nodosa. *Archives of Dermatology,* **110,** 407.

Dyk, T. (1973) Cutaneous polyarteritis. *British Medical Journal,* **i,** 551.

Ketron, L. W. & Bernstein, J. C. (1939) Cutaneous manifestations of periarteritis nodosa. *Archives of Dermatology and Syphilology* (Chicago), **40,** 929.

Kussmaul, A. & Maier, R. (1866) Ueber eine bisher nicht beschriebene eigenthümliche arterien erkrankung (Periarteritis nodosa) die mit Morbus Brightii und rapid fortschreitender allgemeiner Muskellähmung einhergeht. *Deutsches Archiv für klinische Medizin,* **1,** 484.

Lindberg, K. (1931) Ein beitrag zur kenntis der periarteritis nodosa. *Acta Medica Scandinavica,* **76,** 183.

Lindberg, K. (1932) Uber eine subkutane form der periarteritis nodosa mit langwierigem verlauf. *Acta Medica Scandinavica,* **77,** 455, 462.

Lyell, A. & Church, R. (1954) The cutaneous manifestations of polyarteritis nodosa. *British Journal of Dermatology,* **66,** 335.

Melczer, N. & Venkei, T. (1947) Uber die hautformen der periarteritis nodosa. *Dermatologica,* **94,** 214.

Orkin, M. (1970) Cutaneous polyarteritis nodosa. *Archives of Dermatology,* **102,** 571.

Plaut, A. (1951) Asymptomatic focal arteritis of the appendix; eighty-eight cases. *American Journal of Pathology,* **27,** 247.

LIVEDO RETICULARIS

For some authors, the cutaneous manifestations that are most characteristic of polyarteritis nodosa are subcutaneous aneurysms, livedo reticularis, subcutaneous haemorrhage and gangrene (Alarcón-Segovia and Brown, 1964). Of these, subcutaneous aneurysms and subsequent vessel rupture or thrombosis must be exceedingly rare. Livedo reticularis, on the other hand, is common, but it is rarely the end-result of primary arterial disease. Copeman and Ryan (1971) have given reasons for regarding livedo reticularis as a problem of capillary and venular stasis in cooled skin and influenced by anatomical factors and sometimes by arterial vasoconstriction.

The associations of this particular reaction pattern are many and are listed in Table 13.1. Unilateral disease is a not uncommon underlying factor which is sometimes the result of anatomical disturbances or scarring from previous injury or thrombosis, but can also follow unilateral brain injury and resulting unilateral vasomotor instability (Korting and Lachner, 1972).

Table 13.1. List of conditions associated with livedo reticularis.

Physiological	*Intravascular occlusion*
Cutis marmorata	Arterial emboli
Abnormality of artery wall	Thrombocythaemia
Idiopathic	Cryoglobulinaemia
Arteriosclerosis	'Dermite livedoide' of Nicolau (intra-arterial
Hyperparathyroidism	injections of bismuth, etc.)
Arteritis	Compressed air illness
polyarteritis nodosa	Polycythaemia rubra vera
systemic	Hyperviscosity syndromes
benign cutaneous	Cryofibrinogenaemia
'livedo reticularis in children'	Congenital livedo
rheumatoid arteritis	*Eruptions localised by livedo network*
Lupus erythematosus	Erythema ab igne
Dermatomyositis	Various dermatoses demonstrating Köbner
Rheumatic fever	phenomenon
Syphilis	Capillary naevi
Tuberculosis	
Pancreatitis	

When the arteries are primarily involved in an acute obstructive process, the livedo reticularis characteristically has a central blanched area surrounded by blue areas in which no blood flow can be detected. Peripheral embolisation from atheromatous plaques at the lower end of the aorta is one of the commonest causes of this type of acute livedo reticularis affecting the thighs and buttocks. Infarction of the skin, often most severe in the central pale areas, is a consequence (Figure 13.6). This form of livedo reticularis differs from that described by Haxthausen (1930) in perniosis in which the paler areas may have the better blood flow, and the blueness simply represents stasis of blood cooled in the horizontal subpapillary plexus at the periphery of the anatomical network.

Richards, Eliot and Kanjuk (1965) have described a multisystem disease due to cholesterol or atheroma embolism that is similar to polyarteritis nodosa. However, the histology includes clear crystals of cholesterol in the small blood vessels of the lower leg (Fischer and Kistner, 1972).

Another pattern is progressive reticulate ecchymoses with infarction of areas of skin on the legs seen in association with hyperparathyroidism, usually secondary to renal disease. Muscular vessels in the deep dermis or fat show compression and replacement of the media by masses of calcium. Parathyroidectomy cures the condition (Winkelmann and Keating, 1970).

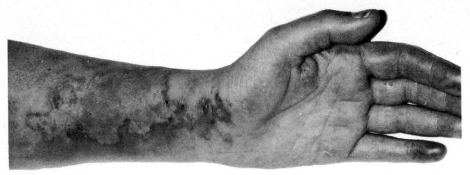

Figure 13.6. Pale infarct from arterial obstruction by emboli. This is one of the few arterial conditions to produce a reticulate infarction of the skin.

References

Alarcón-Segovia, D. & Brown, A. L. (1964) Classification and etiologic aspect of necrotizing angiitis; an analytic approach to a confused subject with a critical review of the evidence for hypersensitivity, in poly-arteritis nodosa. *Proceedings of the Mayo Clinic,* **39,** 205.
Copeman, P. W. M. & Ryan, T. J. (1971) Cutaneous angiitis patterns of rashes explained by 1) flow properties of blood 2) anatomical disposition of vessels. *British Journal of Dermatology,* **85,** 205.
Fischer, D. A. & Kistner, R. L. (1972) Athero-thrombotic emboli in the lower extremities. *Archives of Dermatology,* **104,** 583.
Haxthausen, H. (1930) *Cold in Relation to Skin Diseases.* Copenhagen: Levin & Munksgaard.
Korting, G. W. & Lachner, H. (1972) Zur kenntnis atypischer einseitiger livedo bilder. *Zeitschrift für haut und Geschlechtskrankheiten und deren Grenzgebiete,* **47,** 1.
Richards, A. M., Eliot, R. S. & Kanjuh, V. I. (1965) Cholesterol embolism. A multi-system disease masquerading as polyarteritis nodosa. *American Journal of Cardiology,* **15,** 696.
Winkelmann, R. K. & Keating, F. R. (1970) Cutaneous vascular calcification, gangrene and hyperpara-thyroidism. *British Journal of Dermatology,* **83,** 263.

PAPULAR NECROTIC TUBERCULIDES

The papular necrotic tuberculide is rarely observed in the western world but some of its manifestations have been described by Findlay and Morrison (1973) in Pretoria, South Africa. Arterial infarction is responsible for the acute gangrene of the skin. Clinically the disorder is recognised by the follicular papules and pustules which tend to necrose and to form pock-like scarring (Figure 13.7). Findlay and Morrison (1973) suggested that idiopathic gangrene in African adults (Barr, Roy and Millar, 1972) has the same aetiology, even though disturbances of blood coagulation and fibrinolysis are easily detectable.

A history of tuberculosis, or positive evidence of the disease, or both, is more common in nodular vasculitis which is often limited to the legs; Borrie (1972) described one such case in his series of cutaneous polyarteritis nodosa. Tuberculide-like eruptions are also described in pulseless disease in which the main branches of the aortic arch are narrowed and occluded (Grimaldi, 1970; Takezawa et al, 1966; Amnueilaph et al, 1973).

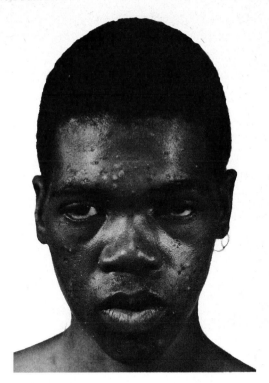

Figure 13.7. Papulonecrotic tuberculid, a 'pock' marking and acneiform eruption that causes peripheral gangrene (see also Figure 8.5).

References

Amnueilaph, P., Charoenvej, R. & Vejjajiva, A. (1973) Pulseless disease presenting with isolated abducens nerve palsy and recurrent cutaneous angiitis. *British Medical Journal,* **iii,** 27.
Barr, R. D., Roy, A. D. & Millar, J. R. M. (1972) Idiopathic gangrene in African adults. *British Medical Journal,* **ii,** 273.
Borrie, P. (1972) Cutaneous polyarteritis nodosa. *British Journal of Dermatology,* **87,** 87.
Findlay, G. H. & Morrison, J. G. L. (1973) Idiopathic gangrene in African adults. *British Medical Journal,* **i,** 173.
Grimaldi, M. G. (1970) Microangioite cutanea con immuno-deposito in corso di sindrome di Takayasu. *Folia Allergologica,* **17,** 134.
Takezawa, H., Sakakura, T., Komada, M., Kotani, Y. & Hamaguchi, T. (1966) Report on two cases of Takayasu's disease complicated with tuberculide or tuberculoderma-like exanthemes. *Japanese Circulation Journal,* **30,** 1045.

ALLERGIC GRANULOMATOSIS (CHURG AND STRAUSS) AND WEGENER'S GRANULOMATOSIS

Granulomata can be produced experimentally using immune complexes in which the antigen and antibody are present in equivalent proportions (Spector and Heeson, 1969). An excess of antibody delays the intracellular degradation of antigen (Sorkin and Boyden, 1959) and the breakdown of phagocytosed bacteria (Cohn, 1963).

In the tissues, a state of antibody equivalence or excess is more likely to occur where there are large collections of immunoglobulin-producing cells and if the antigen either is walled off or reaches a site from the circulation in small amounts at a time. Such granulomata are to be found in the tissues around venules. The hyper-reactivity of the nasal mucosa can be explained by the normal infiltrate in the lamina propria of cells containing IgG, IgA, IgM and IgD (Brandtzaeg, Fjellanger and Gjeruldsen, 1967; Lai A Fat, Cormane and Von Furth, 1974).

It has been explained above that disturbances in blood flow through the capillaries and veins due to an 'allergic' venulitis may lead to ischaemic necrosis of the supplying artery or arteriole. As a result, a picture of necrotising arteritis may supervene on such a venulitis, and for the same reason may be seen in arteries supplying an area of granulomatous venulitis. A picture of this sort is characteristic of Wegener's granulomatosis in which involvement of capillaries and venules is more obvious than in polyarteritis nodosa (Schuh and Herrmann, 1969).

The factors determining the distribution of lesions are the same as those in other forms of vasculitis in which triggering factors interact with local and systemic constitutional factors. The scars of previous respiratory disease are particularly important in this respect as indeed may be the simple scars of skin wounds in, for example, the cutaneous lesions in two cases of Wegener's granulomatosis described by Kraus et al (1965). Immunological factors, ischaemia and intravascular coagulation are involved in these diseases just as much as they are in vasculitis in general. For instance, Lopas, Birndorf and Robboy (1971) described disseminated intravascular coagulation both in patients and in experimental animals with haemoptysis, râles, rhonchi, pulmonary oedema and homogeneous infiltration in the lungs.

The relevance of the Shwartzman phenomenon has been invoked as in other forms of vasculitis (Gonzales, 1969). Fatty tissues such as the breast, thighs and buttocks are sometimes selected for severe infarction (Reed et al, 1963; Pambakian and Tighe, 1971); moreover this is a coagulation necrosis not dissimilar to that seen in coumarin-induced necrosis. Heparin has been recommended in treatment of cases in which fibrin deposition and thrombosis are the main features, although it has produced the occasional disastrous haemorrhage (Roback et al, 1969).

Cases of Wegener's granulomatosis (Wegener, 1939; Walton, 1958) present insidiously with a serous nasal discharge and crusting of the nares, often with intermittent epistaxes, stuffiness of the nose and pain in the antra. Cough, haemoptysis and pleurisy together with general malaise, fever and loss of weight are other common features. Renal involvement, either presenting as haematuria or merely being picked up on routine urinalysis as albuminuria, is the rule and commonly leads to uraemia as a terminal event (Godman and Churg, 1954). Arthralgia, conjunctivitis and peripheral neuropathy are common but do not distinguish it in any way from other vascular disease. Eosinophilia is present in about half of the cases.

Reed et al (1963) reported that 60 (51 per cent) of 118 reported cases had skin signs such as haemorrhagic vesicles and papular necrotic lesions on the extremities, or even pyoderma gangrenosum. Such signs merely indicate that the disease falls into the spectrum of conditions named vasculitis, but apart from the respiratory involvement there is nothing particularly distinctive about it. Indeed, Rose and Spencer (1957), in a review of 111 cases of polyarteritis nodosa, made the point that the majority of cases show neither lung involvement nor granulomatosis, and they therefore separated off a subgroup of 32 cases with lung involvement. This subgroup also had blood and local tissue eosinophilia and vascular lesions that eventually became granulomatous to an extent not seen in the main group of cases of polyarteritis nodosa.

The prominent involvement of the respiratory tract is determined in most cases by a long history of respiratory disease such as bronchitis, asthma or recurrent pneumonia. As Kanan points out in Chapter 9 the nose is a site of predilection for disease processes such as Wegener's granulomatosis partly for developmental reasons, and partly because of a prior adaptation to repetitive insults. The relationship between scar and isomorphic reactions is discussed in Chapter 6, and these phenomena are not confined to the skin.

Churg and Strauss (1951) described the clinical and postmortem findings in patients in whom severe asthma, fever and eosinophilia terminated a necrotising vasculitis. Many of the vascular lesions were granulomatous with epithelioid and giant cells, and among the skin signs were subcutaneous nodules with a similar histology. Braverman (1970) emphasised the long preceding history of respiratory disease and remission of asthma before the final vasculitis phase. It was indicated in Chapter 3 that asthma and urticaria lie in a different part of the disease spectrum from that occupied by necrotising vasculitis. The latter is a destructive no-flow state with severe ischaemia, whereas urticaria is a state of increased vascular permeability in which ischaemia is not a feature; it is therefore not surprising that when necrotising arteritis supervenes, urticaria and asthma cease. Nor is it surprising that prolonged urticaria and asthma may 'prepare' the tissues for a subsequent infarctive process.

Most cases have been described only at postmortem, by which time the initial pathology has been submerged in the terminal state by the severest form with the predominantly secondary arterial pathology. Antemortem cases can be found in reports by Lincoln (1957), Abul-Haj and Flanagan (1961), Sokoloff, Wilens and Bunim (1951) and Varriale, Minogue and Alfenito (1964). McCombs and Dvorak (1971) described a 49-year-old woman with a long history of asthma who developed purpura, fever, eosinophilia, neuropathy and a positive rheumatoid factor, and who clearly had later arterial involvement. The use of the term polyarteritis nodosa for this case was carefully avoided by these authors. The following references give examples of cases in the literature reported as polyarteritis nodosa but which probably were Wegener's or allergic granulomatosis (Wilson and Alexander, 1945; Hennel and Sussman, 1945; Hejtmancik, Schofield and Herrmann, 1949; Rose and Spencer, 1957; Ellman, 1958); cases 1 and 2 (Scadding, 1958); case 3 — a case described by Klinger (1931) referred to by Wegener (1939), Banowitch, Polayes and Charet (1942), Lindsay, Aggeler and Lucia (1944), Weinberg (1946), Howells and Friedmann (1950), Stratton, Price and Skelton (1953), McCallum (1954), Mallory (1950), and Fienberg (1953).

The overlap of various syndromes has been well described by Burton and Burton (1972) and one could add to their 'Chöffler Train' some other diseases such as Behçet's syndrome in which nasal and lung lesions have been described (Decroix et al, 1968; Dawes, 1973).

The role of eosinophilia in these diseases is not known, but it is often a feature of granulomata in which angiolymphoid hyperplasia is prominent (see Chapter 4). It is less a feature of ischaemic infarctive processes and of the more destructive end of the spectrum of vasculitis. Thus, some authors such as Braverman (1970) have not associated eosinophilia with Wegener's granulomatosis. The fibrinolytic activity of eosinophils may well prevent such infarction (see Chapter 4).

Just as limited forms of polyarteritis nodosa with a good prognosis have been described, so Carrington and Liebow (1968) emphasised a subgroup of Wegener's granulomatosis without renal disease; all 11 patients of this subgroup survived. However, more careful study in another otherwise similar series detected focal glomerular disease (Horn, Fauci and Rosenthal, 1974). Other limited and benign forms have been described (Cassan, Coles and Harrison, 1970; Israel and Patchetsky, 1971). A localised variety, restricted to the nose, had to be distinguished from a lymphosarcoma of that site. It is always important to distinguish between neoplastic and inflammatory diseases particularly in sites such as the paranasal sinuses where destructive processes are not amenable to early diagnosis; the mid-line facial granulomas, relevant here, are discussed in Chapter 9. Typical of the diagnostic difficulties encountered in patients presenting with solitary lesions in the nose was a series of ten patients described by Byrd, Shearn and Tu (1969) in which one patient subsequently developed mycosis fungoides, four developed systemic vasculitis, and the others had purely localised lesions for an average of 48 months.

The frequent description of lymphoma associated with respiratory vasculitis is difficult to understand. In 1973 Liebow reviewed 203 cases of pulmonary vasculitis and granulomatosis and subdivided them into: (1) classical Wegener's granulomatosis (24 cases), (2) limited forms of Wegener's granulomatosis (85 cases), (3) lymphomatoid granulomatosis (74 cases), (4) necrotising sarcoid (11 cases), and (5) bronchocentric granulomatosis (9 cases). Of these, the term lymphomatoid granulomatosis was applied to patients in whom lesions were infiltrated with varying numbers of lymphocytes, lymphoblasts, plasma cells, and large mononuclear elements and larger reticulum cells and their derivatives. Mitoses were numerous in some lesions and the atypical cells were similar to plasma cell precursors. The concept they described was similar to that of lymphomatoid papulosis in the dermatological literature (Macaulay, 1968) which is characteristically self-limiting but histologically suggestive of a malignant lymphoma. This pattern of disease has been described in Sjögren's syndrome and in alpha heavy chain disease involving the intestinal tract. Lukes and Collins (1974) designated such conditions as immunoblastic sarcomata.

True lymphoma is a not infrequent outcome. It is doubtful whether the vasculitis associated with such lesions is anything more than the uncontrolled venular proliferation, clotting and leakiness seen in many inflammatory processes in which there is impairment of local clearance of debris and metabolites by the mononuclear phagocytic system. In a case description from the Massachusetts General Hospital (Rytaned et al, 1975) the patient described was variously labelled as "Wegener's granulomatosis — limited forms of 'lymphomatoid granulomatosis' of the lung, and 'malignant lymphoma histiocytic' type of lung". It seems to be difficult for the medical profession to accept that a hypoxic, proliferating and exhausted endothelial system may be the cause or effect of a proliferating and exhausted immunological and macrophage system. The exhaustion manifests itself as a failure to prevent clotting or to clear debris and thus to maintain blood flow.

The difficulties of classifying limited forms of Wegener's granulomatosis are considerable and may be due to inadequate investigation. It is not without relevance that even vasculitis *limited* to the skin may show lung signs. Thus Catterall (1968), who studied lung function in patients with vasculitis of the skin but with no respiratory symptoms, detected a diffusion defect suggesting microvascular pathology and thus indicating that lung involvement may perhaps be a usual feature of all types of vasculitis.

The lung differs from the rest of the body in that pulmonary arterial pressure usually is relatively low. However, in pulmonary hypertension it behaves like any other tissue and develops arteriolar spasm, necrosis of the vessel wall, thrombosis, endothelial proliferation and recanalisation. A hypertrophied muscular pulmonary artery becomes suddenly replaced by a meshwork of small channels which, in turn, leads into a group of dilated arterioles ending in ordinary pulmonary capillaries (Wagenvoort, 1959).

The questions that are asked about perpetuating factors in pulmonary fibrosis are the same as those asked about the post-inflammatory scarring in vasculitis, venous stasis and ischaemia. Thus, Turner-Warwick (1974) asked how far does fibrosis "depend on secondary factors and no longer on the initiating agents — for example, intravascular coagulation or various types of auto-allergy — and what is the nature of the variation of host responsiveness that allows one patient to be affected so much more severely than another?"

Many changes seen in the endothelium in vasculitis are nonspecific or are due to ischaemia. In the lung similar changes can be induced by immunological injury (Bohm et al, 1973), by poisons such as 1-naphthylthiourea (Amringham and Hurley, 1972) or by hyperperfusion following asphyxia (Finlay-Jones and Papadimitriou, 1973).

References

Abul-Haj, S. K. & Flanagan, P. (1961) Asthma associated with disseminated necrotising granulomatous vasculitis. The Churg and Strauss syndrome. *Medical Annals of the District of Columbia,* **50,** 670.

Amringham, A. L. & Hurley, J. V. (1972) Alpha-naphthyl thiourea induced pulmonary oedema in the rat, a topographical and electron microscope study. *Journal of Pathology,* **106,** 25.

Banowitch, M. M., Polayes, S. H. & Charet, R. (1942) Periarteritis nodosa; report of five cases. *Annals of Internal Medicine,* **16,** 1149.

Bohm, G. M., Vugman, I., Valeri, V., Sarti, W., De Carvalho, I. F. & Laus-Filho, J. A. (1973) Ultrastructural alterations to pulmonary blood vessels in acute immunological lung lesions in rats, mice and guinea pigs. *Journal of Pathology,* **111,** 95.

Brandtzaeg, P., Fjellanger, J. & Gjeruldsen, S. T. (1967) Localisation of immunoglobulins in human nasal mucosa. *Immunochemistry,* **4,** 57.

Braverman, I. M. (1970) *Skin Signs of Systemic Disease.* Philadelphia: W. B. Saunders. p. 203.

Burton, J. L. & Burton, P. A. (1972) Pulmonary eosinophilia associated with vasculitis and extra vascular granulomata. *British Journal of Dermatology,* **87,** 412.

Byrd, L. J., Shearn, M. A. & Tu, W. H. (1969) Relationship of lethal granuloma to Wegener's granulomatosis. *Arthritis and Rheumatism,* **12,** 247.

Carrington, C. B. & Liebow, A. A. (1968) Limited forms of angiitis and granulomatosis of Wegener's type. *American Journal of Medicine,* **41,** 497.

Cassan, S. M., Coles, D. T. & Harrison, E. G. (1970) The concept of limited forms of Wegener's granulomatosis. *American Journal of Medicine,* **49,** 366.

Catterall, M. (1968) Lung function in patients with cutaneous vasculitis. *XIII Congressus, Internationalis Dermatologiae.* p. 1215. Amsterdam: Excerpta Medica.

Chajek, T. & Fainaru, M. (1973) Behçets disease with decreased fibrinolysis and superior vena caval occlusion. *British Medical Journal,* **i,** 782.

Churg, J. & Strauss, L. (1951) Allergic granulomatosis, allergic angiitis and periarteritis nodosa. *American Journal of Pathology,* **27,** 277.

Cohn, Z. A. (1963) The fate of bacteria within phagocytic cells. II. The modification of intracellular degradation. *Journal of Experimental Medicine,* **117,** 43.

Dawes, J. D. (1973) Behçets syndrome with haemoptysis and pulmonary lesions. *Journal of Pathology,* **109,** 351.

Decroix, G., Louvier, M., Guillet, P., Lichtenstein, H., Berkman, N. & Sors, C. (1968) Syndrome de Behçet avec manifestations pulmonaires. *Bulletin de la Société Médicale des Hôpitaux,* **19,** 87.

Ellman, P. (1958) Discussion on the lungs as an index of systemic disease. *Proceedings of the Royal Society of Medicine,* **51,** 654.

Fienberg, R. (1953) Necrotising granuloma and angiitis of the lungs and its relationship to cholesterol pneumonitis of the cholesterol type. *American Journal of Pathology,* **29,** 913.

Finlay-Jones, J. M. & Papadimitriou, J. M. (1973) The autolysis of neonatal pulmonary cells in vitro — an ultrastructural study. *Journal of Pathology,* **111,** 125.

Forman, L. (1960) Thrombophlebitis und arteritis in der pathologie des Behçet syndrome. *Hautartz,* **11,** 363.

Godman, G. C. & Churg, J. (1954) Wegener's granulomatosis — pathology and review of the literature. *Archives of Pathology,* **58,** 533.

Gonzales, G. L. (1969) Granulomatosis di Wegener. *Chronache dell idi,* **24,** 357.

Hejtmancik, M. R., Schofield, N. D. & Herrmann, G. R. (1949) Allergic cardiovascular disease with report of two cases of periarteritis nodosa. *American Journal of Medical Sciences,* **217,** 187.

Hennell, H. & Sussman, M. L. (1945) Roentgen features of eosinophilic infiltrations in lungs. *Radiology,* **44,** 328.

Horn, R. G., Fauci, A. S. & Rosenthal, A. S. (1974) Renal biopsy pathology in Wegener's granulomatosis. *American Journal of Pathology,* **74,** 423.

Howells, G. H. & Friedmann, I. (1950) Giant cell granuloma associated with lesions resembling polyarteritis nodosa. *Journal of Clinical Pathology,* **3,** 220.

Israel, H. L. & Patchetsky, A. S. (1971) Wegener's granulomatosis of lung; diagnosis and treatment. Experience with twelve cases. *Annals of Internal Medicine,* **74,** 881.

Klinger, H. (1931) Grenzformen der periarteriitis nodosa. *Frankfurter Zeitschrift für Pathologie,* **42,** 455.

Kraus, Z., Vortel, V., Fingerland, A., Salavec, M. & Krch, V. (1965) Unusual cutaneous manifestations in Wegener's granulomatosis. *Acta Dermato-venereologica,* **45,** 288.

Lai A Fat, R. F. M., Cormane, R. H. & Furth, R. von (1974) An immunohistopathological study on the synthesis of immunoglobulins and complement in normal and pathological skin and the adjacent mucous membrane. *British Journal of Dermatology,* **90,** 123.

Lincoln, C. S. (1957) Disseminated pathergic (allergic) granulomatosis. *Archives of Dermatology,* **75,** 107.

Lindsay, S., Aggeler, P. M. & Lucia, S. P. (1944) Chronic granuloma associated with periarteritis nodosa; report of case with renal failure. *American Journal of Pathology,* **20,** 1057.

Lopas, H., Birndorf, N. I. & Robboy, S. J. (1971) Experimental transfusion reactions and disseminated intra-vascular coagulation produced by incompatible plasma in monkeys. *Transfusion*, **11**, 196.

McCombs, R. P. & Dvorak, H. F. (1971) Case records of the Massachusetts General Hospital. *New England Journal of Medicine*, **284**, 262.

Pambakian, H. & Tighe, J. R. (1971) Breast involvement in Wegener's granulomatosis. *Journal of Clinical Pathology*, **24**, 343.

Reed, W. B., Jensen, A., Konwaler, B. E. & Hunter, D. (1963) The cutaneous manifestations in Wegener's granulomatosis. *Acta Dermato-venereologica*, **43**, 250.

Roback, S. A., Herdman, R. C., Hayer, J. & Good, R. A. (1969) Wegener's granulomatosis in a child. *American Journal of Diseases in Childhood*, **118**, 608.

Rose, G. A. & Spencer, H. (1957) Polyarteritis nodosa. *Quarterly Journal of Medicine*, **26**, 43.

Rytaned, D. A., Castleman, B. & Dorfman, R. F. (1975) Pulmonary mass, cutaneous nodules and fever. *New England Journal of Medicine*, **293**, 292.

Scadding, J. G. (1958) Discussion on the lungs as an index of systemic disease. *Proceedings of the Royal Society of Medicine*, **51**, 649.

Schuh, D. & Herrmann, W. R. (1969) Zur morphologie der vaskulitis bei der Wegenerschen granulomatose. *Angiologica*, **6**, 339.

Sokoloff, L., Wilens, S. L. & Bunim, J. J. (1951) Arteritis of striated muscle in rheumatoid arthritis. *American Journal of Pathology*, **27**, 157.

Sokolov, R. A., Rachmaninoff, N. & Kaine, H. D. (1962) Allergic granulomatosis. *American Journal of Medicine*, **32**, 131.

Sorkin, E. & Boyden, S. V. (1959) Studies on the fate of antigens in vitro. I. The effect of specific antibody on the fate of I^{131} trace labeled human serum albumin in vitro in the presence of guinea-pig monocytes. *Journal of Immunology*, **82**, 332.

Spector, W. G. & Heeson, N. (1969) The production of granulomata by antigen—antibody complexes. *Journal of Pathology*, **98**, 31.

Stratton, H. J. M., Price, T. M. L. & Skelton, M. O. (1953) Granuloma of nose and periarteritis nodosa. *British Medical Journal*, **i**, 127.

Turner-Warwick, M. (1974) A perspective view on widespread pulmonary fibrosis. *British Medical Journal*, **ii**, 371.

Varriale, P., Minogue, W. F. & Alfenito, J. C. (1964) Allergic granulomatosis. *Archives of Internal Medicine*, **113**, 235.

Wagenvoort, C. A. (1959) The morphology of certain vascular lesions in pulmonary hypertension. *Journal of Pathology and Bacteriology*, **78**, 503.

Walton, E. W. (1958) Giant cell granuloma of the respiratory tract (Wegener's granulomatosis). *British Medical Journal*, **ii**, 265.

Wegener, F. (1939) Ueber eine eigenartige rhinogene granulomatose mit besonderer beteiligung des arterien-systems und der nirren. *Beiträge zur pathologischen Anatomie und zur allgemeinen Pathologie*, **102**, 36.

Weinberg, T. (1946) Periarteritis nodosa in granuloma of unknown etiology: report of two cases. *American Journal of Clinical Pathology*, **16**, 784.

Wilson, K. S. & Alexander, H. L. (1945) The relationship of periarteritis nodosa to bronchial asthma and other forms of human hypersensitiveness. *Journal of Laboratory and Clinical Medicine*, **30**, 195.

BEHÇET'S DISEASE

A disease which has so far largely defied explanation (Haim, 1975) was first described by Behçet (1937) as a triad of mouth and genital ulceration and iritis. Arthritis is often a feature, and many cases in the literature have had clear manifestations of a clotting process taking place in veins (Table 13.2). Thus Mowat and Hothersall (1969) described a man with skin nodules of vasculitis type and subsequent gangrene of his foot; and Pallis and Fudge (1956) reported a case with gangrene of the finger tips. Dowling (1961), reviewing the subject, described thrombophlebitis in 12 per cent of patients. France et al (1951) emphasised the histological picture of perivenular infiltrates and found thrombo-phlebitis in 25 per cent of their series. Since then, Carr (1957), Nazzaro (1966) and Haim, Sobel and Friedman-Birnbaum (1974) all have emphasised this association and have found involvement of the veins in 16 of 36 patients. Numerous references to arterial and venous pathology were given in a report by Nazzaro, Di Carlo and Nazzaro (1971).

Vena caval block was described by Prosser-Thomas (1947), Boolukos (1960), Forman (1960), Ishii, Miyata and Yoshitani (1964) and Scave and Cramaressa (1966). Arterial aneurysms have also been reported (Hills, 1967). Enoch's (1969) case of gangrene due to thrombotic occlusion of major arteries and veins, in which bilateral popliteal aneurysms were a feature, showed acute nonspecific arteritis and phlebitis of all layers of the vessels.

Table 13.2. Manifestations in the order of frequency in 36 patients with Behçet's disease.

Symptom	No. of cases	Percentage frequency
Aphthous stomatitis	36	100.0
Ulceration of genitals	34	94.4
Involvement of veins	16	44.4
Ocular symptoms	12	33.3
Erythema nodosum-like lesion	11	30.5
Pustular lesions and furunculosis	11	30.5
Joint pathology	10	26.0
Central nervous system	3	8.3
Orchitis	3	8.3
Gastrointestinal symptoms	3	8.3
Epididymitis, lymphadenopathy, headache and mental disturbances	2 (each)	5.5

Some authors do not make a distinction between Behçet's syndrome and erythema multiforme exudativum major (Stevens—Johnson syndrome), and Alexander and Cope found widespread necrosis with fibrinoid of arterioles and venules in one such patient. According to O'Duffy, Carvey and Deodhar (1971), sub-ungual haemorrhagic lesions can be a manifestation of vasculitis in Behçet's disease, and in Shikano's (1966) opinion the eye lesions too are essentially due to the same process. Chajek and Fainaru (1973) described superior vena caval occlusion in two patients with Behçet's disease who had impaired blood fibrinolysis and who did well with fibrinolytic therapy. Others also have emphasised the role of impaired fibrinolysis in this disease (Chajek, Aronowski and Izak, 1973; Cunliffe, Roberts and Dodman, 1973; Haim, Sobel and Friedman, 1974; Sobel, Tabori and Tatarski, 1974) (Table 13.3). Chajek and Fainaru (1975) reviewing coagulation processing in 41 cases observed that Factor VIII was usually raised in those with high levels of fibrinogen in the blood, a sure sign of endothelial cell injury.

Most authors emphasise the perivenular infiltrates (France et al, 1951). If one accepts as part of Behçet's disease obscure forms of venulitis affecting large veins as well as small, one must agree that identical problems sometimes exist in the absence of mouth or genital ulceration. Steele et al (1973) have described a shortened platelet survival time in patients with idiopathic recurrent anticoagulant-resistant venous thrombosis.

Behçet's original description was of a *limited* form of a disease — venulitis — that often affects organs other than the eye, mouth and genitalia. However, Miki and Kawatsu (1971) recorded the full triad in only 25 per cent of a Japanese series. Monacelli and Nazzaro (1968) stated that even the aphthae are a consequence of a necrotising angiitis. In the opinion of Sakurai and Miyaji (1971), there are more similarities than differences histopathologically between Behçet's disease, polyarteritis nodosa and systemic lupus erythematosus; in their study, fibrinoid necrosis was a feature of all three diseases. Kidney involvement, however, is rare in Behçet's disease.

Table 13.3. Studies of fibrinolytic activity in eleven patients with Behçet's disease.

No.	Age	Venous complications	Fibrinogen (mg/100 ml)[a]	Euglobulin time (hours)[b]	FDP[c] (µg/ml)
1	43		258	3 h	2.12
2	36		475	3 h 30 min	1.06
3	25		348	1 h 50 min	<10
4	28	Calf vein thrombosis	321	2 h 10 min	2.12
5	21		333	3 h	—
6	17		311	3 h 10 min	
7	48		1252	7 h 50 min	2.12
8	22	Saphenous vein thrombosis	377	3 h 55 min	<1.06
9	52	Recurrent thrombophlebitis Calf vein thrombosis	977	5 h 5 min	33.92
10	44	Superior vena cava thrombosis	692	6 h 10 min	4.24
11	53	Inferior vena cava thrombosis	1280	4 h	2.12

[a]Normal range 200—400.
[b]Normal range 3—4 hours.
[c]Fibrin degradation products.

The inclusion of involvement of the large veins in this syndrome makes it a little unlikely that a purely autoimmune attack on mucosae is a major factor. Haemagglutinating, complement fixing and precipitating antibodies to fetal oral mucosa were demonstrated by Lehner (1967), and he postulated a cross-reactivity between oral epithelium and viruses or mycoplasma-like agents in the mouth lesions. Endothelial proliferation, numerous mast cells, mononuclear infiltrates and binding of IgG and IgM to intracellular epithelial material were also described by Lehner (1969).

Behçet's disease has also been described in association with Sjögren's syndrome (Ramirez-Peredo, Cetina and Alarcón-Segovia, 1973). As in other diseases discussed in this book, associated symptoms include myalgia, exacerbation at menstruation and eosinophilia.

One feature of this systemic disorder is the outstanding hyper-reactivity of the skin to any intracutaneous injection or needle prick. Nazzaro (1966) described three types of initial skin lesions: (1) nonspecific aphthae, (2) erythema nodosum, and (3) papular pustules. Fromer (1970) described a patient with arthritis and crops of pustular lesions in the genital area, trunk, extremities and mucous membranes. These were initially intra-epidermal with many neutrophils, and they subsequently scarred. Australian workers liken this response to the Arthus reaction (Cooper, Penny and Fiddes, 1971). Lesions induced by skin testing were infiltrated by large numbers of neutrophils and eosinophils, provided they were examined within 24 hours (Monacelli and Nazzaro, 1968). The outstanding hyper-reactivity in this disorder has been referred to by several authors (Blobner, 1937; Jenson, 1941; Katzenellenbogen, 1968; Sobel et al, 1973). Probably it should be regarded as merely the localisation by trauma of a systemic factor — in other words an isomorphic phenomenon (see Chapter 6) — especially as it is manifest at the height of the outbreak and fades away at the time of remission. In this respect Behçet's disease and pyoderma gangrenosum are very similar (Pierard, De Besaques and Kint, 1960). Furthermore the hypersensitivity to tuberculin in Behçet's syndrome is no more and no less a valid indication of tuberculosis than it is in nodular vasculitis (Miki and Kawatsu, 1971) or in cases 6 and 7 of Sweet's original description of an acute febrile neutrophilic dermatosis (Sweet, 1964).

Basic research into this disease by Romalho and Rodrigo (1973) suggests that changes in permeability with leakage and diapedesis of blood cells occur before any of the grosser vascular changes of phlebitis.

References

Behçet, H. (1937) Uber die rezidivierende aphthöse durch ein virus verursachte geschwüre am mund, am auge und an den genitalien. *Dermatologische Wochenschrift*, **105**, 1152.

Blobner, F. (1937) Zur rezidivierenden hypopion-iritis. *Zeitschrift für Augenheilkunde*, **91**, 129.

Boolukos, V. P. G. (1960) Phlebitiden und thrombosen grosser korpervenen las begleiterschein ungen der Behçet schen krankheit. *Helvetica Medica Acta*, **27**, 264.

Carr, G. R. (1957) Cellulitis and thrombophlebitis in Behçets syndrome. *Lancet*, **ii**, 358.

Chajek, T. & Fainaru, M. (1973) Behçets disease with decreased fibrinolysis and superior vena caval occlusion. *British Medical Journal*, **i**, 782.

Chajek, T. & Fainaru, M. (1975) Behçet's disease. *Medicine* (Baltimore), **54**, 179.

Chajek, T., Aronowski, E. & Izak, G. (1973) Decreased fibrinolysis in Behçets disease. *Thrombosis et Diathesis Haemorrhagica*, **29**, 610.

Cooper, D., Penny, R. & Fiddes, P. (1971) Autologous plasma sensitisation in Behçet's disease. *Lancet*, **i**, 910.

Cunliffe, W. J., Roberts, B. E. & Dodman, B. (1973) Behçet's syndrome and oral fibrinolytic therapy. *British Medical Journal*, **ii**, 488.

Dowling, G. B. (1961) Discussion on Behçet's disease. *Proceedings of the Royal Society of Medicine*, **54**, 101.

Enoch, B. A. (1969) Gangrene in Behçet's syndrome. *British Medical Journal*, **iii**, 54.

Forman, L. (1960) Thrombophlebitis und arteritis in der pathologie des Behçet syndrome. *Hautartz*, **11**, 363.

France, R., Buchanan, R. N., Wilson, M. W. & Sheldon, M. B. Jr (1951) Relapsing iritis with recurrent ulcers of the mouth and genitalia (Behçet's syndrome). *Medicine*, **30**, 335.

Fromer, J. L. (1970) Behçets syndrome. *Archives of Dermatology*, **102**, 116.

Haim, S. (1975) Behçet's disease, etiology and treatment. *Dermatologica*, **150**, 163.

Haim, S., Sobel, J. D. & Friedman-Birnbaum, R. (1974) Thrombophlebitis and a cardinal symptom of Behçets syndrome. *Acta Dermato-venereologica*, **54**, 299.

Hills, E. A. (1967) Behçets syndrome with aortic aneurysms. *British Medical Journal*, **iv**, 152.

Ishii, M., Miyata, M. & Yoshitani, H. (1964) A case of vena caval thrombosis accompanied by Behçets syndrome. *Journal of the Japanese Society of Internal Medicine*, **53**, 575.

Jenson, T. (1941) Sur les ulcérations aphtheuses de la muqueuse de la bouche et de la peau genitale combinés avec les symptômes oculaires (syndrome Behçet). *Acta Dermato-venereologica*, **22**, 64.

Katzenellenbogen, I. (1968) The significance of specific skin hyperreactivity. *XIII Congressus Internationalis Dermatologiae*. Amsterdam: Excerpta Medica, p. 321.

Lehner, T. (1967) Behçet's syndrome and autoimmunity. *British Medical Journal*, **i**, 465.

Lehner, T. (1969) Pathology of recurrent oral ulceration in Behçets syndrome. *Journal of Pathology*, **97**, 481.

Miki, Y. & Kawatsu, T. (1971) Cutaneous manifestations of Behçets syndrome. *Folia Ophthalmologica*, **22**, 898.

Monacelli, M. & Nazzaro, P. (1968) Cutaneous manifestations of Behçet's disease. *XIII Congressus Internationalis Dermatologiae*. Amsterdam: Excerpta Medica. p. 331.

Mowat, A. G. & Hothersall, T. E. (1969) Gangrene in Behçet's syndrome. *British Medical Journal*, **ii**, 636.

Nazzaro, P. (1966) Cutaneous manifestations of Behçet's disease; clinical and histological findings. *Proceedings of the International Symposium on Behçet's Disease*. p. 15. Basle: Karger.

Nazzaro, P., Di Carlo, A. & Nazzaro, P. M. (1971) Le alterazioni venuse et arteriose nella malattia de Behçet. *Bollettino dell Instituto Dermatologico S. Gallicano*, **7**, 45.

O'Duffy, J. D., Carvey, J. A. & Deodhar, S. (1971) Behçet's disease. Report of 10 cases, three with new manifestations. *Annals of Internal Medicine*, **75**, 561.

Pallis, C. A. & Fudge, B. J. (1956) The neurological complications of Behçet's syndrome. *Archives of Neurology and Psychiatry*, **75**, 1.

Pierard, J., De Besaques, J. & Kint, A. (1960) A propos of the pyoderma gangrenosum of Brunsting, Goeckerman and O'Leary. *Archives Belges de Dermatologie et Syphiligraphie*, **16**, 421.

Prosser-Thomas, E. W. (1947) So called triple symptom complex of Behçet. *British Medical Journal*, **i**, 14.

Ramirez-Peredo, J., Cetina, J. A. & Alarcon-Segovia, D. (1973) Sjögren's syndrome in Behçet's disease. *Lancet*, **ii**, 732.

Romalho, P. S. & Rodrigo, F. G. (1973) Vascular permeability and ultrastructural changes in Behçet's disease. 7th European Conference on Microcirculation, Aberdeen 1972. *Bibliotheca Anatomica*, **11**, 364.

Sakurai, M. & Miyaji, T. (1971) Behçet disease from the point of view of vascular pathology. *Folia Ophthalmologica Japonica*, **22**, 903.

Scave, D. & Cramaressa, L. (1966) Superior vena cava syndrome. In *Proceedings of the International Symposium on Behçet's Disease*, p. 137. Basle: Karger.

Shikano, S. (1964) Ocular pathology of Behçet's syndrome. In *Proceedings of the International Symposium on Behçet's Disease* (Ed.) Monacelli, M. & Nazzaro, P. p. 111. Basel: Karger.

Shikano, S. (1966) Ocular pathology of Behçet's syndrome. In *Proceedings of the International Symposium on Behçet's Disease* (Ed.) Monacelli, M. & Nazzaro, P. Basel: Karger.

Sobel, H. D., Haim, S., Shafrir, A. & Gellei, B. (1973) Cutaneous hyperreactivity in Behçet's disease. *Dermatologica,* **146,** 350.

Sobel, J. D., Tabori, S. & Tatarski, I. (1974) Fibrinolysis and thrombosis in Behçet's disease. *Dermatologica,* **148,** 93.

Steele, P. P., Weily, H. S. & Genton, E. (1973) Platelet survival and adhesiveness in recurrent venous thrombosis. *New England Journal of Medicine,* **288,** 1148.

Sweet, R. D. (1964) An acute febrile neutrophilic dermatosis. *British Journal of Dermatology,* **76,** 349.

PYODERMA GANGRENOSUM AND PHAGEDENIC PYODERMA

The terms pyoderma gangrenosum, phagedenic pyoderma and chronic ulcerative dermatitis refer to a pattern of disease which usually involves a localised destruction of the skin (Figure 13.8). There are often neutrophil-containing abscesses and almost invariably clotting in the capillaries and venules in the affected area (Turin, Mandel and Hornstein, 1959). It has been described most commonly in ulcerative colitis, since Brunsting, Goeckerman and O'Leary (1930) first drew attention to their occurrence. Figures of 50 to 60 per cent are given for this association (Perry and Winkelmann, 1972).

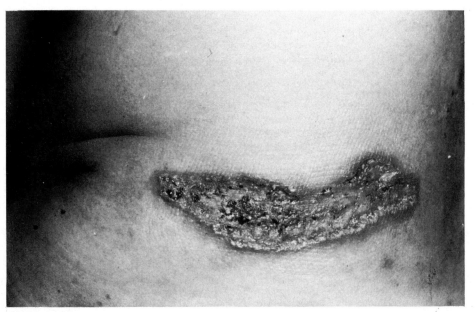

Figure 13.8. Typical superficial ulceration of non-arterial ulcer commonly associated with plasma cell dyscrasia or with ulcerative colitis.

However, it also occurs with regional ileitis. Stathers, Abbot and McGuiness (1967), for example, described a woman who developed tender erythematous nodules that later ulcerated; only much later was regional enteritis diagnosed. Pyoderma gangrenosum has been seen most commonly in association with Crohn's disease of the colon in the author's outpatient clinic held on the same day as the ulcerative colitis clinic supervised by Dr S. Truelove. It has also been described in rheumatoid arthritis (Philpott, Goltz and Park, 1966) and in association with a number of other diseases to be discussed below.

The histological overlap between necrotising vasculitis and pyoderma gangrenosum has been emphasised by Stoleman et al (1975), Samitz (1966), Samitz, Dana and Rosenberg (1970) and Thompson et al (1973).

Sites of skin necrosis show a predilection for the face, buttocks, calves and lateral surfaces of the thighs (Hjort, Rapaport and Jorgensen, 1964). The clinical picture is often identical to erythema nodosum which may also have the same histology (Bishopric and Bracken, 1964). Since erythema nodosum overlaps with chronic panniculitis and with nodular vasculitis, it is not surprising that pyoderma gangrenosum may also show a variety of infiltrating cells including neutrophils, epithelial cells and giant cells (Bishopric and Bracken, 1964).

The overlap with purpura fulminans should also be emphasised. Clinically, the latter is often more widespread and acute but the lesions often look the same and have the same histology. Those who cite the Shwartzman phenomenon in these disorders (Rostenberg, 1953; Goldgraber and Kirsner, 1960; Bishopric and Bracken, 1964) would not separate pyoderma gangrenosum from purpura fulminans. It is in fact difficult not to invoke the Shwartzman phenomenon in cases such as that described by Forsbeck (1962); this was a young man with large areas of ulceration on his skin and with bloody diarrhoea following the administration of an autologous vaccine prepared from boils.

The current interpretation of the Shwartzman phenomenon is that an initial insult or a constitutional disturbance either locally or systemically causes paralysis of the reticuloendothelial system so that it is unable to protect the tissues from the second insult. The blood vessels are the site of insult, and local coagulation is one aspect of the inflammatory process. Proof of coagulation may be difficult to find if the gangrene is not widespread (Perry and Didisheim, 1968), and equally, milder forms show less obvious changes in the blood than do fulminant purpura or gangrene; sequential studies are necessary.

There is an obvious overlap with Behçet's syndrome, as initially described (a triad of mouth and genital ulceration with iritis), but the more generalised venulitis of Behçet's syndrome is now a well recognised feature. Philpott, Goltz and Park (1966) described one patient with pyoderma gangrenosum, rheumatoid arthritis and diabetes mellitus who presented with tongue and scrotal lesions and who later required amputations on account of peripheral vascular disease.

Both Behçet's disease and pyoderma gangrenosum may be heralded by erythema nodosum or by an eruption of multiple vesiculo-pustules which subsequently break down and ulcerate. In both diseases the lesions may be a consequence of trauma such as pressure or venepuncture. Some authors have described patients with polyarteritis and vesiculo-pustules under the heading pyoderma gangrenosum (Ayres and Ayres, 1958; Sluis, 1966), and others under the heading Behçet's syndrome (Fromer, 1970). Vesiculo-pustules are a feature of Sweet's syndrome and sometimes affect the oral cavity (Figure 13.9). This syndrome is gradually collecting the full range of associations like any other vasculitis, and this includes infections, ulcerative colitis, leukaemia, tumours (Matta et al, 1973; Mackie, 1974), as well as a similar range of altered reactivity of the skin (Goldman and Moschella, 1971).

There is a strong suggestion that the reticuloendothelial system is malfunctioning in pyoderma gangrenosum. Long and Uesu (1964) described two patients with multiple vesicular red tender nodules which subsequently ulcerated and scarred; one patient had hypogammaglobulinaemia and the other had ulcerative colitis. Both reacted to inoculation of their leucocytes with an inflammatory lesion 24 hours later, and they also rejected skin autotransplants.

Lazarus et al (1972) have shown that patients with pyoderma gangrenosum fail to react to DNCB, candidin, mumps antigen and streptokinase. Immunological incompetence was further demonstrated by their inability to produce the migration inhibition

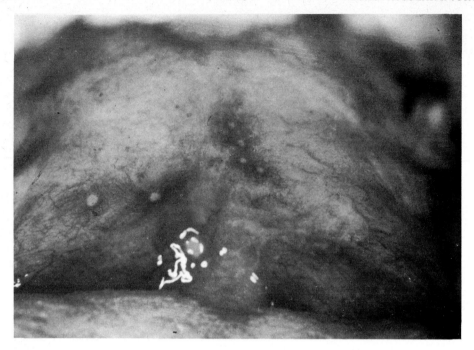

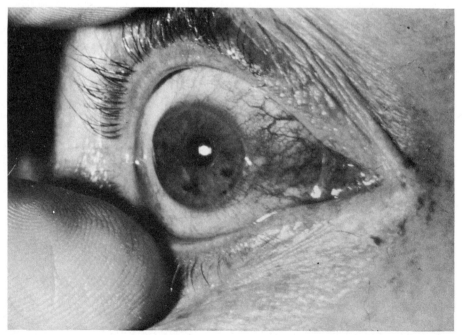

Figure 13.9. Sweet's acute febrile neutrophilic dermatosis. Such cases often show features of overlap with pyoderma gangrenosum. Behçet's syndrome and erythema multiforme. This patient is also illustrated in Figure 2.2.

factors (MIF). These patients also had polyarteritis and one had myasthenia gravis.

Arthritis is not an unusual association in pyoderma gangrenosum whether secondary to ulcerative colitis, regional ileitis, rheumatoid arthritis, Behçet's syndrome or Sweet's disease. Thrombosis of superficial vessels and abscesses with neutrophils have been described in both pyoderma gangrenosum and phagedenic ulcers (Apted, Buntine and Newell, 1971; Lazarus et al, 1972).

The constitutional defect contributing to pyoderma gangrenosum ranges from diabetes mellitus (Philpott, Goltz and Park, 1966) to leukaemia in three cases described by Perry and Winkelmann (1972), Goldin and Wilkinson (1974) and Pegum (1974).

The concept of a disorder of the reticuloendothelial system underlying pyoderma gangrenosum is supported by the increasing number of reports of plasma cell dyscrasia (Thivolet et al, 1964; Jablonska, Stachow and Dabrowska, 1967; Maldonado et al, 1968; Beevers, 1972). Monoclonal gammopathies precede for years overt multiple myeloma (Sluis, 1966; Jablonska, Stachow and Dabrowska, 1967; Thivolet, Perrot and Hermier-Abgrall, 1969), and patients with monoclonal IgA components have been described by several authors (Duperrat, Gougal and Galy, 1962; Rockl, Knedel and Schropl, 1964; Sluis, 1966; Meiers, Orfanos and Schilling, 1967; Schropl, 1967). Figure 13.10 illustrates

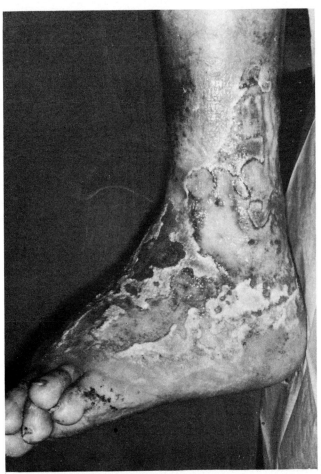

Figure 13.10. Ulceration of the skin in a patient with seronegative arthritis, abnormal plasma cells and a serum IgA of 2300 mg/100 ml.

such a patient with what is probably the more characteristic ulcerative dermatitis and sero-negative arthritis. Patients with IgG gammopathies also have been reported (Degos et al, 1966; Imhof et al, 1969). Cream (1971) described a 71-year-old man with a monoclonal IgM component which could be shown to agglutinate red cells in vitro. The patient had had blind boils which later formed pustules, ulcerated and scarred. These had occurred in various regions over the previous 20 years. The agglutinating factor did not require complement and would clump cells from normal subjects.

Delescluse, de Bast and Achten (1972) described a patient with severe pyoderma gangrenosum of the legs, abdomen, thighs and trunk, beginning as sterile pustules and evolving into large ulcers. They demonstrated dermonecrotic factors in the serum which produced pyoderma gangrenosum in the skin of guinea-pigs. Their patient failed to react to intradermal tuberculin, trichophytin and candidin but streptococcal antigen produced gross ulceration. There was a failure to sensitize with DNCB.

Necrotising vasculitis and myelomatosis (lethal reticuloendothelial disease) were recorded by Mitchell-Sams, Harville and Winkelmann (1968), and more recently the overlap between erythema elevatum diutinum, leucocytoclastic vasculitis and pyoderma gangrenosum with an IgA paraprotein was well illustrated by a case described by Thompson et al (1973). She had a diversity of lesions which were urticarial, papular, vesicular, bullous, plaque-like and purpuric and the ulcers were serpiginous with overhanging violaceous edges; she also had sero-negative arthritis. Biopsy of the edge of the large ulcer revealed marked leucocytoclasia and abundant eosinophils. Lesions could be induced by inoculating bacterial antigen and by a potassium iodide patch test; they were widely infiltrated by fibrin, IgG and complement.

It has been shown that fresh human serum contains a factor which is dermonecrotic when injected into the skin of guinea-pigs (Uhlenhuth, 1897; Lovell, Pryce and Boake, 1954; Ebringer, Doyle and Harris, 1969) and is readily inactivated by heat, storage at room temperature and ageing. This is to some extent a quantitative phenomenon for if enough is injected, serum from nearly all human subjects will induce necrosis. However, the concentration or activity of this agent, which is an IgG, is increased in hypertension (Ebringer, Doyle and Harris, 1969). It is also raised in polyarteritis nodosa, malignancy, peptic ulcer and chronic rheumatic carditis.

Pyoderma gangrenosum has been described in polycythaemia rubra vera (Feuerman and Potruch-Eisenkraft, 1971), and the author has observed it in two cases of myelofibrosis.

References

Apted, J. H., Buntine, D. & Newell, A. C. (1971) Pyoderma gangrenosum. *Medical Journal of Australia*, **2**, 423.
Ayres, S. Jr & Ayres, S. (1958) Pyoderma gangrenosum with an unusual syndrome of ulcers, vesicles and arthritis. *Archives of Dermatology*, **77**, 269.
Beevers, D. G. (1972) Cutaneous lesions in multiple myeloma. *British Medical Journal*, **iv**, 275.
Bishopric, G. A. & Bracken, J. S. (1964) Pyoderma gangrenosum as the presenting sign of regional ileitis. *Southern Medical Journal*, **57**, 675.
Brunsting, L. A., Goeckerman, W. H. & O'Leary, P. (1930) Pyoderma (erythema) gangrenosum. Clinical and experimental observations in five cases occurring in adults. *Archives of Dermatology*, **22**, 665.
Cream, J. J. (1971) Cellulitis and thrombophlebitis in Behçet's syndrome. *Lancet*, **ii**, 358.
Degos, R., Touraine, R., Danon, L., Rigolet, D., Debat, M. & Zilberman, J. (1966) Pyodermite phagedenique avec dysglobulinemie. *Bulletin de la Société Française de Dermatologie et de Syphiligraphie*, **73**, 370.
Delescluse, J., de Bast, Cl. & Achten, G. (1972) Pyoderma gangrenosum with altered cellular immunity and dermonecrotic factor. *British Journal of Dermatology*, **87**, 529.
Duperrat, B., Gougal, A. & Galy, C. (1962) Phagédénisme cutane faisant decouvir une dysglobulinemia latente. *Bulletin de la Société Française de Dermatologie et de Syphiligraphie*, **69**, 11.

Ebringer, A., Doyle, A. E. & Harris, G. S. (1969) Dermonecrotic factor. 1) Nature and properties of a dermonecrotic factor to guinea pig skin found in human serum. *British Journal of Experimental Pathology*, **50**, 559.

Feuerman, E. & Potruch-Eisenkraft, S. (1971) Pyoderma gangrenosum; un cas de polycythemie vrai. *Bulletin de la Société Française de Dermatologie et de Syphiligraphie*, **78**, 260.

Forsbeck, M. (1962) Case for diagnosis. Sanerelli—Schwartzman phenomenon. *Acta Dermato-venereologica*, **41**, 416.

Fromer, J. L. (1970) Behçet's syndrome. *Archives of Dermatology*, **102**, 116.

Goldgraber, M. B. & Kirsner, J. B. (1960) Gangrenous skin lesions associated with chronic ulcerative colitis. A case study. *Gastroenterology*, **39**, 94.

Goldin, D. & Wilkinson, D. S. (1974) Pyoderma gangrenosum with chronic myeloid leukaemia. *Proceedings of the Royal Society of Medicine*, **68**, 1239.

Goldman, G. C. & Moschella, S. L. (1971) Acute febrile neutrophilic dermatosis. *Archives of Dermatology*, **103**, 654.

Hjort, P. F., Rapaport, F. I. & Jorgensen, L. L. (1964) Purpura fulminans report of a case successfully treated with heparin and hydrocortisone. Review of fifty cases. *Scandinavian Journal of Haematology*, **1**, 169.

Imhof, J. W., Schutter, G. J. N. V., Hart, H. & Zegers, B. J. M. (1969) Monoclonal gammopathy (IgG) and chronic ulcerative dermatitis (phagedenic pyoderma). *Acta Medica Scandinavica*, **186**, 289.

Jablonska, S., Stachow, A. & Dabrowska, H. (1967) Entre la pyodermite gangreneuse et le myélôme. *Annales de Dermatologie et de Syphiligraphie*, **94**, 121.

Lazarus, G. S., Goldsmith, L. A., Rucklin, R. E., Pinals, R. S., de Buisseret, J. P., David, J. R. & Draper, N. (1972) Pyoderma gangrenosum altered hypersensitivity and polyarthritis. *Archives of Dermatology*, **105**, 46.

Long, P. I. & Uesu, C. T. (1964) Pyoderma gangrenosum. *Journal of the American Medical Association*, **187**, 336.

Lovell, R. R. H., Pryce, D. M. & Boake, W. C. (1954) Necrotic lesion in guinea pig skin produced by certain human sera. *British Journal of Experimental Pathology*, **35**, 345.

Mackie, R. M. (1974) Sweet's syndrome. *Dermatologica*, **149**, 69.

Maldonado, N., Torres, V. M., Mendez-Cashion, D., Perez-Santiago, E. & de Costas, M. C. (1968) Pyoderma gangrenosum treated with 6-mercapto purine and followed by acute leukaemia. *Journal of Pediatrics*, **72**, 409.

Matta, M., Malak, J., Tabet, E. & Kurban, A. K. (1973) Sweet's syndrome: systemic associations. *Cutis*, **12**, 561.

Meiers, H. G., Orfanos, C. & Schilling, W. H. (1967) Paraproteinamien bei haut kranken. *Hautartz*, **18**, 307.

Mitchell Sams, J., Harville, D. D. & Winkelmann, R. K. (1968) Necrotising vasculitis associated with lethal reticuloendothelial disease. *British Journal of Dermatology*, **80**, 555.

Pegum, J. (1974) Discussion of Goldin, D. & Wilkinson, D. S. (1974) Pyoderma gangrenosum and chronic myeloid leukaemia. *Proceedings of the Royal Society of Medicine*, **67**, 1240.

Perry, H. O. & Didisheim, P. (1968) Consideration of the etiology of pyoderma gangrenosum. *XIII Congressus Internationalis Dermatologiae*. Amsterdam: Excerpta Medica. p. 1108.

Perry, H. O. & Winkelmann, R. K. (1972) Bullous pyoderma gangrenosum and leukaemia. *Archives of Dermatology*, **106**, 901.

Philpott, J. A., Goltz, R. W. & Park, R. K. (1966) Pyoderma gangrenosum, rheumatoid arthritis and diabetes mellitus. *Archives of Dermatology*, **94**, 732.

Rockl, H., Knedel, M. & Schropl, F. (1964) Uber das vorkommen von para proteinaemie bei pyodermia ulcerosa serpiginosa (pyoderma gangraemosum) dermatitis ulcerosa. *Hautartz*, **15**, 165.

Rostenberg, A. Jr (1953) The Shwartzman phenomenon; a review with a consideration of some possible dermatological manifestations. *British Journal of Dermatology*, **65**, 389.

Samitz, M. H. (1966) Cutaneous vasculitis in association with ulcerative colitis. *Cutis*, **2**, 383.

Samitz, M. H., Dana, A. S. & Rosenberg, P. (1970) Cutaneous vasculitis in association with Crohn's disease. *Cutis*, **6**, 51.

Schropl, F. (1967) Dermatitis ulcerosa (pyoderma gangrenosum) mit paraproteinaemie. *Archiv für klinische und experimentelle Dermatologie*, **228**, 430.

Sluis, I. van der (1966) Two cases of pyoderma (ecthyma) gangrenosum associated with the presence of an abnormal serum protein (β_2A-paraprotein) with a review of the literature. *Dermatologica*, **132**, 409.

Stathers, G. M., Abbott, L. G. & McGuiness, A. E. (1967) Pyoderma gangrenosum in association with regional enteritis. *Archives of Dermatology*, **95**, 375.

Stoleman, L. P., Rosenthal, D., Yaworsky, R. & Horan, F. (1975) Pyoderma gangrenosum and rheumatoid arthritis. *Archives of Dermatology*, **3**, 1020.

Thivolet, J., Perrot, H. & Hermier-Abgrall, C. L. (1969) Phagedenisme et dysglobulinémie. *Giornale Italiano di Dermatologiae Sifilografia*, **44**, 48.

Thivolet, J., Pellerat, J., Hermier, C. & Durani, B. (1964) Myelome avec a gammaglobulinemie révélé par une pyodermite phagédénique. *Lyon Médical*, **30**, 161.

Thompson, D. M., Main, R. A., Beck, J. S. & Albert-Recht, F. (1973) Studies on a patient with leucocyto-blastic vasculitis, pyoderma gangrenosum and paraproteinaemia. *British Journal of Dermatology*, **88**, 117.

Turin, R. D., Mandel, S. & Hornstein, L. (1959) Fulminating purpura with gangrene of lower extremity necessitating amputation. *Journal of Pediatrics*, **54**, 206.

Uhlenhuth, P. (1897) Zur kennts der giftigen eigenschaften des blutserums. *Zeitschrift für Hygiene und Infectionskrankheiten*, **26**, 384.

THROMBOANGIITIS OBLITERANS AND DEGOS' MALIGNANT ATROPHIC PAPULOSIS

One of the most puzzling relationships is between progressive systemic sclerosis and malignant atrophic papulosis (Durie, Stroud and Kahn, 1969). That the latter is a thrombotic condition was first emphasised by Degos, Delort and Tricot, (1942) and Degos (1954), while Kohlmeier (1940) and later Lausecker (1949) stressed its fibrinoid features by calling it a form of thromboangiitis obliterans. It is often a lethal multi-system disease, and the characteristic lesion is a pale erythematous papule that later develops a depressed white centre due to an ischaemic scar (Figure 3.3). This is surrounded by erythema or telangiectasis. It has much in common with the scarring of atrophie blanche which usually occurs in the leg in association with a particular pattern of venous stasis, but can also arise in scleroderma of the legs or other areas of the body. The lesion described by Degos, however, has no clear anatomical distribution but is common on the trunk. Infarction of the small intestine is a frequent cause of death in these cases.

Histological and histochemical analysis in scleroderma, atrophic papulosis and atrophie blanche often reveals mucin and usually an acellular picture at least in the late stages; thrombosis of the microvessels is a prominent feature. Roenigk and Farmer (1968) reported raised levels of circulating fibrinogen and cryofibrinogen and Black, Nishioka and Levine (1973) reported diminished fibrinolytic activity in the skin and blood in two cases.

Systemic lupus erythematosus and scleroderma occasionally are responsible for skin lesions resembling both atrophie blanche and malignant atrophic papulosis. They are usually found over bony prominences such as the malleoli, knuckles, knees and elbows, as in a case described by Dubin and Stawiski (1974). These authors stated that the diagnosis of malignant atrophic papulosis should not be made without a thorough attempt to exclude other causes of vasculitis such as 'collagen' disease, for depressed atrophic lesions with porcelain-like centres can be secondary to micro-infarcts due to vasculitis associated with many diseases.

Howard and Nishida (1969), for instance, described a young woman with lesions of this type on her eyelids and conjunctivae, and by reporting lesions in a mother and her child, Hall-Smith (1969) provoked a debate on the relative merits of genetic and environmental (viral) causes.

References

Black, M. M., Nishioka, K. & Levine, G. M. (1973) The role of dermal blood vessels in the pathogenesis of malignant atrophic papulosis (Degos' disease). *British Journal of Dermatology*, **88**, 213.

Degos, R. (1954) Malignant atrophic papulosis, fatal cutaneous intestinal syndrome. *British Journal of Dermatology*, **66**, 304.

Degos, R., Delort, J. & Tricot, R. (1942) Dermite papulo squamous atrophiante. *Bulletin de la Société de Dermatologie et Syphiligraphie,* **49,** 148.

Dubin, H. V. & Stawiski, M. A. (1974) Systemic lupus erythematosus resembling atrophic papulosis. *Archives of Internal Medicine,* **134,** 321.

Durie, B. G. M., Stroud, J. D. & Kahn, J. A. (1969) Progressive systemic sclerosis with malignant atrophic papulosis. *Archives of Dermatology,* **100,** 575.

Hall-Smith, P. (1969) Malignant atrophic papulosis (Degos' disease). Two cases occurring in same family. *British Journal of Dermatology,* **81,** 817.

Howard, R. O. & Nishida, S. (1969) Case of Degos' disease with electron microscopic findings. *Transactions of the Academy of Ophthalmology,* **73,** 1097.

Kohlmeier, W. (1940) Thromboangiitis obliterans mit besonderer Beleilugung der Darmgefasse. I. Intestinale form der von Winiwarter Buergerschen Krankheit. *Frankfurter Zeitschrift für Pathologie,* **54,** 413.

Lausecker, H. (1949) Beiträge zur intestinalen form der thrombangitis obliterans mit hauterscheinungen. *Acta Dermato-Venereologica,* **29,** 369.

Levi, L. (1972) Definition and evaluation of stress. *Thrombosis et Diathesis Haemorrhagica,* Supplement **51,** 7.

Roenigk, H. H. & Farmer, R. G. (1968) Degos' disease (malignant papulosis). *Journal of the American Medical Association,* **206,** 1508.

THROMBOANGIITIS OBLITERANS

This condition was first described by Buerger (1908) particularly among young adult male Polish and Russian Jews. It begins usually in the toes, and these patients have ischaemic pain and coldness of the feet, intermittent claudication and erythromelalgic symptoms. Wessler et al (1960) and Wessler (1969) argued strongly that this disease is neither more nor less than peripheral arterial thrombosis, and it is interesting to return to the earlier literature referred to by Buerger in his original article.

Wilonski (reported by Buerger, 1908) had called the condition arteritis elastica because of multiplication of elastic fibres; in recent years, increased pulsation in arteries has been thought to account for this change. von Manteuffel concluded that the primary change was stripping of endothelium with consequent thrombosis. Cherry, Ryan and Ellis (1974) (see Chapter 5) blamed such stripping on temporary ischaemia followed by reperfusion. Various factors encouraging temporary vasospasm and hence episodic ischaemia could be implicated; these include tobacco smoking, cold exposure, increased blood viscosity or systemic hypercoagulability (reviewed by Juergens, 1972). Most of the literature on this disease is concerned only with relatively late consequences which are in part anatomically determined. The initial events are, in fact, no different from any other form of vasculitis.

References

Buerger, L. (1908) Thrombo-angiitis obliterans: a study of the vascular lesions leading to presenile spontaneous gangrene. *American Journal of the Medical Sciences,* **136,** 567.

Cherry, G., Ryan, T. J. & Ellis, J. (1974) Decreased fibrinolysis in reperfused ischaemic tissue. *Thrombosis et Diathesis Haemorrhagica,* **32,** 659.

Juergens, J. L. (1972) Thromboangiitis obliterans. In *Peripheral Vascular Disease* (Ed.) Fairburn, J. F., Juergens, J. L. & Spittell, J. A. p. 327. Philadelphia: W. B. Saunders.

Wessler, S. (1969) Buerger's disease revisited. *Surgical Clinics of North America,* **49,** 703.

Wessler, S., Ming, S-C., Gurewich, V. & Frieman, D. G. (1960) A critical evaluation of thromboangiitis obliterans. The case against Buerger's disease. *New England Journal of Medicine,* **262,** 1149.

LIVEDOID VASCULITIS, SEGMENTAL HYALINISING VASCULITIS, ATROPHIE BLANCHE, LIVEDO WITH SUMMER OR WINTER ULCERATION

This group of names is one of the more recent inventions of dermatologists (Feldaker, Hines and Kierland, 1956; Bard and Winkelmann, 1967) which must greatly confuse those who are not in this field. It is the same disease process as cutaneous polyarteritis nodosa, has the same associations and creates the same problems for both patient and doctor. It overlaps equally with thrombo-angiitis obliterans which in turn overlaps with scleroderma and with Degos's malignant atrophic papulosis.

The term atrophie blanche describes its distinctive morphology (Figure 12.7). This is a small white depression in the skin initially the size of a papilla but usually not recognised until it is about 2 to 5 mm in diameter. At the borders, and often piercing the centre of the depression, there are enlarged vessels consisting mainly of greatly coiled capillary venules. In so-called livedoid vasculitis the lesions are confined to the lower leg as in cutaneous polyarteritis nodosa. In Degos's malignant atrophic papulosis, similar lesions are scattered over all areas of the body (Figure 13.11). In scleroderma (Figure 13.12), dermatomyositis and discoid lupus erythematosus, similar depressed white scars with surrounding telangiectasis are seen over bony prominences such as the knuckles, knees and malleoli. Stevanovic (1974) describes such associations as due to a partial or complete occlusion of dermal vessels at sites with a relatively poor blood flow.

By far the commonest association is with venous stasis in the leg. It is for this reason that they are commonly seen around the ankle in women and in the left leg more than the right (Favre, Contamin and Martine, 1924; Milian, 1929; Gonin, 1950; Nelson, 1955; Gray et al, 1966; Ryan, 1969; Ryan and Wilkinson, 1972). However, Table 13.4 illustrates other associations in the author's experience. Figure 13.11 is from a patient of Brödthagen who had widespread disseminated coagulation.

Table 13.4. Atrophie Blanche: list of associated diseases.

Pigmented purpuric eruptions
Gravitational stasis
Thrombophlebitis
Thrombo-angiitis obliterans
Polyarteritis nodosa
Diabetes mellitus
Scleroderma
Lupus erythematosus
Dermatomyositis
Rheumatoid arthritis
Hashimoto's disease
Sickle cell anaemia
Anterior poliomyelitis
Sjögren's syndrome
Capillary naevi
Drug eruptions
Trauma, cuts
Carcinoma

In the pathogenesis, dilated coiled papillary vessels adapted to an exceedingly sluggish circulation are important, for in them flow completely ceases from time to time, either spontaneously or as a result of injury from trauma, contact dermatitis, cold, circulating endotoxin or immune complexes and as a result the vessel thromboses (Figure 3.6) and is obliterated. The virtual absence of flow, even before the eventual irreversible cessation, accounts for the absence of white blood cells in the lesion. New vessel formation, which

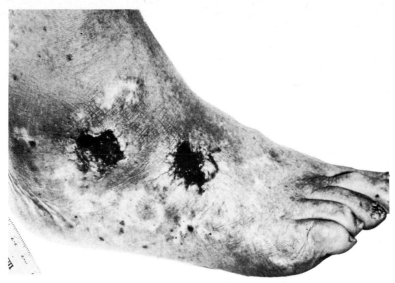

Figure 13.11. Areas of necrosis and white atrophy meriting the name of livedoid vasculitis or atrophie blanche; but in fact it was the presentation in a patient with widespread intravascular coagulation.

would be the response to such a situation in normal skin, does not occur and hence an avascular scar develops. There are a number of reasons why new vessel formation does not occur:

1. There is often a generalised depletion of capillaries such as occurs in 'collagen' disease, old age, atrophic scars, and atherosclerosis (Ryan, 1973).
2. The epidermis is so atrophic that it fails to stimulate (or to demand) new growth (Ryan, 1973).
3. Bypass or alternative channels are so well developed that the skin tends to be deprived by a shunting system (Ryan, 1973): this is equivalent to the brain's 'luxury perfusion' system seen after infarction.

Essentially, therefore, there is a constitutional — local or generalised — defect that discourages normal repair processes and at the same time causes the residual vasculature to dilate and elongate. This type of vasculature, with its gross stasis and exposure to the surface of the skin and the environment is a supreme example of the locus minoris resistentiae, or the 'prepared' state mentioned in other chapters.

A 'skin disease' that is in fact a sign or symptom of a pathological process that can be elicited by many different triggers is often the object of an extraordinary number of treatments. Winklemann et al (1974) list bed-rest, wet dressings, anticoagulants, steroids, nicotinic acid, ganglion blockers, sympathectomy, tetracycline, griseofulvin, methotrexate, sulphapyridine and low molecular weight dextran. Gilliam, Herdon and Prystowsky (1974) prescribed fibrinolytic therapy with successful remission in five patients in whom they diagnosed atrophie blanche (livedo reticularis with summer ulceration).

References

Bard, J. W. & Winkelmann, R. K. (1967) Livedo reticularis, segmental hyalinizing vasculitis of the dermis. *Archives of Dermatology,* **96,** 489.

Favre, M., Contamin, N. & Martine, R. (1924) La dermite pigmentée et purpurique et les phlebites chroniques syphililiques des membres inférieurs. Syphilis et ulceres variqueux. *Lyon Médical,* **133,** 136.

Feldaker, M., Hines, E. A. Jr & Kierland, R. R. (1956) Livedo reticularis with ulcerations. *Circulation,* **13,** 196.

Gilliam, J. N., Herdon, J. H. & Prystowsky, S. D. (1974) Fibrinolytic therapy for vasculitis of atrophie blanche. *Archives of Dermatology,* **109,** 664.

Gonin, R. (1950) Atrophie blanche et ulcère de jambe à douleurs intolérable. *Annales de Dermatologie et Syphiligraphie,* **10,** 633.

Gray, H. R., Graham, J. H., Johnson, W. & Burgoon, C. F. (1966) Atrophie blanche. *Archives of Dermatology,* **93,** 187.

Milian, G. (1929) Les atrophies cutanées syphililiques. *Bulletin de la Société Française de Dermatologie et de Syphiligraphie,* **36,** 865.

Nelson, L. M. (1955) Atrophie blanche en plaque. *Archives of Dermatology,* **72,** 242.

Ryan, T. J. (1969) The epidermis and its blood supply in venous disorders of the leg. *Transactions of the St John's Hospital Dermatological Society,* **55,** 51.

Ryan, T. J. (1973) In *Physiology and Pathophysiology of the Skin* (Ed.) Jarrett, A. New York: Academic Press.

Ryan, T. J. & Wilkinson, D. S. (1972) Diseases of the veins, leg ulcers. In *Textbook of Dermatology* (Ed.) Rook, A., Wilkinson, D. S. & Ebling, F. J. G. p. 996. Oxford: Blackwell.

Stevanovic, D. V. (1974) Atrophie blanche. A sign of dermal blood occlusion. *Archives of Dermatology,* **109,** 858.

Winkelmann, R. K., Schroeter, A. L., Kierland, R. R. & Ryan, T. M. (1974) Clinical studies of livedoid vasculitis (segmental hyalinizing vasculitis). *Mayo Clinic Proceedings,* **49,** 746.

14. Investigation

Investigation of vasculitis begins with adequate history taking and clinical examination to ascertain that there is in fact vascular injury. Efforts should then be made not only to detect triggers such as immune complexes, infection or drugs but also to look for factors enhancing vascular injury such as coagulation, impaired fibrinolysis, gross stasis or hypoxia. In practice, a few simple inexpensive screening tests are usually required before deciding whether more time-consuming or expensive investigations are relevant or necessary, as some require considerable expertise and are not without risk to the patient.

The recognition of relatively distinct clinical patterns of disease such as erythema nodosum or Schönlein—Henoch purpura in a child with a sore throat will act as a guideline; in such cases extensive investigation is usually not justified. However, when such preliminary procedures fail to provide the expected answer, it may be more expedient to regard all types of vasculitis as having broadly the same pathogenesis and to investigate accordingly for other possible mechanisms. Thus, in erythema nodosum it is good sense first to exclude streptococcal infection, tuberculosis or sarcoidosis, and then to follow up any clear clue from the history such as symptoms of ulcerative colitis. But some of these cases will need further study as painful nodules on the shins can be a rare consequence of most infections, may follow the ingestion of many agents, and can herald or complicate malignancy, 'collagen' disease or disseminated intravascular coagulation (Ryan and Wilkinson, 1972). Similar associations in necrotising vasculitis are listed in Table 14.1.

ROUTINE SIMPLE TESTS (Table 14.2)

Full blood count, including platelet count and erythrocyte sedimentation rate

A full blood count, including platelets, supplemented by an estimation of the erythrocyte sedimentation rate should be carried out in every case. The significance of

Table 14.1. Necrotising angiitis; associated diseases in 16 patients and serological abnormalities in another 14 patients without obvious systemic disease.

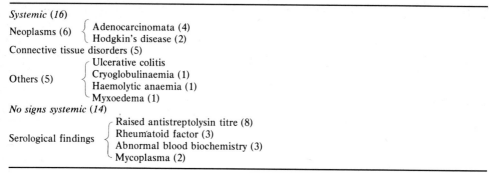

Systemic (16)

Neoplasms (6) { Adenocarcinomata (4)　Hodgkin's disease (2)

Connective tissue disorders (5)

Others (5) { Ulcerative colitis　Cryoglobulinaemia (1)　Haemolytic anaemia (1)　Myxoedema (1)

No signs systemic (14)

Serological findings { Raised antistreptolysin titre (8)　Rheumatoid factor (3)　Abnormal blood biochemistry (3)　Mycoplasma (2)

any one abnormal finding must always be interpreted in terms of the whole patient. Most disease states are a manifestation of a constellation of disorders and most people can tolerate and possibly already possess at least one quantitatively abnormal factor. Most figures quoted as normal for any one laboratory are based on the curve of the universal distribution and a minority lie perfectly innocently at the extremes of that curve and denote no abnormality.

Ward and Reinhard (1971) described as 'normal' a leucocytosis between 10 000 and 20 000/ml in 35 Caucasian patients followed for several years; eleven developed no significant illness. Although the moral of their tale was to avoid making patients unnecessarily anxious about a high white blood cell count, it is worrying that the series ultimately included four cases of significant disease, namely Hodgkin's disease,

Table 14.2. Routine investigation should include a search for triggers of vasculitis as well as for constitutional defects.

Infection:	Streptococcal sore throat Tuberculosis Leprosy 　　　　or any history of recent 'flu'-like illness, cystitis, sinusitis or vaccinations
Foods and drugs:	Aspirin — headache pills, throat lozenges Purgatives Health foods Soft drinks — especially highly coloured and in large quantities Antibiotics Any medicine given for any specific illness Any recent intake of food or drugs to which the patient is known to be allergic
Constitutional:	Undue exposure to extremes of temperature in the environment, to bright sunlight or to cold winds Any known chronic illness such as: diabetes mellitus, blood disorders, rheumatoid arthritis or other form of 'collagen' disease, chronic respiratory disease, disorders of the bowel or liver, or hypertension Malignant disease Recent surgery or pregnancy Any unusual degree of anxiety or an anxious personality
Local constitution:	Trauma, cold exposure, gravitational stasis, changes in vascular anatomy or in cellular infiltration

rheumatoid arthritis, miliary tuberculosis and cryoglobulinaemic vasculitis.

Platelet counts are sometimes omitted by busy laboratories, but if they are abnormally raised or depressed they can be an important clue to accelerated platelet turnover, production or consumption. In polycythaemia rubra vera, an elevated platelet count indicates a greater likelihood of thrombotic and haemorrhagic complications (Dawson and Ogston, 1970). It is not very unusual for a rise in the platelet count to precede changes in the haematocrit (Edwards and Cooley, 1970).

The erythrocyte sedimentation rate, when increased, is an indicator in systemic illness that can be used to monitor therapy. The ESR rises with age (Bottinger and Svedberg, 1967); it is higher in women than in men, especially in those taking an oral contraceptive; and an ESR of 1 to 2 mm per hour is commoner in cool weather (Tromp, 1973). This latter author has claimed that cold weather depresses gamma-globulin production and that this results not only in a lower ESR but an increased susceptibility to infection.

In adults with vasculitis with sufficient pathology to lead one to expect a rise in the ESR, a rate of less than 3 mm per hour Westergren is a clue to the kind of viscosity problem met commonly in vasculitis associated with perniosis, and it is a notable feature of polycythaemia rubra vera. Treatment of the viscosity problem by plasma-pheresis has produced a paradoxically normal ESR (Schwab and Fahey, 1960).

In pyoderma gangrenosum associated with abnormal plasma proteins a typical patient with myelomatosis may have an ESR well over 100 mm per hour Westergren, but when the tissue necrosis is due to a circulating dermatonecrotic factor (Delescluse, de Bast and Achten, 1972) or an agglomerating factor (Cream, 1971) the sedimentation rate may be low. An ESR persistently above 50 mm in vasculitis of the Schönlein—Henoch type in children is unusual and suggests an active underlying infection such as tonsillitis or a complication such as renal disease. Comparison of the Westergren ESR measured at 37°C and at 21°C distinguishes between cold agglutinins and cryoglobulins: cold agglutinins accelerate the sedimentation rate in the cold, whereas cryoglobulins accelerate it in the warm.

In general in vasculitis a haemoglobin level of more than 16 g/ 100 ml or a PCV more than 46 per cent may be of more significance than a haemoglobin of less than 12 g or a PCV less than 38 per cent. This is certainly true of mortality statistics (Elwood et al, 1974; Takkunen and Avomaa, 1974).

Sickle cell anaemia should always be excluded in vasculitis in the North American negro. The sickle cell trait is in itself benign (Petrakis, 1974) but the homozygous disease commonly presents with vasculitis. It can be excluded by haemoglobin electro-phoresis and phosphate buffer solubility (Manning et al, 1973).

The biochemistry of apparently healthy populations has been discussed by Bailey (1974). Screening of large numbers of adults in Sweden, the U.S.A. and the U.K. revealed hypercholesterolaemia, diabetes mellitus and liver disease in up to five per cent of the population. Any one of these could predispose to vasculitis or at least complicate it. While the economics of screening the seemingly healthy is debatable, there need be no doubts about the value of checking the levels of cholesterol, glucose and liver enzymes in the blood of patients with vasculitis.

Electrophoresis of serum proteins will show a reduction in serum albumin and a rise in alpha- and immunoglobulins in all the inflammatory diseases. Quantitative determina-tion of immunoglobulins by radial diffusion techniques is important in the detection of myeloma, Waldenström's macroglobulinaemia or hypergammaglobulinaemia; a few relevant studies have been done in vasculitis in general (Copeman, 1970). Thompson, Main, Beck and Albert-Recht (1973) reported that serum levels of IgA were altered during the disease in cases of leucocytoclastic angiitis associated with pyoderma gangrenosum and paraproteinaemia.

References

Bailey, A. (1974) Biochemistry of well populations. *Lancet,* **ii,** 1436.
Bottinger, L. E. & Svedberg, C. A. (1967) Normal erythrocyte sedimentation rate and age. *British Medical Journal,* **ii,** 85.
Copeman, P. W. M. (1970) Investigations into the pathogenesis of acute cutaneous angiitis. *British Journal of Dermatology,* **82** (Supplement 5), 2.
Cream, J. J. (1971) Pyoderma gangrenosum with a monoclonal IgM red cell agglomerating factor. *British Journal of Dermatology,* **84,** 223.
Dawson, A. A. & Ogston, D. (1970) The influence of the platelet count on the incidence of thrombotic and haemorrhagic complications in polycythaemia vera. *Postgraduate Medical Journal,* **46,** 76.
Delescluse, J., de Bast, Cl. & Achten, G. (1972) Pyoderma gangrenosum with allied cellular immunity and dermonecrotic factor. *British Journal of Dermatology,* **87,** 529.
Edwards, E. A. & Cooley, M. H. (1970) Peripheral vascular symptoms as the initial manifestation of polycythaemia vera. *Journal of the American Medical Association,* **214,** 1463.
Elwood, P. C., Waters, W. E., Benjamin, I. T. & Sweetnam, P. M. (1974) Mortality and anaemia in women. *Lancet,* **i,** 891.
Manning, J. M., Cerami, A., Gillette, P. N., de Furia, F. G. & Miller, D. R. (1973) Cyanate inhibition of red blood cell sickling. In *Sickle Cell Disease* (Ed.) Abramson, H., Bertles, J. F. & Wethers, D. L. p. 177. St. Louis: Moseby.
Petrakis, N. L. (1974) Sickle cell disease. *Lancet,* **ii,** 1368.
Ryan, T. J. & Wilkinson, D. S. (1972) Cutaneous vasculitis (angiitis). In *Textbook of Dermatology* (Ed.) Rook, A., Wilkinson, D. S. & Ebling, F. J. G. p. 920. Oxford: Blackwell.
Schwab, P. J. & Fahey, J. L. (1960) Treatment of Waldenström's macroglobulinemia by plasmapheresis. *New England Journal of Medicine,* **263,** 574.
Takkunen, H. & Aromaa, A. (1974) Mortality and anaemia. *Lancet,* **ii,** 523.
Thompson, D. M., Main, R. A., Beck, J. S. & Albert-Recht, F. (1973) Studies on a patient with leucocytoclastic vasculitis, pyoderma gangrenosum and paraproteinaemia. *British Journal of Dermatology,* **88,** 117.
Tromp, S. W. (1973) Meteorological changes in resistance to infection. *Lancet,* **ii,** 1517.
Ward, H. N. & Reinhard, E. H. (1971) Chronic idiopathic leukocytosis. *Annals of Internal Medicine,* **75,** 193.

RADIOGRAPHY

A routine chest x-ray is a useful screening procedure (Figure 14.1). In this way tuberculosis and malignancy may be detected. Malignancy must otherwise be sought according to clues from clinical examination and history. Intravenous pyelograms and barium studies of the gastrointestinal tract are frequently needed for diagnostic purposes. A prone barium swallow to reveal defective oesophageal peristalsis is an essential investigation of Raynaud's phenomenon, since most patients with systemic sclerosis have oesophageal involvement. Pyoderma gangrenosum usually justifies a barium enema even in the absence of symptoms of ulcerative colitis.

Abnormal serum proteins are one sign of myelomatosis but a radiological skeletal survey should also be requested if this disease is suspected. A sinus x-ray will provide supporting evidence of upper respiratory tract involvement in Wegener's granulomatosis or may reveal a significant focus of infection. Similarly, jaw x-rays may show dental disease or the alveolar changes of scleroderma.

Phlebography is a simple way of demonstrating the presence of a venous thrombus in the leg (Browse, Lea Thomas and Solan, 1967; Browse et al, 1969) especially if there is a good superficial vein on the dorsum of the foot. Arteriograms taken to show atheroma of the lower aorta sometimes explain embolic infarction of the lower leg and buttocks (Figure 14.2). In polyarteritis nodosa of the kidney, arteriograms are the best way to reveal multiple aneurysms in the renal cortex. As they occur in some 60 per cent of cases of polyarteritis nodosa, arteriography is a safer procedure than renal biopsy (Bron and Gajaraj, 1970; Herschman, Blum and Lee, 1970).

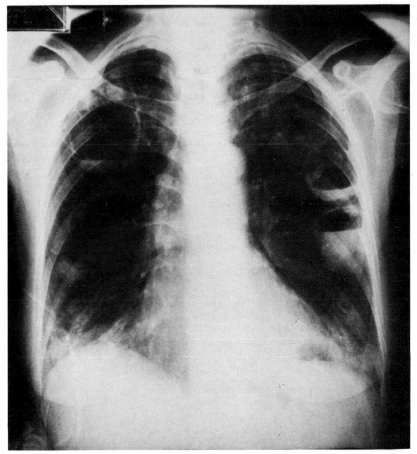

Figure 14.1. Multiple cavitation of the lung with fluid levels detected during investigation of renal disease suggestive of Wegener's granulomatosis.

References

Bron, K. M. & Gajaraj, A. (1970) Arteriographic demonstration of hepatic aneurysms in polyarteritis nodosa. *New England Journal of Medicine,* **282,** 1024.

Browse, N. L., Lea Thomas, M. & Solan, M. J. (1967) Management of the source of pulmonary emboli; the value of phlebography. *British Medical Journal,* **iv,** 596.

Browse, N. L., Lea Thomas, M., Solan, M. J. & Young, A. E. (1969) Prevention of recurrent pulmonary embolism. *British Medical Journal,* **iii,** 382.

Herschman, A., Blum, R. & Lee, Y. C. (1970) Angiographic findings in polyarteritis nodosa. *Radiology,* **94,** 147.

THE SEARCH FOR INFECTION

A degree of common sense or clinical acumen is necessary in assessing every case. It is possible to overdo investigation, and mild cases of vasculitis, especially in children,

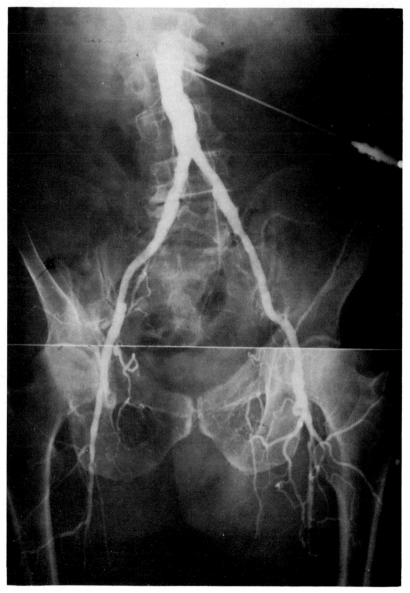

Figure 14.2. Arteriogram lower end of aorta to show atheroma responsible for peripheral infarction.

hardly justify making the patient for ever fearful and tearful in the presence of the medical profession.

The pattern of the disease is only broadly a clue to the likely aetiology; the classic Schönlein—Henoch syndrome and erythema nodosum, however, always justify swabbing the throat and estimating the anti-streptolysin O titre. Classic erythema nodosum and the Bazin type of disease patterns should always merit a chest x-ray. The more vigorous the search for tuberculosis in cases of nodular vasculitis of the calves, the greater the likelihood of finding an active focus. Förstrom, Hannuksela and Rauste (1973) advocated lymphangiograms in every case of panniculitis of the legs, with close scrutiny of the pelvic lymph glands thus revealed. Acute meningococcal septicaemia with its widespread haemorrhagic vasculitis is unlikely to be missed in the presence of meningitis, but chronic septicaemia, whether due to the meningococcus, the gonococcus or to sub-acute bacterial endocarditis, is often missed. It should be suspected when scattered inflammatory skin lesions accompany fever, loss of weight and general ill health. Repeated blood cultures must be done in such cases.

Chronic urinary infection is an occasional cause of vasculitis (Ryan and Wilkinson, 1972).

References

Forstrom, L., Hannuksela, M. & Rauste, J. (1973) Lymphographic investigation of panniculitis of the legs. *Acta Dermato-venereologica*, **53**, 347.
Ryan, T. J. & Wilkinson, D. S. (1972) Cutaneous vasculitis (angiitis). In *Textbook of Dermatology* (Ed.) Rook, A., Wilkinson, D. S. & Ebling, F. J. G. p. 920. Oxford: Blackwell.

DELAYED TYPE BACTERIAL ANTIGEN TESTS

Bacterial tests cause unpleasant skin necrosis but occasionally are of value (Storck, 1951; Rudski et al, 1964; Wilkinson, 1965); they are referred to in Chapter 8. Standard preparations of bacterial extracts are used, e.g. Bencard, 5×10^8 organisms per ml: F_1—F_2 *Staphylococcus aureus, S. albus, Escherichia coli* and control or streptolysin. These are inoculated, 0.1 ml, intradermally. An immediate weal is of little consequence but a delayed response at 24 to 48 hours may have some significance. The histology within the first 12 hours is often leucocytoclastic, as was the case in leucocytoclastic vasculitis, pyoderma gangrenosum with paraproteinaemia (Thompson et al, 1973) and in erythema elevatum diutinum (Cream, Levine and Calnan, 1971) but, by 48 hours, it is usually composed of a perivascular mononuclear infiltrate with fibrinoid changes, and with added ischaemic ulceration in the more strongly positive reactions. As indicated in Chapter 8, the morphology of the response tends to mimic the disease for which the test is being performed. Although a positive result may have a somewhat obscure mechanism and meaning it justifies a more rigorous search for infection. Thus a positive test to *E. coli* led to the successful diagnosis and management of a case of pyelonephritis (Wilkinson, 1965).

Pevny and Metz (1972) re-emphasised that the test in streptococcal infection is of value only when further investigation gives supporting evidence of clinical infection.

References

Cream, J. J., Levene, G. M. & Calnan, C. D. (1971) Erythema elevatum diutinum: an unusual reaction to streptococcal antigen and response to dapsone. *British Journal of Dermatology,* **84**, 393.

Pevny, I. & Metz, J. (1972) Positiver intracutantest, fern und aufflammphanomen mit Streptokokken-Antigen bei vasculitis allergica. *Hautartz*, **23**, 350.

Rudski, E., Moskalewska, K., Leszczynski, W., Maciejowska, E. & Blaszcyk, M. (1964) Bacterial allergy in the skin diseases. I. The methods of evaluation. *Acta Dermato-venereologica*, **44**, 310.

Rudski, E., Maciejowska, E., Leszczynski, W. & Moskalewska, K. (1965) Bacterial allergy in the skin. II. Delayed allergy to streptococci in some skin diseases. *Acta Dermato-venereologica*, **45**, 135.

Storck, H. (1951) Uber hamorrhagische Phanomene in der Dermatologie. *Dermatologica*, **102**, 197.

Thompson, D. M., Main, R. A., Beck, J. S. & Albert-Recht, F. (1973) Studies on a patient with leucocytoclastic vasculitis, pyoderma gangrenosum and paraproteinaemia. *British Journal of Dermatology*, **88**, 117.

Wilkinson, D. S. (1965) Some clinical manifestations and associations of "allergic" vasculitis. *British Journal of Dermatology*, **77**, 186.

URINALYSIS

The prognosis of Schönlein—Henoch purpura depends largely on the degree of renal involvement. The urine should be checked for protein, red cells and casts daily during the acute illness, then at the end of the attack and one to three months after it has subsided. Such testing will be positive at some time in 75 per cent of cases and even the most chronic cases merit an occasional examination of the urine.

Allen, Diamond and Howell (1960) recorded renal involvement in Schönlein—Henoch purpura in 25 per cent of children under two years of age and in 50 per cent of older children. Twenty-eight per cent of this series of 131 children had some evidence of persistent renal disease. Persistent haematuria is a bad sign. Ansell (1970), reporting on 85 attacks in 75 children, recorded that in only one child did renal involvement make its first appearance as late as six weeks after the appearance of purpura, and in 50 per cent it appeared during the first two weeks of the illness. The total incidence of renal involvement was 47 per cent, a figure which is approximately the same as in several other series reviewed. However, persistent renal disease with its sequelae is seen in less than four per cent of children presenting with purpura (Haahr, Thomsen and Sparrevohn, 1974). In adults, death from renal complications is less unusual, there being four out of 10 in one study (Ballard, Eisinger and Gallo, 1970) and three out of 38 in another (Cream, Gumpel and Peachey, 1970). Even when the blood urea has been as high as 100 mg/100 ml or the nephrotic syndrome has developed, complete recovery can occur (Ballard, Eisinger and Gallo, 1970).

Urinary infection is commonplace, affecting some 12 per cent of persons attending their general practitioners (Logan, 1958). An infected urinary tract is a common source of gram-negative septicaemia (Altemeier, Todd and Inge, 1967) and as such it is a likely trigger of vasculitis. Kass (1956) introduced a quantitative method of urine culture to distinguish between the heavy growth from a urine already infected before it is voided and the lighter growth due to contamination during or after voiding. The presence of more than 100 000 bacteria per ml of urine is referred to as 'significant' bacteriuria and is present in three to five per cent of the female population (Asscher, 1974).

Diabetes mellitus is always a possible factor in vasculitis and the glucose oxidase strip test (Clinistix) should not be omitted. It produces false positive reactions because it is not only highly specific for but very sensitive to glucose. By also using the copper reduction tablet method (Clinitest) which is less specific, but also less sensitive, one should identify the true diabetic.

RENAL BIOPSY

This is indicated when there is persistent proteinuria, haematuria or azotaemia, but textbooks on renal disease should be consulted for the interpretation of the results. A poor prognosis is associated with crescent formation (Figure 14.3) and diffuse glomerular lesions. Meadow et al (1972) observed that no child with isolated microscopic haematuria showed more than minor focal lesions.

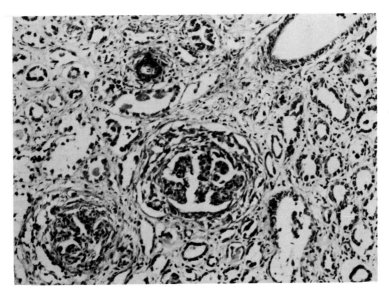

Figure 14.3. Schönlein—Henoch purpura complicated by glomerulonephritis. Epithelial crescent in glomerulus — an appearance associated with a poor prognosis.

References

Allen, D. M., Diamond, L. K. & Howell, D. A. (1960) Anaphylactoid purpura in children (Schönlein—Henoch syndrome). Review with a follow up of renal complications. *American Journal of Diseases of Children*, **99**, 333.

Altemeier, W. A., Todd, J. C. & Inge, W. W. (1967) Gram negative septicaemia: a growing threat. *Annals of Surgery*, **166**, 530.

Ansell, B. M. (1970) Henoch—Schönlein purpura with particular reference to the prognosis of the renal lesion. *British Journal of Dermatology*, **82**, 211.

Asscher, A. W. (1974) Urinary tract infection. *Lancet, ii*, 1365.

Ballard, H. S., Eisinger, R. P. & Gallo, G. (1970) Renal manifestations of the Henoch—Schönlein syndrome in adults. *American Journal of Medicine*, **49**, 328.

Cream, J. J., Gumpel, J. M. & Peachey, R. D. G. (1970) Schönlein—Henoch purpura in the adult. A study of 77 adults with anaphylactoid or Schönlein—Henoch purpura. *Quarterly Journal of Medicine*, **34**, 461.

Haahr, J., Thomsen, K. & Sparrevohn, S. (1974) Renal involvement in Henoch—Schönlein purpura. *British Medical Journal*, **iv**, 405.

Kass, E. H. (1956) Asymptomatic infections of urinary tract. *Transactions of the Association of American Physicians*, **69**, 56.

Logan, W. P. D. & Cushion, A. A. (1958) *Morbidity Statistics from General Practice*, Vol. I. London: H. M. Stationery Office.

Meadow, S. R., Glasgow, E. F., White, R. H., Moncrieff, M. W., Cameron, J. S. & Ogg, C. W. (1972) Schönlein—Henoch nephritis. *Quarterly Journal of Medicine*, **41**, 241.

CAPILLARY MICROSCOPY (Ryan, 1973)

Anyone familiar with this technique will seldom use it in the investigation of vasculitis. It is, however, a useful tool for demonstrating to the inexperienced how distorted the microvasculature becomes in disease. The lower leg and the nail fold are particularly well suited for showing the gross disturbances in vascular pattern and blood flow caused by cooling in perniosis, by gravitational stasis and by collagen diseases such as scleroderma or lupus erythematosus, or even in scars of previous trauma or disease. Figure 14.4 demonstrates some of the distorted patterns responsible for stasis, sludging and silting out of particulate matter in the circulation.

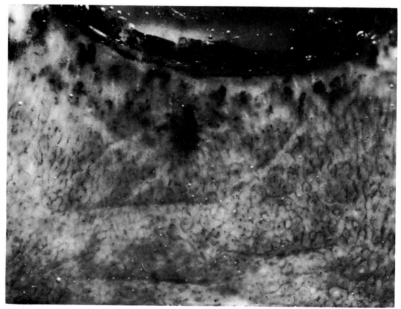

Figure 14.4. Dilated irregular nail fold capillaries in dermatomyositis in a six-year old boy — a usual finding in this disease.

Without microscopy it is not always possible to distinguish between capillary dilatation, haemorrhage or thrombosis; this is especially true of the nail fold where the term 'splinter haemorrhage' may be applied loosely to all three phenomena (Figure 3.12, Chapter 3).

References

Ryan, T. J. (1973) In *Physiology and Pathophysiology of the Skin* (Ed.) Jarrett, A. Volume 2. New York, London: Academic Press.

BLOOD VISCOSITY

The viscosity of a fluid is its ability to resist flow. A simple indication of the viscosity of a fluid is the time taken for a given amount of it to move along a tube of standard bore when subjected to a standard pressure. Being a relatively complex suspension of semisolid material, blood is a non-Newtonian fluid, and this is why one of its main characteristics is that sluggish flow in certain vascular beds makes it disproportionately viscous. Exposure to low temperatures increases the viscosity of all fluids, but especially the non-Newtonian variety; in this way the flow properties of blood in skin are disturbed, especially in areas such as the lower legs where there also is stasis.

In practice it is very difficult to estimate the role of blood viscosity at any one site. One can, however, estimate factors such as a high haematocrit, high fibrinogen levels, or reversed albumin/globulin ratios, all of which increase whole blood viscosity and may be assumed to increase resistance to flow through cooled skin especially where it is already known to be sluggish.

One can also use capillary microscopy to observe *flow* through skin capillaries. Significant ill-effects due to ischaemia should be expected when flow is virtually at a standstill and the blood in consequence is of even higher viscosity (Ryan, 1973).

There are various methods for measuring whole blood or plasma viscosity; some use capillary tubes, others a rotating cone fitted on to a plate into which blood is poured (Dintenfass, 1971). Figure 12.6 illustrates a simple viscometer using four metres of 0.5 mm diameter polythene tubing. Figure 12.5 illustrates the time taken for blood of high or low viscosity to move 1 cm along such tubing when subjected to a pressure of 100 mm of mercury and exposed to temperatures of 15, 20 and 37°C. The more viscous the blood, the greater the effect of moderate cooling. The velocity at which the blood flows in this apparatus is no higher than may be observed in the dilated venules of perniotic skin. Many hospitals now use plasma viscosity as an alternative to the erythrocyte sedimentation rate (ESR). It is a test that takes only 20 seconds, it is suitable for samples sent in the post, it is cheap and it is not influenced by red cell depletion. It is particularly recommended as an alternative to the ESR in the elderly.

Dormandy et al (1973) measured whole blood viscosity at fast and slow shear rates. They found that there was a significant correlation between progressive deterioration in the peripheral circulation and the initial blood viscosity. Patients with intermittent claudication and heart disease had the highest viscosity.

Viscosity is greatest in cooled areas. For this reason a simple estimation of skin temperature should be made. This can be done by touch; significant cooling in perniotic skin or the extremities is easily assessed by the human hand and, in routine management, that is all that is required. The rate of warming of the skin 20 minutes after exposure to a warm atmosphere after previous cooling is also useful; perniotic skin remains cool.

References

Dintenfass, L. (1971) *Viscosity Factors in Blood Flow, Ischaemia and Thrombosis.* London: Butterworths.
Dormandy, J. A., Hoare, E., Khattab, A. H., Arrowsmith, D. E. & Dormandy, T. L. (1973) Prognostic significance of rheological and biochemical findings in patients with intermittent claudication. *British Medical Journal,* **iv,** 581.
Ryan, T. J. (1973) In *Physiology and Pathophysiology of the Skin,* Volume 2. (Ed.) Jarrett, A. New York, London: Academic Press.

COAGULATION AND FIBRINOLYSIS

The minimum of tests required to demonstrate significant intravascular coagulation must at least show that coagulation factors and platelets are being used up. Prolonged prothrombin time and a fall in fibrinogen levels and in the platelet count provide such evidence.

Fibrin degradation products should be measured at the same time since they indicate that fibrin is being formed (Reid and Nkrumah, 1972). Robboy et al (1973) have suggested that clear evidence of intravascular coagulation is most easily secured by a skin biopsy to demonstrate capillaries filled with fibrin (Figure 14.5) and they found it particularly helpful when preliminary coagulation tests were equivocal. In frank disseminated intravascular coagulation a warm steely-blue area of skin which fails to blanch on pressure is a suitable site to biopsy.

To demonstrate that a minor but significant degree of intravascular coagulation is occurring in diseases such as meningococcal septicaemia, it is necessary to measure soluble circulating fibrin (Kisker and Rush, 1973). Such a test is based on the ability of the fibrin stabilising enzyme — plasma transglutaminase (Factor XIII) — to incorporate ^{14}C glycine ethyl ester into fibrinogen after the alpha peptide of fibrinogen has been hydrolysed by thrombin.

The assessment of the relative degrees of coagulation and fibrinolysis is always difficult. Wood et al (1974) believed that, by measuring immunoreactive fibrinogen, heat-precipitable fibrinogen and cryofibrinogen, they could deduce whether there was (a) coagulation balanced by fibrinolysis, (b) predominant coagulation or (c) predominant fibrinolysis; for technical details see Wolf and Farrell (1972). These tests are quite within the capabilities of any laboratory.

Cryofibrinogen levels are given by the difference between the amount of heat-precipitable fibrinogen in a plasma sample left at room temperature for 20 to 24 hours and that in a duplicate left at 4°C. It is regarded as an index of the action of thrombin on fibrinogen, and therefore of coagulation (Shainoff and Page, 1962).

Red cells damaged on passing through strands of fibrin clot will be seen as distorted, fragmented erythrocytes in a blood film (Figure 14.6). Endothelial cells may be liberated into the circulation of patients with vascular injury (Gaynor, Bouvier and Spaet, 1970; Payling-Wright, 1973), and their nuclei may fuse to form larger masses which are trapped in the lung; at one time these were thought to be megakaryocytes (Simpson, Robertson and Stalker, 1973). Buffy coat smears or thick blood films should be stained with aqueous Giemsa or Leishman stains (Goodall, 1973) to demonstrate such nuclei in blood.

Wardle (1974), in a discussion on glomerulonephritis, suggested that if fibrin is seen to be blocking capillaries, then the vascular endothelium has already lost its local fibrinolytic activity and the damage is done. In this case, tests for measuring an earlier stage of coagulation are necessary. He went so far as to suggest that the ESR may one day prove to be the most useful test! In the meantime, he has recommended platelet function tests, including the measurement of platelet factor 4, of radio-fibrinogen catabolism, or chromatographic detection of plasma fibrin monomer complexes.

The typical pattern of laboratory results in disseminated intravascular coagulation may sometimes be due to localised conversion of fibrinogen to fibrin, rather than from a disseminated process. Straub (1973), in a study of patients with arterial aneurysms, recorded elevation of fibrin degradation products and increased turnover in fibrinogen.

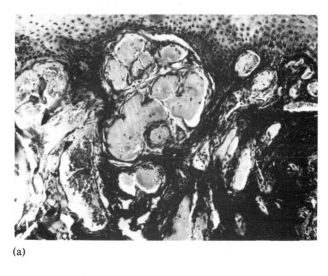

(a)

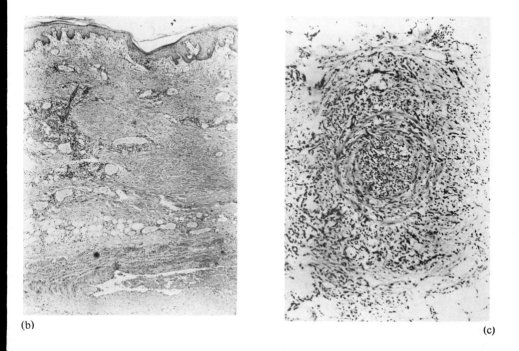

(b)

(c)

Figure 14.5. Examples of the intravascular coagulation in the skin demonstrated by conventional histology: (a) fibrin in capillaries, (b) and (c) recanalised veins in subcutaneous fat.

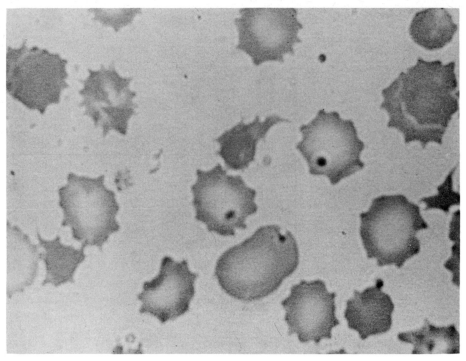

Figure 14.6. Blood film in micro-angiopathic haemolytic anaemia. Such distortion is caused by tearing of the red cell membrane as it flows through strands of fibrin in partially occluded small vessels.

References

Gaynor, E., Bouvier, C. C. & Spaet, T. H. (1970) Vascular lesions: possible pathogenetic basis of the generalised Shwartzmann reaction. *Science,* **170,** 989.
Goodall, H. B. (1973) Giant nuclear masses in the lungs and blood in malignant malaria. *Lancet,* **ii,** 1124.
Kisker, C. T. & Rush, R. (1973) Circulating fibrin and meningococcaemia. *Journal of Pediatrics,* **82,** 787.
Payling Wright, H. (1973) Endothelial injury and repair. *Bibliography of Anatomy,* **12,** 87.
Reid, H. A. & Nkrumah, F. K. (1972) Fibrin degradation products in cerebral malaria. *Lancet,* **i,** 218.
Robboy, S. J., Mihm, M. C., Colman, R. W. & Minna, J. D. (1973) The skin in disseminated intravascular coagulation: Prospective analysis of 36 cases. *British Journal of Dermatology,* **88,** 221.
Shainoff, J. R. & Page, I. H. (1962) Significance of cryoprofibrin in fibrinogen—fibrin conversion. *Journal of Experimental Medicine,* **116,** 686.
Simpson, J. G., Robertson, A. J. & Stalker, A. L. (1973) The effect of immune complexes on coagulation and fibrinolysis. In *Clinical Aspects of Microcirculation, part II; 7th European Conference on Microcirculation* (Ed.) Ditzel, J. & Lewis, D. S. p. 260. Basel: S. Karger.
Straub, P. (1973) Chronic intravascular coagulation: localised or generalised. *Thrombosis et Diathesis Haemorrhagica,* **56,** 1.
Wardle, E. N. (1974) Urinary F.D.P. excretion in glomerulonephritis. *British Medical Journal,* **ii,** 273.
Wolf, P. & Farrell, G. W. (1972) In *Methods in Microcirculation Studies* (Ed.) Ryan, T. J., Jolles, B. & Holti, G. p. 92. London: H. K. Lewis.
Wood, S. M., Burnett, D., Picken, A. M., Farrell, G. W. & Wolf, P. (1974) Assessment of coagulation and fibrinolysis in pre-eclampsia. *British Medical Journal,* **ii,** 145.

RADIOACTIVE ISOTOPES FOR FIBRIN, PLATELETS AND COMPLEMENT

There have been many reports of the use of ^{125}I-labelled fibrinogen to detect fibrin deposition in the leg veins and also in experiments to study coagulation such as those reported on page 104 (Hobbs and Davies, 1960; Atkins and Hawkins, 1965; Nanson et al, 1965; Negus et al, 1968). Human fibrinogen labelled with 100 μCi ^{125}I (which has a half-life of 60 days) is injected intravenously. Potassium iodide in a dose of 150 mg is given by mouth 24 hours earlier and then daily for three days to protect the thyroid from ^{125}I uptake. Counts over the heart are used as a baseline, and a persistent elevation of more than 15 to 20 per cent at any point suggests localisation and conversion of the fibrinogen into fibrin. Such measurements can be continued for several days.

The technique does not indicate the earliest phase of clotting in which only small amounts of fibrinogen are converted, nor does it detect established thrombosis in which conversion has stopped. Oedema, wounds or inflammation will cause localisation of fibrinogen without necessarily indicating its conversion into fibrin.

The technique should not be used in pregnancy; it carries a debatable, slight risk of causing either malignancy in the long term or infective hepatitis.

References

Atkins, P. & Hawkins, L. A. (1965) Detection of venous thrombosis in the legs. *Lancet,* **ii,** 1217.
Hobbs, J. T. & Davies, J. W. L. (1960) Detection of venous thrombosis with I^{131} labelled fibrinogen in the rabbit. *Lancet,* **ii,** 134.
Nanson, E., Palko, P., Dick, A. & Fedorak, S. (1965) Early detection of deep venous thrombosis of the legs using I^{131} tagged human fibrinogen: a clinical study. *Annals of Surgery,* **162,** 438.
Negus, D., Pinto, D. J., LeQuesne, L. P., Brown, N. & Chapman, M. (1968) I^{125}-labelled fibrinogen in the diagnosis of deep vein thrombosis and its coagulation with phlebography. *British Journal of Surgery,* **55,** 835.

IMMUNOFLUORESCENCE FOR FIBRIN COMBINED WITH TODD'S TECHNIQUE FOR ESTIMATING FIBRINOLYSIS

The balance between fibrinolysis and fibrin deposition is altered in vasculitis, and an assessment of both gives some impression of the dynamics of this balance (Ryan, Nishioka and Dawber, 1971; Gebhart and Kraft, 1971). Table 10.5 illustrates the results of such a study by Turner, Ryan and colleagues. Table 14.3 is an outline of Todd's technique as used by Turner, Kurban and Ryan (1969). Figure 14.7 illustrates the technique of applying a film of fibrin over frozen sections prior to incubating them for a few minutes.

References

Gebhart, W. & Kraft, D. (1971) Aussagewert zweier unter suchungs methoden bei gefasz veand errungen: bestimmung der lokalen Fibrinolytischen aktivitat nach Todd und Fibrinogen, nachweiss mittels Immunofluoresz Technik. *Annali Italiani di Dermatologia Clinica e Sperimentale,* **25,** 413.
Ryan, T. J., Nishioka, K. & Dawber, R. P. R. (1971) Epithelial—endothelial interactions in the control of inflammation through fibrinolysis. *British Journal of Dermatology,* **84,** 501.
Turner, R. H., Kurban, A. K. & Ryan, T. J. (1969) Fibrinolytic activity in human skin following epidermal injury. *Journal of Investigative Dermatology,* **53,** 458.

Table 14.3. Fibrinolytic autographic technique.

1. Soak cellophane paper in veronal buffer for at least 2 hours (in bath).
2. Add 10 ml veronal buffer to 0.2 g fibrinogen in a plastic bottle (disposable).
3. Spin for 10—15 min. (or for 1 hour if '4' not carried out).
4. Place in water bath at 37°C for 5—10 min.
5. Filter through funnel containing cotton wool plug.
6. *Thrombin:* Place 0.1 ml of the mixture in a bijou bottle and add 2 ml of veronal buffer.
7. *Cellophane paper (300—400 P.T.):* Lay the paper in the trough and smooth it flat with a glass rod (no air-bubbles under paper).
8. Take 0.1 ml of thrombin/buffer mixture in a bijou bottle and add 3.5 ml of fibrinogen. Spread this immediately onto the paper in the trough and smooth (with glass rod +/− blowing); leave for ¾—1 hour.
9. Prepare the polythene boxes with distilled water.
10. Trim off left and right edges of paper and cut down the middle horizontally. Cut 'coverslip-sized' pieces of the fibrin film and place carefully on the frozen sections (avoiding air-bubbles); put the specimens in the polythene boxes and leave overnight in fridge (12—18 hours).
11. Incubate at 37°C for 20 min.; look every 5—10 min. to observe degree of lysis.
12. Put in 10% formalin fixative for at least 1 hour, remove from formalin, place in water then peel off cellophane paper; wash in water for 20—30 min.
13. Filter haematoxylin solution.
14. Stain for 5 min. then leave in water overnight.
15. Dry specimens and mount on glass slides.

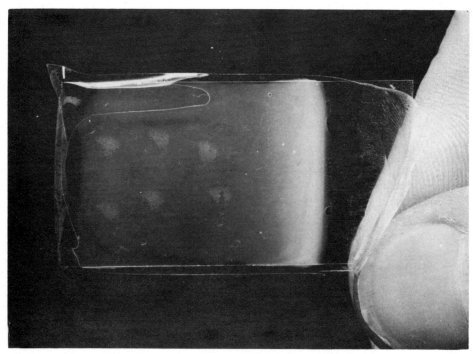

(a)

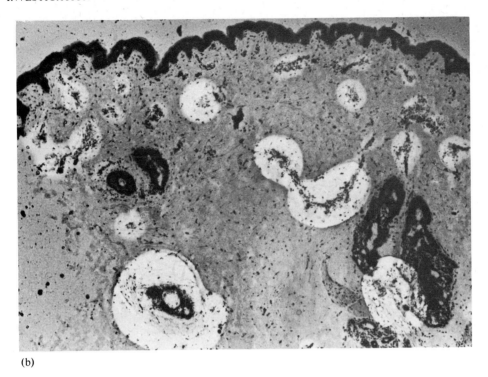

(b)

Figure 14.7. (a) A film of fibrin placed over frozen sections of skin prior to incubation. The fibrin contains plasminogen and this is activated by enzymes released from dermal blood vessels.
(b) Normal skin fibrinolysis — clear areas are lysed fibrin.

IMMUNOFLUORESCENCE FOR IMMUNOGLOBULINS AND COMPLEMENT

Immunofluorescence in vasculitis is discussed in Chapter 7. Several studies on the deposition of immunoglobulins and complement have been made. Their interpretation is often difficult because they are incomplete. In fact to assess the significance of materials deposited in small amounts in the vessel wall one must measure several other indices. Table 7.2 shows that the use of several other agents such as 'Transferrin' gave some idea of the vascular permeability and therefore how specific was the deposition of immunoglobulin.

As an example of full immunological investigations Figure 14.8 (a) and (b) illustrates a patient at present under the care of the Dermatology Department at Oxford who presented with a multi-system disease including nephritis (Powell and McDougall, 1974; Iveson et al, 1975) and, as is so often the case, was initially labelled as polyarteritis nodosa. Muscle biopsy showed him to have leprosy. Figure 14.8 (a) and (b) illustrates endocapillary mesangial proliferation and acid-fast bacilli in the juxtaglomerular region. Immunofluorescence revealed faint scattered linear deposition of IgM, IgG and complement along glomerular capillary walls (Figure 14.9). The significance of this was enhanced by the demonstration of a cryoglobulin (2 mg/100 ml of serum) composed of IgG and IgM which was considered to be polyclonal because both kappa and lambda chains were present. No rheumatoid activity was detected.

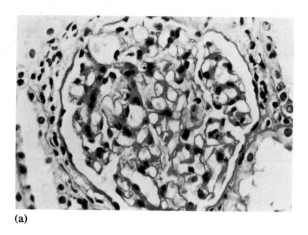

(a)

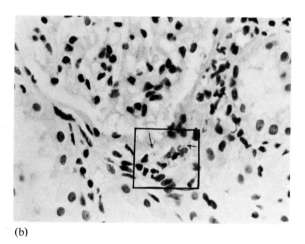

(b)

Figure 14.8. (a) Endocapillary mesangial proliferation in glomerular disease caused by immune complexes in lepromatous leprosy.
(b) Mycobacterium in juxtaglomerular region.

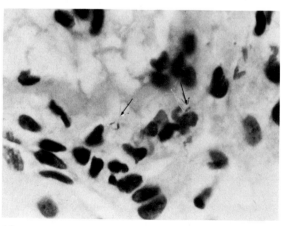

(c)

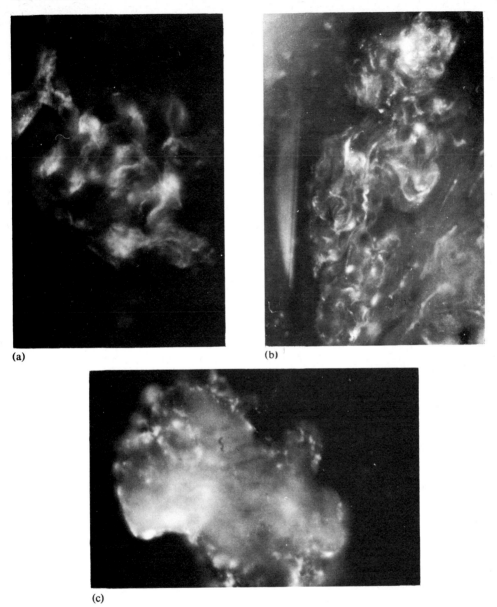

(a)

(b)

(c)

Figure 14.9. Linear deposition of (a) IgG (b) IgM (c) complement in the walls of the capillaries in the glomerulus due to presumed deposition of immune complexes in lepromatous leprosy.

Double infusion in agarose of cryoglobulin against anti-*M. leprae* serum (absorbed with serum and skin) gave a line of precipitation and a line of identity with the original *M. leprae* material but not with the normal serum or skin extract. This suggested an antigen present in the cryoglobulin (cross) reacting with anti *M. leprae* antiserum (although the antiserum probably contained other unspecified antibody also). The suggestion was therefore that the cryoglobulin might contain IgG, IgM and an *M. leprae*-like antigen. Other examples of the value of immunofluorescence in the investigation of vasculitis are illustrated in Figure 14.10a, b, c.

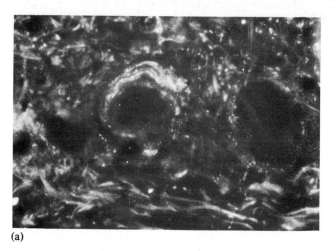

(a)

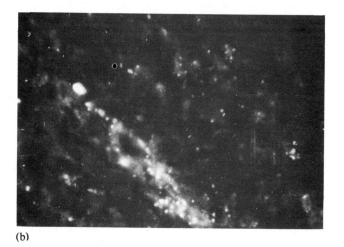

(b)

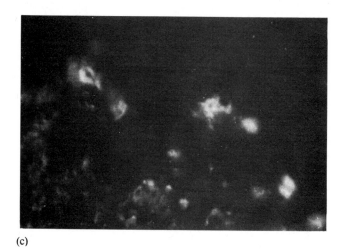

(c)

SOLUBLE IMMUNE COMPLEXES

Soluble immune complexes or aggregated immunoglobulin should be suspected when high molecular weight material is detected by the examination of serum proteins in a Sephadex column. Heating serum to 56°C destroys complement (C1) bound to immune complexes. The complex so freed can be used to bind standard preparations of complement. Estimation of the complement remaining after such complexing is easily done using a red cell lysis system. In one series (Johnson, Mowbray and Porter, 1975) soluble immune complexes were demonstrated in 30 per cent of subjects with urticaria and 50 per cent of 58 subjects with vasculitis. In glomerulonephritis 90 per cent of those patients with fibrinoid necrosis are positive compared to only 22.5 per cent of those without fibrinoid necrosis.

COLD PRECIPITABLE PROTEINS

Cryoglobulins (Grey and Kohler, 1973)

Blood should be collected from the cubital vein preferably with no occlusion of the upper arm and no cooling of the forearm. The syringes and containers for the blood should be pre-warmed in an incubator at 37°C, and after collection the blood is put into dry sterile containers which are kept in the incubator for an hour or so while the blood clots. The serum should be centrifuged in apparatus that is at least at warm room temperature. A small centrifuge that can be placed in the incubator before use is useful for this purpose. Serum should be stored at 4°C.

Monoclonal cryoglobulins, such as are a feature of myelomatosis, usually precipitate within 24 hours, but mixed cryoglobulins that represent immune complexes often take up to five days to precipitate. If the serum gels instantaneously on cooling a monoclonal cryoglobulin may be the cause, but to prove it will necessitate the collection of blood in EDTA, each 10 ml of plasma being treated later with 0.1 ml $CaCl_2$ (16 g/100 ml distilled H_2O). As much as 80 μg/ml of cryoglobulin may be detected in apparently normal individuals and trace amounts are usual (Cream, 1972). The smaller the amount of cryoglobulin the lower the temperature necessary to promote precipitation.

The cryoglobulin concentration can be measured either directly after washing with saline, or by subtracting the concentration of protein in serum after cooling from that present before cooling. Antigenic analysis by immunoelectrophoresis and testing for rheumatoid factor should follow. The incidence of the different types of cryoprecipitate will vary according to the type of disease being studied. Only in recent years have the

---

Figure 14.10. (a) Skin section of a DLE lesion. Blue narrow band illumination, ocular 6 ×, obj. 50 ×, water immersion. DIF method RAHu/IgM/FTC (unitage 4, dilution 1:32). Note: IgM granular deposits partly in a lamellar arrangement in a blood vessel wall of the mid-dermis and to a lesser extent in the perivascular areas. (b) Skin section of the skin adjacent to the lesional skin of a patient with dermatitis herpetiformis. Blue narrow band illumination, ocular 6 ×, obj. 50 ×, water immersion. DIF method RAHu/IgA/FTC (unitage 2, dilution 1:32). Note: IgA granular deposits in the blood vessel wall and to a lesser extent in the perivascular areas. (c) Skin section of the skin adjacent to the lesional skin of a patient with vasculitis (Gougerot syndrome). Blue narrow band illumination, ocular 6 ×, obj. 50 ×, water immersion. DIF method RAHu/IgD/FTC (unitage 2, dilution 1:32). Note: IgD granular deposits closely packed, almost homogeneous fluorescence of the small blood vessels in the superficial layer of the dermis.

smaller amounts of mixed cryoprecipitates been recognised. Patients with Raynaud's phenomenon and large plaques of relatively superficial and painless purpura are more likely to have monoclonal cryoglobulins, whereas those with the tender, palpable, papular or nodular lesions, encountered by dermatologists most commonly in association with arthritis and which have a leucocytoclastic histology, are likely to have mixed cryo-globulins.

Repeated examination for cryoglobulins is necessary in the Schönlein—Henoch type of vasculitis, since they may occur only transiently and tend to disappear as a result of therapy or with spontaneous regression of the disease (Biro, Kaldor and Torok, 1965).

Cold agglutinins

Cold agglutinins are picked up by noticing agglutination of red cells when spreading or examining slides of peripheral blood made at room temperature.

References

Biro, I., Kaldor, I. & Torok, E. (1965) Transient cryoglobulinaemia. *Acta Dermato-venereologica*, **45**, 159.
Cream, J. J. (1972) Cryoglobulins in vasculitis. *Clinical and Experimental Immunology*, **10**, 117.
Grey, H. M. & Kohler, P. F. (1973) Cryoglobulins. *Seminars in Hematology*, **10**, 87.
Iveson, J. M. I., McDougall, A. C., Leatham, A. J. & Harris, H. J. (1975) Lepromatous leprosy presenting with polyarthritis, myositis and immune-complex glomerulonephritis. *British Medical Journal*, **iii**, 619.
Johnson, A., Mowbray, J. F. & Porter, K. A. (1975) Detection of circulating immune complexes in pathological human sera. *Lancet*, **i**, 762.
Powell, S. & McDougall, C. (1974) Clinical recognition of leprosy. Some factors leading to delays in diagnosis. *British Medical Journal*, **i**, 612.

Cryofibrinogen

Cryofibrinogen which is occasionally responsible for skin necrosis in cold weather (Waxman and Dove, 1969) was first described in pregnant women (Morrison, 1946). It was associated transiently with transient indurated skin lesions in infants in one study (Robinson et al, 1966).

Thomas, Smith and van Korff (1954) found it in the Shwartzman reaction and in patients with rheumatic fever or rheumatic disease, and Kalbfleisch and Bird (1960) observed it in malignancy. It is now recognised in many inflammatory diseases including some dermatoses (Fyrand, 1974). It is probably commoner than cryoglobulinaemia and was described in 9 out of 13 cases of vasculitis by German workers (Goring and Gans, 1973).

In about one-third of the normal population, cryoprecipitate is present in the plasma, there being on average 0.16 mg/ml; this may not redissolve on warming. Larger amounts of a more readily soluble cryoprecipitate are found in disease. Blood should be collected in oxalate.

References

Florey, H. (1954) *Lectures in General Pathology*. Philadelphia: W. B. Saunders.
Fyrand, O. (1974) Heparin precipitable fraction (H.P.F.) in an unselected material of dermatological patients. *Acta Dermato-venereologica*, **54**, 293.

Goring, H. D. & Gans, U. (1973) Uber des vorkommen der kryoproteine heparin precipitable fraction. Kryofibrinogen und Kryoglobulin in einem nicht ausgewahlten dermatologischen Krankengut. *Dermatologische Monatsschrift,* **159,** 520.

Kalbfleisch, J. M. & Bird, R. M. (1960) Cryofibrinogenemia. *New England Journal of Medicine,* **263,** 881.

Morrison, I. R. (1946) Quantitative changes in fibrinogen which influence erythrocyte sedimentation rate and clot retraction time. *American Journal of the Medical Sciences,* **211,** 325.

Robinson, M. G., Troina, G., Cohen, H. & Foadi, M. (1966) Acute transient cryofibrinogenemia in infants. *Journal of Pediatrics,* **69,** 35.

Thomas, L., Smith, R. T. & von Korff, R. W. (1954) Cold-precipitation by heparin of protein in rabbit and human plasma. *Proceedings of the Society for Experimental Biology and Medicine,* **86,** 813.

Waxman, S. & Dove, J. T. (1969) Cryofibrinogenemia aggravated during hypothermia. *New England Journal of Medicine,* **281,** 1291.

COMPLEMENT

Hypocomplementaemia is a feature of systemic lupus erythematosus and immune complex diseases; it also occurs in heparin or dextran sulphate therapy or in the absence of a complement inhibitor. In the latter case it is depleted by a low-grade inflammatory process. It is also lowered in mastocytosis (Sbano, Andreassi and Valentino, 1971) and in DIC in malaria (Skrichaikul et al, 1975).

Normal figures for complement components (Royal Postgraduate Medical School, London) are listed in Table 14.4. Sera can be stored at 70°C in 0.1 per cent sodium azide. The dynamics of complement behaviour can be studied using ^{125}I-labelled C_3. Low levels, when accompanied by hypercatabolism, are good evidence of complement activation (Charlesworth et al, 1974).

Table 14.4. Normal serum levels of components of complement expressed as percentages of reference pooled normal human serum (Royal Postgraduate Medical School, London).

Clq	C3	C4	GBG	Properdin	C1 inhibitor
60—136	68—116	50—210	40—210	40—210	70—100

GBG = Glycine rich β glycoprotein.

References

Charlesworth, J. A., Williams, D. G., Sherington, E. L., Lachmann, P. J. & Peters, D. K. (1974) Metabolic studies of the third component of complement and glycine-rich beta glycoprotein in patients with hypocomplementaemia. *Journal of Clinical Investigation,* **53,** 1578.

Sbano, E., Andreassi, L. & Valentino, A. (1971) Contributo allo studio dei rapports fra complementemia ed eparinemia nella mastocitosi. *Giornale Italiano di Dermatologia,* **112,** 492.

Srichaikul, T., Puwasatien, P., Puwasatien, P., Karnjanajetanee, J. & Bokisch, V. A. (1975) Complement changes and disseminated intravascular coagulation in Plasmodium falciparum malaria. *Lancet,* **i,** 770.

ANTINUCLEAR AND RHEUMATOID FACTOR

Antinuclear factor

Rowell (1971) believed that a titre of more than 1 in 64 in a patient with a rash or multi-system disorder is very suggestive of lupus erythematosus or systemic sclerosis and almost certainly rules out dermatomyositis or polyarteritis nodosa. Its help in distinguishing discoid from systemic lupus erythematosus is limited in so far as the titres in the latter are usually but not necessarily higher. A titre of less than 1 in 16 in an otherwise fit person is of little significance.

Table 14.5 lists laboratory abnormalities found on initial examination in 120 patients with discoid lupus erythematosus and 40 patients with systemic lupus erythematosus (Rowell, 1968). Rowell (1971) stated that 15 per cent of patients with undoubted systemic lupus erythematosus had a normal ESR.

Table 14.5. Laboratory abnormalities in lupus erythematosus.

	Discoid	Systemic
No. of cases	120	40
ESR >20 mm/hour	20%	85%
Glubulin >3 g %	29%	76%
LE cell test positive	1.7%	83%
Antinuclear factor(s)	35%	87%
homogeneous	24%	74%
speckled	11%	26%
nucleolar	0%	5.4%
Precipitating autoantibody(ies)	4%	42%
False +ve Wasserman reaction	5%	22%
Rheumatoid factor test positive	15%	37%
Direct Coombs' test positive	2.5%	15%
Leucopenia	12.5%	37%
Thrombocytopenia	5%	21%

Burnham (1972) reported significantly higher titres of antinuclear factor in patients with malignancy and suggested that in the absence of a family history of 'connective tissue' disease or of drug reactions a consistently positive antinuclear factor test should be regarded as an indication of malignancy.

Investigation of lupus erythematosus should include a full blood count including platelets, estimation of serum proteins and serum protein electrophoresis, ESR, Wasserman reaction, Coombs test, examination for serum cold agglutinins, cryoglobulins, and antinuclear factor, LE cell tests and urinalysis (Rowell, 1971). LE cells are present in 80 per cent of patients with systemic lupus erythematosus but, since they are also found in other 'collagen' diseases and in chronic active hepatitis, such tests are becoming obsolete. Antibodies to DNA combined with a fall of serum complement are more specific (Hughes, 1971; Jablonska and Chorzelski, 1974).

Rheumatoid factor

A variety of techniques is used to measure rheumatoid activity. The value of this test lies in the better prognosis of sero-negative disease and the high risk of a complicated course in persons with high titres (Alexander and McCarthy, 1966). It is not necessarily an indication of joint disease, being rather an abnormal response to antigenic stimulus (see page 150). Raised titres of rheumatoid factor are seen in sub-acute bacterial endocarditis, viral illnesses, leprosy, liver disease, lupus erythematosus and chronic hypergammaglobulinaemia.

References

Alexander, W. R. M. & McCarthy, D. D. (1966) In *Modern Trends in Rheumatology* (Ed.) Gardiner-Hill, A. p. 153. London: Butterworths.

Burnham, T. K. (1972) Antinuclear antibodies in patients with malignancies. *Lancet*, **ii**, 436.

Hughes, G. R. V. (1971) Significance of anti-DNA antibodies in systemic lupus erythematosus. *Lancet*, **ii**, 861.

Jablonska, S. & Chorzelski, T. P. (1974) Lupus erythematosus. In *Immunological Aspects of Skin Diseases* (Ed.) Fry, L. & Seah, P. P. pp. 66-152. Lancaster, England: Medical and Technical Publishing Company.

Rowell, N. R. (1968) Polyarteritis nodosa. In *Textbook of Dermatology* (Ed.) Rook, A., Wilkinson, D. S. & Ebling, F. J. G. p. 578. Oxford: Blackwell.

Rowell, N. R. (1971) Laboratory abnormalities in the diagnosis and management of lupus erythematosus. *British Journal of Dermatology*, **84**, 210.

LYMPHOCYTE FUNCTION TESTS (Asherson, 1972)

Lymphocytes can be stimulated in vitro by nonspecific agents such as phytohaemagglutinin (PHA) and concanavalin A or by specific antigen such as purified protein derivative in persons known to be sensitive to the tubercle bacillus. Unfortunately the reactivity of lymphocytes in vitro is not always demonstrable even in subjects with clear evidence of delayed hypersensitivity on skin testing. Thus, with respect to *Candida albicans,* 65 per cent of adults showed blast cell transformation, although it is assumed that all adults will have been exposed to this organism (Folb and Trounce, 1970). While it is not difficult to demonstrate in vitro depression of lymphocyte function, the specificity of such tests is often in doubt.

Transformation of lymphocytes is recognised by their enlargement and by their increased RNA production which is manifested as basophilic and pyroninophilic cytoplasm and can be demonstrated by the use of tritiated thymidine. Such tests are. usually done on blood samples taken from the cubital vein, but these lymphocytes may not be representative because, in severe hypersensitivity, lymphocytes transformed in vivo tend to be sequestered in the target tissues, few being left in the circulation (Francis and Oppenheim, 1970). The tests of lymphocyte function are usually performed in normal human serum or animal serum to avoid inhibition by agents in the patient's own serum (B cells respond by becoming plasma cells and producing antibody).

Lymphocytes transforming in response to specific antigen are usually derived from the thymus (T cells). The identity of T cells can be confirmed by their collection around sheep red cells to form 'rosettes' (Papamichail et al, 1972; Stjernsward et al, 1972) and by immunofluorescence using a specific autoantibody (Thomas, 1972). Stimulated lymphocytes release lymphokines that include a migration inhibition factor for macrophages, a mitogenic factor and various mediators of inflammation (Pick et al, 1970; Schwartz, Catanzaro and Leon, 1971). These lymphocytes can be assayed. B cells can be detected by immunofluorescence techniques designed to demonstrate immunoglobulins on their surface.

References

Asherson, G. L. (1972) The development of lymphocyte function tests. *British Journal of Hospital Medicine*, **8**, 665.

Asscher, A. W. (1974) Urinary tract infection. *Lancet*, **ii**, 1365.

Folb, P. I. & Trounce, J. R. (1970) Immunological aspects of candida infection complicating steroid and immunosuppressive drug therapy. *Lancet*, **ii**, 1112.

Francis, T. C. & Oppenheim, J. J. (1970) Impaired lymphocyte stimulation by some streptococcal antigens in patients with recurrent aphthous stomatitis and rheumatic heart disease. *Clinical and Experimental Immunology*, **6**, 573.

Papamichail, M., Holborow, E. J., Keith, H. & Currey, H. (1972) Sub-population of human peripheral blood lymphocytes distinguished by combined rosette formation and immunofluorescence. *Lancet*, **ii**, 64.

Pick, E., Brostoff, J., Krejci, J. & Turk, J. L. (1970) Interaction between "sensitised lymphocytes" and antigen in vitro. II. Mitogen induced release of skin reactor and macrophage migration inhibitory factors. *Cell Immunology*, **1**, 92.

Schwartz, H. J., Catanzaro, P. J. & Leon, M. A. (1971) An analysis of the effects of skin reactive factor released from lymphoid cells by concanavalin A in vivo. *American Journal of Pathology*, **63**, 443.

Stjernsward, J., Jondal, M., Vanky, F., Wigzell, H. & Sealy, R. (1972) Lymphopenia and change in distribution of human B and T lymphocytes in peripheral blood induced by irradiation for mammary carcinoma. *Lancet*, **i**, 1352.

Thomas, D. H. (1972) Antibodies to membrane antigen(s) common to thymocytes and a subpopulation of lymphocytes in infectious mononucleosis sera. *Lancet*, **i**, 399.

TESTS FOR DEPRESSION OF CELLULAR IMMUNITY

In many countries most adults will have been tested in adolescence for sensitivity to mycobacterial antigen and if negative will have received BCG vaccination. Thus all adults should react to PPD. Similarly, most adults react to *Candida albicans* antigen and to streptokinase/streptodornase. By using a battery of agents one can test T cell function and if depressed discriminate between specific impairment and the nonspecific depression of inflammation. Dinitrochlorobenzene (DNCB) is a strong sensitiser and is commonly used to assess cellular immunity. Normally, 0.1 ml of 5 per cent DNCB painted on the skin sensitises within 7 to 10 days, and to test for such sensitivity 0.1 ml of 0.1 per cent DNCB is used.

In sarcoidosis, after the initial presentation with erythema nodosum, reactions both to tuberculin and to candidin are depressed. This may be a useful guide when aetiology is in doubt, since both tests are unlikely to be negative when the erythema nodosum is due to streptococcal throat infection.

The Kveim test

This test was at one time considered to be specific for sarcoidosis, a view with which few workers would now agree. The procedure entails an intradermal injection of 0.15 to 0.20 ml of a fine suspension in saline of material from lymph glands involved with active sarcoidosis. A positive reaction usually produces a nodule 3 to 8 mm in diameter some four to six weeks later, with a characteristic sarcoid histology.

Israel and Goldstein (1971), studying 37 cases of known sarcoidosis, observed that a positive Kveim test could be correlated with size of hilar lymph glands rather than with disease activity. The test remains positive in chronic inactive disease for up to 26 years from the onset provided the hilar glands remain enlarged. The test was negative in 10 per cent of 11 patients with active sarcoidosis of the skin but with normal chest x-rays. These authors obtained positive results in two cases of chronic lymphatic leukaemia, two cases of tuberculosis and one case of infectious mononucleosis, all with lymphadenopathy. The Kveim test is positive in 50 per cent of cases of Crohn's disease (Mitchell et al, 1970) and can be negative in sarcoidosis of the liver (Maddrey et al, 1970).

Gilroy (1971) reported that in active sarcoidosis typhoid and paratyphoid vaccine produce a histologically acceptable 'positive Kveim reaction'.

Sjögren's syndrome (Hughes and Whaley, 1972)

The full triad of Sjögren's syndrome consists of a kerato-conjunctivitis sicca (dry eyes), xerostomia (dry mouth), and a 'connective tissue' disorder — usually rheumatoid arthritis — and sometimes vasculitis (Bloch et al, 1965). In rheumatoid arthritis, the incidence of drug reactions is three times more common if Sjögren's syndrome also is present (Williams, St Inge and Young, 1969).

Schirmer's test is a standard investigation recommended as routine in all 'rheumatic' diseases. Five 35-mm filter-paper strips (Tilden Yates Labs Inc., Wayne, New Jersey 07470, USA) are bent 5 mm from one end and are hooked over the lower eyelid at the junction of the middle and outer thirds. The length of the wetting is measured at five minutes; less than 15 mm is regarded as abnormal.

A biopsy of the lower lip to look for diffuse lymphocytic infiltration in the labial glands and destruction of salivary tissue is another simple test.

References

Bloch, K. J., Buchanan, W. W., Wohl, M. J. & Bunim, J. J. (1965) Sjögren's syndrome. A clinical patho-logical and serological study of 62 cases. *Medicine*, **44**, 187.
Gilroy, J. (1971) Kveim test. *British Medical Journal*, **iii**, 369.
Hughes, G. R. V. & Whaley, K. (1972) Sjögren's syndrome. *British Medical Journal*, **iv**, 533.
Israel, H. L. & Goldstein, R. A. (1971) Relation of Kveim-antigen reaction of lymphadenopathy. Study of sarcoidosis and other diseases. *New England Journal of Medicine*, **284**, 345.
Maddrey, W. C., Johns, C. J., Boitnott, J. K. & Iber, F. L. (1970) Sarcoidosis and chronic hepatic-disease. A clinical and pathological study of 20 patients. *Medicine*, **49**, 375.
Mitchell, C. G., Eddleston, A. L. W. F., Smith, M. G. M. & Williams, R. (1970) Serum immunosuppressive activity due to azathioprine and its relation to hepatic function after liver transplantation. *Lancet*, **i**, 1196.
Williams, B. O., St. Inge, R. A. & Young, A. (1969) Penicillin allergy in rheumatoid arthritis with special reference to Sjögren's syndrome. *Annals of the Rheumatic Diseases*, **28**, 607.

Defective phagocytosis: the nitroblue tetrazolium test (Segal, 1974) (Table 14.6)

The process of phagocytosis is an active energy-dependent one. Neutrophil leucocytes show an increase in respiratory activity within a few minutes of phagocytosing particles. This requires NADH oxidase, the activity of which can be detected using the dye nitroblue tetrazolium (NBT).

Leucocytes are incubated with inert particles which they phagocytose. The increased respiration and NADH oxidase activity turns the dye from yellow to violet.

The test is negative in chronic granulomatous disease. It may be positive even without the in vitro stimulation of phagocytes in the newborn and in bacterial infection, as well as following abdominal surgery or fractures (Ninane and Schmitz, 1974), possibly because of temporary endotoxaemia (Cocchi, 1974). Numbers of NBT-positive cells above 30 per cent strongly suggest active bacterial infection as against viral infection (Feigin et al, 1971). This method may help to detect secondary infection in immuno-suppressed patients and to screen for aetiologically relevant subclinical infection in vasculitis; however, immune complexes which inhibit phagocytosis are responsible for false negative results (Segal, 1974).

Table 14.6. Some conditions in which false-positive and false-negative NBT test results have been reported.

False negative	False positive
Pyogenic bacterial infection	Non-pyogenic infections
appendicitis	fungal infection
arthritis	leprosy
meningitis	malaria
streptococcal pharyngitis	mycoplasma
systemic bacterial infection	parasitic disease
Drug therapy	toxoplasmosis
antibiotics	viral infections
glucocorticoids	Drugs
phenylbutazone	oral contraceptives
salicylates	Immune deficiency
Immune deficiency	Chédiak—Higashi syndrome
chronic granulomatous disease	Other conditions
glucose-6-phosphate dehydrogenase deficiency	Behçet's syndrome
hypogammaglobulinaemia	haemophilia
lipochrome histiocytosis	inflammatory bowel disease
myeloperoxidase deficiency	lymphoma
Other conditions	myelofibrosis
nephrosis	myocardial infarction
premature infants (infected)	neonates
sickle-cell disease	neoplasia
systemic lupus erythematosus	osteogenesis imperfecta
	polycythaemia vera
	pregnancy
	postoperative period
	psoriasis
	typhoid vaccination

References

Cocchi, P. (1974) N.B.T. test and endotoxaemia. *Lancet,* **ii,** 1322.
Feigin, R. D., Shackelford, P. G., Choi, S. C., Flake, K. K., Franklin, F. A. & Eisenberg, C. S. (1971) Nitro blue tetrazolium dye test as an aid in the differential diagnosis of febrile disorders. *Journal of Pediatrics,* **78,** 230.
Ninane, G. & Schmitz, A. (1974) Specificity of N.B.T. test. *Lancet,* **ii,** 174.
Segal, A. W. (1974) Nitroblue tetrazolium test. *Lancet,* **ii,** 1248.

THE INVESTIGATION OF DRUG AND FOOD SENSITIVITY (Copeman, 1972)

The only way to be *certain* that a particular drug is responsible for a particular eruption is to re-administer it and then see what happens. This is a dangerous practice.

Anaphylaxis is one of the direst of emergencies, and a widespread systemic Arthus reaction, while usually less immediate an emergency, can be equally devastating. Ackroyd's (1949) sedormid thrombocytopenic purpura is another example in which the proven presence of an antibody is an absolute contraindication to readministration of the drug. On the other hand, some rashes, such as a fixed drug eruption, justify retesting with the drug because little pathology results and the entirely predictable response occurs within six hours of ingestion only at the sites of the previous eruption. A battery of drugs commonly responsible for such eruptions can be given in a single test dose; the ingredients are butobarbitone, phenolphthalein, sulphonamide, quinidine, tetracycline and promethazine, each in its therapeutic dose range (Levine, 1972).

The contribution of drugs to vasculitis seems increasingly to be a non-allergic one, and the re-introduction of a drug long after the phase of altered reactivity does not have any ill-effect. Drug reactions such as those demonstrated by Juhlin, Michaelsson and Zetterstrom (1972) using aspirin and tartrazine (see page 192) or drugs responsible for the Shwartzman reaction seem to act only in the presence of an altered constitution during the phase of active disease. Such drugs can be given again a few months after all signs of active disease have regressed when usually there will be no response.

Patch testing

Patch testing is a means of demonstrating cell-mediated hypersensitivity when a contact dermatitis is suspected. It is of relatively little value for non-eczematous eruptions, but positive results in vasculitis, supporting a diagnosis of allergy from parenteral administration, have been reported for sulphonamides and chlorpromazine (Symmers, 1958); its value for practolol, diazepam and meprobamate has been recently re-emphasised by Felix and Comaish (1974) and Houwerzijl, de Gast and Nater (1974). The technique, familiar to all dermatologists, consists of applying the drug to the skin surface at the correct concentration in a suitable vehicle.

Intracutaneous tests

Since most drugs act as haptens which have to be combined with serum or epidermal proteins to become allergenic, it is pointless to inject them into the dermis, where they have little chance of combining with such protein; false negative results would inevitably occur. Similarly, some drugs are allergic only after their structure is altered by digestion and metabolism. Others produce irritation or release histamine in the skin and such reactions should be regarded as falsely positive. Truly allergic immediate reactions from intracutaneous testing are not without risk, since even minute amounts of drugs may produce severe anaphylaxis in the sensitive. For all these reasons the demand for a satisfactory in vitro test for drug allergy is one of the most pressing in present day therapeutics. None is as yet satisfactory.

In vivo tests for platelet interaction

Platelets agglutinate in the presence of specific antibody and lyse if complement also is present; complement fixation in such a test situation can be measured. If addition of a drug to whole blood inhibits clot retraction the presence of specific antibody is implied.

Comaish (1968) measured serotonin release as an indication of platelet response to drugs, whereas others have measured platelet Factor III. Karpatkins (1971) and Miescher (1973) discussed this subject fully and outlined eight tests.

The 'thrombocyte' index

It has long been known that there is a fall in the number of platelets in the peripheral blood in anaphylaxis and allergy. Nilzen (1953), Storck, Hoigne and Koller (1955) and

Berquist and Nilzen (1960) regarded a decrease of 20 per cent as a positive response. In 104 cases of drug reaction — mainly to aspirin, barbiturate or penicillin — 70 per cent showed such a fall (Heijer, Nilzen and Skog, 1960), and similar results were found in bacterial allergy (Berquist and Nilzen, 1960). The platelets are counted before and at one hour after skin testing.

Elimination diets

The value of these are twofold. Firstly patients who continue to develop extensive vasculitis after five days of virtual starvation are unlikely to need to pay much further attention to the problem. This can be valuable information for worried patients suffering from chronic urticaria. The author prescribes a diet of rye biscuit and weak tea without milk (it is not expensive and it is sometimes unexpectedly therapeutic) (see Chapters 8 and 15).

Secondly, it can be used to eliminate and then to retest with likely agents. This is particularly valuable with foods which contain azo dyes and benzoates (Table 14.7) which, as Michaelsson and Juhlin (1973) and Michaelsson, Pettersson and Juhlin (1974) have emphasised, can sometimes aggravate urticaria and vasculitis.

Test doses of these agents (Table 14.7) can be given after an early light breakfast. One agent is prescribed each day and can be given in increasing doses during the day if urticaria is the problem under study. For vasculitis, a much slower introduction of foods in the daily regime is wiser. Smaller doses are prescribed if patients are asthmatic.

Table 14.7. Test doses of food and drug additives as used in a study of urticaria and purpura by Michaelsson et al (1974).

Dye tartrazine FDC yellow No. 5 1 mg in 10—20 ml of water.
Acetylsalicylic acid capsule containing 1 mg, 2.5 mg, 5 mg, 10 mg, 50 mg, 500 mg.
Acetylsalicylic acid anhydride capsule containing 5 mg, 10 mg, 25 mg and 100 mg.
4-hydroxybenzoic acid 50 mg capsule.
Benzoic acid sodium salt 250 mg capsule.

Test every two hours for urticaria.
Test every day for vasculitis.

INTRADERMAL TESTS FOR AUTO-ERYTHROCYTE SENSITISATION — PAINFUL BRUISING

Hersle and Mobacken (1969) used the agents listed in Table 14.8, inoculating 0.1 ml quantities intradermally. A positive result is more likely when skin that has already experienced bruising is chosen as the injection site.

Table 14.8. Agents used for intradermal testing in painful bruising syndrome.

Histamine: 0.1 mg/ml in sterile distilled water
DNA: from calf thymus in concentrations of 0.6 mg/ml and 0.06 mg/ml
Old tuberculin: 1:2000
PPD: 2.0 T.U.
L-Phosphatidyl serum: 10-fold dilution series 12 000 μg/ml to 0.12 μg/ml
Erythrocyte suspensions of saline washed red cells
Plasma from heparinised patients and control blood
Serum from patients and control, taken from blood clotted at 37°C for 2 hours
Autologous white cells and thrombocyte suspension

Some sera contain a dermatonecrotic factor which will produce a pustule and swelling within a few hours of being inoculated into the skin of a guinea-pig (Delescluse, de Bast and Achten, 1972).

References

Ackroyd, J. F. (1949) The pathogenesis of thrombocytopenic purpura due to hypersensitivity to sedormid. *Clinical Science,* **7,** 249.

Berquist, G. & Nilzen, A. (1960) The thrombocyte index after injection of staphylococcus vaccine in man. *Acta Dermato-venereologica,* **40,** 58.

Comaish, S. (1968) The blood platelets in immune hypersensitivity. *Acta Dermato-venereologica,* **48,** 592.

Copeman, P. W. M. (1972) Drug rashes. *British Journal of Hospital Medicine,* **10,** 339.

Delescluse, J., de Bast, Cl. & Achten, G. (1972) Pyoderma gangrenosum with altered cellular immunity and dermonecrotic factor. *British Journal of Dermatology,* **87,** 529.

Felix, R. H. & Comaish, J. S. (1974) The value of patch and other skin tests in drug eruptions. *Lancet,* **i,** 1017.

Heijer, A., Nilzen, A. & Skog, E. (1960) Drug reactions. *Acta Dermato-venereologica,* **40,** 35.

Hersle, K. & Mobacken, H. (1969) Autoerythrocyte sensitisation syndrome (painful bruising syndrome). Report of two cases and review of the literature. *British Journal of Dermatology,* **81,** 574.

Houwerzijl, J., de Gast, G. C. & Nater, J. P. (1974) Tests for drug allergy. *Lancet,* **ii,** 655.

Juhlin, L., Michaelsson, G. & Zetterstrom, O. (1972) Urticaria and asthma induced by food and drug additives in patients with aspirin sensitivity. *Journal of Allergy and Clinical Immunology,* **50,** 92.

Karpatkins, S. (1971) Drug induced thrombocytopenia. *American Journal of the Medical Sciences,* **262,** 68.

Levine, G. M. (1972) Drug rashes, reported by Copeman, P. W. M. *Hospital Medicine,* **10,** 339.

Michaelsson, G. & Juhlin, L. (1973) Urticaria induced by preservatives and dye additives in food and drugs. *British Journal of Dermatology,* **88,** 525.

Michaelsson, G., Pettersson, L. & Juhlin, L. (1974) Purpura caused by food and drug additives. *Archives of Dermatology,* **109,** 49.

Miescher, P. A. (1973) Drug induced thrombocytopenia. *Seminars in Hematology,* **10,** 311.

Nilzen, A. (1953) The thrombocyte decrease in food allergy and the influence of ACTH thereon. *Acta Dermato-venereologica,* **33,** 456.

Storck, H., Hoigne, R. & Koller, F. (1955) Thrombocytes in allergic reactions. *International Archives of Allergy,* **6,** 372.

Symmers, W. St. C. (1958) A symposium organised by the Council for International Organisations of Medical Sciences. In *Sensitivity Reactions to Drugs* (Ed.) Rosenheim, M. L. & Moulton, R. p. 209. Oxford: Blackwell.

15. The Management of Vasculitis

The management of vasculitis includes elimination of known triggers, correction of any constitutional imbalance and attention to and, if possible, elimination of any local factors encouraging the vasculitis at a particular site.

The *triggers* include allergens, drugs and infective agents. The *constitution* includes the complicated humoral and cell-mediated immunological systems, the coagulation and fibrinolytic mechanisms and the mononuclear phagocytic system. Particularly important is the altered reactivity of injured tissues that makes them respond differently to subsequent injury.

Management methods used will depend on the position of the disorder in the spectrum of urticaria, vasculitis and ischaemic necrosis. Attention has been paid to other factors such as hypertension, obesity, anaemia or polycythaemia, and to anxiety and pain which are significant contributors to the psychosomatic aspects of vasculitis. Good management includes advice on cigarette smoking, oral contraception, high blood pressure and hyperlipidaemia.

The *local* factors that must be treated are those contributing to stasis, such as dependency, cold injury and scarring. The tissues must be protected from injury of all kinds — knocks, sunlight, cold winds or constricting bands.

THE DEPENDENCE OF PROGNOSIS ON MANAGEMENT

The prognosis of the diseases discussed in previous chapters depends on the virulence of the trigger, the effectiveness of the tissue reaction to it, including the healing process, the distribution and intensity of any involvement of organs other than the skin, as well as the limitations or complications encountered, both from the disease and from the treatment.

One of the main reasons for discarding eponyms and the classic descriptions of disease is the lack of any easy answer to questions about the prognosis in Schönlein—Henoch purpura or in polyarteritis nodosa. One always has to ask about possible causes, noting a recent episode of streptococcal sore throat and looking for evidence of diabetes mellitus, rheumatoid arthritis, malignant hypertension or underlying neoplasm, as well as finding out if there is renal involvement and, if present, its severity.

The prognosis of vasculitis in general is changing all the time because management is improving, but the morbidity from treatment is great. On the whole, transience of lesions, restriction of the vasculitis to a single organ and the absence of complications all imply a good prognosis, so systemic therapy with, for example, corticosteroids or chemotherapeutic agents should not be rushed into. Monitoring the urine is a simple and essential guide to prognosis, and in the absence of protein, casts or red cells, patients will usually survive even without treatment. Systemic or complicated vasculitis is always difficult to manage, and the kidney is the most commonly affected vital organ.

GENERAL MEASURES

Bed rest

The general management of acute vasculitis, such as the classical Schönlein—Henoch purpura in children, includes putting the patient to bed for rest, elevation of the legs and warmth; this reduces pain and anxiety. If the causative condition is periarticular (Hardisty, 1968), painful joints should be kept in the most comfortable position, but if joint surfaces are clearly involved and permanent deformity a possibility, then the optimal position for function of the limbs should be adopted.

Protection from cold and sunlight

The advisability of protection from cold should be obvious from discussions elsewhere in this monograph (page 290) (Figure 15.1, a and b). Protection from sunlight is less often advocated. Sunlight plays a well known role in lupus erythematosus, in which there seems to be an exaggerated sensitivity to sunburn; this probably also is the case in temporal arteritis, for Kinmont and McCallum (1965) described undue exposure to sunlight and light sensitivity in several such patients. Grice, Ryan and Magnus (1970) have drawn attention to the fact that a minimal erythema dose of short-wave ultraviolet light invariably inhibits fibrinolysis in the skin (Table 15.1). This effect is exemplified by a patient who developed lesions with widespread capillary thrombosis due to plasmin inhibition after exposure to bright sunlight (Figures 15.1 and 15.2) (Brödthagen et al, 1968).

Venous stasis

Venous stasis in the legs makes such a significant contribution to vasculitis (see Chapter 12) that treatment aimed at relieving it is almost always of some benefit. Physicians concerned with leg ulcers and varicose eczema pay great attention to this but often ignore it in other disorders of the legs. Care of the legs and protection from stasis should be ritual. The Lancet in 1958, referring to 'attentiveness' applied to the physiological processes of getting the blood flowing in the legs, stated: "The moment the

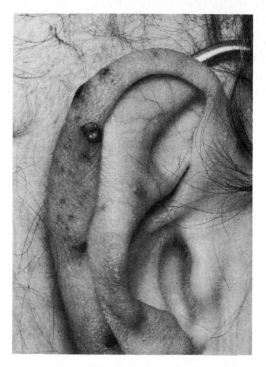

(a)

Figure 15.1. The ears, like other acral areas, should be kept warm. (a) The ears of a patient who had mixed cryoglobulinaemia; (b) the ears of a patient with disseminated intravascular coagulation.

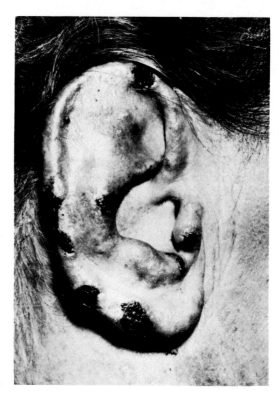

(b)

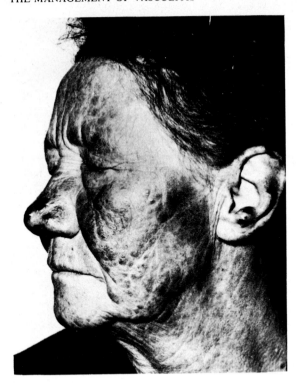

Figure 15.2. The face of the same patient as shown in Figure 15.1 (b). The distribution of the rash is suggestive of exposure to sunlight. Brödthagen et al suggested that sunlight provoked this patient's disease. However, the exact relationship between exposure to sun and previous exposure to cold is always difficult to establish; both cold and sun can be either preparatory or provoking.

patient is put to bed on admission (avoiding tightly tucked in sheets), it must follow him on his stretcher journey to the theatre, it must protect him as he floats limply between stretcher and the operating table, it must inspire the hand which temporarily deprives him of his muscle power, and it must guard over him as he lies acrobatically suspended in poles, hooks and slings. Its arch-priest may not rest content until he has earned the accolade of 'fusspot'". All this was to prevent deep vein thrombosis, but a dedicated 'fusspot' attitude is needed equally for the microvascular compartment of the skin of the legs. This applies particularly to the purpuric and infarctive forms of vasculitis and less to the urticarial element, although prolonged urticarial lesions do often show bruising and purpura restricted to the legs.

The most important single factor in preventing disseminated intravascular coagulation is adequate capillary flow (Hardaway, 1971). So far as the legs are concerned this means elevation well above the level of the heart; merely sitting with the legs on a stool is of little value. Those who cannot raise their legs because of cardiac disease or arthritis benefit from the use of intermittent positive pressure bags (Figure 15.3) (Hills et al, 1972; Roberts et al, 1972; Roberts, 1975), although Ashton (1975) believed that such inflatable splints, when used in fracture clinics, may prevent adequate blood flow. Bourne (1974) insisted that his patients should keep their legs raised vertically for two days before bandages are applied. In practice, a period of complete elevation for two hours is acceptable and is the aim in the leg ulcer clinic supervised by the author.

Treatment of obesity

Obesity contributes to many of the problems to which patients with vasculitis are susceptible; for example, gravitational stasis is all the more difficult to manage, and cold

Table 15.1. Impairment of fibrinolytic activity induced by monochromatic light.

Skin condition	No. of cases	Wavelength	Time of biopsy (hour)	Type of lesion	Fibrinolytic activity	
Normal	3	300	24	Erythema	Diminished	(3)
				Papule	Absent	(1)
Polymorphic light eruption	5	300—307.5	1	Erythema	Present	(1)
			2	Erythema	Present	(1)
			6	Papule	Absent	(1)
			24	Erythema	Diminished or absent	(2)
						(1)
Actinic, reticuloid	6	300	24	Papule	Absent	(5)
			1	Papule	Diminished	(1)
			3	Papule	Absent	(1)
			24	Erythema	Absent	(1)
				Papule	Absent	(1)
		340	24	Papule	Absent	(2)
		360	24	Erythema	Present	(1)
					Absent	(1)
		380	24	Papule	Absent	(1)
Porphyria	7	300	24	Papule	Absent	(1)
		360	24	Papule	Present	(1)
		400	3	Erythema	Diminished	(1)
			24	Erythema	Diminished	(1)
			2.5	Papule	Diminished	(1)
			3	Papule	Present	(1)
			4	Papule	Present	(2)
			6	Papule	Present	(1)
			7	Papule	Present	(1)
			24	Papule	Present	(1)
					Absent	(1)
		500	24	Papule	Present	(1)
Solar urticaria	2	300	0.5	Weal	Present	(1)
			3.6	Papule	Absent	(1)
		White fluorescent lighting	5	Weal	Present	(1)
		400	0.75	Weal	Present	(1)

fat pads over the upper arms and lower legs are the sites of chilblains and nodular vasculitis.

Unfortunately, patients in whom obesity is sufficiently gross to complicate the management of leg ulcers or nodular vasculitis are not usually dieted effectively. Less unfortunate patients manage to lose weight with relatively simple but disciplined dieting.

Obesity in some females, and more so in males, may be due to an abnormally low level of spontaneous activity; in such cases exercise, which promotes venous flow, encourages fibrinolysis and prevents cooling of the tissues, is one of the measures that is of undisputed advantage and is simple and inexpensive. Weight loss in itself increases mobility and this facilitates activity which is important in the obese and in the tall who have an increased susceptibility to deep-vein thrombosis (Naide, 1952; Little, Loewenthal and Mills, 1966; Richards, 1966; Vessey and Doll, 1969).

Rigorous starvation in hospital results in the elimination of three to five litres of body fluid which may account for a considerable initial weight loss. In the management of obesity group therapy is helpful, not only in the initial stages but also in subsequent months when defaulting is common. Knowledge that defaulting is ultimately very likely should not deter the physician if significant obesity is contributing to the failure of leg

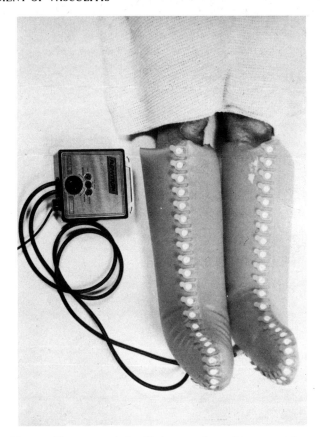

Figure 15.3. Intermittent positive-pressure inflatable bags can be used to prevent deep vein thrombosis and stimulate local fibrinolytic activity. Such bags fill with air at regular intervals and compress the calf veins. The procedure is an advantage only in those patients who are immobile or who cannot raise their legs well above the level of the heart.

ulcers to heal; even a short period of accelerated healing offers distinct advantages. Munro et al (1970) suggested that it is a useful goal to get the weight down to a level which is no higher than 25 per cent above the 'ideal weight'. However, inpatient fasting to do this necessarily occupies beds for at least three months (Innes et al, 1974). As pointed out by Miller and Parsonage (1975) failure to lose weight can be associated with a low metabolic rate; such patients may not be fat. In myxoedema, for instance, weight gain is due to an increase in ground substance.

Protection and support from paste bandages

Repeated or prolonged involvement of the legs by superficial or nodular vasculitis tends to be aggravated by injury to the skin from minor knocks, ill-fitting clothing or bandaging, and by cold exposure. Carefully applied paste bandages are not only protective, but also counteract gravitational stasis and oedema. Such bandages are commonly reserved for obvious venous disorders, and yet the fact that there is often a superimposed vasculitis, and that vasculitis of the legs is a predominantly venous disorder is ignored.

Faulty bandaging technique is, however, a not infrequent cause of injury by pinching and irregular compression and by rucks within footwear, and especially by nicking the skin when the bandages are removed. Figure 15.4 demonstrates how to fold a paste bandage to facilitate its removal above the ankle and shows it being cut at each turn below the ankle. Figure 15.5 demonstrates the use of a single strip of Lestreflex round the heel with no more than three turns of the bandage covering the entire foot and ankle.

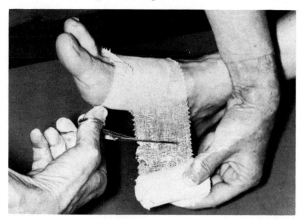

Figure 15.4. The correct application of bandages results in protection without damage to the skin. (a) To avoid wrinkles and an excess of bandage around the foot and ankle it is best to cut the bandage at the completion of each turn. (b) Folding the bandage back on itself in front of the skin instead of repeatedly winding it around the leg facilitates removal.

(a)

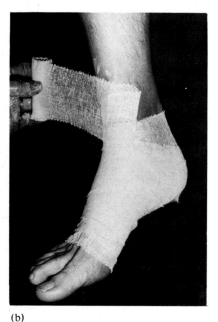

(b)

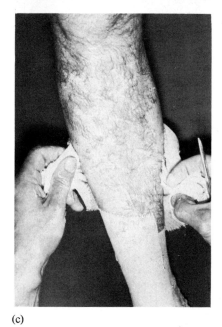

(c)

Treatment of high blood pressure

Hypertension contributes to arteritis (see page 299). Treatment by rest, peace and quiet can be included in the list of general measures recommended for all cases of vasculitis. The management of severe hypertension is the subject of many monographs (see Pickering (1974) and a symposium in the *British Journal of Hospital Medicine* (1974)).

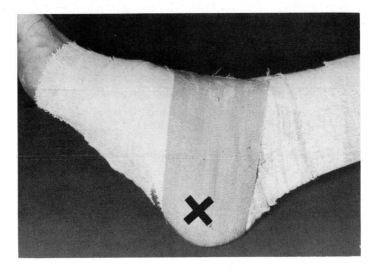

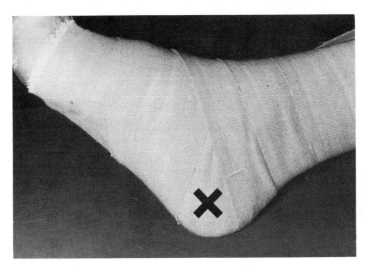

Figure 15.5. The use of Lestreflex (elastic Diachylon, BPC) to bandage the leg. (a) The application of a single strip (X) allows (b) the completion of the bandaging with as little as three turns around the foot. Bandaging done thus protects the skin from the rim of the shoe, does not injure the skin from ridges in the bandage, nor does it so encumber the foot that shoes will not fit.

Several practitioners have advocated hypotensive therapy for everyone with a diastolic blood pressure above 90 mm Hg (Ciba Symposium, 1973), claiming that even the slightest elevation of blood pressure carries an increased risk of cardiovascular morbidity and mortality (Chicago Society of Actuaries, 1959; Kannel and Dawber, 1974). Patients with a diastolic pressure in the range 90 to 114 mm Hg, when given effective hypotensive therapy, suffer less cardiovascular morbidity and mortality than a comparable group treated with a placebo (Veterans Administration Cooperative Study Group, 1970), although it can be argued that this effect is completely convincing only when the diastolic blood pressure is above 115 mm Hg in young persons (Short, 1974).

References

Ashton, H. (1975) Critical closure of blood vessels. *Biorheology,* in press.
Bourne, I. H. J. (1974) Vertical leg drainage of oedema in treatment of leg ulcers. *British Medical Journal,* **ii,** 581.
British Journal of Hospital Medicine (1974) Symposium on hypertension. *British Journal of Hospital Medicine,* **2,** 508.
Brödthagen, H., Larsen, V., Brøckner, J. & Amris, C. J. (1968) Manifestations in capillary dilatation and endovascular fibrin deposits. *Acta Dermato-venereologica,* **48,** 277.
Chicago Society of Actuaries (1959) *Build and Blood Pressure Study.*
Ciba Symposium (1973) Hypertension. *Scottish Medical Journal,* **18,** 119.
Grice, K., Ryan, T. J. & Magnus, I. A. (1970) Fibrinolytic activity in lesions produced by monochromatic ultraviolet irradiation in various photodermatoses. *British Journal of Dermatology,* **83,** 637.
Hardaway, R. M. (1971) Disseminated intravascular coagulation. *Thrombosis et Diathesis Haemorrhagica,* **46,** 209.
Hardisty, R. M. (1968) Treatment of non-thrombocytopenic purpuras. In *Treatment of Haemorrhagic Disorders* (Ed.) Ratnoff, O. D. p. 223. New York: Harper and Row.
Hills, N. H., Pflug, J. J., Jeyasingh, K., Boardman, L. & Calnan, J. S. (1972) Prevention of deep vein thrombosis by intermittent pneumatic compression of calf. *British Medical Journal,* **i,** 131.
Innes, J. A., Campbell, I. W., Campbell, C. J., Needle, A. L. & Munro, J. F. (1974) Long term follow up of therapeutic starvation. *British Medical Journal,* **ii,** 356.
Kannel, W. B. & Dawber, T. R. (1974) Hypertension as an ingredient of a cardiovascular risk profile. *British Journal of Hospital Medicine,* **11,** 508.
Kinmont, P. D. C. & McCallum, D. I. (1965) The aetiology, pathology and course of giant cell arteritis. *British Journal of Dermatology,* **77,** 193.
Little, J. M., Lowenthal, J. & Mills, F. H. (1966) Venous thrombo-embolic disease. *British Journal of Surgery,* **53,** 657.
Miller, D. S. & Parsonage, S. (1975) Resistance to slimming, adaptation or illusion? *Lancet,* **i,** 773.
Munro, J. F., Maccuish, A. C., Goodall, J. A. D., Fraser, J. & Duncan, L. J. P. (1970) Further experience with prolonged therapeutic starvation in gross refractory obesity. *British Medical Journal,* **iv,** 712.
Naide, M. (1952) Spontaneous venous thrombosis in the legs of tall men. *Journal of the American Medical Association,* **1481,** 1202.
Pickering, G. W. (1968) *High Blood Pressure.* London: J. & A. Churchill.
Pickering, Sir George (1974) *Hypertension; Causes, Consequences and Management,* 2nd edition. Edinburgh: Churchill Livingstone.
Richards, R. L. (1966) Venous thrombosis. *British Medical Journal,* **ii,** 217.
Roberts, V. C. & Cotton, L. T. (1975) Failure of heparin to improve efficacy of preoperative intermittent calf compression in preventing postoperative deep vein thrombosis. *British Medical Journal,* **iii,** 458.
Roberts, V. C., Berguer, R., Clark, A. W. & Cotton, L. T. (1972) Prevention of deep vein thrombosis. *British Medical Journal,* **i,** 628.
Short, D. (1974) Diagnosis and treatment of hypertension. *Lancet,* **ii,** 645.
Vessey, M. P. & Doll, W. R. S. (1969) Oral contraceptives and thromboembolic disease. Further report of MRC Statistical Research Unit. *British Medical Journal,* **ii,** 651.
Veterans Administration Cooperative Study Group on Antihypertensive Agents (1970) *Journal of the American Medical Association,* **213,** 1143.

REASSURANCE AND PSYCHIATRY

Many patients with vasculitis are anxious and in pain, for even the smallest area of vasculitis is sometimes intensely painful, as is the case with atrophie blanche. Anxiety can often be relieved by simple good management and a programme of therapy. Just seeing that something is being done by someone who looks competent is reassuring.

There are subgroups of vasculitis, such as psychogenic purpura, that are much more difficult to manage. Sometimes it is hard to distinguish between an artefact induced by mechanical means — burns, scratches or pinches — and that rarer group of spontaneous urticarial or purpuric lesions described in Chapter 11 which can be induced by somewhat obscure mental processes. In the author's experience there is little difference in the psychosocial pattern of these two groups. The prognosis tends to be bad for the lesion but good for survival.

As Sneddon and Sneddon (1975) have pointed out, in young girls the artefactual lesion may be 'a cry for help' which a good social worker can deal with. In older patients multiple admissions to a variety of units are a usual feature. Sneddon and Sneddon (1975) recalled several patients with artefacts who suddenly recovered in spite of rather than because of medical supervision, and it must be admitted that the treatment of this subgroup of vasculitis is not one in which psychiatrists or dermatologists have made great progress.

In general, jogging the patients along and supporting them in their attitude of grin and bear it is the most that can usefully be done (Agle and Ratnoff, 1962). Such patients are often quite pleased to be told that it is a misfortune for them to have such painful lesions but that their life is not in danger. They react warmly to being told that they have an excess of sensibility and an anxious personality.

The families which support these patients often have their own complexes and may be dotingly dependent on the affected members. Disturbing interrelationships of this sort are not always in the best interests of the family unit. On the other hand, some patients have their lives ruined by parents with personality defects, and in trying to steer children from assuming the hysterical bent of their mothers, child guidance clinics may help to avert such tragedies.

The psyche is only one factor in disease. While allergy to prunes could be relieved by prolonged psychoanalysis, it is perhaps cheaper, simpler and wiser not to give the prunes! (Osborn, 1974).

References

Agle, D. P. & Ratnoff, O. D. (1962) Purpura as a psychosomatic entity: a psychiatric study of autoerythrocyte sensitisation. *Archives of Internal Medicine,* **109,** 685.
Osborn, M. L. (1974) Inadequate mothers. *Lancet,* **ii,** 1322.
Sneddon, I. & Sneddon, J. (1974) What happens to artefacts? *British Journal of Dermatology,* **91** (Supplement 10), 13.

ELIMINATION OF TRIGGERS

Elimination of triggers is not always easy. It is possible for the patient to avoid or be protected against some of the antigens, such as drugs to which he is known to be sensitive and infections like malaria and typhoid. Moreover, persons with a family history of intolerance to drugs such as hydrallazine should avoid them. The vasculitis of drug addicts is also clearly an avoidable disease.

Elimination of antigen

At present there is no satisfactory way of eliminating antigen in those who have auto-immune disease or viral infections. However, bacterially induced diseases such as bacterial endocarditis, streptococcal sore throats or leprosy are treatable, and levels of antigen can thus be reduced. Elimination of *Mycobacterium tuberculosis* is particularly relevant in some papulonecrotic and nodular forms of vasculitis. Occasional reports of effective removal of malignant tissue justify attention to this approach when applicable.

Induction of tolerance

Cameron (1972) discussed the treatment of glomerulonephritis and wrote hopefully of restoring the balance between the T and B cells. Encouraging T cell activity probably would reduce the activity of B cells and thereby diminish excessive antibody production. Cyclophosphamide suppression of lupus erythematosus is quoted as an example of this effect.

Elimination of infectious agents

Adequate elimination of all causative organisms is often difficult and does not necessarily rid the system of the autoantibody production that these organisms have triggered.

The role of streptococcal sore throats in Schönlein—Henoch purpura seems less important than was once supposed (see Chapter 8). Only if a pathogenic organism has been isolated from the nose, throat or sputum, should the appropriate antibiotic be prescribed. Hardisty (1968) considered that antibiotics sometimes aggravate purpura.

The treatment of infection is undergoing reappraisal. In general it is wise to treat acute infection in every case, but the treatment and prophylaxis of occult or supposed chronic infection is more debatable. In chronic infections, when the host fails to eliminate an organism, any amount of antibacterial drugs will often fail to do the same. This is a particularly puzzling and depressing aspect of the management of mycobacterial infections such as tuberculosis, leprosy, or from BCG.

Resistance of organisms such as the meningococcus is perhaps more serious than that of the tubercle bacillus because less time is available for changing therapy. The best advice is to make sure that the current status of infection in the patient and the resistance of organisms are known. There is nothing to be lost and everything to be gained by swabbing the throat, nose and skin and recording in the patient's notes the current sensitivities of the organisms isolated so that acute illness can be treated appropriately when it develops, but not necessarily before.

Sensitivities vary not only from patient to patient but also geographically. In 1974, for instance, the meningococcus was sulphonamide-resistant in Brazil, and this seemed to be so in Scotland but not in the United Kingdom as a whole (Leader, *Lancet,* December 14th, 1974).

The use of auto-vaccines and microbial desensitisation is generally a more favoured method of treatment for vasculitis on the continent of Europe than it is in the U.K. or the U.S.A. Ky, Hazard and Laroche (1968) used the method and reported inprovement in the hypersensitivity of 13 patients considered to be sensitive to the streptococcus. Longhin and Ene-Popescu (1968) while recognising the contribution of the nonspecific Shwartzman phenomenon considered that pyoderma gangrenosum should be treated with auto-vaccines as well as corticosteroids and antibiotics.

Fedotov and Bazyka (1967) reported from Russia the use of repeated intradermal injections of pyococcal vaccines for some 90 cases of nodular vasculitis. The lesions disappeared in 41 (46 per cent) and improved in the rest. However, as nodular vasculitis does not last for ever, this apparently beneficial result might be regarded as normal spontaneous remission.

Severe necrosis of the skin sometimes is a consequence of inoculation with vaccines, and in a mild form, it is in fact the expected isomorphic response (Chapter 6). However, pyoderma gangrenosum and purpura fulminans have been recorded following such inoculations (Forsbeck, 1961). Boulton-Jones et al (1974) described a nurse who repeatedly injected herself with diphtheria, pertussis and tetanus (triple) vaccine; she developed a severe proliferative glomerulonephritis, hypocomplementaemia and cryo-globulinaemia. The speed with which this patient recovered after withdrawal of the vaccine demonstrates how elimination of foci of infection can result in successful cure of vasculitis (see Chapter 8).

Miedzinki (1957) controlled Weber—Christian disease by surgical treatment of a suppurative otitis media, and Wereide (1963) cured vasculitis by treating osteomyelitis of a facial bone.

The problem of whether all cases of nodular vasculitis should have anti-tuberculous therapy is discussed in Chapter 8 together with reports of its successful use.

Elimination of drugs and harmful foods

The role of drugs is discussed in Chapter 8. They are occasionally the cause of vasculitis and in these cases they should be withdrawn if possible.

Elimination diets are sometimes indicated. Allen, Diamond and Howell (1960), for example, described a patient who improved after omission of milk from the diet, and Gairdner (1948) reported a case improving after avoiding tomatoes. Michaelsson, Petersson and Juhlin (1974) have done much to show the part played by food additives in purpura (see Chapter 8), where it seems to be an aggravating factor rather than a clearcut allergic state. The elimination of salicylates, benzoates and tartrazine was helpful in their series (see Chapter 8).

The 1975 annual meeting of the National Schizophrenic Association of Great Britain was devoted to this subject. Skin is not the only organ to be cured dramatically of its diseases by a five-day fast. However, it is doubtful whether too much attention should be given to this aspect except in persistent or recurrent episodic forms of vasculitis. There is a strong placebo effect in rigorous dieting — but even this is sometimes worth achieving, and dieting is an economical and harmless way of doing it.

Special diets are listed in Table 15.2. When drugs are being withdrawn, cross sensitivities should be taken into account; a well known example is carbromal purpura which can be evoked by meprobamate (Marcussen, 1958).

Table 15.2. Foods that may aggravate or possibly even initiate urticaria and vasculitis.

Foods to be avoided	Suitable alternatives
Low tartrazine diet	
Fish/shellfish (canned)	Fresh/frozen fish
Yoghurt	Cream, milk
Fruit squash and cordial	Water, soda water
Fruit juice — canned/bottled	Tea, coffee
Fizzy lemonade	
Coca-cola, etc.	
Vinegar, pickles	Salt, pepper
Curry powder, mustard	herbs, spices
Bottled sauces	
Salad cream	
Cakes — shop bought	Home-made cakes and pastries
Cake mix, e.g. Mary Baker	
Biscuits	Ryvita, Ryking, Macvita
	cream crackers, water biscuits, home-made biscuits
Yellow pasta	White macaroni, spaghetti

Table 15.2.—*continued*

Foods to be avoided	Suitable alternatives
Jam and marmalade	Honey, home-made jam, marmalade and lemon curd
Packet and canned soups	Home-made soup
Ice-cream, ice lollies Jelly Custard Blancmange Instant puddings	Rice, sago, tapioca pudding Cold sweets made with gelatine
Packet, tinned and shop puddings Semolina	Home-made sponge and fruit puddings Home-made tart/crumble
Coloured toothpaste	White toothpaste, e.g. Colgate
All coloured sweets and filled chocolates	White sweets, e.g. peppermints, glacier mints Plain and milk chocolates (unfilled)
Food colourings Manufactured convenience-type foods containing food colourings, e.g. instant puddings, cake mixes, etc.	Try to use fresh or home-prepared foods
Low sodium benzoate diet Bottled fruit squash and cordial Bottled natural fruit juice Tinned natural fruit juice[a] All carbonated beverages, i.e. fizzy pop P.L.J. Instant coffee and instant tea[a] Drinking chocolate Chicory essence Cider Beer — some brands[a]	Tea, ground coffee Water Spirits Milk
Jam, marmalade, jelly jam[a]	Home-made jam and marmalade Honey, syrup
Mustard, curry powder Horseradish sauce Pickled food Bottled sauces French dressing Tomato, pulp, paste and purée Rennet	Salt, pepper Herbs, spices
Cranberries, prunes, greengage plums Cinnamon, cloves	All other fruit
Tinned fruit[a]	Fresh fruit (other than those above)
Shop-bought cakes and pastries	Home-made cakes and pastries yeast breads and buns and rolls
Artificial cream	Fresh cream
Low salicylate diet Peas Soups and mixes containing peas	All other vegetables Home-made or tinned soup without peas (check label on tins)
Blackcurrants Apples Bananas Grapes Rhubarb	Oranges, pears, peaches, grapefruit, gooseberries, plums, etc. — tinned *or* fresh
Blackcurrant, rhubarb *or* apple jam/jelly	Lemon curd, honey, marmalade *or* other jam or jelly

Table 15.2.—*continued*

Foods to be avoided	Suitable alternatives
Beer	Spirits
Wine	Soda water, tonic water
Cider	Orange, lemon *or* grapefruit drinks
Apple drinks	Tea, coffee
Blackcurrant squash, e.g. Ribena	Water
Dried fruits — sultanas, raisins, currants, prunes	Fresh *or* tinned fruit (other than those mentioned above)
Cakes, biscuits and chocolate containing dried fruit, e.g. Christmas pudding, fruit cake, Garibaldi biscuits, fruit and nut chocs	Sponge cakes and puddings Plain, cream *or* chocolate biscuits
Muesli-type cereal containing dried fruit, e.g. Alpen, etc.	Home-made muesli omitting dried fruit *or* any other breakfast cereal
Vinegar Bottled sauces containing vinegar, e.g. tomato sauce, brown sauce, salad cream, french dressing Pickles	Salt, pepper, herbs, spices

[a]May or may not contain sodium benzoate.

References

Allen, D. M., Diamond, L. K. & Howell, D. A. (1960) Anaphylactoid purpura in children (Schönlein—Henoch syndrome). Review with a follow up of renal complications. *American Journal of Diseases of Children,* **99,** 333.

Boulton-Jones, J. M., Sissons, J. G. P., Naish, P. F., Evans, D. J. & Peters, D. K. (1974) Self induced glomerulonephritis. *British Medical Journal,* **ii,** 387.

Cameron, J. S. (1972) Bright's disease today: the pathogenesis and treatment of glomerulonephritis III. *British Medical Journal,* **iv,** 217.

Fedotov, V. P. & Bazyka, A. P. (1967) Immunologic reactions in patients with allergic nodular dermohypodermal lesions. *Vestnik Dermatologii e Venerologii,* **41,** 22.

Forsbeck, M. (1961) Case for diagnosis? Sanarelli Shwartzman phenomena. *Acta Dermato-venereologica,* **41,** 416.

Gairdner, D. (1948) The Schönlein—Henoch syndrome (anaphylactoid purpura). *Quarterly Journal of Medicine,* **17,** 95.

Hardisty, R. M. (1968) Treatment of non-thrombocytopenic purpuras. In *Treatment of Hemorrhagic Disorders* (Ed.) Ratnoff, O. D. p. 223. New York: Harper and Row.

Ky, N-T., Hazard, J. & Laroche, C. (1968) Allergies vasculaires cutanées d'origine streptococcus — a propos de vingt observations. *Press Médicale,* **76,** 247.

Longhin, S. & Ene-Popescu, C. (1968) Uber einem fall von pyoderma gangraenosum. *Hautartz,* **19,** 135.

Marcussen, P. V. (1958) Cross sensitisation between carbromal and meprobamate. *Acta Dermato-venereologica,* **38,** 398.

Michaelsson, G., Petersson, L. & Juhlin, L. (1974) Purpura caused by food and drug additives. *Archives of Dermatology,* **109,** 49.

Miedzinski, F. (1957) Some remarks about Weber—Christian disease. *Acta Dermato-venereologica,* **37,** 88.

Tindall, J. P., Whalen, R. E. & Burton, E. E. (1974) Medical uses of intra-arterial injections of reserpine, treatment of Raynaud syndrome and of some vascular insufficiencies of the lower extremities. *Archives of Dermatology,* **110,** 233.

Wereide, K. (1963) Hypersensitive vasculitis of the skin: report of a case caused by focal infection of the facial bone. *Acta Dermato-venereologica,* **43,** 109.

MISCELLANEOUS DRUGS USED IN THE TREATMENT OF VASCULITIS

It must be admitted that in the whole field of vasculitis there have been no adequate trials of drugs. The main reason for this is the difficulty in selecting patients with relatively homogeneous disease. If one considers vasculitis as a spectrum ranging from urticaria to ischaemia, much depends on the position of the disease in that spectrum at the time of administration of the drug. Easier aspects to assess are the age and sex incidence and the degree to which patient and doctor expect a particular result, but such delineation reduces the number of patients admitted to the trial, so that in most instances the average physician will see inadequate numbers in the required period. But even if several centres are involved in a trial, they often fail to agree about the clinical criteria for admission to it.

It is necessary always to take into consideration the idiosyncratic, the unique or the unusual trigger or constitution; this ensures that a drug seemingly effective in a single case will not be ruled out simply because it is not proven to have a beneficial effect in a larger trial. Dermatologists are open to criticism in this respect because they are thought to rely overmuch on single case reports. However, trial experts have a habit of giving notoriety to bizarre side-effects of drugs while at the same time ignoring bizarre successes. Some aspects, like the relief of pain, rely on subjective impressions and a good witness may be particularly valuable.

Vasodilator drugs

Before prescribing vasodilators, the patient should be left in no doubt that stopping smoking is even more effective.

Vasodilator drugs are indicated for vasospastic conditions such as Raynaud's phenomenon and acrocyanosis, whenever simple measures to promote warmth and to protect from cooling are not successful. They are helpful for perniosis in which a degree of vasospasm may contribute to the stasis of blood in cooled skin. There are no drugs which can be relied on consistently to increase blood flow through ischaemic tissue, and the more potent the vasodilator the greater the risk of blood being shunted away from areas of fixed blockage (Gillespie, 1966).

Tolazoline hydrochloride (Priscol), which is the most commonly prescribed drug, acts by counteracting adrenaline and noradrenaline. The alpha-receptor blocker thymoxamine (Opilon) acts similarly. Inositol hexanicotinate (Hexopal) or bamethan sulphate (Vasculit) act mainly on the vessel wall as a local vasodilator. Acetomenaphthone with nicotinic acid (Pernivit) is advocated for chilblains. Intra-arterial reserpine is in vogue: Tindall, Whalen and Burton (1974) treated 102 patients with Raynaud's disease and phenomenon by injecting 1.0 to 1.5 mg of this drug in 2.5 ml physiological saline into the brachial artery over a period of 60 seconds. Two-thirds of their patients had a good or excellent response. Intra-arterial prostaglandin E_1 may yet prove to be the most effective vasodilator for use in severe peripheral vascular disease (Carlson and Eriksson, 1973) (Table 15.3).

Table 15.3. Results from a pilot study of the effect of intra-arterial prostaglandin E_1 on peripheral vascular disease.

Case	Age (years)	Athero-sclerosis	Earlier amputa-tion	Gangrene	Rest pains	Immediate effects of PGE	Side effects
1	77	+++	−	++	++	Disappearance of pain	0
2	84	+++	+	++	++	Disappearance of pain	0
3	70	+++	−	+	++	No change	0
4	79	+++	+	−	++	Disappearance of pain	0

+++ severe.
++ moderate.
+ mild.

The advice of a vascular surgeon and appropriate vascular surgery should always be considered in obliterative peripheral vascular disease.

Anti-inflammatory agents

The effect of corticosteroids, azathioprine and cyclophosphamide will be discussed in relation to humoral antibody; however, such drugs have a complex action, at least some of which is a nonspecific anti-inflammatory effect.

The mediators of inflammation, which include acetylcholine, histamine and kinins, are permeability producing agents acting at the urticarial end of the spectrum of vasculitis. On the one hand, they probably protect the tissues from thrombotic and ischaemic changes since, amongst other actions, they encourage endothelial secretion of plasminogen activator and increase fibrinolysis. On the other hand, increased permeability allows immune complexes to be deposited outside the vessels where they cause further irritation.

The typical histamine-mediated lesion develops quickly and rapidly resolves, but urticarial lesions which persist for several hours not only show leucocytoclasis but usually also have evidence that fibrinolytic activity is exhausted with consequent fibrin deposition. Such lesions might conceivable be made worse by antihistamines. The author uses long-acting antihistamines and cyproheptadine hydrochloride in recurrent urticarial-type lesions, delayed pressure urticaria and anaphylactoid purpura provided there is little purpura and no tendency to necrosis.

The fact that drugs may have such opposite effects in different parts of the spectrum is one explanation of the variable response to them, particularly in disease of mixed morphology. Long-lasting urticarial lesions with a leucocytoclastic histology are suppressed by indomethacin or aspirin provided some antihistamine cover is given. Patients with urticaria and hypocomplementaemia sometimes do well with this combination. One such patient of the author was referred to and reported by Sissons et al (1974), and another was presented to the British Association of Dermatology (1969) by Ryan and Levene.

Aspirin and indomethacin both enhance urticaria, but their roles as inhibitors of prostaglandins, as enhancers of fibrinolysis, and as inhibitors of platelet aggregation (Table 15.4) put them amongst the most useful drugs for vasculitis with more persistent or necrotic lesions.

Table 15.4. Actions of aspirin and indomethacin.

Action	Reference
Inhibition of chemotactic neutrophil migration	Phelps and McCarty, 1967
,, ,, haemolysis of red cells	Brown and MacKay, 1968
,, ,, phagocytosis by human leucocytes	Kvarstein and Stormorken, 1971
,, ,, histamine contraction of smooth muscle	Northover, 1971
Reduction of salt and water retention; inhibition of calcium uptake by cells	Northover, 1971
Inhibition of prostaglandin synthesis	Vane, 1971
Inhibition of ADP or collagen-induced platelet aggregation	O'Brien et al, 1970
Inhibition of platelet release reaction; reduction of fibrin degradation products in urine in glomerulonephritis	Clarkson et al, 1972
Increased fibrinolysis; inhibition of the tetrafurfuryl nicotinate reaction in the skin	Truelove and Duthie, 1959

Enhanced fibrinolysis is probably a factor in some of the more urticarial types of response. ε-Aminocaproic acid is advocated in the anaphylactic type of responses for this reason, and it is particularly valuable in hereditary angio-oedema (see page 385).

Heparin is anticomplementary but probably also has other anti-inflammatory effects (Dolowitz and Dougherty, 1965). These authors emphasise its role as an antihistamine.

Analgesic and anti-inflammatory drugs

Aspirin remains the cheapest and possibly the most reliable of effective drugs. A four-gram daily dose is necessary to achieve an anti-inflammatory effect in arthritis but prolonged administration at this dosage gives rise to a high incidence of gastrointestinal bleeding. Encapsulated forms, while causing less gastric irritation, may be less well absorbed. Aspirin and paracetamol are combined in benorylate (Benoral) which causes little gastric irritation and is absorbed and released slowly.

Phenylbutazone (Butazolidin), or the related but less toxic oxyphenbutazone (Tanderil), besides being anti-inflammatory, seemed particularly valuable for thrombophlebitis and hence for nodular vasculitis. Side-effects such as rashes, dyspepsia, aplastic anaemia and leucopenia have been commonly reported but are relatively rare when related to the frequency with which these drugs are prescribed in general practice. These drugs enhance the anticoagulant effect of warfarin and phenindione and the hypoglycaemic effect of tolbutamide and chlorpropamide.

Ibuprofen (Brufen) seems to have fewer side-effects and is relatively quick-acting; it is receiving increasingly wide usage by rheumatologists.

Acute anaphylaxis

The patient with anaphylaxis should be laid supine with his legs raised vertically. A subcutaneous injection of 1 ml of adrenaline 1:1000 should be given, followed by chlorpheniramine (Piriton) 10 mg with 100 mg of hydrocortisone hemisuccinate intravenously. This combination should relieve bronchospasm and reduce the vascular permeability. Patients remaining shocked require intravenous fluid, and should signs of impending laryngeal obstruction appear the ear, nose and throat surgeon must be alerted and preparations made for tracheotomy.

Dapsone

Dapsone (4,4'-diaminodiphenyl sulphone) has been successfully employed in the treatment of several cases of vasculitis, in particular erythema elevatum diutinum (Kalkoff, 1967; Vollum, 1968; Wells, 1969; Cream, Levene and Calnan, 1971). Thompson et al (1973) also successfully managed a patient with leucocytoclastic angiitis, pyoderma gangrenosum and paraproteinaemia using dapsone.

Sulphonamides

Sulphapyridine has been used in erythema elevatum diutinum (Johnston, 1964), for pyoderma gangrenosum (Jablonska, Stachow and Dabrowska, 1967), and in pemphigus vulgaris (Winkelmann and Roth, 1960; Seah et al, 1973). It was also used successfully by Diaz-Perez and Winkelmann, 1974) in two cases of so-called polyarteritis nodosa. No serious studies of the use of this drug in vasculitis have so far been undertaken, although this should be qualified in so far as some believe that dermatitis herpetiformis is a form of vasculitis.

Sulphamethoxypyridazine was used for erythema elevatum diutinum by Kalkoff (1967).

It is current practice among dermatologists to try dapsone in difficult cases.

Penicillamine

This expensive drug was initially used in Wilson's disease and is a well-known chelating agent. A multicentre trial (Andrews et al, 1973) has shown that it undoubtedly benefited patients with severe acute rheumatoid arthritis and that it has a particular place in the management of vasculitis in patients with high titres of rheumatoid factor.

The usual practice is to give one tablet (250 mg of D-penicillamine B.P.) or two capsules (each 150 mg of D-penicillamine hydrochloride B.P.) by mouth daily. Day et al (1974) suggested that the drug should be introduced slowly, one 150 mg capsule per day for four weeks, and the maintenance dose kept as low as 300 to 600 mg if the response is sufficiently good. On low dosage, serious blood changes were not observed, and the dose was not reduced until proteinuria was more than 2 g/day. The urine should be checked regularly for proteinuria because the penicillamine forms complexes which often cause nephritis. Rashes, loss of taste, nausea and vomiting are other complications.

The makers of this drug (Merck, Dista) have emphasised the absolute necessity (1) of starting with a small dose and (2) of doing white blood cell and platelet counts weekly or fortnightly at first and monthly thereafter for as long as the patient is maintained on the drug (Lyle, 1973). About 30 per cent of patients on this drug have to discontinue it because of intolerance (Andrews et al, 1973; Leader, *Lancet,* May 17, 1975).

Complete relief of the cold intolerance and bleeding tendency in macroglobulinaemia has followed a sustained decrease in blood viscosity produced by this drug (Bloch and Maki, 1973).

Barnett et al (1970) advocated such therapy in cryoglobulinaemic immune complex disease as it suppresses immunoglobulin synthesis and is cytotoxic. However, the exact mechanism of its action is not known. It takes about three weeks to produce its effect and its concentration in the blood is not high enough to influence cryoglobulins by disrupting disulphide bonds.

Iodides

Iodides have long been used to reduce fibrosis. In some varieties of vasculitis affecting the subcutaneous tissue, fat is replaced by thick fibrous tissue; the migratory sub-acute nodular forms that overlap with erythema nodosum respond in this way (Pierini, Abulafia and Wainfield, 1965).

Iodides have long been used to reduce fibrosis and Perry and Winkelmann (1964) gave potassium iodide 1.5 g four times daily for their cases of sub-acute nodular migratory panniculitis.

Iodides themselves, however, are sometimes a cause of vasculitis (Figure 4.25).

References

Andrews, F. M., Golding, D. N., Freeman, A. M., Golding, J. R., Day, A. T., Hill, A. G. S., Camp, A. V., Lewis-Faning, E. & Lyle, W. H. (1973) Controlled trial of D-penicillamine in severe rheumatoid arthritis. *Lancet,* **i,** 275.
Barnett, E. V., Bluestone, R., Cracchiolo, A., Goldberg, L. S., Kantor, G. L. & McIntosh, R. M. (1970) Cryoglobulinemia and disease. *Annals of Internal Medicine,* **73,** 95.

Bloch, K. J. & Maki, D. G. (1973) Hyperviscosity syndromes associated with immunoglobulin abnormalities. *Seminars in Hematology,* **10,** 113.

Brown, J. H. & Mackey, H. K. (1968) Further studies on the erythrocyte anti-inflammatory assay (33051). *Proceedings of the Society for Experimental Biology and Medicine,* **128,** 504.

Carlson, L. A. & Eriksson, I. (1973) Femoral artery infusion of prostaglandin E₁ in severe peripheral vascular disease. *Lancet,* **i,** 155.

Clarkson, A. R., Macdonald, M. K., Cash, J. D. & Robson, J. S. (1972) Modification by drugs of urinary fibrin/fibrinogen degradation products in glomerulonephritis. *British Medical Journal,* **iii,** 255.

Cream, J. J., Levene, G. M. & Calnan, C. D. (1971) Erythema elevatum diutinum: an unusual reaction to streptococcal antigen and response to dapsone. *British Journal of Dermatology,* **84,** 393.

Day, A. T., Golding, J. R., Lee, P. N. & Butterworth, A. D. (1974) Penicillamine in rheumatoid disease: a long term study. *British Medical Journal,* **i,** 180.

Diaz-Perez, J. L. & Winkelmann, R. K. (1974) Cutaneous periarteritis nodosa. *Archives of Dermatology,* **110,** 407.

Dolowitz, D. A. & Dougherty, T. P. (1965) The use of heparin in the control of allergies. *Annals of Allergy,* **23,** 309.

Gillespie, J. A. (1966) An evaluation of vasodilator drugs in occlusive vascular disease by measurement. *Angiology,* **17,** 280.

Jablonska, S., Stachow, A. & Dabrowska, H. (1967) Entre la pyodermite gangreneure et le myelôme. *Annales de Dermatologie et de Syphiligraphie,* **94,** 121.

Johnston, E. N. M. (1964) Erythema elevatum diutinum. *British Journal of Dermatology,* **76,** 90.

Kalkoff, K. W. (1967) Erythema elevatum diutinum. *Proceedings of the 13th International Dermatological Congress, Munich,* Vol. 3, p. 79.

Kvarstein, B. & Stormorken, H. (1971) Influence of acetyl-salicylic acid, butazolidine, colchicine, hydro-cortisone, chlorpromazine and imipramine on the phagocytosis of polystyrene latex particles by human leucocytes. *Biochemistry and Pharmacology,* **20,** 119.

Leader (1975) *O*-Penicillamine in rheumatoid arthritis. *Lancet,* **i,** 1123.

Lyle, W. H. (1973) Penicillamine in rheumatoid arthritis. *Lancet,* **ii,** 235.

Northover, B. J. (1971) Mechanism of the inhibitory action of indomethacin on smooth muscle. *British Journal of Pharmacology,* **41,** 540.

O'Brien, J. R., Finch, W. & Clark, E. (1970) A comparison of an effect of different anti-inflammatory drugs on human platelets. *Journal of Clinical Pathology,* **23,** 522.

Perry, H. O. & Winkelmann, R. K. (1964) Subacute nodular migratory panniculitis. *Archives of Dermatology,* **89,** 170.

Phelps, P. & McCarty, D. J. (1967) Suppressive effects of indomethacin on crystal induced inflammation in canine joints and on neutrophilic motility in vitro. *Journal of Pharmacology and Experimental Therapeutics,* **158,** 546.

Pickering, G. W. (1968) *High Blood Pressure,* 2nd edition. London: J. & A. Churchill.

Pierini, L. E., Abulafia, J. & Wainfield, S. (1965) Las hypodermitis. *Archives Argentinos de Dermatologia,* **15,** 1.

Ryan, T. J. & Levene, G. (1969) *Proceedings and Case Histories of the Annual Meeting of the British Association of Dermatology.*

Seah, P. P., Fry, L., Cairns, R. J. & Feiwel, M. (1973) Pemphigus controlled by sulphapyridine. *British Journal of Dermatology,* **89,** 77.

Sissons, J. G. P., Evans, D. J., Peters, D. K., Eisinger, A. J., Boulton-Jones, J. M., Simpson, I. J. & Macanovic, M. (1974) Glomerulonephritis associated with antibody to glomerular basement membrane. *British Medical Journal,* **iv,** 11.

Thompson, D. M., Main, R. A., Beck, J. S. & Albert-Recht, F. (1973) Studies on a patient with leucocyto-clastic vasculitis, 'pyoderma gangrenosum' and paraproteinaemia. *British Journal of Dermatology,* **88,** 117.

Tindall, J. P., Whalen, R. E. & Burton, E. E. Jr (1974) Medical uses of intra-arterial injections of reserpine. Treatment of Raynaud's syndrome and of some vascular insufficiencies of the lower extremities. *Archives of Dermatology,* **20,** 119.

Truelove, L. H. & Duthie, J. J. R. (1959) Effect of aspirin on cutaneous response to the local application of an ester of nicotinic acid. *Annals of the Rheumatic Diseases,* **18,** 137.

Vane, J. R. (1971) Inhibition of prostaglandin synthesis as a mechanism of action for aspirin-like drugs. *Nature, New Biology,* **231,** 232.

Vollum, D. I. (1968) Erythema elevatum diutinum, vesicular lesions and sulphone response. *British Journal of Dermatology,* **80,** 178.

Wells, G. C. (1969) Allergic vasculitis (trisymtôm of Gougerot) treated with dapsone. *Proceedings of the Royal Society of Medicine,* **62,** 665.

Winkelmann, R. K. & Roth, H. L. (1960) Dermatitis herpetiformis with acantholysis or pemphigus with response to sulphonamides. *Archives of Dermatology,* **82,** 385.

Heparin

Several authors have expressed their belief that heparin is the drug of choice in disseminated intravascular coagulation (DIC). In local coagulation it is not always so effective because ischaemia results in acidosis and a low pH inactivates heparin (Hardaway, 1971). Heparin is thus effective only in conditions where there is some blood flow and hypoxia is not too prolonged. It is only the second best treatment when the cause is known and can be remedied. Thus in DIC, due for example to malaria or trypanosomiasis, adequate chemotherapy for the infection is usually sufficient (Barrett-Connor, Ugoretz and Braude, 1973).

Heparin is the most potent, reliable and effective antagonist of coagulation. Pre-treatment with heparin prevents endotoxin-induced DIC in rabbits (Crowell and Read, 1955) and vascular injury from virus infections such as haemorrhagic fever (Weiss, Halstead and Russ, 1965).

Besides being an anticoagulant, heparin has anti-inflammatory and anticomplementary actions (Ecker and Gross, 1929). It protects rabbits from anaphylactic shock (Johansson, 1961), it is particularly effective in antigen—antibody reactions associated with hyperacute renal allograft rejection (Starzl et al, 1970; Colman et al, 1972), and it inhibits not only the ocular tuberculin reaction (Wood and Bick, 1959) but also delayed hypersensitivity reactions in general (Nelson, 1965; Cohen et al, 1967). As it reduces wealing (Thompson, 1968), it has been used for urticaria (Meyer De Schmid and Neumann, 1952). It also clears the rash of dermatitis herpetiformis (Alexander, 1963).

Where platelet aggregation is the primary event, as in microangiopathic haemolytic anaemia, heparin is especially effective (Brain et al, 1968), but as others have found this to be untrue (Thompson et al, 1973), platelet de-aggregating agents may be preferred. However, its role in prolonging graft survival is believed to be due to its effect on platelet aggregation (Amery et al, 1973).

Colman, Robboy and Minna (1974) pointed out that controlled trials are lacking for most diseases treated by heparin, but the numerous case reports and data on decreased morbidity or dramatic improvement in some chronically diseased patients bear witness to its value.

Bleeding caused by heparin therapy occurred in 7.6 per cent of patients in one series, but bleeding from DIC itself occurs in 85 per cent. To incriminate heparin rather than the disease as the cause of haemorrhage occurring within the first 24 hours of starting therapy is highly presumptuous (Colman, Robboy and Minna, 1974) because it takes at least that time for effective anticoagulation to be achieved.

Colman et al (1974) used rigid criteria to assess improvement, including a rise in the platelet count and prothrombin time and a fall in fibrin degradation products, and they reported that in 54 per cent of 45 cases complete improvement occured in 54 episodes of DIC studied. They had administered heparin intravenously every four hours in doses ranging from 45 to 135 USP units/kg body weight (0.36 to 1.1 mg/kg body weight). Side-effects are rare but include alopecia and anaphylaxis (Colman, Robboy and Minna, 1974), and prolonged heparinisation for several months can cause severe osteoporosis.

Patients observed by the author have been principally under the care of Dr Alan Sharp (Oxford) who at times has used continuous infusions of heparin and who, like Colman et al (1972), has expressed his belief that heparin is frequently given in too small amounts and for too short a period. Those who have recorded failures or severe bleeding and have argued against the use of heparin (Didisheim, 1971; Green et al, 1972) probably have included cases that have been irreversibly injured by infection or neoplasia or in-adequately anticoagulated; at least, this view has been expressed by Robboy of Colman's group (personal communication, 1974).

Dudgeon, Kellog and Gilchrist (1971) considered that inadequate doses of heparin accounted for two deaths in their five cases of purpura fulminans. Though one must agree with Didisheim that treatment of the underlying disorder is the most effective way to control chronic intravascular coagulation, such as is observed in vasculitis, the cause is unfortunately either unknown in most cases or detectable only after prolonged investigation.

Heparin is particularly valuable in vasculitis at a stage when infarction is becoming a possibility, as in a case of anaphylactoid purpura progressing to gangrene described by Kisker, Glueck and Kauder (1968). It is essential treatment of the gangrene that sometimes follows the use of dicoumarol (see Chapter 8) (Everett and Overholt, 1969; Nalbandian et al, 1971), and it is life-saving in purpura fulminans (Cram and Soley, 1968; Benoit et al, 1969).

One of the more interesting aspects of the use of heparin is whether or not it has a therapeutic effect in low dosage. Several reports on the value of subcutaneous heparin, 5000 units given at 12-hourly intervals for the prevention of deep vein thrombosis, have emphasised its safety and lack of bleeding complications (Kakkar et al, 1972; Nicolaides et al, 1972; Van Vroonhoven, Van Zijl and Muller, 1974). Van Vroonhoven, Van Zijl and Muller (1974), in a controlled trial using the ^{125}I-fibrinogen test observed that giving low doses of subcutaneous heparin was more effective prophylaxis of postoperative deep vein thrombosis than was routine oral anticoagulation. Warlow et al (1973) found it to be similarly effective after myocardial infarction, but although Lahnborg et al (1974) reported that it produced significant reduction in pulmonary embolism, Tibbutt et al (1974) found it inferior to streptokinase in this respect. There seems also to be a marked reduction in the frequency of acute duodenal ulceration found at postmortem on patients who have been having such therapy (Margaretten and McKay, 1971; Sharnoff, 1974).

The use of heparin in this way requires no laboratory control, with the important exception that any sort of heparin therapy must be monitored in patients undergoing major surgery (Bonnar and Denson, 1974).

Renewed interest and debate about the value of heparin is referred to in the literature on meningococcal septicaemia. Gerard et al (1973), for instance, reported death in only two of 19 patients with purpura treated with heparin, and they gave 15 references to intravascular coagulation observed in this disorder; the effective use of heparin was reported in 10 of these papers.

Perhaps more relevant to vasculitis is the literature on renal disease. Kincaid-Smith, Saker and Fairley (1968) reported that heparin, given as part of a regime that included corticosteroids and immunosuppressive drugs, greatly improved the urine output of six cases of 'irreversible' acute renal failure due to glomerulonephritis. Other groups also have reported favourable effects of heparin on the course of glomerulonephritis (Shires et al, 1966; Conte et al, 1970; Cade et al, 1971; Wardle and Uldall, 1972) and on transplant rejection (McMillan, 1968; MacDonald et al, 1970; Wardle and Uldall, 1972). Kleinerman (1954) and Halpern et al (1958) inhibited renal damage in animals given anti-kidney antibody by treating them with heparin, and Vassalli and McCluskey (1965) showed that warfarin also was effective. Dolowitz and Dougherty (1965) advocated the use of heparin in a wide range of allergic and inflammatory processes, pointing out that it binds histamine.

For continuous infusion heparin should be in saline. Hydrocortisone hemisuccinate with 5 per cent dextrose, for instance, reduces its potency.

The case against heparin is argued by Straub (1974) who believes it is too frequently prescribed for disseminated intravascular coagulation.

Ancrod (Arvin)

This purified fraction of the venom of the Malayan pit viper acts by converting plasma fibrinogen into a form that is more readily cleared by fibrinolysis and cannot be clotted by physiological thrombin. The blood viscosity in patients receiving Arvin is progressively reduced and this is an advantage in vascular occlusive disease. It is usually administered intravenously and the incidence of a haemorrhagic tendency seems to be low. Maintenance therapy by subcutaneous injection has been used by the author but antibody to the drug soon develops and within a few weeks maintenance therapy has to be discontinued. It is, however, recommended in some forms of vasculitis in which heparin might cause bleeding.

It has been used in sickle cell crises (Gilles et al, 1968), in central retinal vein thrombosis (Bowell, Marmion and McCarthy, 1970), in priapism (Bell and Pitney, 1969), and for vasculitis with acral vascular occlusion (Chesterman, Sharp and Ryan, personal communication, to be published).

Aminocaproic acid (epsilon-aminocaproic acid, EACA)

Hyperfibrinolytic states have been reported as a cause of vasculitis with a particularly haemorrhagic element (Haustein, 1969), and Kurban and Ryan (1969) also found that vasculitis with normal euglobulin lysis tended to be more haemorrhagic. There is also some evidence that in vasculitis in skin the more permeable, urticarial, early inflammatory phase is associated with increased fibrinolysis (Ryan, Nishioka and Dawber, 1971). For this reason EACA has a place in the therapy of some forms of vasculitis (Haustein, 1969).

Reiss (1971) has reviewed the literature reporting the use of EACA to inhibit anaphylactic shock, chronic urticaria, atopic and contact dermatitis, and allergy to drugs. Above all, this drug has become one of the most respected treatments for hereditary angio-oedema (Champion and Lachmann, 1969; Hadjiyannaki and Lachmann, 1971; Frank et al, 1972).

It can be taken by mouth in the form of cachets, the dose being 8 to 16 g per day for many months. Nausea and stuffiness of the nose are common side-effects. Severe side-effects, though rare, include extensive muscle necrosis (Shae and Miller, 1974), peripheral gangrene, thrombosis in coronary, gastrointestinal and glomerular vessels, pulmonary embolism from deep vein thrombosis (Naeye, 1962; Charytan and Purtilo, 1969), cerebral arteritis (Sonntag and Stein, 1974), and thrombosis of the inferior vena cava (Rowell, 1974).

Hydroxychloroquine sulphate

As a pre-operative dose of 1200 mg over 24 hours and 800 mg daily postoperatively this drug has reduced deep vein thrombosis from 16 per cent to 5 per cent as assessed by ^{125}I-tagged fibrinogen (Carter and Eban, 1974). It has also been prescribed successfully for autosensitivity to deoxyribonucleic acid (Levine and Pinkus, 1961).

References

Alexander, J. O'D. (1963) The treatment of dermatitis herpetiformis with heparin. *British Journal of Dermatology*, **75**, 289.

Amery, A. H., Pegrum, G. D., Risdon, R. A. & Williams, G. (1973) Nature of hyperacute rejection in dog renal allografts and effect of heparin rejection process. *British Medical Journal*, **i**, 455.

Barrett-Connor, E., Ugoretz, R. J. & Braude, A. L. (1973) Disseminated intravascular coagulation in trypanosomiasis. *Annals of Internal Medicine*, **131**, 574.

Bell, W. R. & Pitney, W. R. (1969) Management of priapism by therapeutic defibrination. *New England Journal of Medicine*, **280**, 649.

Benoit, P., Raymond, R. & Glorieux, F. H. (1969) Purpura fulminans. *Canadian Medical Association Journal*, **101**, 42.

Bloch, K. J. & Maki, D. G. (1973) Hyperviscosity syndromes associated with immunoglobulin abnormalities. *Seminars in Hematology*, **10**, 113.

Bonnar, J. & Denson, K. W. (1974) Subcutaneous heparin. *Lancet*, **ii**, 956.

Bowell, R. E., Marmion, V. J. & McCarthy, C. F. (1970) Treatment of central retinal vein thrombosis with ancrod. *Lancet*, **i**, 173.

Brain, M. C., Baker, L. R. I., McBride, J. A., Rubenbeg, M. L. & Cadie, J. V. (1968) Treatment of patients with micro-angiopathic haemolytic anaemia with heparin. *British Journal of Haematology*, **15**, 603.

Cade, J. R., de Quesada, A. M., Shires, D. L., Levin, D. M., Hackett, R. L., Spooner, G. R., Schlein, E. M., Pickering, M. J. & Holcomb, A. (1971) The effect of long term high dose heparin treatment on the course of chronic proliferative glomerulonephritis. *Nephron*, **8**, 67.

Carter, A. E. & Eban, R. (1974) Prevention of postoperative deep venous thrombosis in legs by orally administered hydroxychloroquine sulphate. *British Medical Journal*, **iii**, 94.

Champion, R. H. & Lachmann, P. J. (1969) Hereditary angio-oedema treated with epsilon-aminocaproic acid. *British Journal of Dermatology*, **81**, 763.

Charytan, C. & Purtilo, D. (1969) Glomerular capillary thrombosis and acute renal failure after epsilon amino caproic acid therapy. *New England Journal of Medicine*, **280**, 1102.

Cohen, S., Benacerraf, B., McCluskey, R. T. & Ovary, Z. (1967) Effect of anticoagulants on delayed hyper-sensitivity reactions. *Journal of Immunology*, **98**, 351.

Colman, R. W., Robboy, S. J. & Minna, J. D. (1972) Disseminated intravascular coagulation (DIC). An approach. *American Journal of Medicine*, **52**, 679.

Colman, R. W., Robboy, S. J. & Minna, J. D. (1974) Heparin should be used in the therapy of clinically significant disseminated intravascular coagulation. In *Controversies in Internal Medicine* (Ed.) Inglefinger, F. J. Philadelphia: W. B. Saunders.

Colman, R. W., Girey, G., Galvanek, E. G. & Busch, G. (1972) Human renal allografts: the protective effects of heparin, kallikrein, activation and fibrinolysis during hyperacute rejection. In *Coagulation Problems in Transplanted Organs* (Ed.) Von Kaulla, K. N. p. 87. Springfield, Illinois: Charles C. Thomas.

Conte, J., That, H. T., Mignon-Conte, M. & Suc, J. M. (1970) In *Proceedings of the European Dialysis and Transplant Association*, **7**, 273.

Cram, D. L. & Soley, R. L. (1968) Purpura fulminans. *British Journal of Dermatology*, **80**, 323.

Crowell, J. W. & Read, W. L. (1955) In vivo coagulation. A probable cause of irreversible shock. *American Journal of Physiology*, **183**, 565.

Didisheim, P. (1971) The intravascular coagulation and fibrinolysis (I.C.F.) syndrome. *Thrombosis et Diathesis Haemorrhagica*, Supplement **46**, 119.

Dolowitz, D. A. & Dougherty, T. P. (1965) The use of heparin in the control of allergies. *Annals of Allergy*, **23**, 309.

Dudgeon, D. L., Kellog, D. R., Gilchrist, G. S. & Wooley, M. W. (1971) Purpura fulminans. *Archives of Surgery*, **103**, 351.

Ecker, E. E. & Gross, P. J. (1929) Anticomplementary power of heparin. *Journal of Infectious Diseases*, **44**, 250.

Everett, E. D. & Overholt, T. L. (1969) Haemorrhagic skin infarction, secondary to oral anticoagulants. *Archives of Dermatology*, **100**, 588.

Frank, M. M., Sergeant, J. S., Kane, M. A. & Alling, D. W. (1972) Epsilon-aminocaproic acid and therapy of hereditary angioneurotic oedema. A double blind study. *New England Journal of Medicine*, **286**, 808.

Gérard, P., Moriau, M., Bachy, A., Malvaux, P. & De Meyer, R. (1973) Meningococcal purpura report of 19 patients treated with heparin. *Journal of Pediatrics*, **82**, 780.

Gilles, H-M., Reid, H. A., Odutola, A., Ransome-Kuti, O. & Ransome-Kuti, S. (1968) Arvin treatment for sickle cell crisis. *Lancet*, **ii**, 542.

Green, D., Seeler, R. A., Allen, N. & Alavi, I. A. (1972) The role of heparin in the management of consumption coagulopathy. *Medical Clinics of North America*, **56**, 193.

Hadjiyannaki, K. & Lachmann, P. J. (1971) Hereditary angio-oedema: a review with particular reference to pathogenesis and treatment. *Clinical Allergy*, **1**, 221.

Halpern, B., Milliez, P., Lagrue, G., Fray, A. & Morard, J. C. (1958) Protective action of heparin in experimental immune nephritis. *Nature*, **205**, 257.

Hardaway, R. M. (1971) Disseminated intravascular coagulation. *Thrombosis et Diathesis Haemorrhagica*, Supplement **46**, 209.

Haustein, U. F. (1969) Purpura hyperfibrinolytica als pathogenetisches prinzipeines haemorrhagieschen mikrobides miescher. *Dermatologische Monatsschrift,* **155,** 771.

Johansson, S-A. (1961) The protective effect of heparin in cases of anaphylactic shock. *Acta Dermato-venereologica,* **41,** 500.

Kakkar, V. V., Corrigan, T., Spindler, J., Fossard, D. P., Flute, P. T., Crellin, R-Q. Wessler, S. & Yin, E. T. (1972) Efficacy of low doses of heparin in prevention of deep vein thrombosis after major surgery. A double blind randomised trial. *Lancet,* **ii,** 101.

Kincaid-Smith, P., Saker, B. M. & Fairley, K. F. (1968) Anticoagulants in irreversible acute renal failure. *Lancet,* **ii,** 1360.

Kisker, C. T. & Rush, R. (1973) Circulating fibrin and meningococcaemia. *Journal of Pediatrics,* **82,** 787.

Kisker, C. T., Glueck, H. & Kauder, E. (1968) Anaphylactoid purpura progressing to gangrene and its treatment with heparin. *Journal of Pediatrics,* **73,** 748.

Kleinerman, J. (1954) Effects of heparin on experimental nephritis in rabbits. *Laboratory Investigation,* **3,** 495.

Kurban, A. K. & Ryan, T. J. (1969) Fibrinogen titre, fibrinolysis and platelet stickiness correlated with capillary bleeding; or block in the skin. *Transactions of the St John's Hospital Dermatological Society,* **55,** 218.

Lahnborg, G., Friman, L., Bergstrom, K. & Lagergren, H. (1974) Effect of low dose heparin on incidence of postoperative embolism detected by photoscanning. *Lancet,* **i,** 329.

Levine, M. B. & Pinkus, H. (1961) Autosensitivity to desoxyribonucleic acid (DNA). Report of a case with inflammatory skin lesions controlled by chloroquine. *New England Journal of Medicine,* **264,** 533.

MacDonald, A., Busch, G. J., Alexander, J. L., Pheteplace, E. A., Menzoian, J. & Murray, J. E. (1970) Heparin and aspirin in the treatment of hyperacute rejection of renal allografts in presensitized dogs. *Transplantation,* **9,** 1.

Margaretten, W. & McKay, T. (1971) Thrombotic ulcerations in the gastrointestinal tract. *Archives of Internal Medicine,* **127,** 250.

McMillan, R. (1968) Heparin in delayed transport function. *Lancet,* **i,** 1178.

Meyer de Schmid, J. J. & Neuman, A. (1952) Le traitement de l'urticaire chronique par l'heparine. *Bulletin de la Société Française de Dermatologie et de Syphiligraphie,* **59,** 286.

Naeye, R. L. (1962) Thrombotic state after haemorrhagic diathesis: possible complication of therapy with epsilon aminocaproic acid. *Blood,* **19,** 697.

Nalbandian, R. M., Beller, F. K., Kamp, A. K., Henry, R. L. & Wolf, P. L. (1971) Coumarin necrosis of skin treated successfully with heparin. *Obstetrics and Gynecology,* **38,** 395.

Nelson, D. S. (1965) The effects of anticoagulants and other drugs on cellular and cutaneous reactions to antigen in guinea pigs with delayed type hypersensitivity. *Immunology,* **9,** 219.

Nicolaides, A. N., Dupont, P. A., Desai, S., Lewis, J. D., Douglas, J. N., Dodsworth, H., Fourides, G., Luck, R. J. & Jamieson, C. W. (1972) Small doses of subcutaneous sodium heparin in preventing deep venous thrombosis after major surgery. *Lancet,* **ii,** 890.

Reiss, F. (1971) The therapeutic effect of epsilon-aminocaproic acid with special reference to atopic dermatitis. *British Journal of Dermatology,* **85,** 76.

Rowell, N. R. (1974) A painful bleeding syndrome associated with increased fibrinolytic activity. *British Journal of Dermatology,* **91,** 591.

Ryan, T. J., Nishioka, K. & Dawber, R. P. R. (1971) Epithelial—endothelial interactions in the control of inflammation through fibrinolysis. *British Journal of Dermatology,* **84,** 501.

Sharnoff, J. G. (1974) Low dose heparin and stress ulceration. *Lancet,* **ii,** 1319.

Shaw, M. D. M. & Miller, J. R. (1974) E-aminocaproic acid and subarachnoid haemorrhage. *Lancet,* **ii,** 847.

Shires, D., Holcomb, A., Cade, R. & Levin, D. (1966) Treatment of chronic proliferative glomerulonephritis with heparin. *Clinical Research,* **14,** 387.

Sonntag, V. K. H. & Stein, B. M. (1974) Arteriopathic complications during treatment of subarachnoid haemorrhage with epsilon-aminocaproic acid. *Journal of Neurosurgery,* **40,** 480.

Starzl, T. E., Boehmig, H. J., Amemiya, H., Wilson, C. B., Dixon, F. J., Giles, G. R., Simpson, K. M. & Halgrimson, C. G. (1970) Clotting changes, including disseminated intravascular coagulation during rapid renal homograft rejection. *New England Journal of Medicine,* **283,** 383.

Straub, P. W. (1974) A case against heparin therapy of intravascular coagulation. *Thrombosis et Diathesis Haemorrhagica,* **33,** 107.

Thompson, J. S. (1968) Urticaria and angio-oedema. *Annals of Internal Medicine,* **124,** 129.

Tibbutt, D. A., Davies, J. A., Anderson, J. A., Fletcher, E. W. L., Hamill, J., Holt, J. M., Thomas, M. L., Lee, G. de J., Miller, G. A. H., Sharp, A. A. & Sutton, G. C. (1974) Comparison by controlled clinical trial of streptokinase and heparin in treatment of life threatening pulmonary embolism. *British Medical Journal,* **i,** 343.

Truelove, L. H. & Duthie, J. J. R. (1959) Effect of aspirin on cutaneous response to the local application of an ester of nicotinic acid. *Annals of the Rheumatic Diseases,* **18,** 137.

Van Vroonhoven, T. J. M. V., Van Zijl, J. & Muller, H. (1974) Low dose subcutaneous heparin versus oral anticoagulants — the prevention of postoperative deep-venous thrombosis. *Lancet,* **i,** 375.

Vassalli, P. & McCluskey, R. T. (1965) Editorial. The coagulation process and glomerular disease. *American Journal of Medicine,* **39,** 179.

Wardle, E. N. & Uldall, P. R. (1972) Effect of heparin on renal function in patients with oliguria. *British Medical Journal,* **iv,** 135.

Warlow, C., Terry, G., Kenmure, A. C. F., Beattie, A. G., Ogston, D. & Douglas, A. S. (1973) A double blind trial of low doses of subcutaneous heparin in the prevention of deep vein thrombosis after myocardial infarction. *Lancet,* **ii,** 934.

Weiss, H. J., Halstead, S. B. & Russ, S. B. (1965) Hemorrhagic disease in rodents caused by chikungunya virus 1) Studies of hemostasis. *Proceedings of the Society for Experimental Biology and Medicine,* **119,** 427.

Wood, R. M. & Bick, M. W. (1959) The effect of heparin on the tuberculin reaction. *Archives of Ophthalmology,* **61,** 709.

FIBRINOLYTIC THERAPY

Cunliffe (1968) reported three patients with a persistently reduced fibrinolytic activity which was revealed by a prolonged euglobulin lysis time and which returned to normal in two cases as the vasculitis spontaneously healed. Subsequently Turner and Ryan (1969) reported focal loss of fibrinolytic activity in vasculitis. Cunliffe and Menon (1971) then found that 32 out of 52 patients with vasculitis had low plasma fibrinolytic activity and that nine out of ten such patients receiving phenformin hydrochloride and ethyloestrenol improved over a period of six to 36 weeks. Isaacson et al (1970) also found impaired blood fibrinolytic activity in four patients with chronic vasculitis of the legs, and Parish (1972) reported another eight patients.

Kurban and Ryan (1969), however, could find evidence of impaired fibrinolysis in those patients who also had a degree of vessel block or infarction; but those who had no block often had better than normal fibrinolytic activity. Cunliffe and Menon (1971) also recorded increased fibrinolytic activity in three patients with purpura without necrosis, and Haustein described a patient with purpura and accelerated fibrinolytic activity.

Dodman et al (1973) reported a controlled trial in which eight of 13 patients showed considerable clinical improvement on either phenformin and ethyloestrenol or stanozolol, but they did not distinguish between infarctive and non-infarctive forms of vasculitis. This is important because some forms of vasculitis clearly have increased fibrinolysis and then treatment by antifibrinolytic agents is successful. A patient reported by Haustein (1969) is one such example and the author has a collection of biopsy material from vasculitis in which fibrinolysis was active.

Fibrinolytic therapy is indicated in those conditions in which thrombosis and infarction are features (Swan, Williams and Cooke, 1970). Phenformin and ethyloestrenol clearly can achieve this by enhancing fibrinolytic activity (Nilsson and Isaacson, 1972; Chakrabarti, 1974b). Gilliam, Herdon and Prystowsky (1974) prescribed phenformin and ethyloestrenol with success in five patients with atrophie blanche. Phenformin also has an anti-inflammatory action as was demonstrated in adjuvant induced polyarthritis in the rat (Gorog and Kovacs, 1972). Brödthagen et al (1968) described a 64-year-old woman who had widespread capillary thrombosis and high blood levels of fibrinolysis inhibitors (Figures 15.1 and 15.2). Her lesions cleared after infusions of plasmin, but she died of haemorrhage from a gastric ulcer.

Phenformin hydrochloride 50 mg b.d. and ethyloestrenol 2 mg q.i.d. are usually prescribed (Fearnley and Chakrabarti, 1964). Such therapy usually produces amenorrhoea. Stanozolol 5 mg b.d. is a less potent androgen but equally effective in combination with phenformin hydrochloride. Nausea, fluid retention, obesity, acne and lactic acidosis are other side-effects. If anything, the success of these drugs seems least disputable in chronic deep nodular varieties of vasculitis. Cunliffe, Roberts and Dodman (1973) have also reported successful treatment of Behçet's syndrome using these drugs. The patient whose skin lesions of malignant atrophic papulosis are depicted in Figures 3.3 and 4.30 also improved on fibrinolytic therapy (Delaney and Black, 1975).

Chajek and Fainaru (1973) reported the successful use of varidase in the treatment of two cases of Behçet's syndrome which presented with superior vena caval occlusion (Varidase, 12 tablets daily by mouth, each tablet containing streptokinase 10 000 units and streptodornase, 2500 units).

In assessing the overall effect of fibrinolytic therapy in vasculitis, it is important to distinguish between pre-menopausal women on the one hand, in whom fibrinolysis is variable, and post-menopausal women and men on the other. It is also important to realise that injury in general causes an immediate activation of fibrinolysis which is later exhausted, perhaps through the influence of emotion and stress (Innes and Sevitt, 1964; Fearnley, 1974) and acute situations must be distinguished from those with chronic reduction of fibrinolysis (Fearnley, 1974). Drugs such as phenformin and ethyloestrenol may have a more significant effect on small vessels than on large veins. Thus deep vein thrombosis following surgery is not prevented by therapy that effectively increases blood fibrinolysis (Fossard et al, 1974), whereas superficial thrombophlebitis is benefited (Nilsson et al, 1974). The enhanced fibrinolysis produced by phenformin and ethyl-oestrenol does not prevent the rise in fibrinogen that follows surgery (Chakrabarti, 1974b), but they reduce platelet stickiness (Chakrabarti and Fearnley, 1967; Chakrabarti, Evans and Fearnley, 1970). The latter authors also reported that Raynaud's phenomenon is relieved by fibrinolytic therapy, but Paolino et al (1972) found that it produced no improvement in eight patients with scleroderma.

In view of the common association between vasculitis and rheumatoid arthritis, the reduction of plasma fibrinogen and the ESR in 60 per cent of patients on fibrinolytic therapy is of interest (Fearnley and Chakrabarti, 1965).

Innerfield (1974) has proposed that low dosage of systemic kinases or proteases has an effect opposite to that of high dosage. Low dosage enhances coagulation and is anti-inflammatory in the early phases of acute injury, while high dosage enhances fibrinolytic permeability and is effective in the later phases of inflammation.

Thrombolytic therapy using streptokinase is increasingly advocated and is favoured by those in whose experience heparin has failed. Thus Preston and Edwards (1973) described a case of postpartum purpura fulminans which failed to respond to intravenous heparin 10 000 units four-hourly (possibly an inadequate dose) but which responded to streptokinase (initial dose, over 30 minutes, of 250 000 units, followed by 100 000 units hourly by continuous intravenous infusion). Chajek and Fainaru (1973) used such infusions in one case of superior vena caval occlusion in Behçet's disease. It is the treatment of choice for pulmonary embolism (Tibbutt et al, 1974).

Fibrinolysis is activated by endothelial secretions acting on plasminogen. The local enhancement of such activity is encouraged by a number of procedures to increase blood flow including external pneumatic intermittent compression (Allenby et al, 1973) and sauna baths (Britton et al, 1974).

Ekert (1974) found that the incidence of chronic renal disease following the haemolytic-uraemic syndrome is reduced by a combination of streptokinase and heparin together with aspirin or dipyridamole or both.

References

Allenby, F., Boardman, L., Pflug, J. J. & Calnan, J. S. (1973) Effects of external pneumatic intermittent compression on fibrinolysis in man. *Lancet,* **ii,** 1412.

Britton, B. J., Hawkey, C., Wood, W. G., Peele, M., Kaye, J. & Irving, M. H. (1974) Adrenergic, coagulation and fibrinolytic responses to heat. *British Medical Journal*, **iii**, 139.

Brodthagen, H., Larsen, V., Brøckner, J. & Amris, C. J. (1968) Cutaneous manifestations in capillary dilatation and endovascular fibrin deposits. *Acta Dermato-venereologica*, **48**, 277.

Chajek, T. & Fainaru, M. (1973) Behçet's disease with decreased fibrinolysis and superior vena caval occlusion. *British Medical Journal*, **i**, 782.

Chakrabarti, R. (1974a) Generalised capillary and arteriolar platelet thrombosis. *American Journal of the Medical Sciences*, **213**, 585.

Chakrabarti, R. (1974b) Fibrinolytic activity and post-operative deep-vein thrombosis. *Lancet*, **i**, 868.

Chakrabarti, R. & Fearnley, G. R. (1967) Reduction of platelet stickiness by phenformin plus ethyloestrenol. *Lancet*, **ii**, 1012.

Chakrabarti, R., Evans, J. F. & Fearnley, G. R. (1970) Effects on platelet stickiness and fibrinolysis of phenformin combined with ethyloestrenol or stanozolol. *Lancet*, **i**, 591.

Cunliffe, W. J. (1968) An association between cutaneous vasculitis and decreased blood fibrinolytic activity. *Lancet*, **i**, 1226.

Cunliffe, W. J. & Menon, I. S. (1971) The association between cutaneous vasculitis and decreased blood fibrinolytic activity. *British Journal of Dermatology*, **84**, 99.

Cunliffe, W. J., Roberts, B. E. & Dodman, B. (1973) Behçet's syndrome and oral fibrinolytic therapy. *British Medical Journal*, **ii**, 486.

Delaney, T. J. & Black, M. M. (1975) Effect of fibrinolytic treatment in malignant atrophic papulosis. *British Medical Journal*, **iii**, 415.

Dodman, B., Cunliffe, W. J., Roberts, B. E. & Sibbald, R. (1973) Clinical and laboratory double blind investigation on effect of fibrinolytic therapy in patients with cutaneous vasculitis. *British Medical Journal*, **ii**, 82.

Ekert, E. (1974) Thrombolytic therapy in haemolytic uraemic syndrome. *British Medical Journal*, **iv**, 533.

Fearnley, G. R. (1974) Fibrinolysis and deep vein thrombosis. *Lancet*, **i**, 455.

Fearnley, G. R. & Chakrabarti, R. (1964) Pharmacological enhancement of fibrinolytic activity of blood. *Journal of Clinical Pathology*, **17**, 328.

Fearnley, G. R. & Chakrabarti, R. (1965) Phenformin in rheumatoid arthritis, a fibrinolytic approach. *Lancet*, **i**, 9.

Fossard, D. P., Field, E. S., Kakkar, V. V., Friend, J. R., Corrigan, T. P. & Flute, P. T. (1974) Fibrinolytic activity and postoperative deep vein thrombosis. *Lancet*, **i**, 9.

Gilliam, J. N., Herdon, J. H. & Prystowsky, S. D. (1974) Fibrinolytic therapy for vasculitis of atrophie blanche. *Archives of Dermatology*, **109**, 664.

Gorog, P. & Kovács, I. B. (1972) Inhibitory effect of phenformin in adjuvant arthritis of rats. *Pharmacology*, **7**, 96.

Haustein, U. F. (1969) Purpura hyperfibrinolytica als pathogenetisches prinzip eines haemorrhagieschen mikrobides miescher. *Dermatologische Monatsschrift*, **155**, 771.

Innerfield, I. (1974) Enhancement of fibrinolytic activity. *Lancet*, **i**, 632.

Innes, D. & Sevitt, S. (1964) Coagulation and fibrinolysis in injured patients. *Journal of Clinical Pathology*, **17**, 1.

Innes, J. A., Campbell, I. W., Campbell, C. J., Needle, A. L. & Munro, J. F. (1974) Long term follow up of therapeutic starvation. *British Medical Journal*, **ii**, 356.

Isaacson, S., Linell, F., Moller, H. & Nilsson, I. M. (1970) Coagulation and fibrinolysis in chronic panniculitis. *Acta Dermato-venereologica*, **50**, 213.

Kurban, A. K. & Ryan, T. J. (1969) Fibrinogen titre, fibrinolytic and platelet stickiness correlated with capillary bleeding or block in the skin. *Transactions of the St John's Hospital Dermatological Society*, **55**, 218.

Nilsson, I. M. & Isaacson, S. (1972) New aspects of the pathogenesis of thrombo-embolism. *Progress in Surgery*, **11**, 46.

Paolino, J. S., Kaplan, D., Lazarus, R., Emmanuel, G. & Damond, H. S. (1972) Phenformin and ethyl-oestrenol in scleroderma. *Lancet*, **ii**, 1023.

Parish, W. E. (1972) Cutaneous vasculitis: antigen—antibody complexes and prolonged fibrinolysis. *Proceedings of the Royal Society of Medicine*, **65**, 276.

Preston, F. E. & Edwards, I. R. (1973) Postpartum purpura fulminans: successful management with streptokinase. *British Medical Journal*, **iii**, 329.

Swan, C. H., Williams, J. A. & Cooke, W. T. (1970) Fibrinolysis in colonic disease. *Gut*, **11**, 588.

Tibbutt, D. A., Davies, J. A., Anderson, J. A., Fletcher, E. W. L., Hamill, J., Holt, J. M., Thomas, M. L., Lee, G. de J., Miller, G. A. H., Sharp, A. A. & Sutton, G. C. (1974) Comparison by controlled clinical trial of streptokinase and heparin in treatment of life threatening pulmonary embolism. *British Medical Journal*, **i**, 343.

Turner, R. H. & Ryan, T. J. (1969) Fibrinolytic activity in human skin. *Transactions and Reports of the St John's Hospital Dermatological Society*, **55**, 212.

PLATELET AGGREGATION

Platelet aggregation is reduced by dipyridamole or cyproheptadine hydrochloride. These drugs reduce the frequency of arterial embolism in patients with prosthetic heart valves (Harker and Slichter, 1970). According to Harker and Slichter (1972), vasculitis, immune complex disease and arterial disease may be more dependent on platelet embolisation than on fibrin. They recommended oral dipyridamole 100 mg q.d.s., acetylsalicylic acid 4 g daily and prednisone 1 to 2 mg per kg body weight daily.

Wilding and Flute (1974) recommended dipyridamole for peripheral arterial occlusion, and it may have a place in the treatment of embolism from severe atheroma of the lower end of the aorta which causes skin gangrene.

Giromini et al (1972) reported considerable improvement in thrombotic micro-angiopathy when using aspirin and dipyridamole in cases in which heparin and aspirin had had little effect. Kincaird-Smith (1970) also recommended these drugs in acute glomerulonephritis, malignant hypertension and kidney transplant rejection.

Indomethacin, 75 to 175 mg per day, also inhibits platelet aggregation. It has been suggested (Gaetano et al, 1974) that intrarenal inhibition of platelet aggregation reduces subsequent intrarenal fibrin deposition in glomerulonephritis. In a proportion of such patients fibrin degradation products in the urine are reduced in amount. In glomerulonephritis, aspirin similarly reduces the urinary content of fibrin degradation products (Clarkson et al, 1972).

Gaetano et al (1974) believed that there is, however, a subgroup of patients who are non-responders, and that in these platelet aggregation is less strongly inhibited.

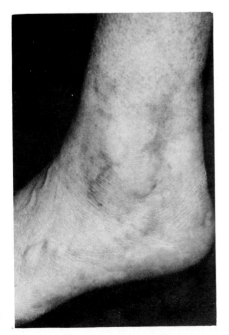
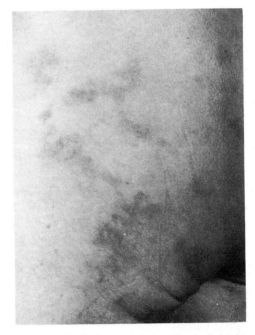

Figure 15.6. Areas of tender dusky erythema and slight palpable nodularity in two patients with raised platelet counts preceding the development of polycythaemia rubra vera. Their pain was strikingly relieved for up to three days by a 300 mg tablet of aspirin.

Elevated platelet counts account for haemorrhagic and thrombotic episodes in polycythaemia rubra vera (Dawson and Ogston, 1970). Edwards and Cooley (1970) found that 16 of 26 patients with this disease had presented with red or cyanotic fingers or toes, erythromelalgia or thrombophlebitis; six of them had a raised platelet count and a normal haematocrit.

Two patients presented to the author in 1972 with nodular vasculitis (Figure 15.6) and their pain was relieved by one aspirin tablet every three days. They all had a similarly elevated platelet count but did not develop measurable changes in their red cell or white cell counts over the subsequent six months.

As is often stated in this book, vasculitis is not a homogeneous disease; this is germane to the use of aspirin, indomethacin or fibrinolytic enhancers, for the author, in an uncontrolled series, has found that patients with more infarctive lesions or with deep nodular lesions do benefit, but that some patients with more urticarial lesions are made worse and occasionally their urticarial element is severely exacerbated — a well-known phenomenon in urticaria (Warin and Champion, 1974).

The speed with which pain is relieved by aspirin is diagnostic and was referred to by Preston et al (1974) who successfully treated six patients with essential thrombocythaemia and peripheral gangrene.

References

Clarkson, A. R., MacDonald, M. K., Cash, J. D. & Robson, J. S. (1972) Modification by drugs of urinary fibrin/fibrinogen degradation products in glomerulonephritis. *British Medical Journal,* **iii,** 255.
Dawson, A. A. & Ogston, D. (1970) The influence of the platelet count on the incidence of thrombotic and haemorrhagic complications in polycythaemia vera. *Postgraduate Medical Journal,* **46,** 76.
Edwards, E. A. & Cooley, M. H. (1970) Peripheral vascular symptoms as the initial manifestation of polycythaemia vera. *Journal of the American Medical Association,* **214,** 1463.
Gaetono, G. de, Vermylen, J., Donati, M. B., Dotremont, G. & Michielsen, P. (1974) Indomethacin and platelet aggregation in chronic glomerulonephritis; existence of non-responders. *British Medical Journal,* **ii,** 301.
Giromini, M., Bouvier, C. A., Dami, R., Denizot, M. & Jeannet, M. (1972) Effect of dipyridamole and aspirin in thrombotic microangiopathy. *British Medical Journal,* **i,** 545.
Harker, L. A. & Schlichter, S. J. (1970) Platelets and fibrinogen in patients with prosthetic heart valves. *New England Journal of Medicine,* **283,** 1302.
Harker, L. A. & Schlichter, S. J. (1972) Platelet and fibrinogen consumption in man. *New England Journal of Medicine,* **287,** 999.
Kincaird-Smith, P. (1970) The pathogenesis of the vascular and glomerular lesions of rejection in renal allografts and their modification by antithrombotic and anticoagulant drugs. *Australian Annals of Medicine,* **19,** 199.
Preston, F. E., Emmanuel, I. G., Winfield, D. A. & Malia, R. G. (1974) Essential thrombocythaemia and peripheral gangrene. *British Medical Journal,* **iii,** 549.
Warin, R. P. & Champion, R. H. (1974) *Urticaria.* London: W. B. Saunders.
Wilding, R. T. & Flute, P. T. (1974) Dipyridamole in peripheral upper limb ischaemia. *Lancet,* **ii,** 999.

CYTOTOXIC AGENTS

Azathioprine, mercaptopurine and corticosteroids have a part to play in the suppression of immune complex disease. In drug-induced disease, immunosuppression may be especially valuable after the withdrawal of the offending drug; acute reactions which should be short-lasting can be even more quickly suppressed. It is more difficult to suppress reactions occurring in diseases such as leprosy or tuberculosis, in which the infection is slow to be eliminated and may even be encouraged by immunosuppression.

Unbridled infection unleashed by immunosuppression is the commonest cause of death after transplantation.

Drugs such as methotrexate, mercaptopurine, chlorambucil, cyclophosphamide and azathioprine are used to suppress many of the diseases discussed in this book. That they have some beneficial effect is not disputed, but it is by no means always clear that the good they do is greater than that achieved by allowing spontaneous remission which at least has fewer side-effects. These drugs are antimetabolites and in particular they interfere with cell turnover. The activity of lymphocytes and plasma cells is thereby reduced, but so also is the activity of numerous other cells either caught or playing an essential role in the inflammatory process.

In recent years, achievement of an immunosuppressive effect has been the usual aim of prescribers of these drugs, but in practice it has to be admitted that it is not dramatic, and that the nonspecific anti-inflammatory action of these drugs may be just as important. There are few studies on the effects of these drugs in vasculitis of the skin, so most of the information of any use to dermatologists comes from the trials of antimetabolites in renal disease and in 'connective tissue' disorders.

In rheumatoid arthritis the beneficial effect of a drug like azathioprine is at best 'modest' and its side-effects frequent, troublesome and occasionally dangerous (Currey, 1971).

In systemic lupus erythematosus, a controlled trial was undertaken in which 16 patients took prednisolone plus azathioprine while 19 comparable patients took only prednisolone; over the one to four years of the trial a significantly improved prognosis was demonstrated in the group taking azathioprine. It is a usual finding that immuno-suppressive drugs permit a reduction in the dose of prednisolone (Sztejnbok et al, 1971). Often they also produce a reduction in, for example, rheumatoid factors and immuno-globulins, but this effect is not necessarily linked with clinical improvement. In lupus erythematosus, it is more important to assess the clinical response and renal function than the gamma-globulin, complement components, cryoglobulins, serum DNA and RNA antibodies, LE cells and antinuclear factor; yet a complete assessment must include them all.

Three other trials of azathioprine in lupus nephritis and systemic lupus erythematosus showed no benefit compared to steroids alone (Cade, Spooner and Schlein, 1973; Donaldio, Holley and Wagoner, 1974; Hahn, Kantor and Osterland, 1975).

The main indication for immunosuppressive drugs is as alternative therapy for patients intolerant of large doses of corticosteroids. In this respect, their use in vasculitis differs very little from that in other skin diseases such as pemphigus vulgaris (Jablonska, Chorzelski and Blaszczyk, 1970), and the complications of treatment are no less common.

It should be remembered that liver and renal function are sometimes impaired in vasculitis, particularly in the very ill, and in such patients, detoxication and excretion of immunosuppressive drugs are reduced and side-effects are more troublesome (Swanson and Schwartz, 1967; Mitchell et al, 1970).

An overall view of the value of these drugs in vasculitis is difficult to obtain, and to some extent vasculitis includes such a varied mixture of processes that it makes nonsense to lump them all together for the purpose of therapy. Yet nobody has attempted to separate these diseases and to assess therapy according to mechanisms. It does appear, however, that the milder forms of vasculitis have an urticarial element and show little necrosis, and that the prognosis in the absence of necrosis is good. Diseases that have progressed to infarction and ulceration, like polyarteritis nodosa, Wegener's granuloma-tosis or even Behçet's disease, have a higher mortality, which immunosuppressive drugs do not reduce.

At the present time, several reports suggest that the drugs of first choice in Wegener's granulomatosis are the immunosuppressive agents, including azathioprine (Bouroncle, Smith and Cuppage, 1967; Kaplan, Hayslett and Calabresi, 1968; Norton, Suki and Stunk, 1968; Peermohamed and Shafar, 1969; Aldo et al, 1970; Raitt, 1971), methotrexate (Aldo et al, 1970; Capizzi and Bertino, 1971), cyclophosphamide (Greenspan, 1965; Fauci, Wolff and Johnson, 1971; Raitt, 1971; Novack and Pearson, 1971) and chlorambucil (McIlvanie, 1966; Hollander and Manning, 1967). However, some limited forms of vasculitis have a good prognosis without such drugs (Carrington and Liebow, 1968; Cassan, Coles and Harrison, 1970).

Azathioprine

Azathioprine, derived from mercaptopurine, has a greater immunosuppressive action, but an equal antimitotic effect (Bach, Dardenne and Fournier, 1969). It is converted to mercaptopurine in the body. No adequate trials of its use in vasculitis have yet been carried out so any assessment depends somewhat on the evaluation of the drug by clinicians using it for nephritis, lupus erythematosus and related diseases.

The Medical Research Council (1971) controlled trial showed no benefit from azathioprine and prednisolone in glomerulonephritis, although Michael et al (1967) reported their effectiveness when used in a higher dosage in a series which included three cases of nephritis in Schönlein—Henoch purpura. McIntosh et al (1972) observed favourable responses in glomerulonephritis only in patients with clinical and morphological findings similar to those seen in patients who recover spontaneously. In their trial they used azathioprine 4 mg/kg body weight with prednisolone 60 mg/m² of body surface each on alternative days.

The drug is not dramatically successful in ulcerative colitis (Jewell and Truelove, 1972). However, Goldbloom and Drummond (1968) reported a case of anaphylactoid purpura with nephrosis not responding to steroids but which improved dramatically on azathioprine. Steroids in combination with azathioprine are recommended by Hutas, Miklos and Fenyes (1969), Kustner et al (1971), and Wishart (1975). Schopf, Schultz and Schultz (1969) provided a convincing account of localised gangrene of the breast healing on azathioprine, and Maldonado et al (1968) used mercaptopurine in a similar case. Azathioprine has been used successfully for livedo with ulceration (Braun-Falco and Meigel, 1972), and Behçet's disease (Rosselet, Soudan and Zenklusen, 1968; Nethercott and Lester, 1974).

Zarem and Dimitrievich (1970) studied the effect of azathioprine on the microvasculature of full-thickness skin allografts in the mouse. The maturation of the blood vessels was delayed and the sticking of white cells to the endothelium was minimised. Moreover, the endothelium was less swollen and blood flow was maintained for seven days longer than in control mice.

The hazards of using these drugs, apart from causing depression of leucopoiesis, may include a long-term risk of neoplasia. This is an unresolved question raised by animal experiments (Doell, De Vaux and Grabar, 1967; Casey, 1968a, 1968b), and arising in man after renal transplantations (Karnofsky, 1967; Schneck and Penn, 1971).

There have been a number of reports of malignancy appearing and then quickly disseminating in patients on azathioprine, and although this is a problem particularly in renal transplantation (Hoover and Traumeni, 1973), it has been described also in skin diseases (Burton and Greaves, 1974). In addition, Sneddon and Wishart (1972) reported a reticulosarcoma of the vulva occurring in a patient receiving azathioprine for dermatomyositis. However, some very large surveys have not given much support to this association (McEwan and Petty, 1972). Furthermore, Mason et al (1973), discussing immunosuppression in young persons of child-bearing age, suggested that, from their experience of six cases, this drug has little effect on sperm counts compared to cyclophosphamide, which not only depresses it drastically — albeit reversibly (Buchanan et al, 1975) but also causes amenorrhoea (Feng et al, 1973; Snaith et al, 1973). Chlorambucil also produces amenorrhoea.

Cyclophosphamide and chlorambucil

Cyclophosphamide has the theoretical advantage of inducing immune tolerance (Dukor and Dietrich, 1968) and acts in a suppressive fashion on experimental autoimmune disease (Gerebtzoff et al, 1972). It is more effective than other alkylating agents in suppressing antibody production (Crabbe et al, 1969; Lemmell, Hurd and Ziff, 1971), and it depresses T cell as well as B cell functions (Ziff, Hurd and Stastny, 1974).

Crawford, Sherman and Favara (1967) reported that cyclophosphamide induced a sustained remission in cases of pyoderma gangrenosum that had failed to respond to intensive adrenocorticosteroid therapy. Behçet's disease had also responded to cyclophosphamide (Buckley and Gills, 1969). Mathison et al (1971) treated purpura, arthralgia and glomerulonephritis due to mixed cryoglobulinaemia by splenectomy as well as cyclophosphamide in the belief that the spleen produced much of the abnormal protein.

Feng et al (1973) have treated 42 cases of systemic lupus erythematosus with this drug for more than seven years without severe complications; and response to therapy is often very good. Hill and Scott (1964), Cameron et al (1970), Steinberg et al (1971) and Fauci, Wolff and Johnson (1971) have recommended its use in Wegener's granulomatosis. White, Cameron and Trounce (1966) reported improvement in three children in whom nephrosis followed Schönlein—Henoch syndrome, and later, in 1971, suggested that cyclophosphamide was the drug of choice in the steroid-dependent nephrotic child following Schönlein—Henoch nephritis.

The toxic effects of cyclophosphamide become apparent within two to four weeks of starting oral administration. They are reversible but the white cell count may continue to fall for 10 days after stopping the drug (Goodman and Gilman, 1965). For young patients the loss of hair caused by cyclophosphamide may be intolerable. Another unpleasant side-effect is sterile haemorrhagic cystitis, but it is quickly reversible. Vasculitis, presenting as purpura and skin ulceration with Raynaud's phenomenon and not responding to steroids, nevertheless responded well to chlorambucil in a series of patients with systemic lupus erythematosis including nephritis (Snaith et al, 1973). These authors recommended chlorambucil rather than azathioprine and cyclophosphamide because side-effects are few.

Swanson and Schwartz (1967) found that some immune responses were suppressed and others enhanced. Clinical response, however, did not correlate with the immune suppressive effect, therefore they considered that drugs such as azathioprine and methotrexate act through their anti-inflammatory effect.

References

Aldo, M. A., Benson, M. D., Comerford, F. R. & Cohen, A. S. (1970) Treatment of Wegener's granulomatosis with immunosuppressive agents; description of renal ultrastructure. *Archives of Internal Medicine,* **126,** 298.
Bach, J. F., Dardenne, M. & Fournier, C. (1969) In vitro evaluation of immunosuppressive drugs. *Nature,* **222,** 998.
Bouroncle, B. A., Smith, E. J. & Cuppage, F. E. (1967) Treatment of Wegener's granulomatosis with Imuran. *American Journal of Medicine,* **42,** 314.

Braun-Falco, O. & Meigel, W. (1972) Zur Azathioprin-Therapie der idiopathischen Livedo Racemosa mit Ulcerationen. *Hautartz*, **23**, 136.

Buchanan, J. D., Fairley, K. F. & Barrie, J. U. (1975) Return of spermatogenesis after stopping cyclophosphamide therapy. *Lancet*, **i**, 156.

Buckley, G. E. & Gills, J. P. Jr (1969) Cyclophosphamide therapy of Behçet's disease. *Journal of Allergy*, **43**, 273.

Burton, J. L. & Greaves, M. W. (1974) Azathioprine for pemphigus and pemphigoid — a four year follow up. *British Journal of Dermatology*, **91**, 103.

Cade, R., Spooner, G. & Schlein, E. (1973) Comparison of azathioprine, prednisolone and heparin alone or combined in treating lupus nephritis. *Nephron*, **10**, 37.

Cameron, J. S., Boulton-Jones, M., Robinson, R. & Ogg, C. (1970) Treatment of lupus nephritis with cyclophosphamide. *Lancet*, **ii**, 846.

Capizzi, R. L. & Bertino, J. R. (1971) Methotrexate therapy of Wegener's granulomatosis. *Annals of Internal Medicine*, **74**, 74.

Carrington, C. B. & Liebow, A. A. (1968) Limited forms of angiitis and granulomatosis of Wegener's type. *American Journal of Medicine*, **41**, 497.

Casey, T. P. (1968a) The development of lymphomas in mice with autoimmune disorders treated with azathioprine. *Blood*, **31**, 396.

Casey, T. P. (1968b) Azathioprine (Imuran) administration and the development of malignant lymphomas in NZB mice. *Clinical and Experimental Immunology*, **3**, 305.

Cassan, S. M., Coles, D. T. & Harrison, E. G. (1970) The concept of limited forms of Wegener's granulomatosis. *American Journal of Medicine*, **49**, 366.

Crabbe, P. A., Nash, D. R. & Bazin, W. (1969) Antibodies of the IgA type in intestinal plasma cells of germ free mice after oral or parenteral immunization with ferritin. *Journal of Experimental Medicine*, **130**, 723.

Crawford, S. E., Sherman, R. & Favara, B. (1967) Pyoderma gangrenosum with response to cyclophosphamide therapy. *Journal of Pediatrics*, **71**, 255.

Currey, H. L. F. (1971) *Modern Trends in Rheumatology*, 2nd edition (Ed.) Hill, A. G. S. p. 174. London: Butterworths.

Doeglas, H. M. G. & Bleumink, E. (1974) Familial cold urticaria. *Archives of Dermatology*, **110**, 382.

Doell, R. G., De Vaux St. Cyr, C. & Grabar, P. (1967) Immune reactivity prior to development of thymic lymphoma in C57 BL mice. *International Journal of Cancer*, **2**, 103.

Donaldio, J. V., Holley, K. E. & Wagoner, R. D. (1974) Further observations on the treatment of lupus nephritis and prednisolone and combined prednisolone and azathioprine. *Arthritis and Rheumatism*, **17**, 573.

Dukor, P. & Dietrich, F. M. (1968) Characteristic features of immunosuppression by steroids and cytotoxic drugs. *International Archives of Allergy*, **34**, 32.

Fauci, A. S., Wolff, S. M. & Johnson, J. S. (1971) Effect of cyclophosphamide upon the immune response in Wegener's granulomatosis. *New England Journal of Medicine*, **285**, 1493.

Feng, P. H., Jayaratnam, F. J., Tock, E. P. C. & Seah, C. S. (1973) Cyclophosphamide in treatment of systemic lupus erythematosus. Seven years experience. *British Medical Journal*, **ii**, 450.

Gerebtzoff, A., Lambert, P. H. & Miescher, P. A. (1972) Immunosuppressive agents. *Annual Review of Pharmacology*, **12**, 287.

Goldbloom, R. B. & Drummond, K. N. (1968) Anaphylactoid purpura with massive gastrointestinal haemorrhage and glomerulonephritis. *American Journal of Diseases of Children*, **116**, 97.

Goodman, L. S. & Gilman, A. (1965) *The Pharmacological Basis of Therapeutics*, 3rd edition. New York: Macmillan.

Greenspan, E. M. (1965) Cyclophosphamide and prednisone therapy of lethal midline granuloma. *Journal of the American Medical Association*, **193**, 74.

Hahn, B. H., Kantor, O. S. & Osterland, C. K. (1975) Azathioprine plus prednisolone alone in the treatment of systemic lupus erythematosus. Report of a prospective controlled trial in 24 patients. *Annals of Internal Medicine*, **83**, 597.

Hill, R. D. & Scott, G. W. (1964) Cytotoxic drugs for systemic lupus. *British Medical Journal*, **i**, 370.

Hollander, D. & Manning, R. T. (1967) The use of alkylating agents in the treatment of Wegener's granulomatosis. *Annals of Internal Medicine*, **67**, 393.

Hoover, R. & Traumeni, J. F. Jr (1973) Risk of cancer in renal transplant recipients. *Lancet*, **ii**, 55.

Hutas, I., Miklos, G. Y. & Fenyes, D. (1969) Immunosuppressive therapia Wegener Granulomatosisban. *Orv Hetilap*, **110**, 2164.

Jablonska, S., Chorzelski, T. & Blaszczyk, M. (1970) Immunosuppressants in the treatment of pemphigus. *British Journal of Dermatology*, **83**, 315.

Jewell, D. P. & Truelove, S. C. (1972) Azathioprine in ulcerative colitis. Final report on a controlled therapeutic trial. *British Medical Journal*, **iv**, 627.

Kaplan, S. R., Hayslett, J. P. & Calabresi, P. (1968) Treatment of advanced Wegener's granulomatosis with azathioprine and diazomycin. *New England Journal of Medicine*, **278**, 239.

Karnofsky, D. A. (1967) Symposium on immunosuppressive drugs. Late effects of immunosuppressive anti-cancer drugs. *Federation Proceedings*, **26**, 925.

Kustner, W., Lubbers, P., Uthgenannt, H. & Wegener, F. (1971) Die Wegenersche Granulomatose diagnostische probleme und klinische verlaub unter immunosuppressiver Therapie. *Schweizerische medizinische Wochenschrift*, **101**, 1137.

Lemmel, E., Hurd, E. R. & Ziff, M. (1971) Differential effects of 6-mercaptopurine and cyclophosphamide on autoimmune phenomena in N.Z.B. mice. *Clinical and Experimental Immunology*, **8**, 355.

Maldonado, N., Torres, V. M., Mendez-Cashion, D., Perez-Santiago, E. & de Costas, M. C. (1968) Pyoderma gangrenosa treated with 6-mercaptopurine and followed by acute leukaemia. *Journal of Pediatrics*, **72**, 409.

Mason, M., Brown, John A. M., Harris, J. & Woodland, J. (1973) Treatment of systemic lupus erythematosus. *British Medical Journal*, **ii**, 422.

Mathison, D. A., Condemi, J. J., Leddy, J. P., Callerame, M. L., Panner, B. J. & Vaughan, J. H. (1971) Purpura, arthralgia and IgM and IgG cryoglobulinaemia with rheumatoid factor activity: response to cyclophosphamide and splenectomy. *Annals of Internal Medicine*, **74**, 383.

McEwan, A. & Petty, L. G. (1972) Oncogenicity of immunosuppressive drugs. *Lancet*, **i**, 326.

McIlvanie, S. K. (1966) Wegener's granulomatosis; successful treatment with chlorambucil. *Journal of the American Medical Association*, **197**, 90.

McIntosh, R. M., Griswold, W., Smith, F. G., Kaufman, D. B., Urizar, R. & Vernier, R. L. (1972) Azathioprine in glomerulonephritis: a long term study. *Lancet*, **i**, 1085.

Medical Research Council Working Party (1971) Controlled trial of azathioprine and prednisone in chronic renal disease. *British Medical Journal*, **ii**, 239.

Michael, A. F., Vernier, R. L., Drummond, K. N., Levitt, J. L., Herdmann, R. C., Fish, A. M. & Good, R. A. (1967) Immunosuppressive therapy for chronic renal disease. *New England Journal of Medicine*, **276**, 817.

Mitchell, C. G., Eddleston, A. L. W. F., Smith, M. G. M. & Williams, R. (1970) Serum immunosuppressive activity due to azathioprine and its relations to hepatic function after liver transplantation. *Lancet*, **i**, 1196.

Nethercott, J. & Lester, R. S. (1974) Azathioprine therapy in incomplete Behçet syndrome. *Archives of Dermatology*, **110**, 432.

Norton, W. L., Suki, W. & Stunk, S. (1968) Combined corticosteroid and azathioprine therapy in two patients with Wegener's granulomatosis. *Archives of Internal Medicine*, **121**, 554.

Novack, S. N. & Pearson, C. M. (1971) Cyclophosphamide therapy in Wegener's granulomatosis. *New England Journal of Medicine*, **248**, 938.

Peermohamed, A. R. & Shafar, J. (1969) Sustained azathioprine induced remission in Wegener's granulomatosis. *British Medical Journal*, **iv**, 600.

Raitt, J. W. (1971) Wegeners granulomatosis: treatment with cytotoxic agents and adrenocorticosteroids. *Annals of Internal Medicine*, **74**, 344.

Rosselet, E., Soudan, Y. & Zenklusen, G. (1968) Les éffêts de l'azathrioprine (Imuran) dans la mâladie de Behçet. *Ophthalmologica*, **156**, 218.

Schneck, S. A. & Penn, I. (1971) De novo brain tumours in renal transplant recipients. *Lancet*, **i**, 983.

Schopf, E., Schultz, H. J. & Schultz, K. H. (1969) Azathioprin Behandlung der Dermatitis ulcerosa (Pyoderma Gangrenosum). *Hautartz*, **20**, 558.

Snaith, M. L., Holt, J. M., Oliver, D. O., Dunnill, M. S., Halley, W. & Stephenson, A. C. (1973) Treatment of patients with systemic lupus erythematosus, including nephritis, with chlorambucil. *British Medical Journal*, **ii**, 197.

Sneddon, I. & Wishart, J. M. (1972) Immunosuppression and malignancy. *British Medical Journal*, **iii**, 238.

Steinberg, A. D., Kattreider, H. B., Staples, P. J., Goetzz, N. T., Talal, N. & Decker, J. L. (1971) Cyclophosphamide in lupus nephritis; a controlled trial. *Annals of Internal Medicine*, **75**, 165.

Swanson, M. A. & Schwartz, R. S. (1967) Immunosuppressive therapy, the relation between clinical response and immunologic competence. *New England Journal of Medicine*, **277**, 163.

Sztejnbok, M., Stewart, A., Diamond, H. & Kaplan, D. (1971) Azathioprine in the treatment of systemic lupus erythematosus. A controlled study. *Arthritis and Rheumatism*, **14**, 639.

White, R. H. R., Cameron, J. S. & Trounce, J. R. (1966) Immunosuppressive therapy in steroid resistant proliferative glomerulonephritis accompanied by the nephrotic syndrome. *British Medical Journal*, **ii**, 853.

Wishart, J. M. (1975) Wegener's granulomatosis controlled by azathioprine and corticosteroids. *British Journal of Dermatology*, **92**, 461.

Zarem, H. A. & Dimitrievich, G. S. (1970) In vivo observations of effects of imuran on microvasculature within full thickness mouse skin allografts. *Plastic and Reconstructive Surgery*, **45**, 51.

Ziff, M., Hurd, E. R. & Stastny, P. (1974) B and T lymphocytes in rheumatoid synovitis and the effect of cyclophosphamide. *Proceedings of the Royal Society of Medicine*, **67**, 536.

Corticosteroids

Cameron (1972) stated that no adequately controlled trials had ever shown that corticosteroids, azathioprine or cyclophosphamide, alone or in combination, could produce any long term beneficial effect whatsoever in any variety of glomerulonephritis that does not have a marked tendency to remit or to heal spontaneously. The same can be said with certainty about forms of vasculitis that affect the skin, though on present evidence one suspects that there are some complicated systemic variants, Wegener's granulomatosis being one, that might form a significant subgroup in respect of therapy. Indeed, some of the most acute forms of vasculitis, and in particular some specific complications affecting the eye, joints or gut, are quickly alleviated by large doses of steroids.

Steroids revolutionised the treatment of many of the diseases described in this monograph. However, there are few instances in which they are the essential and undisputed therapy for the disease. Temporal arteritis with incipient blindness is one example. Jennings (1973), for instance, believed that prednisolone should be prescribed immediately to anyone over 60 years of age who has slight tenderness and thickening of a temporal artery, accompanied by malaise, 'rheumatic' symptoms and a raised ESR.

Allen, Diamond and Howell (1960), reviewing 131 cases of Schönlein—Henoch purpura in children, claimed that steroids were chiefly of value for severe and uncomfortable localised soft tissue oedema, particularly of the scalp, eyes, joints or intestine. About one-third of cases lost this oedema and discomfort within the first 24 hours of administration. Abdominal colic was relieved in approximately 50 per cent of cases within about 72 hours. Such findings have not been confirmed in a controlled trial, and one might expect significant spontaneous improvement within three days in a high proportion of children. Allen, Diamond and Howell (1960) recorded no intussusception in those treated with steroids whereas it occurred in four cases not so treated. Ramsay and Fry (1969) found that patients responded to as little as 25 mg of prednisolone daily, but it was not possible to withdraw the drugs within six weeks.

The dangers of short-term prescription of steroids are negligible compared to the dangers of prolonged massive intestinal bleeding caused by the disease; therefore, cases sufficiently severe to require transfusion should also be given a high dose of steroids, intravenously if necessary (Stefanini and Martino, 1956; Cohen et al, 1967; Goldbloom and Drummond, 1968). High dosage was also recommended by Hardisty (1968) who gave oral prednisolone in a dose of 2 mg/kg of body weight per day up to a maximum of 60 mg t.d.s.

Jansen et al (1971) produced experimental evidence that the vasculitis from the bite of the Brown Recluse Spider is less severe if steroids are prescribed (Figure 15.7).

There is nothing to be gained from continuing steroids if there has been no symptomatic relief within three to four weeks and, in the author's opinion, no advantage is likely after one week's failure to respond to adequate dosage. As far as the skin is concerned, corticosteroids have least effect on necrotising or infarctive forms of vasculitis once the lesion has developed. The infarctive lesions of Wegener's granulomatosis, for example, do poorly on steroids compared to immunosuppressive drugs (Walton, 1958; Beidleman, 1963; Aldo et al, 1970) (Table 15.5). Their maximum effect is on deep tender swellings in which blood flow is still maintained, such as deep pressure urticaria, erythema nodosum, early pyoderma gangrenosum or Behçet's disease. When these deep lesions are associated with ulcerative colitis or regional enteritis, the response to steroids is particularly satisfactory, whereas the gangrene associated with the purpura fulminans picture of disseminated intravascular coagulation is not so responsive.

Experimental studies on the Shwartzman phenomenon suggest that steroids prepare

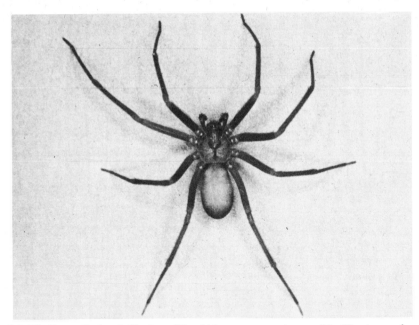

Figure 15.7. The Brown Recluse Spider has a bite which causes an acute vasculitis. The degree of necrosis is minimised when methyl prednisolone is administered within six hours of the bite.

Table 15.5. Comparison of results of steroids and immunosuppressive therapy.

	Controls	Steroids	Azathioprine and alkylating drugs
Average lifespan	5	12.5	18.7+
One-year survival rate %	18	34	80

for the generalised Shwartzman reaction. In skin diseases they generally have a suppressive or an initially stabilising action on endothelium, but this is only short-term and is replaced by an unstable sensitivity of the microcirculation associated with stimulation of the alpha-adrenergic receptor sites (Latour, Prejean and Margaretten, 1971). In this respect they are most valuable in the short-term management of vasculitis when the trigger is a transient one, but when the trigger persists the gradual dependence and instability that steroids induce in the tissues may make them more vulnerable. Other authors have expressed their belief that they have little effect on the duration of the illness, the frequency of recurrences or the renal consequences; or for that matter on the vasculitis (Allen, Diamond and Howell, 1960; Goldbloom and Drummond, 1968; Hardisty, 1968).

Some low-grade chronic forms of pyoderma gangrenosum respond to intralesional triamcinolone (Moschella, 1967; Gardner and Acker, 1972), and systemic steroids have been used with sulphapyridine to control pyoderma gangrenosum associated with myeloma (Jablonska, Stachow and Dabrowska, 1967).

Corticotrophin (ACTH) is recommended for patients who will tolerate regular injections since it is free from the dangers of adrenal suppression and rarely causes gastric ulceration. Tetracosactide is free from foreign protein but may nevertheless, like corticotrophin, cause the occasional allergic reaction.

Many patients with leg lesions are immobile and, particularly if they are in the older age groups, they are liable to develop severe osteoporosis. Conversely, young patients with corticosteroid-treated allergic disorders such as asthma or atopy seem to tolerate steroids extraordinarily well (Klein, Villaneuva and Frost, 1965). Hosking and Chamberlain (1973) suggested that any tendency to produce osteoporosis may be more than compensated for by the return of well-being and mobility produced by this form of therapy. Steroid purpura is a useful clue to the development of osteoporosis; about one-third of patients who develop steroid purpura do so early but the rest may not show it for years (McConkey, 1973).

THE MANAGEMENT OF ACUTE GLOMERULONEPHRITIS

Dermatologists should be familiar with the early management of acute glomerulo-nephritis caused by systemic vasculitis, but renal failure and chronic glomerulonephritis are best managed in renal units. In the initial stages, bed rest and fluid restriction to 0.5 litres per day should be prescribed, and the volume lost in urine and vomitus during the previous 24 hours should be estimated and replaced. The diet should be low in protein, salt and potassium (chocolate, fruit, vegetables and brown sugar are rich in potassium).

Anuria, uraemia and hypertension are indications for referral to a renal unit. However, as the blood urea is a relatively insensitive test, it is best to monitor the plasma creatinine which is less influenced by diet and glomerular filtration rate; this test can be done in most laboratories. Normal values range from 0.4 mg/100 ml at two years of age to 1 mg/100 ml at adolescence. Autoanalysers usually give slightly higher figures.

References

Aldo, M. A., Benson, M. D., Comerford, F. R. & Cohen, A. S. (1970) Treatment of Wegener's granulomato-sis with immunosuppressive agents; description of renal ultrastructure. *Archives of Internal Medicine,* **126,** 298.

Allen, D. M., Diamond, L. K. & Howell, D. A. (1960) Anaphylactoid purpura in children (Schönlein—Henoch syndrome). Review with a follow up of renal complications. *American Journal of Diseases of Children,* **99,** 333.

Beidleman, B. (1963) Wegener's granulomatosis. Prolonged therapy with large doses of steroids. *Journal of the American Medical Association,* **186,** 827.

Burton, J. L. & Greaves, M. W. (1974) Azathioprine for pemphigus and pemphigoid — a four year follow up. *British Journal of Dermatology,* **91,** 103.

Cameron, J. S. (1972) Bright's disease today: the pathogenesis and treatment of glomerulonephritis III. *British Medical Journal,* **iv,** 217.

Cohen, S., Benacerraf, B., McCluskey, R. Y. & Ovary, Z. (1967) Effect of anticoagulants on delayed hyper-sensitivity reactions. *Journal of Immunology,* **98,** 351.

Gardner, L. W. & Acker, D. W. (1972) Triamcinolone and pyoderma gangrenosum. *Archives of Dermatology,* **106,** 599.

Goldbloom, R. B. & Drummond, K. N. (1968) Anaphylactoid purpura with massive gastrointestinal haemorrhage and glomerulonephritis. *American Journal of Diseases of Children,* **116,** 97.

Hardisty, R. M. (1968) Treatment of non-thrombocytopenic purpura. In *Treatment of Hemorrhagic Disorders* (Ed.) Ratnoff, O. D. p. 223. New York: Harper and Row.

Hosking, D. J. & Chamberlain, M. J. (1973) Osteoporosis and long-term corticosteroid therapy. *British Medical Journal,* **iii,** 125.

Jablonska, S., Stachow, A. & Dabrowska, H. (1967) Entre la pyodermite gangreneuse et le myélôme. *Annales de Dermatologie et de Syphiligraphie,* **94,** 121.

Jansen, G. T., Morgan, P. N., McQueen, J. N. & Bennett, W. E. (1971) The brown recluse spider bite — controlled evaluation of treatment using the white rabbit as an animal model. *Southern Medical Journal,* **64,** 1194.

Jennings, G. H. (1973) Blindness in granulomatous arteralgia. *British Medical Journal*, **i**, 415.

Klein, M., Villaneuva, A. R. & Frost, H. M. (1965) A quantitative histological study of rib from 18 patients treated with adrenal corticosteroids. *Acta Orthopaedica Scandinavica*, **35**, 171.

Latour, J. G., Prejean, J. P. & Margaretten, W. (1971) Corticosteroids and the generalised Shwartzman reaction. *American Journal of Pathology*, **65**, 189.

Levin, M. B. & Pinkus, H. (1961) Autosensitivity to desoxyribonucleic acid (DNA). Report of a case with inflammatory skin lesions controlled by chloroquine. *New England Journal of Medicine*, **264**, 533.

McConkey, B. (1973) Osteoporosis and long term corticosteroid therapy. *British Medical Journal*, **iii**, 498.

Moschella, S. L. (1967) Pyoderma gangrenosum. A patient successfully treated with intralesional injection of steroid. *Archives of Dermatology*, **95**, 121.

Ramsay, C. & Fry, L. (1969) Allergic vasculitis, clinical and histological features and incidence of renal involvement. *British Journal of Dermatology*, **81**, 96.

Stefanini, M. & Martino, M. B. (1956) Use of prednisone in the management of some hemorrhagic states. *New England Journal of Medicine*, **254**, 313.

Walton, E. W. (1958) Giant cell granuloma of the respiratory tract (Wegener's granulomatosis). *British Medical Journal*, **ii**, 265.

LOW MOLECULAR WEIGHT DEXTRAN

Cunliffe and Menon (1969) studied 22 patients with peripheral vascular disease of the small vessel type associated with systemic sclerosis, systemic lupus erythematosus, rheumatoid arthritis, dermatomyositis, idiopathic Raynaud's phenomenon and chilblains. Eighteen had decreased blood fibrinolytic activity, but following an infusion of low molecular weight dextran, fibrinolytic activity rose to normal levels and remained there for several weeks. Subsequently, Issroff and Whiting (1971) reported the success of this treatment in livedo reticularis with ulceration. The author also has used low molecular weight dextran on several occasions for chronic ulceration of the legs associated with gross microvascular stasis. In some patients it quickly relieves pain and promotes healing. But occasionally deeper shunting channels are opened up instead of the capillaries that supply the epidermis, and then diffuse, dark, punctate lesions can be seen, caused by a total cessation of flow through engorged papillary vessels. However, this is not necessarily disastrous, possibly because the skin as a whole may have improved oxygenation. Nevertheless, prolonged observation of the microvasculature of mouth ulcers has led to the suggestion that low molecular weight dextran is less effective than heparin in relieving congestion in the papillary vessels (Ryan, 1966).

Myers and his group in New Orleans claimed that Dextran 40 seemed to augment survival of skin flaps subjected to pure venous occlusion (see Chapter 5), but the drug had little effect on cutaneous flaps in dogs. The original idea was that Dextran 40 would thin the blood, but some workers have suggested that it thickens it (Myers, 1975).

Tables 15.6, 15.7 and 15.8, taken from studies of 150 patients by Holti (1973), report the use of low molecular weight dextran, illustrating the action and clinical response, and listing the precautions to be taken.

Table 15.6. Low molecular weight dextran effects upon blood and blood vessels.

1. Increase of colloid osmotic pressure
2. Decrease of blood viscosity
3. Disaggregation of red cell clumps and fibrinogen—fibrin complexes; decrease of platelet aggregation and adhesiveness
4. Decrease of abnormally prolonged fibrinolysis
5. Decrease of abnormally increased serum cholesterol and phospholipids
6. Coating of vascular endothelium interfering with adhesion of circulating cells to vessel walls
7. Increase in lymphatic flow

Table 15.7. Objective response to intermittent infusions of low molecular weight dextran of 150 patients with peripheral vascular diseases.

Diagnosis	No. of patients	Peak increase in finger temperature more than (°C)			Clinical response		
		1.0	0.5—1.0	0.5	Good	Fair	None
Systemic sclerosis	48	46	2	—	44	4	—
Lupus erythematosus	14	14	—	—	14	—	—
Dermatomyositis	4	4	—	—	4	—	—
Polyarteritis nodosa	5	4	1	—	5	—	—
Arteriosclerosis obliterans	33	21	10	2	21	12	—
Rheumatoid arthritis	6	5	1	—	6	—	—
Familial Raynaud's phenomenon of early onset	4	—	—	4	—	—	4
Chilblains	36	—	6	30	36	—	—

Table 15.8. Precautions during infusions with low molecular weight dextran.

1. Rate of infusion 1 l/24 h
2. Urinary output above 1.5 l
3. Specific gravity of urine not to rise above 1045
4. Blood urea below 60 mg/100 ml
5. 4-hourly temperature and pulse record during waking hours
6. Frequent inspection of the infusion site

HYPERBARIC OXYGEN THERAPY

An increase in partial pressure of oxygen in the lungs from 100 mm to 1500 to 2000 mm will result in a proportionately greater quantity of oxygen being taken up by the arterial blood in physically dissolved form. This blood with an increased oxygen content delivers more oxygen to the tissues. To make use of this principle in treatment requires special chambers in which the entire patient can be exposed to 2 to 3 atmospheres absolute pressure. Treatment consists of two-hour periods in the chamber three or four times per day. Periods longer than this cause sickness, cramps, and if used over a prolonged period, cataracts develop (Barr, Enfors and Eriksson, 1972).

The method has been used to reduce bacterial infection of the skin (McAllister et al, 1963; Irvin and Smith, 1968) and for various types of leg ulcers (Illingworth, 1962; Bird and Telfer, 1965; Slack, Thomas and De Jode, 1966; Barthelemy, Parc and Mathé, 1967; Besznyak, Nemes and Sebsetény, 1970; Mantz and Temple, 1968; Shaldin, 1969; Barr and Benson, 1970; Bass, 1970; Kidokoro et al, 1970; Lefebvre et al, 1970).

Local oxygen therapy can be applied to leg ulcers by enclosing the leg in a bag into which oxygen is delivered, and although this procedure is often drying and painful, it has been used in dermatology clinics in South Africa and by the author.

Wadell et al (1965), Kuzemko and Loder (1970), Barr, Enfors and Eriksson (1972) and Thomas, Crouch and Guastello (1974) all have reported the value of hyperbaric oxygen in pyoderma gangrenosum. The author of this monograph noted immediate improvement in the colour of the skin lesions of one such patient on each of repeated treatments, but to secure the return of the circulation, heparin therapy was necessary. Several patients of dermatologists in the Oxford region have received hyperbaric oxygen at the R.A.F. Hospital, Wroughton, with considerable benefit.

Dowling, Copeman and Ashfield (1967) described improvement of Raynaud's phenomenon in scleroderma, and Barr, Enfors and Eriksson (1972) reported improvement of the whole skin as well as ulcers in one severe case of scleroderma. Roding, Groeneveld and Boerema (1972) have treated 130 patients with clostridial gas-producing infections; after five treatments each for two hours within the first 48 hours no deaths occurred.

Studies of sickle cell anaemia are informative, since in this disease hypoxia at a local site on the leg may follow quite mild inflammation or injury and be sufficient to produce severe sickling (Moschella in discussion of Parish, 1972).

For a discussion of the relative merits of different sizes of chambers readers are referred to the correspondence columns of the *British Medical Journal* (23rd September, 1972) that followed a leading article on this subject.

AMPUTATION

Especially when the factors contributing to chronic vasculitis are localised predominantly to the lower leg, the disablement may be out of all proportion to the local lesion. One is sometimes faced with the problem of a seemingly irreparable limb which is grossly ulcerated and ischaemic and is causing intolerable pain and prolonged immobilisation. Such a limb is useless and even were healing to take place, further breakdown would be likely; under these circumstances the question of amputation should be considered. A good stump is painless and with a good prosthesis amputation causes very little restriction to a normal life.

A distinction must be made between the ulcer that is a consequence of microvascular disease and that due to generalised arterial disease. The prognosis for a life of good quality from the latter is poor (Little, 1975), and Little, Petrisi-Jones and Kerr (1974) painted a gloomy picture of loss of employment and social activity in such cases. Women are more likely to be concerned by the cosmetic aspects of amputation. One also has to be aware of religions in which wholeness of the body in this life and later life is considered important.

References

Barr, P. O. & Benson, F. (1970) Clinical application of OPH in Sweden. In *Proceedings of the 4th International Congress on Hyperbaric Medicine* (Ed.) Wada, J. & Iwa, T. p. 531. London: Bailliere, Tindall and Cassall.

Barr, P. O., Enfors, W. & Eriksson, G. (1972) Hyperbaric oxygen therapy in dermatology. *British Journal of Dermatology*, **86**, 631.

Barthelemy, L., Parc, J. & Mathé, P. (1967) L'oxygène hyperbaré dans le cadre de la marine nationale expérience de dix ans. *Anesthésie, Analgésie, Réanimation*, **24**, 375.

Bass, B. H. (1970) The treatment of varicose leg ulcers by hyperbaric oxygen. *Postgraduate Medical Journal*, **46**, 407.

Besznyak, I., Nemes, A. & Sebsetény, M. (1970) The use of hyperbaric oxygen in the treatment of experimental hypoxaemic skin ulcers of the limb. *Acta Chururgica Academiae Scientiarum Hungaricae*, **11**, 15.

Bird, A. D. & Telfer, A. B. M. (1965) The effect of hyperbaric oxygen on limb circulation. *Lancet*, **i**, 355.

Cunliffe, W. J. & Menon, I. S. (1969) Blood fibrinolytic activity in diseases of small blood vessels and the effect of low molecular weight dextran. *British Journal of Dermatology*, **81**, 220.

Dowling, G. B., Copeman, P. W. M. & Ashfield, R. (1967) Raynaud's phenomenon in scleroderma treated with hyperbaric oxygen. *Proceedings of the Royal Society of Medicine*, **60**, 1268.

Holti, G. (1973) Intermittent low molecular weight dextran infusion in the management of ischemic skin disorders. *Bibliographia Anatomique*, **11**, 359.

Illingworth, C. (1962) Treatment of arterial occlusion under oxygen at two-atmosphere pressure. *British Medical Journal,* **ii,** 1271.

Irvin, T. T. & Smith, G. (1968) Treatment of bacterial infections with hyperbaric oxygen. *Surgery* (St Louis), **63,** 363.

Issroff, S. W. & Whiting, D. A. (1971) Low molecular weight dextran in the treatment of livedo reticularis with ulceration. *British Journal of Dermatology* (Supplement 7), **85,** 26.

Kidikoro, H., Sakakibara, K., Takao, J., Nibei, M., Hibi, Y., Sakakibara, B., Kawamura, M., Kobayashi, S. & Konishi, S. J. (1970) Experimental and clinical studies upon hyperbaric oxygen therapy for peripheral vascular disorders. In *Proceedings of the 4th International Congress on Hyperbaric Medicine* (Ed.) Wada, J. & Iwa, T. p. 462. London: Bailliere, Tindall and Cassell.

Kuzemko, J. A. & Loder, R. E. (1970) Purpura fulminans treated with hyperbaric oxygen. *British Medical Journal,* **iv,** 157.

Lefebvre, F., Dossa, J., Serre, L., Joyeux, R. & du Cailer, D. J. (1970) Résultats thérapeutiques de l'oxygène hyperbaré dans les ulcères variqueux. *Seminaine des Hôpitaux de Paris,* **46,** 127.

Little, J. M. (1975) *Major Amputations for Vascular Disease.* Edinburgh: Churchill Livingstone.

Little, J. M., Petrisi-Jones, D. & Kerr, C. (1974) Vascular amputees; A study in disappointment. *Lancet,* **i,** 793.

McAllister, T. A., Stark, J. M., Norman, J. M. & Ross, R. M. (1963) Inhibitory effect of hyperbaric oxygen on bacteria and fungi. *Lancet,* **ii,** 1040.

Mantz, J. M. & Temple, J. D. (1968) Die Sauerstoff-uberdruck behandlung. *Munchener medizinische Wochenschrift,* **110,** 2186.

Myers, B. (1975) *Skin Flaps.*

Parish, L. C. (1972) Sickle cell leg ulcer. *Archives of Dermatology,* **106,** 754.

Roding, B., Groenveld, P. H. A. & Boerema, I. (1972) The years of experience in the treatment of gas gangrene with hyperbaric oxygen. *Surgery, Gynecology and Obstetrics,* **134,** 579.

Ryan, T. J. (1966) Periadenitis mucosae necroticans. *Proceedings of the Royal Society of Medicine,* **59,** 255.

Shaldin, I. (1969) Oxygen therapy in pressure chamber in trophic ulcers and persistently non-healing wounds of the extremities. *Vestnik Khirurgii, Grekova,* **102,** 46.

Slack, W. K., Thomas, D. A. & De Jode, L. R. J. (1966) Hyperbaric oxygen in the treatment of trauma, ischaemic disease of limbs and varicose ulceration. In *Proceedings of the 3rd International Symposium on Hyperbaric Medicine, Washington.* p. 621. Washington: National Academy of Sciences.

Thomas, C. Y., Crouch, J. A. & Guastello, J. (1974) Hyperbaric oxygen therapy for pyoderma gangrenosum. *Archives of Dermatology,* **110,** 445.

Wadell, W. B., Saltzman, H. A., Fuson, R. L. & Harris, J. (1965) Purpura gangrenosa treated with hyperbaric oxygenation. *Journal of the American Medical Association,* **191,** 971.

PLASMAPHERESIS

Plasmapheresis is used to remove abnormal plasma components. It was first used by Adams, Blahd and Bassett (1952) for a patient with myelomatosis from whom they removed 30 g of plasma protein daily for more than a month. The technique was developed by Solomon and Fahey (1963), and later Bloch and Maki (1973) recommended the removal of 500 ml of blood which was then centrifuged at 5000 rev/min for 7.5 minutes at 4°C, and the red cells then resuspended in a small amount of saline for reinfusion. This procedure is repeated immediately so that the plasma from 1000 ml of blood is removed in one session. Patients are treated in this fashion once or twice weekly. Anaemic patients should first be transfused so that their haemoglobin is at least 10 g/100 ml, although the inevitable rise in the haematocrit is not without hazard.

Improvement of retinopathy and vision, resolution of severe oral and other mucosal bleeding, improvement in cold tolerance, remission of seizures, improvement of gait and hearing, lessening of anaemia and healing of chronic ulcers all are beneficial effects which have been observed (Solomon and Fahey, 1963; Bloch and Maki, 1973).

One patient with severe cold urticaria due to a monoclonal cryoprotein with rheumatoid factor activity was rendered asymptomatic for three years (Grey and Kohler, 1973).

Plasmapheresis is of particular value in monoclonal cryoglobulinaemia of the IgM type since most of the macroglobulin is intravascular. Removal of 1000 ml of plasma reduces the IgM levels by 15 to 20 per cent. If oedema develops because of hypo-albuminaemia, then albumin may be added to the reinfusion. Haemorrhagic manifestations should improve; if they do not, coagulation studies should be done to see whether depletion of clotting factors is occurring and, if necessary, requisite replacement therapy should be given (Perkins, MacKenzie and Fudenburg, 1970).

Sanderson (1972), however, reported that plasmapheresis failed to improve the skin lesions of a patient in whom a monoclonal cryoglobulin gelled between 31 and 34°C and produced gross sludging in venules.

References

Adams, W. S., Blahd, W. H. & Bassett, S. H. (1952) A method of human plasmapheresis. *Proceedings of the Society for Experimental Biology and Medicine,* **80,** 377.

Bloch, K. J. & Maki, D. G. (1973) Hyperviscosity syndromes associated with immunoglobulin abnormalities. *Seminars in Hematology,* **10,** 113.

Grey, H. M. & Kohler, P. F. (1973) Cryoglobulins. *Seminars in Hematology,* **10,** 87.

Perkins, H. A., MacKenzie, M. R. & Fudenburg, H. H. (1970) Hemostatic defects in dysproteinemias. *Blood,* **35,** 695.

Sanderson, K. (1972) In discussion of Cream, J. J. & Ramsey, C. (1972) Single component cryoglobulinaemic vasculitis. *Proceedings of the Royal Society of Medicine,* **65,** 765.

Solomon, A. & Fahey, J. L. (1963) Plasmapheresis therapy in macroglobulinaemia. *Annals of Internal Medicine,* **58,** 789.

Index

407